D1254415

# Eye signs and symptoms in brain tumors

# Eye signs and symptoms in brain tumors

**ALFRED HUBER, M.D.**

Professor of Ophthalmology and Consultant Ophthalmologist, Neurosurgical Clinic, University of Zurich, Switzerland

*Third edition edited and newly written material translated by*

**FREDERICK C. BLODI, M.D.**

Professor and Head, Department of Ophthalmology, University of Iowa College of Medicine, Iowa City, Iowa

*Foreword by*

**PROF. H. KRAYENBÜHL**

Formerly Director of the Neurosurgical Clinic, University of Zurich, Switzerland

*English translation of the first edition by*

**STEFAN VAN WIEN, M.D.**

Formerly Associate, Department of Ophthalmology, Northwestern University Medical School, Chicago, Illinois

*Foreword to the first English translation by*

**DERRICK VAIL, B.A., M.D., D.Oph. (Oxon.), F.A.C.S., F.R.C.S. (Hon.)**

Formerly Professor and Director, Department of Ophthalmology, Northwestern University Medical School, Chicago, Illinois

**THIRD EDITION**

*with 233 illustrations*

**THE C. V. MOSBY COMPANY**

*Saint Louis 1976*

German edition by Dr. Alfred Huber entitled *Augensymptome bei Hirntumoren* published by Medizinischer Verlag Hans Huber, Bern and Stuttgart

**THIRD EDITION**

**Library of Congress Cataloging in Publication Data**

Huber, Alfred, 1918-
    Eye signs and symptoms in brain tumors.

    Translation of Augensymptome bei Hirntumoren.
    Bibliography:  p.
    Includes index.
    1.  Brain—Tumors—Diagnosis.  2.  Ocular manifestations of general diseases.  I.  Title.  [DNLM: 1.  Brain neoplasms—Diagnosis.  2.  Eye manifestations.  WL358 H877a]
RC280.B7H83    1976        616.9′92′81        76-28437
ISBN 0-8016-2302-2

CB/CB/B    9    8    7    6    5    4    3    2    1

**Dedicated to the sick**

*Whose suffering has contributed to the discovery of new methods for better treatment of others*

# FOREWORD

In 1918 Dandy performed ventriculography for the first time, and in 1927 Moniz introduced cerebral angiography, that is, the visualization of cerebral vessels using radiographic contrast medium. Both methods have been gradually accepted as very important diagnostic tools and finally widely used. It has become possible to explore the brain in some detail preoperatively, and neurosurgery has advanced dramatically.

These two discoveries diminished the muteness of the brain to x-ray examination to a certain extent, but until very recently Moniz's dictum that the brain is "mute to X-rays" still held. The breakthrough was made by Hounsfield (1973), a research engineer and physicist working in England at the Central Research Laboratories of EMI, Ltd. He was interested in methods by which information about patterns could be stored. It became apparent that x-ray examination was one area wherein improved methods of retrieving and storing usable information might greatly improve the efficiency of the technique.

Hounsfield's method employs the property of crystal scintillation to measure a scanning x-ray beam. The very large number of readings taken are handled by a computer programmed to reconstruct the anatomic configuration of the slice of brain scanned. By employing crystal x-ray photon detectors in conjunction with tomographic principles and a computer to store and process the very large amount of data, it is estimated that a hundred times more information can be obtained from x-ray examination of the brain than conventional methods permit.

In this way, Hounsfield has brought Moniz's dream to fruition—the brain is no longer mute to x-ray examination. By this technique, computerized axial tomography with the EMI scanner is achieved. The system was first evaluated by Ambrose at Atkinson Morley's Hospital, and it became clear that many different pathologic processes affecting the brain could be identified.[*] This method allows a detailed study of intracranial neoplasms in the very short time of 20 to 30 minutes. In addition, normal and abnormal structures of the orbit may be identified by computerized axial tomography.

---

[*]Gawler, J., et al.: Computerized axial tomography. In Krayenbühl, H., editor: Advances and technical standards in neurosurgery, vol. 2, Heidelberg, 1975, Springer Verlag.

Furthermore, in special cases, ultrasonic scanning of the carotid arteries has become an indispensable diagnostic tool. Directional Doppler sonography of the ophthalmic artery is applied to the measurement of direction of flow through this artery and allows the recognition of flow reversal in the periorbital branches of this vessel. This method furnishes important information on carotid and orbital circulation.

Despite these outstanding technical advances, I must emphasize that the most important diagnostic procedure is still an accurate history and clinical examination. Only if all these clinical factors are taken into consideration will it be possible to decide what other ancillary methods should be employed for a more detailed differential diagnosis.

Dr. Huber is well aware of this, and especially from this point of view, his work is to be welcomed. It had its origin in his need to follow an explicit method for his neuro-ophthalmologic technique of examination. Based on his neuro-ophthalmologic findings and thanks to his profound training in neurology, his observation of individual signs and symptoms merely serves as a foundation to present a fascinating and comprehensive picture of all essential factors involved. Just the same, certain details that are of equal interest to the ophthalmologist and the neurosurgeon (as, for instance, the differential diagnosis of the choked disc or the significance of the blood pressure in the retinal vessels) are treated with detailed consideration. This volume is particularly stimulating and important because neurosurgical diagnostic procedures are enriched by the wealth of experience of an ophthalmologist.

**H. Krayenbühl**
*Zurich, Switzerland*

# FOREWORD
## to first English translation

The author of this book, Alfred Huber, a neurologist and ophthalmologist, is a distinguished younger member of the remarkable group of Swiss ophthalmologists whose names are known throughout the world for their contributions (to name but a few of these in our time, Vogt, Gonin, Amsler, Brückner, Streiff, Goldmann, and Franceschetti).

Prof. H. Krayenbühl, Director of the Neurosurgical Clinic at the University of Zurich, is as well known in his field of activity as the aforementioned are in ophthalmology. It is in this renowned clinic that Dr. Huber has obtained the necessary experience to write this extraordinarily good book on *Eye Symptoms in Brain Tumors*.

There are a number of good books on brain tumors. The majority of these have been written by neurologists and neurosurgeons. The others have been written by the very few ophthalmologists who have had the required neurologic interest, knowledge, training, and experience to interpret properly the multiple signs and symptoms that are so frequently encountered.

Because early symptoms of a patient with a brain tumor are primarily ocular, he is almost always first seen by the ophthalmologist. As a result of the modern training of ophthalmologists in this country, more and more of them are becoming excellent neurologists, competent to cope with the involved diagnostic problems. However, there is still much room for improvement, it seems to me, in this regard. It is for this reason that Dr. Huber's beautifully written and adequately illustrated work should receive a warm welcome not only by ophthalmologists but also by neurologists and neurosurgeons; in fact, by physicians in every branch of medicine.

Stefan Van Wien, of the Northwestern University Medical School, has performed an important service for us by translating Dr. Huber's text carefully, scientifically, and in a lucid style. He shows an unusual talent for clearly giving us what the author means to say, at the same time avoiding the involved and the cumbersome that tend to creep into translated manuscripts.

I consider it a great honor to have been asked by Dr. Huber to write this brief foreword and to help in the launching of his work. I am grateful to him for this, but particularly for giving to us all the fruits of his many years of intelligent and diligent studies on the eye symptoms of brain tumors.

**Derrick Vail**
*Chicago, Illinois*

# PREFACE

Since the appearance of the first edition of this book, the disciplines of ophthalmology, neurosurgery, and especially neuro-ophthalmology have made great and unexpected progress. Thus there was no doubt that the book would have to be carefully and extensively revised in the second and now the third editions.

Several portions of the chapter on methods of neuro-ophthalmologic examination have been completely rewritten, especially the section on eye motility and nystagmus. The introduction of static perimetry to the study of visual fields has added new information, and electromyography has contributed many new concepts and diagnostic possibilities to the subject of extraocular muscle palsies. A review of the new techniques of dynamometry, dynamography, and Doppler ultrasound has been added in the section on the ocular fundus. One of the most important additions, however, is the presentation of the new method of fluorescein angiography of the fundus and the demonstration of angiographic patterns of the optic disc under normal and pathologic conditions. Red-free fundus photography for the evaluation of retinal nerve fiber abnormalities in optic nerve disease receives special consideration with corresponding illustrations.

In the chapter on general symptoms of increased intracranial pressure, fluorescein angiographic photographs have been added, especially in the discussion of papilledema and its differential diagnosis. Special care was taken to renew some photographs showing early and chronic papilledemas and also to add some new illustrations concerning edema of the disc resulting from conditions other than increased intracranial pressure, such as ischemic papillitis, leukemia, spinal cord tumor, or metastatic tumor within the optic nerve.

In the chapter on local symptoms of brain tumors, new schematic drawings have been introduced, especially of sellar and suprasellar tumors. In some places, computer tomograms of tumors have been added in order to demonstrate the value of this promising new x-ray technique. The chapter on the relationship between the type of tumor and ocular signs and symptoms has been enriched by some new statistics. The chapter on subdural hematomas, brain abscesses, and aneurysms has been expanded to include information on cerebral pseudotumors, with corresponding illustrations of papilledemas not caused by intra-cranial neoplasms. In the section on intracranial aneurysms, some new concepts and newer classifications have been adopted. Here, too, new illustrations have been included.

The literature has been brought up to date to include the most recent textbooks, monographs, and individual articles. As in the first edition, only a selected choice of the vast literature can be given. The third edition of *Clinical Neuro-Ophthalmology* by Walsh and Hoyt is referred to frequently for information on subjects not discussed in detail in this book.

As a consultant at the Neurosurgical Clinic of the University of Zurich, I would like to thank Professor H. Krayenbühl and his successor Professor G. Yasargil for their interest in this book and especially for having given me the opportunity to use all the clinical data necessary for preparing the new edition. I would especially like to thank Professor Yasargil for allowing me to publish once again the excellent human brain section he prepared. I am also indebted to Professor G. Weber (St. Gallen), as well as to the many present and former residents at the Neurosurgical Clinic for their valuable suggestions and advice. Special credit is also due Mr. H. P. Weber, artist at the Neurosurgical Clinic, for surgical drawings and numerous new sketches.

The University Eye Clinic and its chairman Professor R. Witmer also made my task easier. I especially wish to thank Professor Witmer for giving me the opportunity to publish the wonderful fluorescein angiographic photographs of the normal and pathologic disc. I am grateful to Mr. A. Würth, the photographer of the University Eye Clinic at Zurich, who prepared the excellent fundus photographs with the able assistance of Mrs. Kleinhäny. The visual field sketches, as well as a number of other drawings, are the creation of Mr. Glitsch, artist of the University Eye Clinic in Zurich; my special thanks are extended for the care he took in this time-consuming labor. My secretary, Miss A. Brunner, typed the entire manuscript, and I am greatly indebted to her for her untiring efforts.

My sincere appreciation is offered to Dr. Frederick C. Blodi of the University of Iowa for having kindly taken over the important task of translating the newly written chapters and revising the old text, which was originally translated by Dr. Stefan Van Wien. By his time-consuming effort, Dr. Blodi has made a great contribution to the second and third editions.

**Alfred Huber**
*Zurich, Switzerland*
*July, 1976*

# CONTENTS

## 2  General signs and symptoms of increased intracranial pressure in patients with brain tumors, 92

## 3  Local signs and symptoms of brain tumors, 167

## 4   Relationship between type of tumor and ocular signs and symptoms, 303

## 5   Pseudotumor cerebri, subdural hematomas, brain abscesses, and aneurysms, 310

## 6   Summary, 338

## Literature, 341

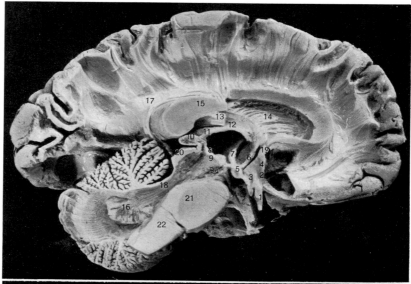

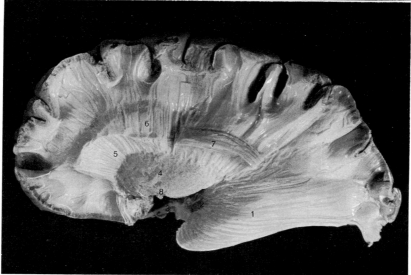

Mesial longitudinal section through human brain demonstrating *fiber* systems of visual radiation, external and internal capsules. **Top:** *1*, Optic chiasm; *2*, chiasmal recess; *3*, infundibular recess; *4*, lamina terminalis; *5*, mamillary body; *6*, anterior column of fornix; *7*, mamillothalamic tract; *8*, habenular-intercrural tract; *9*, red nucleus; *9a*, substantia nigra; *10*, pineal body; *11*, habenular commissure; *12*, stria medullaris and thalamus; *13*, fornix; *14*, internal capsule; *15*, splenium of corpus callosum; *16*, dentate nucleus; *17*, cingulum; *18*, cerebellocerebral tract; *19*, anterior commissure; *20*, quadrigeminate bodies; *21*, pons; *22*, medulla oblongata. **Bottom:** *1*, Optic radiation; *2*, lateral geniculate body; *3*, optic tract; *4*, putamen; *5*, external capsule; *6*, internal capsule; *7*, superior longitudinal bundle; *8*, anterior commissure. (Fiber specimen prepared by Prof. G. Yasargil, M.D., Neurosurgical Clinic. University of Zurich.)

# Introduction

Eye symptoms and ocular signs appear with significant frequency in patients with brain tumors. As a general statement based on other publications and our own series of 8100 cases, it can be said that *some form* of ocular symptom or sign can be observed in *somewhat more than 50% of patients with brain tumors.* These eye symptoms and signs are not merely insignificant accompanying features. The following statistical data show that this actually is not the case. In about 60% of our series, *ocular symptoms were among the initial complaints in the early stages.* In about 60% of the patients, papilledema was found, generally a sign permitting a diagnosis of increased intracranial pressure or a space-consuming lesion. Furthermore, because of the close anatomic relationship between the eye and the brain, the ocular signs and symptoms alone allow fairly accurate localization of a tumor in about 25% of the patients if it is situated near the visual pathways.

On the basis of these facts, there can be no doubt that *the majority of eye symptoms and signs in brain tumors actually are of diagnostic and even localizing significance.* Although the ocular signs and symptoms of brain tumors are the main point of interest in this book, we should not lose sight of other neurologic signs and symptoms. To avoid a distortion of the actual clinical picture, the significant manifestations will be considered in their totality in the discussion of the various sites of tumors.

This book is primarily intended for the ophthalmologist, who frequently finds himself in a position of being the first to make a decision as to whether or not there is an increase in intracranial pressure or to make a diagnosis as to whether an impairment of the visual pathways or of the extraocular muscles is caused by a tumor. The tremendous *responsibility of the ophthalmologist who has to make an early diagnosis of a brain tumor needs no further emphasis* if one considers that ocular symptoms are among the early findings in brain tumors in 60% of such patients. This also demonstrates the *importance of close cooperation between the various specialties.* The discovery of minute and early ocular signs by means of suitable technical equipment should remain within the realm of the ophthalmologist despite a more generalized awareness by others of the signifi-

cance of some of these signs in brain tumors. At the same time the ophthalmologist should never evaluate his findings as isolated facts, but should always co-
ordinate them with those of the neurologist, the radiologist, the internist, the
otologist, and the neurosurgeon.

Eye signs and symptoms in brain tumors are discussed in a number of publications on neuro-ophthalmology (Rea; Walsh and Hoyt; Lyle; Kestenbaum; Bing
and Brückner; Kyrieleis; Smith; Glaser; Brégeat; Dubois-Poulsen; Guillaumat, Morax, and Offret; Ashworth; Sachsenweger) as well as in the standard texts on
neurosurgery (Cushing; Bailey; Dandy; Olivecrona; Tönnis; Krayenbühl). Most of
these publications are part of the English literature. Still we do not believe that this
book is superfluous. Perhaps our method of presentation, limited to the field of brain
tumors with its ever-increasing importance, is as novel as is the fact that it is *based
on the large material of an up-to-date neurosurgical department,* which was made
available to me through the courtesy of Professor Krayenbühl and Professor Yasargil. The great privilege of being associated with such an institution as consulting
ophthalmologist also invokes a certain obligation. The large number of patients
examined and followed up by me personally may justify this addition to an already ample literature on the subject. *Personal experience in the evaluation of
this material* seems to us to be of the utmost importance.

Regarding terminology, we include among ocular signs and symptoms not
only changes involving the eye itself, but also anomalies of the oculomotor
system and disorders of the visual sensory system (optic nerve, chiasm, higher
visual pathways, visual cortex, and higher visual centers). Thus the phrase
"ocular signs and symptoms" is used in its broadest sense; it would perhaps
be more appropriate to speak of "signs and symptoms of the visual organ."
In this book, we have limited ourselves to the neoplasms of the meninges
and the brain tissue proper. However, a concluding chapter with a brief separate presentation of ocular signs and symptoms typical of aneurysms and other
tumorlike lesions (pseudotumors, abscesses, hematomas, etc.) has been included.

In view of the tremendous wealth of literature dealing with brain tumors
and their neuro-ophthalmologic aspects, the bibliography should be considered
only as a random selection, especially of the more recent publications. Whenever an author is quoted, the appropriate reference is listed. In addition, the
bibliography includes a number of references and publications not expressly
cited in the book. The bibliography has been divided according to the individual
chapters and divisions to facilitate its use.

# ONE

## Methods of neuro-ophthalmologic examination in patients with suspected brain tumors

The neuro-ophthalmologic methods of examination have been discussed in general in numerous older as well as some more recent publications (Wilbrand and Saenger; Lyle; Kestenbaum; Rea; Bing and Brückner; Brégeat; Dubois-Poulsen; Guillaumat, Morax, and Offret; Walsh and Hoyt; Ashworth). The excellent book by Kestenbaum is arranged according to the principles of the techniques of examination; the pathologic changes are discussed in individual chapters according to important ocular signs. Many valuable references to neuro-ophthalmologic diagnostics in brain tumors can be found in numerous articles (see bibliography) as well as in textbooks on neurosurgery (Cushing; Bailey; Dandy; Sachs; Krayenbühl; Olivecrona; Tönnis) and ophthalmology (Schieck and Brückner; Bailliart, Coutela, Redslob, and Velter; Duke-Elder and Scott; Amsler, Brückner, Franceschetti, Goldmann, and Streiff).

In view of the large amount of material available, it would almost seem superfluous to present a separate discussion on the methods of examination at this point. However, we are anxious to give *our own experience* with and *our evaluation* of various methods and their usefulness in the neuro-ophthalmologic diagnosis of brain tumors. In general the neuro-ophthalmologic method of examination in patients with brain tumors does not differ from that in patients with other morbid changes of the central nervous system. However, we intend to elaborate on some of the peculiarities of these methods and the interpretation of their results. These aims may justify the following rather condensed presentation of methods of examination.

### HISTORY AND SYMPTOMS

Even the most detailed neuro-ophthalmologic examination carried out with the most refined ancillary instruments has to be preceded by a carefully taken history, an unavoidable procedure, as in any other clinical diagnostic problem. This may not always be an easy task in patients with a brain tumor if increased intracranial pressure has dimmed or completely abolished consciousness or if

3

the tumor has caused a motor or sensory aphasia. In such patients, it is frequently imperative to obtain additional data concerning the course of the disease from relatives of the patient. In a large number of patients the spontaneous history has to be supplemented with leading questions by the examining physician. The severity and importance of the ocular signs and symptoms may easily be outweighed by other neurologic signs or symptoms. It should be stated emphatically that *the patient may be quite unaware of certain visual sensations and defects.*

### Visual field defects

With regard to the previous statement, we want to recall particularly homonymous hemianopic field defects that, in one fourth of all patients, either are not appreciated at all or are not disturbing, especially in symmetric defects and defects that spare the central fixation. Critchley, in particular, concerned himself with the interesting phenomenon of *"awareness and nonawareness" of hemianopic field defects,* concluding that the defective perceived object is frequently "filled in," that is, an interpolation, so to speak, causes the patient not to be aware of the field defect. We know of numerous patients who had a resection of the occipital lobe because of a tumor and who hardly noticed a complete homonymous hemianopic defect (without sparing of the macula) except (in right-sided cases) when reading. Such a patient, for instance, sees not just one half of the face in a mirror (or at least one half covered by a veil), but rather sees the entire face. In part, this may be caused by a constant lateral wandering of the eyes toward the side of the hemianopia. However, the "visual completion" realized by the higher visual centers is a necessary complementary factor (Poppelreuter; Goldstein and Gelb). In some patients, this phenomenon can be explained by the fact that the *hemianopia* caused by the tumor *is only relative in the sense of a so-called unilateral visual inattention.* Only qualitative partial functions of the visual perception (dyschromatopsia, spatial disorientation, retarded form recognition, indistinct outlines, or changes in the perception of movements) are disturbed in the involved halves of the visual field. The patient is not aware of these defects in everyday life. However, even a superficial simultaneous testing of both fields (for instance, with both hands) will demonstrate such a hemianopic disturbance of attention, whereas perimetry does not reveal any field defects. This diagnostically important phenomenon of "visual inattention" will be discussed further on p. 176. Other conditions that frequently are not realized by the patient are bitemporal defects or concentric constrictions of the field.

*Pseudohemianopia,* which occurs in unilateral gaze palsies, together with absence of visual attention in the missing "field of gaze" will be discussed in detail in connection with tumors of the frontal lobe (p. 175).

The patient may be unaware of the visual field defect as such, but not of its consequences in everyday experiences. In addition to patients who are not at all aware of such defects, there are others *who complain, either spontaneously or when questioned, that they frequently collide to one (homonymous hemianopia) or both (bitemporal hemianopia) sides with persons or objects without any apparent reason.* Such statements strongly suggest hemianopia. The motorist hits the wall of the garage. The cyclist overlooks a pedestrian on one side of the street. A patient hurriedly writes past the margin of the paper. These are some examples selected from case histories to demonstrate the consequences of hemianopia in everyday life. Some patients do not even mention such details in their histories. Their hemianopia is masked by the complaint of cloudy or poor vision (they blame insufficient lighting at their place of work) or the statement that one or both eyes are visually disturbed. (A homonymous hemianopia is projected by the patient to the eye corresponding to the side of the hemianopia; bitemporal hemianopia is projected to both eyes.)

## Disturbance of simple and higher visual functions

A history of *loss of vision* is an important symptom in tumors near the optic nerve, the chiasm, or the optic tract. The patient, however, does not always make such a specific statement. If not alert, the patient does not appreciate a deterioration of visual acuity for quite a while. We can cite from our material numerous patients with pituitary tumors who suspected at first that their glasses were not adequate and consulted the optician or ophthalmologist for stronger lenses! Loss of vision is not necessarily the result of direct pressure of a tumor on the distal visual pathways. It could be the precursory symptom of an imminent optic atrophy resulting from a chronic papilledema, prognostically a particularly unfavorable situation. The *early stages of progressive loss of vision* are not always easy to detect. However, just these stages are of enormous importance to the neurosurgeon. In taking a careful history, one may learn of *loss of vision only under poor lighting* (impaired dark adaptation as an early sign of damage to the optic nerve!) or of certain changes or *disturbances of the color sensation* (also symptoms of damaged fibers of the optic nerve). Occasionally, patients report a veil, fog, or smoke before the eyes in early stages of optic atrophy caused by a tumor. Not infrequently, loss of vision in one eye is not appreciated because the other eye functions well and vicariously substitutes for the other. Thus amaurosis in one eye may develop without the patient being aware of it. Only a deterioration of vision in the second eye causes alarm and unexpectedly brings forth this catastrophic situation. One should always interpret somewhat skeptically subjective complaints of a sudden visual disturbance and particularly a sudden decrease in vision. As a rule, defects of the conductivity of the visual pathways resulting from a tumor show a progressive development. It is often only the patient who suddenly discovers the loss! We shall discuss the so-called *amblyopic attacks* in patients with brain tumor in greater detail later; these brief attacks of blackout or fogginess (not infrequently associated with violent headaches) are well-known accompanying symptoms of papilledema (especially in its chronic form) and should not be missed (p. 123).

*Photopsia* (that is, the sensation of sparks, lightning, luminous rings, etc., mostly in both visual fields) is not likely to be missed in taking the history because it is quite an impressive and actually frightening phenomenon. According to Ethelberg and Jensen, it occurs mostly in association with the attacks of amblyopia or obscurations already mentioned—happening as a prodromal symptom, simultaneously with these attacks, rarely after the attack, or as an isolated symptom. Photopsia caused by retinal disease in all these cases has to be ruled out, of course.

Various forms of photopsia show an imperceptible transition to *visual hallucinations* that should always be sought if a brain tumor is suspected. In principle, visual hallucinations may occur as a consequence of a lesion anywhere along the visual pathway, namely, the retina, the optic nerve, the chiasm, the optic tract, or the higher visual pathways (Weinberger and Grant). We are not in agreement with Weinberger and Grant's opinion that the type of hallucination is completely useless for purposes of localization. Rather, we agree with Walsh and Hoyt and with Parkinson, Rucker, and McCraig in the belief that the customary classification of optic hallucinations is more or less correct: *unformed crude light sensations* (fiery globes, luminous rings, stripes, circles, discs, blinking lights) are typical for *occipital lesions,* whereas *formed, differentiated,* and *complex sensations* (objects, animals, persons, entire scenes), not infrequently associated with dreamy states and olfactory or gustatory hallucinations, are more typical for *tumors of the temporal lobe.* If the occurrence of such hallucinations is revealed while taking the history, their nature may be of some value in localizing the site of the tumor. This is all the more welcome because tumors in the temporal and occipital lobes develop in relatively "silent" zones. In the majority of patients the hallucinations occur in the region of the hemianopic field defects (Wilbrand; Henschen; Cushing; Horrax). Depending on the nature and topography of the hallucinations, the site of the tumor can be hypothesized with some degree of probability. Only the proof of hemianopia, however, will provide certainty, because time and again reports indicate hallucinations either in the intact half of the visual field or on both sides (Weinberger and Grant; Sanford and Blair). Unfortunately, visual hallucinations do not occur very frequently. According to Horrax and Putnam and to Parkinson, Rucker, and McCraig, their frequency in patients with occipital tumors varies between 15% and 20%. In our own series, their occurrence in patients with tumors of the temporal lobes as well as the occipital lobes was even rarer (only a few percent).

*Micropsia* and *macropsia* are occasionally mentioned by patients with brain tumors. Such symptoms should be further analyzed (peripheral causes such as affections of the macula or disturbances of refraction and accommodation must be ruled out) before they can be interpreted and evaluated as phenomena of central origin. Bender and Savitsky are of the opinion that, in addition to affections of the parietal and occipital regions, other lesions of the visual pathways (for instance, tumors near the chiasm) may be responsible for micropsia and macropsia; in other words, these symptoms are not of localizing value. We have observed micropsia in a patient with glioblastoma multiforme of the occipital lobe. From time to time this patient saw objects in her surroundings (especially furniture in her home) strikingly smaller than usual. She reported this sensation simultaneously with a homonymous loss of the visual field. Hemimacropsia in the right halves of the visual field (without hemianopia) has been observed in a patient with a tumor of the left occipital lobe.

The visual hallucinations and the phenomena of micropsia and macropsia actually bring us to the symptomatology of *disorders of the higher visual functions* that may also have to be considered in taking the history (Fig. 1-1).

Tumors in the occipital cortex, especially in the calcarine fissure, result in sensory disturbances of the true *cortical blindness* type if the involvement is bilateral. Characteristic findings are loss of all visual sensations, including the differentiation between light and dark, preservation of the pupillary reaction to light and convergence, and loss of the lid reflex to bright light or finger movements before the eyes. Occasionally cortical blindness is accompanied by unformed visual hallucinations. A particularly interesting phenomenon in cortical blindness is the fact that the *patients frequently are not aware of the loss of visual sensations,* as if they were "blind for their blindness" (anosognosia, Anton's syndrome). The patients behave as if they actually could see and describe (as in hallucinations) their surroundings, which they believe they see in the most minute and fanciful detail. We have done follow-up studies of two such patients with cortical blindness. In one the cause was an x-ray necrosis of both occipital

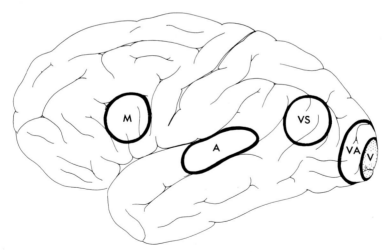

**Fig. 1-1.** Sketch of dominant hemisphere demonstrating position of visual centers and centers for reading, speech, and understanding of symbolic expression. Lesions of some of these areas may lead to different forms of central disorders of visual integration. *V,* Visual cortex (cortical blindness); *VA,* visual associational area (visual object agnosia or mind blindness); *VS,* visual speech area (alexia, word blindness); *A,* auditory speech area (sensory aphasia); *M,* motor speech area (motor or verbal aphasia).

lobes following irradiation after extirpation of a temporal tumor; it remained irreversible until death. The other patient showed cortical blindness that appeared suddenly following a bilateral ventriculography performed through the occipital lobes. Obviously, it was caused by an acute local edema. On recovery, this patient had complete restitution of the visual functions. As a rule, this recovery is not complete at once, but progresses from the stage of mere light-dark perception to the recognition of form and finally to color perception and all the other attributes of normal vision. Generally, tumors involve the optic radiation rather than the visual cortex and, at that, more often only one side. Thus the phenomenon of cortical blindness in patients with neoplasms of the brain is rarely encountered.

Lesions at a higher level of the optognostic pathways (the border area between the occipital, temporal, and parietal lobes) may cause central disorders of visual integration of the type of so-called *mind blindness* or *visual object agnosia,* which is the inability to appreciate the meaning of a visual perception. The patients are able to describe details of objects, but are unable to classify the objects in their totality in the storeroom of their memories and to identify them accordingly. However, the moment they are aided by another sense (for instance, when they touch the object they could not identify), they recognize it instantly. Since most objects in everyday life are identified by means of the visual sense, mind blindness means an unpleasant and even disastrous condition and one that patients are hardly able to dissimilate. There is no unanimity of opinion as to the exact localization of this higher visual disturbance. Probably it is in the parietooccipital region near the angular gyrus (Wernicke; Wilbrand). Other schools of thought do not believe that there are precise centers for higher cortical functions: they explain such disorders by the interruption of association pathways at certain sites related with certain functions. The lesion can be unilateral. It does not seem to make any difference whether the dominant (as a rule, the left) or the other side of the brain is involved. This type of visual disturbance is also found infrequently in patients with cerebral tumors.

Tumors in the area of the angular gyrus and in the border area between the parietal and occipital lobes of the dominant hemisphere (mostly on the left side) are more likely to result in *sensory-aphasic disturbances* of the type of *word blindness* or *alexia.* Although vision is intact, the patient is unable to read. In other words, the patient is unable to comprehend the significance of written or printed words, musical notes, or digits. (This special form of "visual agnosia" is limited to the partial function of the process of reading.) Since the motor function depends on the sensory function and its evaluation, alexia is almost perforce combined with a motor-aphasic phenomenon, namely, *agraphia* (the inability to write, either spontaneously or in dictation). The combination of alexia and agraphia occurs particularly in patients with so-called cortical alexia. In lesions of the left occipital lobe and of the splenium of the corpus callosum (disconnection syndrome), one finds pure alexia without marked disturbance of the ability to write—the patient is unable to read what he has written. Usually this condition is found in combination with a disturbance of conductivity in the optic radiation, that is, with right-sided homonymous quadrantanopia or hemianopia. We have frequently observed alexia with agraphia either as isolated disorders or in combination with apractic as well as other sensory-aphasic disturbances in patients with tumors of the parietal and occipital lobes (Fig. 1-2).

*When the history is taken, alexia and agraphia must be carefully differentiated from peripheral disturbances of the function of the visual organ.* As a rule, such a differentiation should cause no difficulties. The situation will only become complicated and difficult if, for instance, because of a chronic papilledema with optic atrophy, the vision has already become so impaired that reading and writing are no longer possible. If it is taken into consideration, however, that *alexia and agraphia rarely occur alone* but are *frequently combined with other sensory-aphasic disturbances* such as *the inability to understand speech in the presence of intact hearing, the inability to understand gestures and mimic actions,* and *particularly the inability to express thoughts in words, gestures,* or *mimic actions,* it is difficult not to evaluate such conditions properly.

### Disturbances of extraocular muscles

*Paralysis of extraocular muscles* usually causes a very disturbing *double vision,* especially if the vertical muscles are involved. Thus as a rule the patients mention diplopia spontaneously. *In patients with a less severe paresis, especially of the horizontal rotators (medial rectus and lateral rectus),* there usually is no

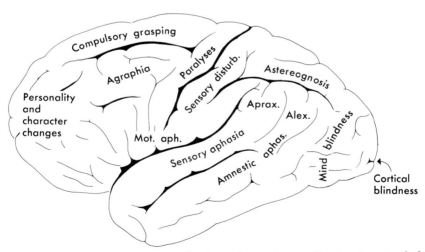

**Fig. 1-2.** Sketch of left lateral surface of the brain hemisphere indicating functional disturbances that occur if certain areas or connections to them are damaged. Of special interest are cortical blindness as the result of lesions of both visual occipital cortex areas and mind blindness and alexia as the result of damage to the parieto-occipital region.

double vision at all in parts of the field of gaze. Even if the patient looks toward the side of the paretic muscle, there may perhaps be no true double vision but merely a complaint of an *uncertain blurring of objects* or a glimmer that it is difficult to describe. This is, so to speak, an expression of a minimal disparity of the two images, a minimal displacement of contours without complete lateral or vertical separation of the objects. In patients with brain tumor, such slight pareses quite frequently are the sequelae of the general increase of the intracranial pressure (involving especially the sixth nerve). In taking a careful history, one should suspect that such pareses may be masked by vague statements on the part of the patient.

In cases of manifest diplopia, one should inquire whether the images are separated in the vertical, in the horizontal, or in both planes. Furthermore, one should determine in *which direction of gaze is the maximal horizontal or vertical separation of the two images.* On the basis of these data ascertained from the history, one is frequently in the position to diagnose the paretic muscle with the aid of a simple diagram (Fig. 1-14), provided only one muscle is responsible for the diplopia.

As a rule, patients are not aware of supranuclear *gaze palsy* or *paresis* unless, in the course of the examination, attention is called to the inability to shift the gaze sideways or up. This fact can be understood if one considers that such palsies can be easily compensated for in everyday life by certain movements or positions of the head. A certain exception is the vertical palsy present in patients with *Parinaud's syndrome.* Among eight such cases, usually caused by tumors in the region of the roof of the midbrain, we were able to obtain a history of *vertical diplopia* in six—obviously an expression of the disparity in the vertical impairment of the individual eye (or a consequence of an additional nuclear third nerve paralysis). This type of diplopia, in combination with pupillary disturbances (of the Argyll Robertson type) and the unmistakable vertical gaze palsy, permits the definite diagnosis of Parinaud's syndrome, pathognomonic for lesions in the region of the mesencephalic tegmentum. A few times we have seen Parinaud's syndrome combined with so-called *paralysis of convergence.* Distant objects were seen as single; at *close range* there was *crossed diplopia* with only a slight horizontal disparity of images that showed little change during lateral conjugate movements. Paralysis of convergence, like Parinaud's syndrome, suggests a mesencephalic lesion. (Perlia's nucleus is the hypothetical center of convergence.) We find *uncrossed diplopia* with a corresponding convergent position of the eyes *for distance* but not for near in the so-called *paralysis of divergence.* The horizontal separation of the images in all directions of gaze remains unchanged. The ability to converge is intact. There is an impairment of the divergence, although each lateral rectus muscle functions properly. A number of autopsy findings (Savitsky and Madonick; Lippmann) suggest lesions (including tumor) in the area of the brain stem near the sixth nerve nuclei.

*Gaze nystagmus* or *central vestibular nystagmus,* usually occurring in patients with brain tumors, practically never causes symptoms. Only the peripheral vestibular nystagmus (either resulting from a lesion in the inner ear or in the region of the vestibular nucleus) may cause ocular disturbances such as vertigo with whirling of the surroundings around the patient, associated headaches, nausea, and a general sensation of insecurity (the well-known symptoms of Ménière's disease).

In the history given by patients with neuro-ophthalmologic problems, symptoms of a disturbance of vision or ocular motility are quite preeminent because they are appreciated relatively early and distinctly. Other ocular symptoms in patients with brain tumors may give rise to subjective sensations that, in the overall picture, are less important for diagnosis and localization, but will be discussed briefly.

## Pain

Headache, as a symptom of increased intracranial pressure, occasionally radiates into the eyes and is interpreted as an associated eye ache. However, it is minor compared with the general cephalalgia. *If the eye ache is the outstanding symptom, a localized disease of the eye has to be considered,* which in turn may cause radiating pain into various regions of the head. *Acute or subacute glaucoma,* in addition to a deep-seated eye ache, may cause diffuse headaches, nausea, or even vomiting, symptoms that could easily be mistaken for those of a general increase in intracranial pressure. The ocular signs are increased intraocular pressure, ground-glass appearance of the cornea, a relatively dilated pupil, ciliary congestion of the globe, and possibly glaucomatous excavation of the disc, signs that usually pose no diagnostic problems.

The eye is within the area of distribution of the ophthalmic branch of the trigeminal nerve; thus tumors affecting this cranial nerve may cause ocular pain. However, an isolated pain in the eye is rare. Rather, there are neuralgias within the entire area of distribution of the first branch and possibly also in those of the other two branches, that is, the maxillary and mandibular nerves. In the *superior orbital fissure syndrome* and the *cavernous sinus syndrome* affecting the third, fourth, fifth, and sixth cranial nerves, there may be referred pain, especially in the area of the first branch of the trigeminal nerve involving the upper face and eye. Unlike idiopathic trigeminal neuralgia, there is no paroxysmal onset of pain in the case of a tumor or an aneurysm of the internal carotid artery within the cavernous sinus. The pain is rather persistent and sharply localized within the area of distribution of one of the trigeminal branches, occasionally with sensory disturbances registered on corresponding skin areas. A similar type of pain, also radiating into the eye, may be caused by a tumor within the gasserian ganglion itself (a neurinoma of the trigeminal nerve), a tumor in the middle fossa (cavum of Meckel), or a tumor in the posterior fossa (meningioma, acoustic neurinoma, and others) if there is a corresponding involvement of the trigeminal nerve. One should not forget that ocular pain in the area of distribution of the first branch of the trigeminal nerve is frequently accompanied by increased *lacrimation* and painful *photophobia*.

### Photophobia

Excessive sensitivity to light in the form of photophobia is often painful and so annoying that the patient will mention it spontaneously. The *peripheral* form referred via the trigeminal nerve has already been discussed in connection with pain. We have seen abnormal photophobia in a few patients with tumor of the midbrain, especially combined with Parinaud's syndrome. One of these patients would cover his eyes with a dark cloth, even indoors, so the photophobia would not annoy him. It disappeared completely after a course of x-ray treatments. Milder forms of photophobia, according to our own observations, occur quite commonly in any type of increased intracranial pressure, even in cases of subdural hematomas. This type of photophobia should be regarded as *central* in origin and should be differentiated from the peripheral trigeminal form. It is possible that in the production of "central photophobia" the entire central mechanism of the sensory trigeminal nerve (including the mesencephalic root and nucleus) together with the optic nerve (pathways entering the midbrain) is involved. This hypothesis for a central form of photophobia is supported by the observation of a type that may occasionally be quite severe, occurring after minor but more frequently after severe trauma to the skull, in meningitis, in migraine, and in subarachnoid hemorrhage.

### Observations made by the patient when looking into a mirror

Patients will often mention observations they have made while looking into a mirror, observations that will assume considerable importance during the course of the examination.

A unilateral *widening of the lid fissure* will be quite conspicuous to the patient. It is the result of central or peripheral facial palsy, a frequent phenomenon in brain tumor that is not only caused by localized pressure, but also by a generalized increase in intracranial pressure. A complete lagophthalmos (that is, the inability to close the eye) occurs much more rarely, except as a surgical complication; for instance, during extirpation of an acoustic neurinoma, damage to the facial nerve sometimes cannot be avoided for technical reasons (Fig. 1-3).

Widening of the lid fissure may also be an early sign of *exophthalmos*. In the initial stage of exophthalmos, only the change in the width of the lid fissure, not the proptosis, will be obvious to the patient. An exophthalmos does not necessarily have an orbital cause. We have observed numerous cases of unilateral exophthalmos caused by intracranial tumors. It is most common in meningiomas of the sphenoid wing (Fig. 1-5). Less frequent causes are sellar, parasellar, and suprasellar tumors and occasionally even a tumor of the frontal or temporal lobe. In the advanced stages, exophthalmos may cause symptoms such as pressure sensation or even dull pain in the orbit in addition to eventual diplopia.

*Narrowing of the lid fissure* may be noticed by the patient even earlier. A *ptosis* (even of the slightest degree) will always be considered a blemish and will certainly be mentioned in the history. Ptosis may be a part of *Horner's syndrome* (miosis, ptosis, enophthalmos). Damage to the central sympathetic system caused by tumors may occur in the cervical region, the medulla oblongata, the pons, and occasionally the thalamus. Much more frequent and pronounced, even with a complete inability to raise the upper lid, is the ptosis in patients with *paresis* or *paralysis of the oculomotor nerve.* If combined with a paralytic mydriasis, a slight ptosis may be part of the transtentorial herniation syndrome, a syndrome that may be characteristic for a generalized increase in intracranial pressure caused by tumors. According to Fischer-Brügge, displaced brain substance presses the oculomotor nerve at the site of its emergence from the brain stem either against the clivus ridge of the tentorial notch or against the superior cerebellar artery, thus causing its damage (p. 161). However, the transtentorial herniation syndrome may be of localizing value in tumors of the temporal lobe with direct pressure on the oculomotor nerve caused by a herniation of the lobe through the tentorial notch. Pareses or paralyses of the oculomotor nerve causing a ptosis may be caused by pressure resulting from tumors anywhere along the entire course of the nerve from the brain stem to the orbit. Their localizing value will be discussed in greater detail on p. 38. In the subjective

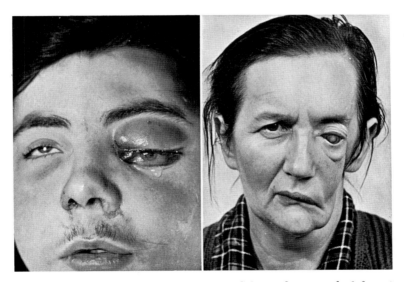

Fig. 1-3. Lagophthalmic corneal ulcer. In patient on left, condition resulted from incomplete lid closure caused by poor general condition and stupor. Thrombosis of the cavernous sinus, exophthalmos, lid edema, chemosis of the conjunctiva, and hypopyon are present. In patient on right, condition resulted from incomplete lid closure caused by peripheral facial palsy. Loss of physiologic folds of face, drooping of angle of mouth and of lower lid, and widening of lid fissure may be noted.

symptomatology, it is important to remember that even an incomplete ptosis *(as long as the upper lid covers the pupil)* will eliminate the eye from the act of binocular vision, *thus masking diplopia caused by paresis of the oculomotor nerve.* In such an instance, one is tempted to talk about a "rational" protective mechanism on the part of nature that makes it unnecessary for the physician to prescribe occlusion. In such a severe ptosis, it is imperative to raise the upper lid in order to analyze the diplopia (Fig. 1-19).

Differences in the size of the pupil will also be mentioned by an observant patient. Of course, in most instances the patient will be unable to distinguish between an abnormal dilation on one side or an abnormal constriction on the other side. *Unilateral miosis* as part of Horner's syndrome causes no subjective sensations. In the history of patients with brain tumors a *unilateral mydriasis* is of greater importance. If the pupil is fixed, *dazzling* and even photophobia (an abnormally large amount of light entering the eye) and *blurring of vision* (the spherical and chromatic aberration of the crystalline lens is greater with a large than with a small pupil) will almost always be in evidence. If the unilateral mydriasis is caused by an impairment of the oculomotor nerve, it will usually be associated with a more or less distinct *paresis of accommodation* (Fig. 1-8). The patient will have fairly good distance vision if the dazzling is not too annoying. However, the near vision at 20 to 30 cm will be blurred to the extent that the patient will be unable to read without the aid of a 3- or 4-diopter convex lens.

The simultaneous involvement of the pupillary reaction and the accommodation results from the fact that the iris sphincter and the ciliary muscle are both innervated by the efferent parasympathetic fibers of the oculomotor nerve. Unilateral impairment of accommodation may also cause micropsia or macropsia of the involved eye. Unilateral mydriasis as a result of peripheral damage to the third nerve has already been discussed in connection with the transtentorial herniation syndrome. In the *differential diagnosis of unilateral mydriasis*, we have to consider, in addition to lesions of the oculomotor nerve, *the effect of certain drugs* (homatropine, atropine, epinephrine), a *congenital anisocoria*, and in particular, *Adie's syndrome* (abolished light reaction of the mydriatic pupil, tonic reaction and relaxation in convergence, and tonic accommodation).

The patient may be able to discover a *paralytic strabismus* when looking into a mirror if the third, fourth, or sixth cranial nerve is involved, as happens quite frequently with cerebral neoplasms. However, in the majority of patients the subjective sensation of double vision will be the dominating factor and will consequently be stressed by the patient. Patients are unable to notice nystagmus by themselves; someone else has to call to their attention such a disturbance of ocular motility. Likewise, it is impossible for patients to observe gaze palsies.

From our dissertation so far it should seem amazing *how many important diagnostic clues can be gained merely from the history of patients with brain tumors.* It pays to "lose time" and take a detailed history! We have therefore elaborated on this material because, in our opinion, it is very important.

## OBJECTIVE EXAMINATION
### External aspect of the eyes

Some aspects included in this section have been treated in the preceding discussion of the symptoms because external changes of the eyes may be conspicuous to the patient. One should listen to the patient's side of the story, but should not make the mistake of depending on it too much. A careful glance at the eyes and their surroundings may yield diagnostic clues in the course of the neuro-ophthalmologic examination.

*Unilateral widening of the lid fissure,* as mentioned before, *is primarily the result of a facial paresis* or more rarely of an irritation of the ocular sympathetic fibers. The central and peripheral forms of Bell's palsy are frequent signs in brain tumors. The frontal branch is not involved in the central but only in the peripheral form. The orbicularis oculi may be slightly or not at all involved in a supranuclear paresis. The loss of tone may cause raising of the upper lid and sagging of the lower lid; the sclera above and below the limbus is not covered by the lids and thus is visible. In testing the strength of the active lid closure the patient is asked to close the eyes as forcefully as possible. The examiner attempts to open the lids with the fingers and should be able to diagnose a paresis from the weak or missing resistance and by a comparison with the opposite side. A total paralysis of the orbicularis muscle leads to *lagophthalmos,* the inability to close the eyes completely. It is seen only in peripheral Bell's palsy. If the patient attempts to close the eye, it characteristically rotates upward (Bell's phenomenon). A deficiency in the moistening of the cornea by the conjunctiva of the upper lid in patients with lagophthalmos may lead to a lagophthalmic corneal keratitis manifested by a perilimbal ciliary congestion as well as by cloudiness and infiltration of the lower part of the cornea. The early damage to the corneal epithelium caused by the exposure can be demonstrated by a positive stain after instillation of 2% fluorescein. It may progress to ulcer formation of the cornea and after a secondary infection may produce the severe picture of a serpiginous ulcer with accumulation of pus (hypopyon) in the anterior chamber. We have observed lagophthalmic keratitis in stuporous or unconscious patients with a brain tumor when, even in the absence of a facial paralysis or perhaps one of a minor degree, no proper lid closure was possible as a result of the poor general condition (lagophthalmos in sopor), increasing the danger of corneal exposure. A particularly serious situation exists in patients who have been operated on for a tumor of the cerebellopontine angle. In addition to a facial palsy, there is usually a lesion of the trigeminal nerve. The exposure of the cornea is complicated by neurotrophic disturbances—a combination of lagophthalmic keratitis and neuroparalytic keratitis (Figs. 1-3 and 1-7).

If there is a difference in the width of the two lid fissures, it is not always easy to decide whether there is a pathologic widening on one side or narrowing on the other side. Testing the active tone of the orbicularis muscle will usually facilitate such a decision. An examination of the pupils (p. 22) should supply additional data. A widening of the lid fissure in patients with Bell's palsy will not be associated with pupillary disturbances. A narrowing of the lid fissure, on the other hand, will often be combined with a pathologic miosis (impairment of the sympathetic fibers) or mydriasis (paresis of the oculomotor nerve).

A *unilateral narrowing of the lid fissure* is usually caused by an abnormal drooping of the upper lid, that is, a *ptosis*. This may be caused either by a paresis of the oculomotor nerve or a lesion of the sympathetic fibers. In the first instance the ptosis results from a paresis of the levator muscle. In the latter the ptosis is caused by involvement of the superior tarsal muscle (Müller's muscle). Associated signs may help in the differential diagnosis. According to a classic rule, *a wider pupil on the side of the ptosis indicates a paresis of the oculomotor nerve, and a narrower pupil on the side of the ptosis* (Horner's syndrome) *means a sympathetic lesion.* Relatively often a ptosis will occur without pupillary changes. In that event the evaluation of the position of the lower lid will be of importance (Kestenbaum). It will be normal in "oculomotor ptosis." In "sympathetic ptosis," however, the lower lid on the involved side is somewhat higher than on the normal side. (The downward pull of the sympathically innervated inferior tarsal muscle is missing.) In other words the lower lid margin covers a larger segment of the limbus on the involved eye. Thus "sympathetic ptosis" can be diagnosed on the basis of the difference in the limbus segmented covered by the lower lid, which will be larger on the involved side. "Oculomotor ptosis" plays a more important role in brain tumors. It has already been mentioned as a manifestation of a general increase in intracranial pressure if associated with mydriasis (transtentorial herniation syndrome) or of a localized pressure caused by tumors of the temporal lobe (Fig. 2-48).

In the differential diagnosis of ptosis, *unilateral blepharospasm* must be ruled out. It may be a sign of a local irritative process in the eye, or it may be an idiopathic phenomenon (generally the case in elderly persons) occasionally associated with a facial spasm. Charcot's "eyebrow sign" is occasionally of some value. In actual ptosis the eyebrow is at the level of the upper orbital margin, whereas it is distinctly lower in blepharospasm.

Under certain conditions, *exophthalmos* may simulate a widening of the lid fissure. A unilateral proptosis of the globe can be recognized only by comparison with the other side. The following method is suitable for a preliminary examination. The examiner stands behind the patient and studies the prominence of the globes by looking down from above; he raises the upper lids and directs the patient to look straight ahead. Quantitative measurements can be obtained with a *ruler,* using a simple test suggested by Kestenbaum. A ruler is held vertically so it touches both the superior and the inferior orbital rims. With the eye closed and the globe in a normal position, the ruler will just touch the skin of the upper lid over the corneal apex. In the patient with exophthalmos the ruler will be in contact with the inferior orbital rim, but will miss the superior orbital rim by a distance dependent on the prominence of the globe. The distance of the ruler from the superior orbital rim is measured and the amount divided by two. The value obtained represents the extent of the exophthalmos. More reliable figures are obtained with the *Hertel* or *Krahn exophthalmometer*. The principle of these instruments is based on the determination of the relative distance between the apex of the cornea and the lateral orbital rim. This is accomplished by an ingenious arrangement of mirrors. If the readings are repeated on the same patient, it is important to always employ the same baseline between the mirrors. Since there are considerable individual variations in the anatomic configuration of the lateral orbital rims, the figures obtained with Hertel's instrument are not absolute values. In normal eyes, they vary between 12 and 17 mm. The method is, however, suitable for comparative exophthalmometry (that is, for a comparison between the two eyes and also for repeated measurements on the same patient on different occasions). Variations or differences of less than 1 mm are not significant (Figs. 1-4 and 1-5).

Exophthalmos is the cardinal symptom of an orbital tumor (Fig. 3-96). The exophthalmos is unilateral. Characteristically, a distinct resistance is felt if one attempts to push the globe into the orbit. Tumors of the anterior and middle fossa may cause exophthalmos by direct invasion of the orbit or by compression of the cavernous sinus. Exophthalmos is an almost constant sign in patients with *meningiomas of the sphenoid wing* (especially of the medial and middle thirds)

Fig. 1-4 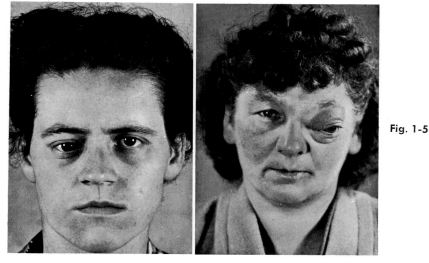 Fig. 1-5

**Fig. 1-4.** Exophthalmos of right eye with downward displacement, the result of extradural dermoid cyst of right frontal region with pressure atrophy of corresponding orbital roof.
**Fig. 1-5.** Exophthalmos of left eye with downward and outward displacement of globe ("chameleon eye") as the result of recurrence of meningioma of left sphenoid ridge (mesial and middle thirds) with invasion into orbit. Enormous lid swelling, extensive impairment of motility of globe, and complete optic atrophy with amaurosis and amaurotic mydriasis are present. This is a recurrence 12 years after first surgical intervention.

(Fig. 3-81). It is seen less frequently with large olfactory meningiomas or pituitary tumors. Actually, brain tumors in almost any location can cause an exophthalmos that is usually bilateral. This is not just a simple proptosis of the globe, but rather an "extrusion" of the orbital contents—obviously the result of an extension of the increased intracranial pressure through the orbital fissures. The frequency of exophthalmos in brain tumors is reported to be between 2% and 8% (Cushing; Uhthoff; Elsberg, Hare, and Dyke), usually caused by meningiomas (which, according to Cushing, may frequently cause a unilateral exophthalmos) and tumors at the base of the brain. Exophthalmos of a lesser degree may occur in patients with tumors of the posterior fossa, a sign of increased pressure. This complication may result in part from the relatively frequent and early development of an internal hydrocephalus in patients with brain tumors. Such an exophthalmos is of little value for purposes of localization; only if it is unilateral may it point out the site of the tumor.

Pareses of the extraocular muscles, a frequent event with brain tumors, may create some degree of proptosis because of the missing retraction of the globe. In such instances, it may be difficult to rule out "pressure exophthalmos."

One should not forget *Graves' disease* in the differential diagnosis of exophthalmos. Although as a rule there is a bilateral proptosis, an asymmetrical or even unilateral exophthalmos is not unusual. Numerous characteristic signs (Graefe, Moebius, Stellwag) as well as the determination of the basal metabolic rate, protein-bound iodine, radioactive iodine uptake, and the Werner triiodothyronine suppression test should help make the correct diagnosis in most cases.

An *intermittent exophthalmos* (proptosis of the globe on bending or on extreme turning of the head) is caused by varicose veins or a varix within the orbit. *Pulsating exophthalmos* is an important sign of an aneurysm of the internal carotid artery within the cavernous sinus (Fig. 5-22). The pulsation can be demonstrated by the rhythmic movements of the reflex to a source of light focused on the cornea. In addition to the pulsation, a marked stasis of the episcleral veins (which should not be confused with a conjunctivitis) is frequently conspicuous in the involved eye. The grave picture of an inflammatory *thrombosis of the cavernous sinus* can easily be differentiated from other forms of exophthalmos. Usually there is a bilateral proptosis with lid edema and severe chemosis, immobilized globes, corneal anesthesia, and general signs of septicemia (Fig. 1-3).

*Swelling of the lids with or without chemosis of the conjunctiva* is not necessarily caused by an inflammatory process in the orbit or the cavernous sinus. We have observed patients with meningiomas of the sphenoid ridge in whom this sign was quite prominent in addition to a pronounced exophthalmos. Obviously, there is an impediment of the circulation of the ophthalmic veins or the cavernous sinus or lymphedema caused by tumor compression (Fig. 3-82).

By definition, exophthalmos is merely a proptosis of the globe in the anteroposterior direction. There may also be a *vertical* or *lateral displacement of the eye.* Intraorbital tumors or tumors invading the orbit from the middle fossa frequently cause a grotesque displacement of the globe downward (Fig. 1-4) or downward and outward ("chameleon eye") (Fig. 1-5). The motility of such eyes is, of course, severely impaired. As a result of such a displacement, pseudolagophthalmos (possibly with signs of keratitis), chemosis, and lid edema are frequent accompanying signs.

The sclera and its vessels may be of some importance in the evaluation of the external aspect of the eye. As mentioned, pressure caused by a tumor in the region of the cavernous sinus or of the ophthalmic vein may cause a *stasis of the episcleral* and *scleral* or even the *conjunctival veins.* The veins in the "white" of the eye are dilated, tortuous, more conspicuous (thus appearing more numerous), and occasionally distinctly prominent. Such a condition can easily be mistaken for aconjunctivitis or episcleritis. We have observed a patient with a post-traumatic carotid-cavernous fistula that was not recognized at first and was treated as chronic conjunctivitis in the presence of obvious signs of stasis (Fig. 1-6).

Corneal changes have been listed in the discussion of lagophthalmos and the resulting *keratitis.* The ulcer seen in this type of keratitis has a typical shape. The upper border is a more or less horizontal line that corresponds approximately to the position of the upper lid margin during sleep. The lower border is a curved line parallel to the limbus. It is difficult to differentiate this form of ulcer from *neuroparalytic ulcer* (Fig. 1-7). Here we also have a perilimbal ciliary or mixed injection, a superficial cloudy zone (consisting mostly of delicate vesicles) in the center of the cornea or slightly below it, positive staining of the damaged epithelium with 2% fluorescein, and eventually outright ulceration. In contrast to lagophthalmic keratitis, the annoying symptoms of foreign body sensation, photophobia, and blepharospasm are missing in patients with neuroparalytic keratitis because the impairment of the trigeminal nerve has caused a loss of sensitivity. The testing of *corneal sensitivity* (p. 21) should be particularly helpful in the differential diagnosis. On the other hand, in cases of lagophthalmic keratitis a paresis or paralysis of the orbicularis muscle should be taken into con-

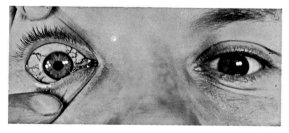

**Fig. 1-6.** Venous stasis of conjunctival and episcleral vessels of right eye in patient with aneurysm of internal carotid artery in cavernous sinus (carotid-cavernous fistula).

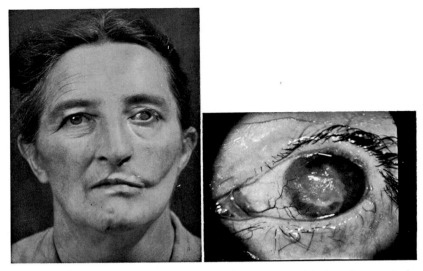

**Fig. 1-7.** Neuroparalytic keratitis of left eye caused by trigeminal lesion after surgical removal of acoustic neurinoma. (A coexisting facial palsy has been greatly compensated by plastic surgery.) Illustration on right is enlargement of ulcerated, dense, central corneal opacity with superficial vascularization originating from limbus.

sideration. *A combination of a lesion of the facial nerve with one of the first branch of the trigeminal nerve,* as seen frequently in patients with tumors of the cerebellopontine angle, especially postoperatively, will cause a *particularly severe* involvement of the cornea. If one does not perform an early tarsorrhaphy in such patients, the corneal ulceration may spread, the stroma may undergo a dense, snow-white infiltration, and the cornea may show superficial and deep vascularization—complications that may reduce the central vision to mere light perception. A superimposed infection or perforation of such ulcers may lead to the complete functional loss of the eye and necessitate enucleation. We have been fortunate to have observed such cases only on rare occasions. However, the gravity of such a complication and the failure of our therapeutic measures has always made a deep impression on us. Corneal transplants are usually out of the question because of the severe neurotrophic disturbances and the extensive vascularization.

*Disturbances of motility* as well as *pupillary changes,* some of the most important changes in the external aspects of the eyes and of great diagnostic significance, will be discussed separately.

### Corneal sensitivity

Corneal sensitivity, one of the attributes of the first branch of the trigeminal nerve in its area of distribution, plays an extremely *important part* in the neuro-ophthalmologic examination for a group of brain tumors, mainly because diagnostically valuable disturbances occur before the appearance of hyperesthesia or hypoesthesia of the skin.

Corneal sensitivity is tested with a small paper strip, a small bead on the end of a pencil (Kearns), or preferably a small, moist, pointed wisp of cotton. The examiner carefully touches the upper and lower halves of the corneas of both eyes with these objects without touching the cilia and the lid margins and compares the force of the orbicularis reflex in the various areas of contact. The direct as well as the consensual corneal reflex on the opposite side should be examined. In testing the upper quadrants of the cornea, one cannot avoid, as a rule, lifting the upper lids a bit with the finger and asking the patient to look down. This is desirable because the force of the closure reflex of the lids can be felt with the finger. It is also important to ask the patient on which side the touch of the test object is felt less distinctly. If the difference between the two sides is slight, the test may be equivocal. In brain stem lesions, it is important to differentiate fifth (sensory) from seventh (motor) nerve impairment of the corneal reflex. Examining the sensitivity of the conjunctiva, the skin of the lids, or even the remainder of the skin in the area of distribution of the first branch of the trigeminal nerve (particularly the frontal and temporal area) or even of the second trigeminal division may possibly supply additional information. A more exact method employs the use of Frey's hairs. For clinical purposes, only the modifications suggested by Boberg-Ans working with a standardized nylon filament might be suitable.

In a unilateral hypoesthesia or anesthesia of the cornea, it may be necessary to rule out local conditions (status after trauma or herpes zoster or simplex of the cornea). *The unilateral absence* or *diminution of the corneal reflex* may represent an *important sign of a tumor in the cerebellopontine angle.* We have noted this condition in practically every case of acoustic neurinoma in our series of patients. We have emphasized that the branch of the ophthalmic division of the trigeminal nerve supplying the skin need not necessarily be involved. Disturbances of corneal sensitivity, combined with lesions of other branches of the trigeminal nerve, are found in the *cavernous sinus,* the *superior orbital fissure,* and the *orbital apex syndromes* (various combinations of involvement of the third, fourth, fifth, and sixth cranial nerves; in the case of the apex syndrome, additional involvement of the optic nerve, occasionally associated with exophthalmos).

## Pupils and pupillary reactions

The true significance of pupillary disturbances caused by brain tumors is based on the protracted course of the reflex arc and the central position of the pupillary center in the midbrain. Even more important, the afferent part of this reflex arc follows the optic nerve and optic tract and the efferent part follows the oculomotor nerve, both structures quite frequently involved by cerebral neoplasms (Fig. 1-11).

During the examination the *size* of the pupils should be observed first. Even under normal conditions, it varies with age (wider pupils in children), the color of the iris (wider pupils in blue eyes), the refractive state (wider pupils in myopic persons), and the tone of the autonomous system (wider pupils in sympatheticotonic persons). A relatively symmetric dilatation of both pupils varying from moderately wide to maximally wide occurs in the terminal stage of increased intracranial pressure. This phenomenon may be caused by damage of both oculomotor nerves immediately after their emergence from the brain stem or occur on the basis of midbrain damage in connection with uncal herniation; some (Scharfetter) have interpreted it to be a consequence of irritation of the sympathetic nervous system. An abnormal bilateral miosis is occasionally a sign of a pontine tumor.

More important for diagnostic and localizing purposes are *differences in the size of the pupils* (anisocoria). It is advisable in such cases to measure the size of the pupils in order to have some data on record for the sake of comparison at a later date. It is best to use a *pupillometer,* a small ruler with graduated circles indicating pupillary sizes from 2 to 8 mm. The actual size of the pupil examined can be determined by comparing it with a circle of the corresponding size of the ruler. For repeated examinations on subsequent occasions a constant illumination (possibly with the aid of a light meter) is, of course, essential. Obviously it is not always easy to decide whether a difference in size of the pupils indicates a pathologic mydriasis on one side or an abnormal miosis on the other side. Usually there are other signs that should make a differential diagnosis easier, and these will be stressed in the discussion to follow.

A *unilateral mydriasis* is caused either by *stimulation of the sympathetic fibers* or by *paralysis of the sphincter of the pupil* secondary to an *involvement of the oculomotor nerve.* A unilateral irritation of the sympathetic branches is rarely caused by pontine and medullary tumors. It is evidenced by a widening of the lid fissure, hyperrhidiosis of the face, and exophthalmos, signs that are occasionally observed only unilaterally in Graves' disease. Paralytic mydriasis, however, plays an important part in brain tumors. In describing subjective symptoms, we have already mentioned that it is frequently associated with a more or less complete paralysis of accommodation. The *impairment of accommodation* can be determined by testing the near vision. The patient is asked to read the smallest print possible at a distance of 20 to 25 cm—first with the good eye, next with the eye involved. If there is an inability to read small print with the latter, perhaps even at an increased distance, a paresis of accommodation can be assumed. This can be compensated by a convex lens (up to 4 diopters), which allows the patient to read at a normal near point. *Mydriasis* and *paresis of accommodation* are typical *signs of a lesion of the oculomotor nuclei* in the midbrain. Tumors, including pineal tumors, may cause such a lesion in this area, usually in combination with a vertical gaze palsy (Parinaud's syndrome) and loss of convergence. A unilateral mydriasis (with or without paresis of accommodation) may also occur in patients with a peripheral oculomotor lesion. It has been mentioned repeatedly as one of the signs of the transtentorial herniation syndrome (Fig. 2-51). This may be either the *manifestation of a generalized increase in the intracranial pressure* or a *localizing sign of a temporal lobe tumor* (may be early slight homolateral ptosis) caused by pressure on the peripheral oculomotor nerve against the clivus ridge by displaced brain substance (transtentorial herniation of the hippocampal gyrus). In the early stage of this syndrome the mydriatic pupil will still react slightly to light. During the course of the disease the reaction will become increasingly more sluggish. Once the patient has lapsed into unconsciousness, the pupil will be fixed. In this connection, we should like to mention the importance of unilateral mydriasis for the localization of epidural or subdural hematomas (Krayenbühl and Noto). A *unilateral mydriasis in combination with paresis of the extraocular muscles supplied by the oculomotor nerve* plus ptosis is seen in even more distal lesions of the oculomotor nerve, as, for instance, in the syndromes of the cavernous sinus, the superior orbital fissure, or the orbital apex—all of which could be caused by tumors, including aneurysms, in addition to other factors (Fig. 1-8). There are also numerous reports of pituitary tumors that may cause peripheral oculomotor pareses with mydriasis and ptosis during the course of an extrasellar lateral expansion.

In the differential diagnosis of a unilateral mydriasis the following conditions

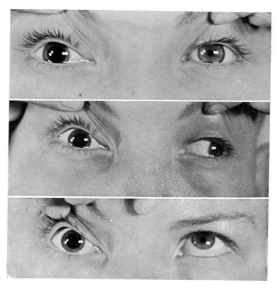

**Fig. 1-8.** Unilateral mydriasis with no pupillary reaction to light and on convergence; paresis of accommodation. This is absolute pupil rigidity in patient with right basal oculomotor paralysis caused by intracavernous aneurysm of internal carotid artery. Lower photographs illustrate inability of right eye to adduct (paresis of medial rectus muscle) and to elevate (paresis of superior rectus muscle).

should be ruled out: *congenital anisocoria, drug mydriasis* (homatropine, atropine, cocaine, adrenaline), and in particular *Adie's syndrome* (a wide pupil that does not react to light and that will dilate even more in subdued light, a pupil with a tonic convergence reaction and prolonged, slow redilation when looking at distance, and a tonic accommodation; this syndrome is mostly unilateral and occurs more frequently in females). Local conditions of the eyes (such as iritis, glaucoma, iris coloboma, and traumatic sphincter tears) can, as a rule, be easily excluded by a closer inspection of the eye.

A *unilateral miosis* is caused either by a stimulation of the iris sphincter or by a *paralysis* of the dilator. The former occurs rarely with brain tumors. Fischer-Brügge describes the unilateral miosis as a quasi first stage of the transtentorial herniation syndrome. There is at first a stimulation of the oculomotor nerve, which later gives way to a partial and, in the end, a complete palsy. We have not observed a unilateral miosis as an early sign of a general increase in the intracranial pressure among our patients. It is seen early in the course of massive subdural or subarachnoid hemorrhage or rapidly expanding aneurysms. The other possibility, a *paralysis of the sympathetic fibers*, results in a *Horner syndrome* characterized by the triad of miosis, ptosis, and apparent enophthalmos (Fig. 1-9). Occasionally, the skin of the forehead on the same side is paler and drier than on the opposite side as a result of the loss of the ability to sweat. In young individuals with brown irides a unilateral lesion of the cervical sympathetic fibers may be followed by a depigmentation of the iris, causing the involved eye to appear lighter or bluish (heterochromia). It may become necessary to differentiate an "oculomotor" from a "sympathetic" miosis, especially if there are no distinctive accompanying symptoms. The *cocaine test* (Jackson) is particularly useful for this purpose. One instills a few drops of a 4% cocaine solution into each eye and observes the behavior of the pupil. If the pupil fails to dilate or dilates poorly, there must be a lesion in the sympathetic pathway to the eye. For a precise localization of a sympathetic lesion with a Horner syndrome the pharmacodiagnostic scheme of Thompson is recommended (Table 1).

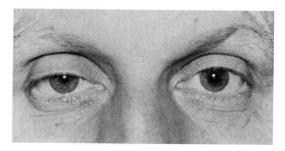

**Fig. 1-9.** Horner syndrome on right side, showing distinct ptosis, miosis, and slight depigmentation of iris (heterochromia).

**Table 1.** Scheme for localization of break in chain of three neurons of sympathetic system°

| Testing substance | Mydriatic effects | | | |
|---|---|---|---|---|
| | First neuron | Second neuron | Third neuron | Normal |
| Cocaine, 4% | + | – | – | + |
| Epinephrine, 0.1% | – | – | ++ | – |
| Phenylephrine, 2% | + | ++ | +++ | + |
| Hydroxyamphetamine, 1% | + | + | – | + |

°Prepared by H. S. Thompson, M.D., Iowa City, Iowa.

The first neuron (hypothalamus to ciliospinal center) is the one most likely to be affected by brain tumors. We have reviewed our series of patients with tumors or with pressure symptoms in the hypothalamic region (craniopharyngiomas). Despite the fairly large number of patients, there was only one with a slight miosis, but none with a fully developed Horner syndrome. More distal would be the region of the pons. A unilateral or bilateral "pinpoint-sized" miosis has been mentioned as typical for pontine and intrapontine tumors. There was no case of a pontine tumor with such miosis in our series. Primary or metastatic tumors located in the medulla oblongata, in the upper cervical spine, or directly in the ciliospinal center (lowest part of the cervical or highest part of the dorsal spine) are also possible sites for a Horner syndrome. An intracranial lesion of the sympathetic system supplying the eye could, however, also occur in the most distal part, that is, in the third neuron; sympathetic fibers accompany the internal carotid and ophthalmic arteries in their course through the cavernous sinus and the superior orbital fissure. Such neoplasms usually cause a simultaneous oculomotor paresis or paralysis, resulting in additional extraocular muscle pareses, a ptosis, and a homolateral mydriasis; in other words, the sympathetic miosis would be superseded by the parasympathetic mydriasis. It is not easy in such cases to demonstrate the sympathetic lesion because the miosis, the outstanding sign, is missing. Instillation of homatropine will cause a less extensive mydriasis of the homolateral pupil than of the normal contralateral one because of the additional damage to the sympathetic fibers.

An *Argyll Robertson* pupil is the primary consideration in the differential diagnosis of a unilateral miosis. It is also known as *reflex pupillary paralysis,* or pupillary "light-near dissociation," and is characterized by its inactivity to light and the preserved reaction to convergence as well as by miosis and anisocoria.

After noting any possible difference in the size of the two pupils, the *reaction to light* is tested. A small but bright pencil flashlight serves quite well for clinical purposes. It is rapidly moved from one eye to the other, with the light beam in the visual axes. It is best if the examining room is not too brightly illuminated so that the light source of the flashlight furnishes the differential threshold for testing the pupillary reaction. The room should not be completely dark, since this makes the evaluation of the consensual light reaction difficult or impossible.

In testing the direct reaction to light, the opposite eye should be covered by hand or, even better, by a black cloth, lest a consensual reaction interfere with the test, giving a false result. Note the rate of speed of the pupillary contraction, the extent of the contraction, whether the contraction is uniform or limited only to parts of the pupillary margin, and the length of time the contraction is sustained. Electronic pupillography (eventually with infrared light) may be used to measure accurately pupillary size, to detect differences in size, and to evaluate abnormal pupillary reactions, but this technique is still largely a research method. Even under normal conditions the light reaction shows considerable variations. It is less active in older than in younger persons, less active in more darkly pigmented irides, and less active in small pupils. The consensual reaction normally is exactly equal to the direct reaction.

Disturbances of the pupillary reaction to light are of considerable importance in brain tumors. In patients with *amaurotic pupil rigidity* the pupil on the blind side is not wider than that on the other side. If the amaurotic eye is exposed to light, neither pupil will react. Both pupils will react if the healthy side is exposed to light. Amaurotic pupil rigidity occurs in patients with tumors of the optic nerve and its sheaths, with pituitary tumors, with tumors of the tuberculum sellae, and with meningiomas of the sphenoid ridge—provided the function of one optic nerve has been destroyed completely by one of these tumors. If the interruption of the optic nerve is partial rather than complete, the direct reaction to light on the involved side and the consensual reaction on the other side are distinctly diminished (afferent pupillary defect). Generally, there is a correlation between the impairment of the visual function and the degree of the pupillary reaction to light. Occasionally, however, there is still a trace of light reaction in a blind eye with a secondary optic atrophy after papilledema. It is considered evidence in favor of the hypothetical separate pupillomotor fibers of the optic nerve, which are supposed to be more resistant. If only one of the optic nerves has been damaged anywhere between the globe and the chiasm (for instance, by the type of

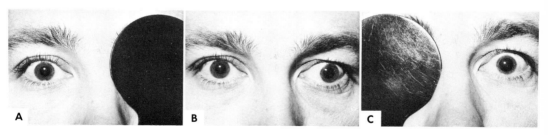

**Fig. 1-10.** Positive left Marcus Gunn pupillary sign after traumatic lesion of left optic nerve (white pallor of whole disc, amaurosis). Pupil of affected eye with normal eye covered is larger, **C,** than pupil of normal eye with affected eye covered, **A. B,** Both eyes under uniform illumination of face. Note equal size of both pupils and left affected eye in slight divergent deviation (concomitant squint).

tumors just mentioned), Kestenbaum's modification of the *Marcus Gunn pupillary sign* may be significant; under uniform illumination of the face the pupil of the affected eye will be larger with the normal eye covered than the pupil of the normal eye with the affected eye covered. The test can also be performed with a swinging flashlight that alternates the stimulus from one eye to the other (Levatin). The light is passed several times across the tip of the nose from one eye to the other while the patient looks into the distance. It is important to wait 5 to 10 seconds on each side for the pupils to redilate (Fig. 1-10). The pupillo-motor strength of the eye involved, with identical illumination, is weaker than that of the healthy eye. If one is able to rule out a purely local cause (such as lens or vitreous opacities or some retinal involvement) in a patient with uni-lateral decrease of vision, a positive Marcus Gunn pupillary sign is rather definite proof of a retrobulbar interference in the conductivity of the prechiasmal afferent pupillary pathway and thus of the homolateral optic nerve between the disc and chiasm (Thompson).

An interruption within the optic tract is known to cause a homonymous hemianopia. If the defect is located between the chiasm and the point where the pupillary reflex fibers branch off just distal to the lateral geniculate body, there is necessarily an impairment of the pupillary reaction of the Wernicke type (*homonymous hemianopic pupil rigidity*). Neither pupil will react if the light falls on the blind retinal halves, but both pupils will react promptly if the light falls on the intact halves. The Wernicke sign is of some importance in cases of homonymous hemianopia caused by a tumor if one wishes to decide whether the lesion is located in the optic tract or in the optic radiation. Actually, it is enormously difficult to demonstrate hemianopic pupil rigidity because of the problem of projecting the light strictly on one half of the retina; there is inter-ference both by the scattering of the refractive media and by the transparency of the sclera. Furthermore, a physiologic factor has to be taken into considera-tion as a possible source of error in testing for hemianopic pupil rigidity: the nasal half of the retina always shows a more distinct pupillomotor effect than the temporal half. The significance of Wernicke's sign can be summarized as follows: if it is definitely positive, the lesion is situated in the optic tract; if it is equivocal, the lesion may be either in the tract or in the radiation. Certain observations by Harms tend to make this question even more confusing. He was able to demonstrate by static perimetry a hemianopic pupil rigidity even in certain hemianopias caused by lesions of the occipital cortex. This should be further proof that Wernicke's phenomenon, or rather the influence of the higher visual centers on the pupillary reflexes, should be carefully reevaluated. One would expect a *bitemporal hemianopic pupil rigidity* in patients with bitemporal hemianopia caused by pituitary tumors. However, we have never observed it in a fairly large number of patients (Fig. 1-11).

In addition to the reaction to light, the pupillary *reaction on convergence* should always be tested. Its presence or absence may be of importance not only

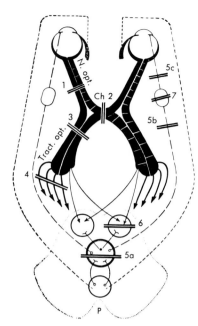

**1,**  Lesion in optic nerve = Amaurotic pupil paralysis

**2,**  Lesion in chiasm = Bitemporal hemianopic pupil rigidity

**3,**  Lesion in optic tract = Homonymous pupil rigidity (right)

**4,**  Lesion in optic radiation = Homonymous hemianopia (right) without hemianopic pupil rigidity

**5a,** Lesion in sphincter nucleus (Edinger-Westphal nucleus) = Absolute pupil rigidity

**5b and 5c,** Lesion of sphincter fibers in oculomotor nerve = Absolute pupil rigidity

**6,**  Lesion in synapsis between sensory and motor part of reflex arc = Light rigidity of pupil (Argyll Robertson)

**7,**  Lesion in ciliary ganglion = Adie's pupil

**Fig. 1-11.** Pathways for pupillary reflexes. Circle *(P)* below sphincter nucleus, *5a*, indicates center of convergence (Perlia's nucleus?). It is point of origin for impulses for convergence of eyes to near point, for accommodation, and for near reflex of pupils.

from the point of etiology, but also for the purpose of localization. The illumination of the room should be even and not too bright. The patient, after having gazed into the distance, is asked to fix on an object (such as a finger or a pencil) held close to his nose. The examiner should note the contraction of the pupils that occurs normally and observe any deviation from this normal reaction, such as diminution, complete absence, or a difference between the two sides as well as the dilatation of the pupils when decreasing the convergence.

The so-called *light rigidity of the pupil*, or pupillary "light-near dissociation" (Argyll Robertson), is characterized by a usually bilateral absence of any reaction to light in the presence of a well-preserved or even exaggerated reaction on convergence (Fig. 1-11). A unilateral or bilateral miosis (caused by a superimposed sympathetic lesion?) is an important additional sign. It is essential to demonstrate (if necessary, with the aid of a loupe or slit lamp) the complete absence of the reaction to light. In its typical form (associated with anisocoria, miosis, and the failure to dilate after the instillation of atropine) the Argyll Robertson pupil is pathognomonic for syphilis of the central nervous system, tabes as well as general paresis being present. The exact site of the lesion is still quite controversial, although it is very likely the region surrounding the Sylvian aqueduct in the rostral midbrain, causing an interruption of the afferent pupillomotor input to the Edinger-Westphal nucleus.

We have purposely described the typical picture of the Argyll Robertson pupil in such detail because *atypical forms* are observed in *tumors of the midbrain,* especially those of the anterior quadrigeminate plate, the third ventricle, and the sylvian aqueduct. Among 10 patients with tumors in this location, we saw eight with bilateral pupillary disturbances of the Argyll Robertson type and one with a unilateral case. Half of these patients had pinealomas. The disturbances were atypical either because the pupils were not completely refractory to light or because there was an incomplete or even complete absence of reaction on convergence. If the pupils, in addition to being totally or partially fixed to light, show a complete or partial loss of convergence reaction, it would be more correct to speak of a *complete* or *incomplete general pupil rigidity.* It is more appropriate to use these terms for the pupillary reactions of some of the tumors in the midbrain than to talk about an atypical Argyll Robertson pupil. For practical clinical purposes, these differences are of a more academic interest because the nuclei for the light and near reaction in the midbrain are very close together. Neoplasms may damage both nuclei or involve just one. Furthermore, such tumors only rarely cause an isolated involvement of the pupillary nuclei in the midbrain, but rather additional (and not less characteristic) signs, such as isolated nuclear palsies of extraocular muscles innervated by the oculomotor nerve, vertical gaze palsies, and paralysis of convergence—all signs that, in their entirety, form *Parinaud's syndrome.*

A *general pupil rigidity* (that is, absence of light and near reaction, together with mydriasis and perhaps even paralysis of accommodation, so-called fixed pupil) suggests most of all a focus involving the sphincter nucleus (Edinger-Westphal). We have seen such a case of an isolated unilateral pupillary disturbance following encephalography. We made a tentative diagnosis of encephalitis or multiple sclerosis activated by the diagnostic procedure. The complete or incomplete general pupil rigidity may, however, be caused by lesions localized in other areas, *lesions involving the efferent pupillary reflex arc (that is, the oculomotor nerve).* The various forms of insults to the oculomotor nerve in its distal portion caused by tumors are discussed in the section on unilateral mydriasis (clivus ridge, cavernous sinus, superior orbital fissure, and orbital apex syndromes). The degree of involvement of the individual factors that form the general pupil rigidity (light reaction, near reaction, mydriasis) may vary. In the more severe and in the complete lesions, there will be a greater tendency toward a complete paralysis to light with maximal mydriasis on convergence (for instance, in the transtentorial herniation syndrome in the advanced stage of unconsciousness). For the sake of completeness, it should be stated that damage to the peripheral oculomotor nerve may cause any combination of pareses or palsies of extraocular muscles in addition to the pupillary impairment (Fig. 1-8).

The differentiation of a light or general pupil rigidity from *Adie's syndrome* usually presents no difficulty. The observation of a tonic convergence reaction and a slow redilation on divergence will help to establish the diagnosis. There are, however, atypical forms of the Adie pupil (for instance, if it is bilateral) that are not so easy to differentiate from the pupillary anomalies just discussed. Certain pharmacologic tests may then be helpful. Topical instillation of 2.5% methacholine (Mecholyl), a cholinergic substance, usually causes contraction of the Adie pupil, but not of the normal pupil (Scheie). Atropine will cause dilation of the Adie pupil, but not the Argyll Robertson pupil.

Testing the pupillary reaction to light may be of importance in yet another respect in the case of brain tumors. It may allow the *differentiation of cortical blindness* and *peripheral amaurosis* (for instance, one caused by a pituitary lesion). In cortical blindness the pupils are of normal width and show a perfectly normal direct and consensual reaction to light. In bilateral peripheral amaurosis the pupils are rather large and show a complete absence of reaction to light in both eyes (or at the most a minimal reaction). The presence of a pupillary reaction to light enabled us to make a rather definite diagnosis of cortical blindness in the case of a bilateral x-ray necrosis of the occipital lobes cited on p. 193.

### Motility of the eyes

Even though certain motor anomalies are merely general signs of increased intracranial pressure (Chapter 2) and scarcely of diagnostic value, there are other anomalies (accompanying especially tumors located at the base of the brain) that actually point to a definite area, thus making a specific diagnosis possible. The more or less sudden appearance of *diplopia,* the subjective equivalent of a motor anomaly, is quite frequently one of the first symptoms of a brain tumor in its initial stage and, as such, important for a topical diagnosis. Pareses of the extraocular muscles in the later stages should be regarded rather as manifestations of a general increase in the intracranial pressure and should be evaluated with caution. In the discussion of history and symptoms, it was emphasized that *motor anomalies do not always cause diplopia,* especially if they are slight or if they are of the supranuclear type. One of the objects of the clinical examination is to discover motility disturbances, even though they might be latent, and to analyze them in detail. Such an analysis includes not only the determination of the muscle involved, but also the evaluation of secondary disturbances of the muscle equilibrium such as overaction and contractures of the antagonists. Such secondary changes are known to modify greatly and mask the original picture in pareses of long standing. The localization of certain disturbances of motility is facilitated if we classify them as extraocular muscle palsies, gaze palsies (that is, palsies of the conjugate eye movements), and nystagmus.

### Extraocular muscle palsies or pareses

Extraocular muscle palsies indicate a *disturbed function of a single or several extraocular muscles caused by a process in the muscle itself, the neuromuscular junction or its nerve, or by a nuclear lesion in the brain stem* (Fig. 1-12).

One begins the test for a possible muscle paresis or paralysis by observing the *position of the eyes* in the primary position. The more obvious palsies result in a change in position of the eyes already in the primary position—less an effect of the muscle paresis than secondary to an overaction of one or more antagonists. In patients with unilateral sixth nerve paresis, for instance, the involved eye frequently turns in because of the overaction of the homolateral medial rectus muscle. In a paresis of the medial rectus muscle the eye turns out as a result of overaction of the lateral rectus muscle. In the first instance, there seems to be a convergent strabismus; in the second instance, a divergent strabismus. In pareses of the vertical rotators, there is also a compensatory torsion, depression, or inclination of the head (ocular torticollis), signs that are generally neglected. It should be stated quite emphatically that these are cases of *paralytic strabismus* that should be strictly differentiated from nonparalytic strabismus or concomitant

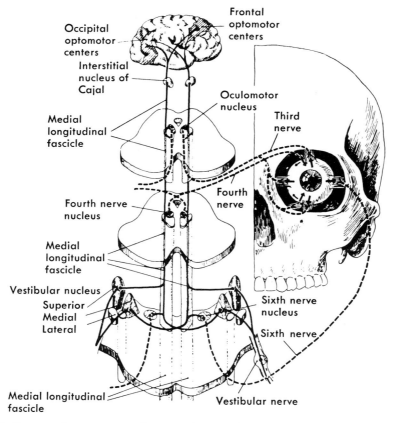

**Fig. 1-12.** Pattern of innervation of extraocular muscles. Cortical optomotor centers, supranuclear centers for conjugate movements in brain stem, medial longitudinal fascicle, nuclei of vestibular nerves, Cajal's nuclei, oculomotor nuclei, oculomotor nerves, and effective organs (six extraocular muscles). (After Netter.)

squint. The mere inspection of the position of the eyes permits no such differentiation, especially if performed only when the eyes are in the primary position. Only a careful study of the excursion of the eyes in the various directions of gaze will help to clarify the situation.

In testing the *motility of the eyes,* one asks the patient to look at or follow an object to the *six cardinal positions* that are of diagnostic significance (to the right, to the left, up and to the right, down and to the right, up and to the left, down and to the left, Fig. 1-13). This simple test may elicit extremely valuable information and may establish the diagnosis of the paretic muscle in some cases. For one thing, it will generally rule out a concomitant strabismus. If the angle of squint (the angle formed by the axes of the two eyes) varies in different directions of gaze, this indicates a paralytic strabismus. If the angle does not vary (in other words, if the degree of convergence or divergence remains constant in the various directions of gaze), this indicates a concomitant strabismus. Testing the excursions in the six cardinal directions should yield another result in the case of a paralytic strabismus: it will indicate the *limitation of movement in a definite direction of gaze that corresponds to the direction of the primary action of the paretic or paralytic muscle.* The diagnosis of the involved muscle can be made by means of a simple diagram (Fig. 1-14) if a limitation of excursion is observed in one of the cardinal directions. If the function of several muscles is impaired, the picture is more complicated. It is not always easy to judge the limitation of excursion of one eye in a certain direction. For one thing, this limitation may be quite minute and may be missed during a casual examination. We have observed this repeatedly in patients with sixth nerve pareses caused by tumors as well as in those with pareses of the vertical rotators. For

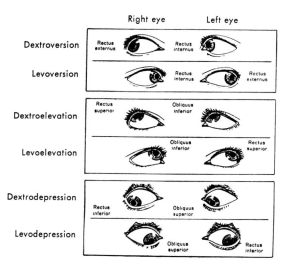

**Fig. 1-13.** Diagnostically important six cardinal directions of gaze with indication of which individual muscles of each eye are involved in each instance. (After Lyle.)

a more accurate and quantitative evaluation of the excursions the *limbus test* elaborated by Kestenbaum is suitable.

   A transparent millimeter ruler is held directly in front of the eye to be tested. The patient is asked to look straight ahead and to fix on the pupil of the examiner. For the determination of abduction the examiner finds the position of the nasal border of the limbus and makes a note of this figure. The patient is then asked to look to the temporal side as far as possible. The position of the nasal border of the limbus is again recorded. The difference between these two figures indicates the amplitude of abduction in millimeters. Similarly, in testing adduction the temporal border of the limbus is used as a point of reference. For the measurements of elevation and depression the lower and upper borders of the limbus are used. Based on a large number of observations, Kestenbaum determined a figure of 9 to 10 mm as normal for abduction and adduction. Figures of 8 mm, or less should be regarded as pathologic. The normal values for depression are 9 to 10 mm, and for elevation, 5 to 7 mm. Differences of 1 mm or more also should be considered as pathologic. These values are outlined more precisely as follows (see also Fig. 1-15)*:

|  |  |
|---|---|
| Maximal abduction | 9-10 mm |
| Maximal adduction | 9-10 mm |
| Maximal depression | 9-10 mm |
| Maximal elevation | 5- 7 mm |

*Values 1 mm or more below those given are pathologic.

**Right eye**

| | Right | Up | Left |
|---|---|---|---|
| **Temporal** | Superior rectus | Superior rectus + inferior oblique | Inferior oblique |
| | Lateral rectus | | Medial rectus |
| | Inferior rectus | Inferior rectus + superior oblique | Superior oblique |
| | Right | Down | Left |

**Nasal**

**Left eye**

| | Right | Up | Left |
|---|---|---|---|
| **Nasal** | Inferior oblique | Superior rectus + inferior oblique | Superior rectus |
| | Medial rectus | | Lateral rectus |
| | Superior oblique | Inferior rectus + superior oblique | Inferior rectus |
| | Right | Down | Left |

**Temporal**

**Fig. 1-14.** Diagram of principal action of individual muscles of both eyes, disregarding torsion. Analysis of impairment of motility of eye according to this diagram should permit determination of paretic or paralytic extraocular muscle in simple cases. (After Franceschetti.)

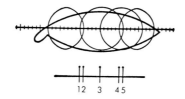

12  3  45

**Fig. 1-15.** Limbus test, according to Kestenbaum, for measurement of excursion capacity of eye: 5-2, normal internal rotation (9 to 10 mm); 1-4, normal external rotation (9 to 10 mm); 1-3, diminished external rotation (5 mm). Horizontal graduated line represents millimeter graduation of transparent ruler.

In partial muscle pareses the limitation of motility may be difficult to visualize. In such patients the demonstration of the so-called *muscle paretic nystagmus* may be a valuable adjuvant. In the terminal position of action of the paretic muscle, there are some jerky nystagmoid movements. These are caused by an alternating complete exhaustion (slow component) and partial recovery (quick component) of the muscle. This nystagmus manifests itself almost exclusively on the side of the involved eye; occasionally, it is bilateral if the healthy eye also responds to the alternating nervous impulses with jerky nystagmoid movements.

The third result of testing the limits of excursion of the eyes should be the *proof of diplopia,* one of the most important symptoms of a paralytic strabismus. The tests for diplopia will in most instances permit one to make a conclusive diagnosis of the paralyzed muscle. Frequently the patient will have complained of double vision during the simple testing of the eyes in the six cardinal directions. To render a latent diplopia manifest and to create a more distinct dissociation of the images of the two eyes, it is advisable or occasionally even necessary to hold a red glass in front of one of the patient's eyes or to use one of the commercially available red-green spectacles (the so-called diplopia goggles). The examiner holds a light source (flashlight, lighted candle, etc.) at a distance of 1 to 2 meters in front of the patient's eyes and moves it in the six cardinal directions. The patient is instructed to follow the light with the eyes, without moving the head, and to indicate in which direction a double image is seen; whether the two images are side by side or vertically displaced; how the horizontal and vertical disparity of the images changes in the various directions of gaze; and how the relative position (right or left) of the two differently colored images changes.

This so-called red glass or *red-green glass test* is extraordinarily well suited for clinical purposes and furnishes absolutely reliable results by simple means and in a relatively short time. It is best to record the position of the double images as indicated by the patient on a diagram of nine squares with colored crayons. In addition to representing the six cardinal positions, these squares also represent the straight up, straight down, and primary positions. Analysis of this *diplopia diagram* permits the diagnosis of the paretic muscle in a simple manner if the following three points are take into consideration (Table 2):

1. *The direction in which the double images show their maximal separation* (horizontal or vertical) *corresponds to the principal function of the paretic muscle in question* (Fig. 1-14).
2. This observation already limits the diagnosis to a single pair of muscles, leaving two possibilities: one muscle for one eye, another muscle for the other eye. The determination of the eye and thus the muscle involved is simple. *In the direction of maximal separation of the two images the one more peripherally seen belongs to the eye involved.* The red glass or red-green glass goggles permit this differentiation with ease.
3. Actually, points 1 and 2 suffice for the diagnosis of the paretic muscle.

**Table 2.** Franceschetti's diagram for examination and interpretation of diplopia with red-green glass goggles or with the Maddox test

| Differential diagnosis of double images in the horizontal plane | | |
|---|---|---|
| Type of separation (first criterion) | Maximum of separation (second criterion) | Diagnosis |
| Uncrossed (homonymous) diplopia | To the right | Paralysis of right lateral rectus muscle |
| | To the left | Paralysis of left lateral rectus muscle |
| | To the right as well as to the left | Paralysis of both lateral rectus muscles |
| | In the primary position | Paralysis of divergence or convergence spasm |
| | No maximum Diplopia rare | Convergent concomitant strabismus |
| Crossed (heteronymous diplopia) | To the right | Paralysis of left medial rectus muscle |
| | To the left | Paralysis of right medial rectus muscle |
| | To the right as well as to the left | Paralysis of both medial rectus muscles |
| | In the primary position | Convergence paralysis |
| | No maximum Diplopia rare | Concomitant divergent strabismus |

| Differential diagnosis of double images in the vertical plane | | | |
|---|---|---|---|
| Type of separation (first criterion) | Increase in vertical separation (second criterion) | Maximum of vertical separation (third criterion) | Diagnosis (paralyzed muscle) |
| Positive vertical separation (position of right eye higher; image of left eye seen higher) | Up | To the right and up | Left inferior oblique muscle |
| | | To the left and up | Left superior rectus muscle |
| | Down | To the right and down | Right inferior rectus muscle |
| | | To the left and down | Right inferior oblique muscle |
| Negative vertical separation (position of right eye lower; image of left eye seen lower) | Up | To the right and up | Right superior rectus muscle |
| | | To the left and up | Right inferior oblique muscle |
| | Down | To the right and down | Left superior oblique muscle |
| | | To the left and down | Left inferior rectus muscle |

In the differential diagnosis within the group of the two elevators and the two depressors the following rule may be useful for a clearer distinction between the recti and the oblique muscles: *if the vertical separation of the two images reaches its maximum with the involved eye in abduction, the muscle in question is a rectus (superior or inferior); if the maximum occurs with adduction of the involved eye, the muscle in question must be an oblique (superior or inferior).*

The more or less distinct inclination of the images as well as a slight horizontal disparity that occurs in pareses of the vertical rotators should be disregarded in these tests.

In our opinion, these methods are perfectly adequate to arrive at a fairly accurate qualitative decision during a bedside examination. For quantitative purposes and for a repetition of the examination on different occasions, more exact methods have to be employed. The same is true for palsies of long-standing duration and for those with pronounced secondary changes (overaction of the homolateral antagonist or the contralateral synergist; secondary paresis of the contralateral antagonist). Such changes may be difficult to elicit with the simple clinical tests.

The *Hess screen* or coordinometer is ideally suited for this purpose. Also based on subjective diplopia, the separation of the two images is accomplished with the use of red-green glass goggles. The great advantage of this method is that at the end of the test the result can be read immediately from a diagram. It gives information on the paretic muscles as well as the overaction of the ipsilateral antagonists and contralateral synergists. If *several ocular pareses overlap,* as is likely to occur in patients with brain tumors, we have used the Hess screen as the *method of choice.* Actually we use a modified Hess screen with a green and red dot projected by an electric flashlight on a tangent screen divided into squares (Lancaster red-green projection test). The examiner points one dot (for instance, red) successively to the various squares on the screen. He directs the patient, whose head is in a fixed position and who wears the red-green glass goggles, to move his flashlight in such a manner that the other dot (for instance, green) seems to cover the first one. In the case of a muscle paresis the patient will project his dot in certain directions incorrectly, thus modifying the Hess

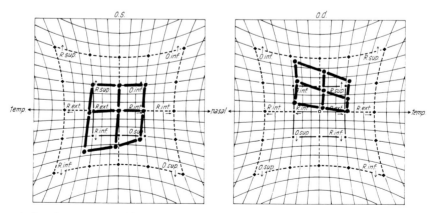

**Fig. 1-16.** Graphic account of disturbances of ocular motility obtained with Hess coordinometer. Example demonstrates paresis of right superior oblique with overaction of left inferior rectus and contracture of right inferior oblique.

diagram in such a manner that it will allow the determination of the type of muscle disturbance. The smaller "field of gaze" always belongs to the eye with the paretic muscle (Fig. 1-16). For further details of the Hess-Lancaster method, refer to the various textbooks of ophthalmology as well as to Lyle and Jackson's *Practical Orthoptics in the Treatment of Squint.*

For a quantitative and even more accurate analysis of motility disturbances, we have used the *Maddox rod test* as an additional method. It is performed at a distance of 5 meters and is based on the method and interpretation elaborated by Franceschetti. We have examined patients with minute pareses that were not manifest on the Hess screen, but could be demonstrated without difficulty on the Maddox cross.

The Maddox test utilizes a tangent scale arranged in the form of a cross with a small source of light in its center. The patient fixes on this light, at a distance of 5 m, with the Maddox rod glass in front of one eye. This changes the point source of light to a streak that runs at a right angle to the direction of the rod glass. The patient should indicate whether the streak of light passes directly through the light seen by the other eye or whether there is a lateral or a vertical displacement. According to the position of the light streak, the lateral or vertical deviation can be read directly in angle degrees on a properly calibrated tangent scale. With paralyzed horizontal rotators, the displacement has to be determined only in the primary position and in dextroversion and levoversion. With paralyzed vertical rotators, it is advisable to measure the vertical displacement in the nine cardinal directions, with the head turned in the appropriate position. The diagram thus obtained is analyzed according to Franceschetti's suggestions (Table 2).

According to the literature as well as our own material, muscle pareses occur in 10% to 15% of patients with brain tumors. Sixth nerve pareses are by far the most frequent, with those of the oculomotor nerve in second place. Pareses of the superior oblique muscle are rare.

As a second part of the test for an ocular paresis, one should attempt to obtain an exact *localization of the basic lesion,* an important factor in brain tumors. It is almost impossible to pinpoint a lesion solely based on the type of ocular paresis found. It is rather the accompanying neurologic signs that might supply such

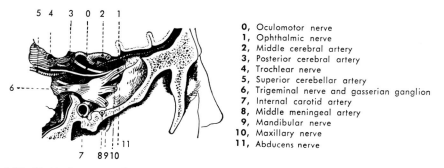

0, Oculomotor nerve
1, Ophthalmic nerve
2, Middle cerebral artery
3, Posterior cerebral artery
4, Trochlear nerve
5, Superior cerebellar artery
6, Trigeminal nerve and gasserian ganglion
7, Internal carotid artery
8, Middle meningeal artery
9, Mandibular nerve
10, Maxillary nerve
11, Abducens nerve

Fig. 1-17. Vertical section through base of brain and base of skull, illustrating intracranial course of oculomotor, trochlear, abducens, and trigeminal nerves.

important clues. The following criteria may serve as guides in the examination of the various innervational disturbances of the nerve supplying the extraocular muscles (Fig. 1-17).

**Abducens nerve (VI).** The characteristic sign of the motility disturbance is a horizontal diplopia with maximal separation of the images in lateral rotation to the involved side. The eye will assume a convergent position if the paresis is severe. Because of the long and exposed intracranial course of the sixth nerve, it may suffer from distant effects of brain tumors in a variety of locations, perhaps as a result of displacement of the brain stem. For that reason an isolated sixth nerve paresis is of little interest as far as localization is concerned. Only in combination with other neurologic defects will it permit certain conclusions (Fig. 1-18).

*Nuclear and fascicular types*
*Millard-Gubler syndrome.* Paresis of the lateral rectus muscle, homolateral peripheral facial palsy, crossed hemiplegia (including crossed hypoglossal paresis).
*Foville's syndrome.* Paresis of the lateral rectus muscle, homolateral peripheral facial palsy, homolateral horizontal gaze palsy (caused by additional damage to the homolateral posterior longitudinal bundle), possibly combined with a Horner syndrome.

*Root types*
Paresis of the lateral rectus muscle usually combined with a homolateral peripheral facial palsy.

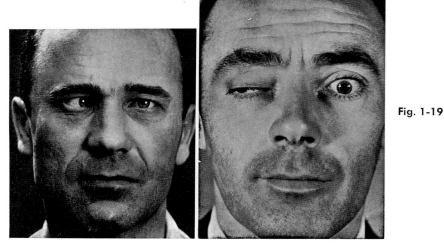

**Fig. 1-19**

**Fig. 1-18**

**Fig. 1-18.** Abducens nerve palsy on right side. Paresis of right lateral rectus muscle. Convergent position of right eye is caused by overaction of homolateral medial rectus muscle.
**Fig. 1-19.** Complete right oculomotor paresis including ptosis, globe turns out and down, and mydriatic absolute pupil rigidity (not visible because of ptosis).

*Basal types*

Paresis of the lateral rectus muscle combined with a varying combination of the third, fourth, fifth, sixth, seventh, and eighth homolateral cranial nerves.

*Clinical picture in cerebellopontine tumors* (acoustic neurinomas!)

*Gradenigo's syndrome.* Homolateral paresis of the lateral rectus muscle and trigeminal lesion (pain, hypesthesia), eventually facial paresis, usually affection of the apex of the petrous bone (otitis, tumor).

*Syndromes of the cavernous sinus, superior orbital fissure, and orbital apex.* Paresis of the lateral rectus muscle combined with pareses of the third, fourth, and fifth cranial nerves; perhaps also the optic nerve in the apex syndrome (tumors, especially metastases and aneurysms, in the cavernous sinus; pituitary adenomas with lateral extension; meningiomas of the middle fossa; trigeminal neurinomas; meningiomas of the sphenoid ridge).

**Oculomotor nerve (III).** Characteristic signs of the motility disturbance include, in the fully developed picture, ptosis, paralysis of the superior rectus, medial rectus, inferior rectus, and inferior oblique muscles, and mydriasis as well as a more or less sluggish pupillary reaction to light and on convergence. In the primary position the involved eye turns out and down. There is horizontal and vertical diplopia in the primary position. The vertical diplopia increases in elevation and depression. The horizontal diplopia increases in rotation to the side of the uninvolved eye (Figs. 1-8 and 1-19).

*Nuclear and fascicular types*

Simultaneous pareses of single extraocular muscles supplied by the oculomotor nerve in both eyes. There may or may not be pupillary disturbances (mydriasis, sluggish pupillary reaction), paresis of accommodation, and severe symmetric ptosis. In tumors within or near the midbrain (pinealomas), there is a combination of isolated muscle pareses with *vertical gaze palsy*, possibly a disturbance of convergence, and nystagmus retractorius (Parinaud's syndrome, sylvian aqueduct syndrome, pineal syndrome).

*Fascicular types*

*Dorsal form.* Unilateral oculomotor paresis with crossed hemitremor *(Benedict's syndrome)*, possibly also with crossed hemianesthesia.

*Ventral form.* Unilateral, mostly complete oculomotor palsy with crossed hemiplegia *(Weber's syndrome)*, possibly with crossed central facial and hypoglossal palsies.

*Root types*

Unilateral oculomotor paresis with crossed hemiplegia *(Weber's syndrome)*.

*Basal types*

A localized lesion shows a monosymptomatic oculomotor paresis with varying affections of the sphincter of the pupil and the ciliary muscle (aneurysms of the posterior communicating artery or rather at the site of its branching off from the internal carotid artery) (Figs. 1-8 and 5-11). A large diffuse lesion at the base of the skull (tumors, basal meningitis) is characterized by an additional involvement of the fourth, fifth, sixth, and possibly the seventh and eighth cranial nerves.

*Cavernous sinus syndrome.* Unilateral oculomotor paresis (mostly with mydriasis and general rigidity of the pupil) combined with pareses of the fourth, fifth, and sixth cranial nerves (Fig. 3-101) (tumors, especially metastases and aneurysms in the cavernous sinus; laterally extending pituitary adenomas; meningiomas of the middle fossa; trigeminal neurinomas). Posterior form: first and second (possibly also third) branches of trigeminal nerve involved. Anterior form: first branch of trigeminal nerve involved.

*Superior orbital fissure syndrome.* Unilateral oculomotor paresis combined with a paresis of the fourth, fifth (first branch) and sixth cranial nerves (Fig. 1-20).

*Apex syndrome.* Pareses, the third, fourth, fifth (first branch), and sixth cranial nerves combined with lesions of the optic nerve (central scotoma; peripheral visual field defects; optic atrophy; or possibly papilledema). Exophthalmos in the case of tumors.

**Trochlear nerve (IV).** Characteristic signs of the motility disturbance include slight upward deviation of the involved eye that increases with inward rotation and depression (a predominantly vertical deviation, with the maximum

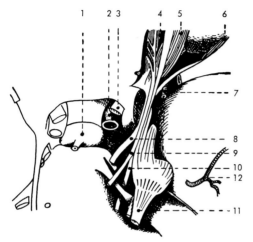

1, Pituitary gland and infundibulum
2, Internal carotid artery
3, Optic nerve
4, Superior oblique muscle
5, Levator muscle of upper lid
6, Lateral rectus muscle
7, Ophthalmic vein
8, Oculomotor nerve
9, Trochlear nerve
10, Abducens nerve
11, Trigeminal nerve
12, Middle meningeal artery

**Fig. 1-20.** Schematic illustration of area of chiasm and cavernous sinus, showing course of nerves supplying extrinsic ocular muscles as they enter orbit from middle cranial fossa.

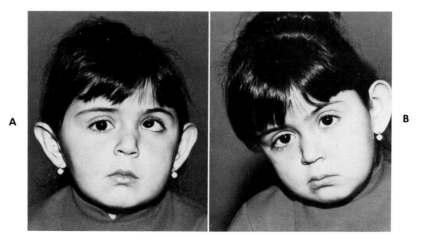

**Fig. 1-21.** Trochlear nerve palsy on left side, showing, **A,** upshoot of left eye in adduction, limitation of downward movement of left eye in gaze down and right, and, **B,** tilting of head to right to eliminate diplopia.

in the in and down position), a compensatory torsion, and a tilting of the head to the opposite side (Fig. 1-21).

An isolated trochlear paresis is rare. It is of no localizing significance because the lesion could be nuclear, somewhere in the brain stem, or affecting the peripheral nerve.

### Nuclear types

A trochlear paresis combined with a homolateral oculomotor paresis, occasionaly in association with vertical gaze palsies, convergence spasm or convergence palsy, and pupillary disturbances is seen in tumors of the *roof of the midbrain* or *pinealomas* (pineal syndrome).

### Peripheral types

See discussions of cavernous sinus, superior orbital fissure, and apex syndromes in association with oculomotor lesions.

• • •

It is obvious that in the differential diagnosis of the extraocular muscle pareses many other causes in addition to tumors have to be considered that were not discussed in detail (encephalitis, meningitis, neuritis, syphilis, tuberculosis, exogenous poisons, diabetes, vascular accidents, trauma, multiple sclerosis, syringobulbia, and others). Although a large number of etiologic factors have to be ruled out by whatever special type of investigation is indicated, there is one in particular that should always be considered and that we have encountered time and again in connection with patients suspected of brain tumors—namely, *myasthenia gravis.* Even though there is an actual involvement of the neuromuscular junction, the resulting picture can easily be mistaken for muscle pareses of neurogenic origin. As a rule the muscle disturbances in patients with myasthenia show conspicuous fluctuations in degree. In the morning, after the patient has had a good night's rest, they may be missing completely, only to return (together with a ptosis of the upper lid!) during the course of the day. Signs of fatigue in other muscle groups (muscles of speech and mastication, muscles of the extremities) may be completely missing initially. The disease may even remain limited to the ocular muscles. The edrophonium (Tensilon) test (intravenous injection of 5 to 10 mg edrophonium), which is almost specific for myasthenia gravis, will in many cases cause the paresis and, with it, the subjective diplopia to disappear for a short time. This is not always the case. We have observed one patient with myasthenia gravis who had several bilateral multiple ocular pareses that did not respond to edrophonium (Fig. 1-22). This patient had been referred to the department of neurosurgery because a tumor in the brain stem had been suspected!

The electromyographic examination of an extraocular muscle during the edrophonium test is indispensable in patients suspected of having myasthenia gravis but in whom neither the ptosis nor the extraocular paresis improved clinically after the administration of edrophonium. The electromyogram (EMG) can give a positive edrophonium effect (transient improvement of the neuromuscular

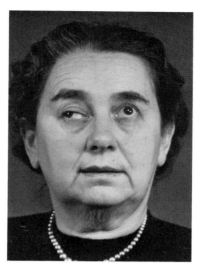

**Fig. 1-22.** Multiple pareses of extraocular muscles (right medial rectus muscle, left medial and inferior rectus muscles, intermittent ptosis of right eye) in myasthenia gravis. In this patient, involvement of ocular muscles was only manifestation of disease.

junction block and activation of motor units) even when no visible effect on the extraocular muscles is observed clinically (Fig. 1-23).

*Electromyography* plays an important role today in the diagnosis of paresis of the extraocular muscles (Breinin; Huber; Esslen and Papst; Blodi and Van Allen; Tamler and Jampolsky). This examination method makes it possible to differentiate between myopathies (myositis, muscular dystrophy, endocrine ophthalmopathy, myotonia), myasthenia (disturbances of the neuromuscular junction), peripheral neurogenic paresis, and supranuclear disturbances (gaze palsies, internuclear ophthalmoplegia, convergence palsies) (Fig. 1-23). This differentiation is of the utmost importance when dealing with ocular muscle paresis produced by cerebral tumors. In these cases we are dealing most often either with a peripheral neurogenic or with a supranuclear form. These have to be differentiated from myopathies or myasthenia. Depending on the case, the electric response has to be obtained from one or several of the extraocular muscles, occasionally even at different time intervals.

In patients with an isolated paresis of the sixth nerve (less frequently in those with pareses of the third or fourth nerve), *multiple sclerosis* always has to be considered. Occasionally it causes ocular symptoms long before the occurrence of other typical neurologic symptoms. If such a paresis is accompanied by vague chronic headaches (we have seen such cases), a brain tumor may be rightly suspected. With the modern diagnostic methods that are available to the neurosurgeon, brain tumor usually can be ruled out with a great degree of probability. Examination of the spinal fluid and perhaps the demonstration of other very

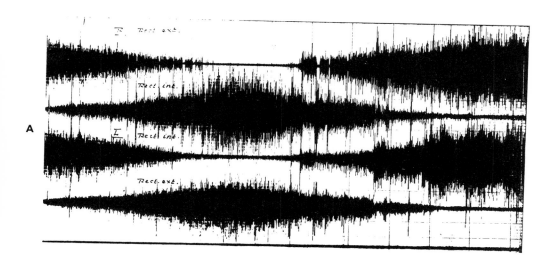

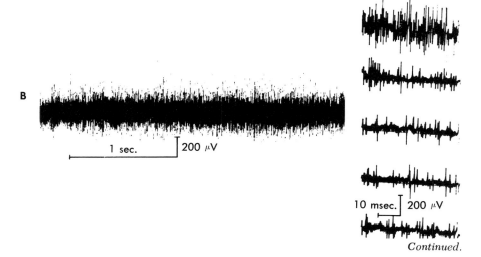

*Continued.*

**Fig. 1-23. A,** EMG's of four horizontal recti of both eyes. Augmentation of activity in agonist is accompanied by concomitant parallel decrement of activity in antagonist. On rotation out of field of action, reduction of electric activity to firing of a few motor units; on rotation into field of action, increase of frequency of discharge and appearance of new motor units (interference pattern). **B,** EMG of ocular myopathy. Intensive interference pattern on effort despite little or no movement of affected muscle and increased number of polyphasic potentials (see curves on right).

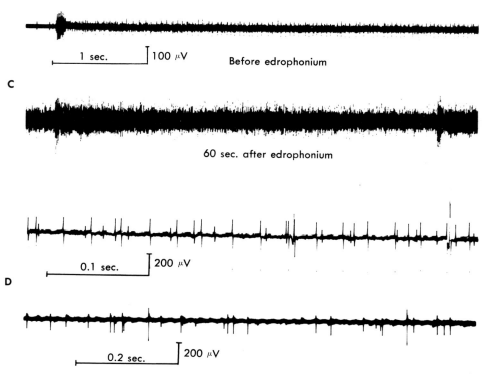

Fig. 1-23, cont'd. **C**, EMG of myasthenia gravis. Note progressive decrease in electric activity of the muscle during sustained effort (fatigue pattern, neuromuscular block) (top curve) and prompt building up of electric activity to interference pattern after intravenous injection of edrophonium (Tensilon) (bottom curve). Reaction pathognomonic for myasthenia! **D,** EMG of neurogenic palsy. There is irregular or sparse recruitment and falling out of motor units, poorly sustained discharge, and loss of interference pattern (top curve) with appearance of fibrillations (discharge of single muscle fiber potentials without relation to volition) as cardinal sign of denervation after 2 to 3 weeks (bottom curve).

minute early signs of multiple sclerosis (unilateral temporal or general pallor of the disc with a history of visual disturbances, bilateral internuclear ophthalmoplegia) are helpful in establishing the diagnosis.

Next to the possibility of a brain tumor, an isolated peripheral oculomotor palsy with involvement of all the corresponding extrinsic muscles, mydriasis, and sluggishness of the pupillary reactions should arouse suspicion of an existing *aneurysm at the base of the brain* (cavernous sinus, posterior communicating artery). Aneurysms, in the broadest sense of the word, are tumors and therefore will be briefly discussed in Chapter 5. (See p. 328 and Figs. 1-8 and 5-15.)

### Palsies of conjugate eye movements

In contrast to the isolated extraocular palsies, with a disturbance of one or several individual muscles, *gaze palsies are disturbances of the supranuclear*

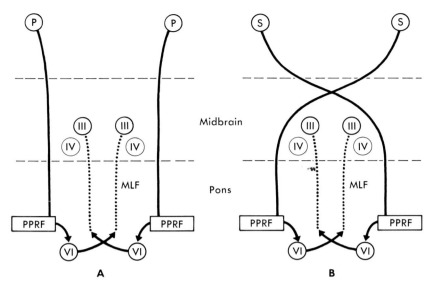

**Fig. 1-24.** Schematic representation of occipito-mesencephalic-pontine pathways serving pursuit movements (pursuit system) and fronto-mesencephalic-pontine pathways serving saccadic movements (saccadic system). *P*, Occipitoparietal representation of pursuit system; *S*, frontal representation of saccadic system; *PPRF*, paramedian pontine reticular formation or pontine gaze center; *VI*, abducens nerve nucleus; *IV*, trochlear nerve nucleus; *III*, oculomotor nerve nucleus; *MLF*, medial longitudinal fascicle. For didactic reasons the double decussation of the pursuit system (*P*) is not shown on **A**.

*centers involving movements that combine the two eyes, so to speak, into a single visual organ that makes uniform movements in space* (directing the fovea to an object of interest, pursuing a moving target, aligning the eyes with respect to one another, and adjusting for movements of the head and body).

For the execution of these eye movements, there exist five supranuclear systems: the *saccadic system* for all fast eye movements (including the fast phases of optokinetic and vestibular nystagmus), the smooth *pursuit system* for the eyes to follow a slowly moving object, the *vergence system* for the alignment of the eyes on an object at any distance, the *vestibular system* for regulating the position of the eyes with respect to the head and body, and the *position maintenance system* for keeping the eyes on target or in a specific position.

The *saccadic system* for fast (also called voluntary or command) movements has its cortical representation diffusely in the *frontal lobes* (including Brodmann's area 8); it is located in the right frontal lobe for horizontal conjugate gaze to the left, in the left frontal lobe for horizontal gaze to the right, and in both frontal lobes together for vertical gaze (Fig. 1-24). The projection fibers from the frontal eye field for horizontal movements, after passing through the internal capsule and the subthalamus, decussate at the level of the trochlear nucleus and terminate in the contralateral paramedine pontine reticular formation (pontine gaze center). The fibers for vertical movements pass from both frontal lobes to the pretectal area (vertical gaze center). The *saccadic system is tested by asking the patient to look rapidly from one object to another or from one gaze position to another,* and the way the eyes react to these instructions is observed (including eventual slight refixation).

In contrast, the smooth *pursuit system* for slow eye movements (serving the functions of fixation and pursuit) has its cortical representation in the occipitoparietal visual association area (including Brodmann's areas 18 and 19); it is located in the right occipital pole for pursuit to the right, in the left occipital pole for pursuit to the left, and in both occipital lobes together for vertical pursuit (Fig. 1-24). The occipitopontine pathways for horizontal pursuit movements run centrifugally from the occipitoparietal lobe in the stratum sagittale internum of the visual radiation through the pulvinar, the pretectal area to the mesencephalic reticular formation (joining the frontal lobe projections), and after double crossing in the midbrain and later at the pontomesencephalic junction to the pontine gaze center (pontine paramedian reticular formation). The axons for vertical pursuit movements use the same pathway to the pretectal area, where they communicate with the oculomotor nuclei and the descending frontomesencephalic pathways for vertical saccades. *The smooth pursuit system is tested by having the patient follow a slowly moving object* (such as a pencil or a finger) *in front of the eyes and across the field of vision.*

The *vergence system* is also cortically represented in the occipitoparietal area; its occipitopretectal pathways descend together with the pursuit paths to the pretectal region and from there to the oculomotor nuclei and other areas of the mesencephalic-pontine junction. *This system is tested by asking the patient to fixate on a pencil or finger, which is moved toward him until touching the nose.* (A simultaneous pupillary constriction will persuade the examiner that a convergence effort is realized!)

The *vestibular system* comprises the vestibular nuclei and their projections, the eighth cranial nerves, and the semicircular canals and otoliths. The fast phase of vestibular nystagmus is generated in the pontine reticular formation and requires for its discharge intact frontomesencephalic pathways (the same as for saccades and the fast phase of optokinetic nystagmus). The slow phase of vestibular nystagmus, generated in the vestibular apparatus, uses as a pathway the eighth nerve, the vestibular nuclei, the medial longitudinal fascicle, and the pontine reticular formation up to the oculomotor nuclei. *The vestibular system is examined by moving the patient's head quickly in one direction and then observing whether or not there is a compensatory reflex of the eyes in the opposite direction (doll's head phenomenon). Another method consists of observing eye movements (jerk nystagmus) while irrigating the external auditory canals with cold or warm water.*

The *position maintenance system* is probably represented in the same anatomic areas as the other systems, that is, in the fronto- and the occipitomesencephalic pathways (Gay et al.). *It is tested by asking the patient to fix for several seconds first on a near and then on a distant object.* Steady fixation on both objects should be possible for a minimum of 5 seconds.

Other tests for evaluating eye movements such as optokinetic nystagmus and electronystagmography will be discussed later.

*Gaze palsy* is the inability to look in a given direction (that is, to the side, up, or down) or to converge the eyes and fix on a near object. As an example, in a right horizontal gaze palsy the right lateral and left medial rectus muscles do not function in an attempted movement to the right. If these muscles are tested individually or in connection with a different type of movement (for instance, convergence or divergence), they appear intact; they fail only if called on to act within the higher function of the conjugate lateral movement.

Although gaze palsies are caused by lesions in various rather centrally located areas of the brain (midbrain, pons, frontal and occipital hemispheres), they rarely occur in patients with brain tumors. Their frequency varies between 3% and 6%.

From a clinical and in particular from a diagnostic point of view, it is expedient to subdivide the gaze palsies into horizontal, vertical, convergence, and divergence types.

A *horizontal gaze palsy*, by definition, is the inability to look to one side with both eyes together. It should be stated quite emphatically that a pure horizontal gaze palsy does not cause diplopia, because the impairment is equal in both eyes, thus causing no change in the relative position of the two eyes. On the basis of a detailed analysis of the lateral conjugate movements (saccadic, pursuit, vergence, and vestibular movements, eventually optokinetic nystagmus), it is quite possible to decide whether, in a given patient, the lesion is located in the frontal hemisphere, the frontomesencephalic pathway, or the pontine gaze center.

An isolated palsy of fast voluntary eye movements (saccades) with preservation of the pursuit and vestibular system is suggestive of a location in the *frontal lobe* (cortex or hemispheric white matter) or in the *frontomesencephalic pathway*. In a unilateral process the gaze palsy is toward the side opposite the lesion: there is a characteristic inability to initiate saccades (including the fast phase of optokinetic nystagmus) to the side opposite the lesion ("saccadic palsy"). Usually there is simultanously a *conjugate tonic deviation of the eyes toward the side of the lesion.* (The patient looks at the lesion!) As a rule, such a horizontal gaze palsy is associated with facial palsy as well as hemiparesis or hemiplegia toward the side of the gaze palsy. Even if caused by a neoplasm the gaze palsy is of relatively short duration (days or weeks), beause obviously the opposite hemisphere vicariously compensates for the lost functions, and normal voluntary saccades may return. The tonic deviation, however, will persist if the opposite hemisphere has already suffered from previous damage. Numerous cases of frontal lobe tumors or conditions after lobectomy because of such a tumor have been reported in which the patients showed this form of gaze palsy and resulting conjugate tonic deviation. In accordance with Tönnis, we were unable to observe a lateral gaze palsy in the form just described among a fairly large number of patients with frontal lobe tumors. However, focal epileptic attacks with conjugate deviation of the eyes can be observed in frontal neoplasms. The so-called *adversive seizure* is actually a focal motor epilepsy of the jacksonian type involving, in part, the frontal center for lateral gaze; it is observed as tonic and clonic contractions of the extraocular muscles that *move both eyes away from the discharging cerebral focus.* It is commonly accompanied by a facial twitching on the affected side and turning of the head to the side opposite the focus. Often a jacksonian progression of motor epilepsy over the extremities of the side contralateral to the lesion follows or precedes this event. Termination of the seizure is characteristically followed by paralysis of the muscles involved in the ictus, including a transient loss of lateral gaze in that direction, with the result that the eyes are often temporarily deviated to the side of the irritative lesion.

The distinguishing feature of lesions in the *occipital lobe* (peristriate area) and the *occipitomesencephalic pathway* is a pronounced involvement of the smooth pursuit system, eventually also of the vergence and position maintenance systems. Instead of an ordinary smooth pursuit movement with the eyes following a slowly moving object, there is in conjugated gaze toward the side of the lesion a series of jerky intervals, a *saccadic pursuit or cogwheel movement.* This "cogwheeling" generally is parallel with a corresponding impairment of the op tokinetic nystagmus toward the side opposite the lesion. (See also the discussion of nystagmus.) If pursuit movements are affected bilaterally, one always has to take into consideration factors of nonlocalizing value such as decreased state of alertness, inattention, or the effect of sedative drugs. Since lesions involving the occipitomesencephalic pathway usually are connected with *homonymous hemianopia* of the contralateral side, the test for smooth pursuit movement in the case of homonymous hemianopia may therefore give some indication concerning the site of the lesion causing the hemianopia (Kestenbaum). If the normal pursuit toward the side opposite the heminanopia is changed into saccadic pursuit, the lesion is most probably in the middle or posterior part of the optic radiation (that is, in the parietal or occipital lobes). A normal pursuit is of no value in localizing the lesion. Still, the proof of cogwheeling may in certain cases facilitate at least the differential diagnosis of a tract and radiation hemianopia. Also, in the occipital lobe there may originate *adversive seizures,* producing conjugate ocular deviations toward the side opposite the epileptic focus.

The horizontal gaze palsies caused by lesions in the *pontine center for horizontal conjugate gaze* (pontine paramedian reticular formation) are much more frequent and definitely of importance in the diagnosis of tumors in this area. If in a lateral gaze palsy *all the individual systems of gaze movements are involved,* that is the saccadic, the pursuit, and the vestibular systems, the focus in question can be assumed to be located in the pons at the level of the sixth nerve nuclei. If the process is unilateral, the resulting gaze palsy is toward the side of the lesion; if there is a conjugate tonic deviation, it is to the side opposite the lesion. Bilateral lesions produce complete paralysis of horizontal conjugate gaze to both sides, occasionally associated with "spastic convergence." Even though the gaze palsies in pontine lesions are of a lesser degree than those of cortical or subcortical foci, as a rule they appear to be more enduring and usually are not compensated for in the course of time. The supranuclear gaze centers in the pons are relatively close together; thus bilateral horizontal gaze palsies are much more likely to occur in supranuclear lesions than in cortical lesions. *Whereas bilateral lesions of the frontomesencephalic system produce complete bilateral saccadic palsy, most often together with loss of vertical saccades, bilateral lesions* (especially of the chronic type) *in the pons usually cause only paralysis of all horizontal versions, but no impairment of the vertical movements.* The convergence center being situated in a higher part of the brainstem (between the oculomotor nuclei), *many pontine lesions, particularly tumors, are notable because of a horizontal gaze palsy with an intact convergence mechanism.* We have observed a patient with a glioma of the pons who had a bilateral horizontal gaze palsy. A command to look to the side or up caused a distinct convergence spasm (Fig. 3-122). The close proximity of the nuclei of the sixth and seventh nerves as well as of the pyramidal tracts to pontine lesions results frequently in important accompanying symptoms in addition to the horizontal gaze palsies. A horizontal gaze palsy with a homolateral peripheral facial palsy, a homolateral abducens nerve palsy, and a hemiplegia of the opposite side (the patient looks to the paralyzed side!) form the so-called *Foville-Millard-Gubler syndrome* (p. 38). It is caused by a paramedian lesion in the lower pons. Among the etiologic factors involved in supranuclear horizontal gaze palsies, tumors of the pons play an important part, occurring especially frequently in children. In judging the localizing value of horizontal gaze palsies, one should not lose sight of the fact that a compression and lesion of the pons and its structures may be caused by neighboring processes. Tumors of the cerebellopontine angle (we have observed a patient with an acoustic neurinoma with horizontal gaze palsy to the side of the tumor), the cerebellum, or the medulla oblongata may occasionally cause horizontal gaze palsies that, however, are usually less distinct and can easily be overlooked. *In some cases the sign of a slight horizontal gaze impairment caused by a pontine lesion may be only a nystagmus evoked by having the patient look to the side* of the lesion (p. 59). Although vertical gaze palsy does rarely occur in pontine lesions, vertical gaze–evoked nystagmus is common. Lateral lesions of the pontine tegmentum produce vertical divergence of the eyes in the sense of *skew deviation* (Hertwig-Magendie's squint position): one eye deviates downward (and sometimes inward) and the other eye upward (and sometimes outward) with the patient experiencing vertical diplopia. The eye on the side of the lesion is generally lower than the other one. As lesions in many different areas of the brain stem and the cerebellar system can produce skew deviation, this phenomenon cannot be regarded as pathognomonic for pontine affections.

It might be of interest to discuss in just a few words the *differential diagnosis of conjugate horizontal gaze palsies from frontal hemispheric and pontine lesions.* Frontal lesions are characterized by loss of contralateral saccadic eye movements with conjugate deviation toward the side of the lesion of short duration (contralateral paralysis of extremities and face); pontine lesions manifest absence of all (saccadic, pursuit, vestibular) ipsilateral eye movements with conjugate deviation toward the opposite side of the lesion of rather permanent duration (paralysis of extremities contralateral and of facial nerve homolateral). *In lesions of both frontal hemispheres, there is bilateral absence of horizontal saccadic eye movements and of vertical saccades* (global saccadic paralysis), whereas *in pontine lesions of both sides, there is paralysis of side-to-side movements without impairment of vertical movements.*

A *vertical gaze palsy* is distinguished by the patient's inability to look up or down (or both). There is usually an inability to look up, less frequently an inability to look up and down. The rarest form is an inability to look down only. The supranuclear nature of a vertical gaze impairment can be demonstrated by observing a positive Bell's phenomenon (elevation of the eyes on closing the lids or during sleep). Vertical gaze palsies point to *lesions in the vertical supranuclear gaze center of the tectal and pretectal area of the midbrain.* Isolated vertical disturbances of gaze practically never occur with cortical hemispheric lesions. (In bilateral frontal lesions, absence or defect of both horizontal and vertical saccades can be observed!) This can be neglected for clinical considerations. As the pathways for vertical saccades and vertical pursuit converge in the tectal area, both systems may be damaged at the same time, the saccades generally before pursuit movements. Upward gaze generally becomes impaired before downward gaze. The immediate proximity to the oculomotor nuclei is responsible for lesions in the mesencephalic tegmentum frequently giving rise to pupillary disturbances (light-near dissociation of the Argyll Robertson type or general pupil rigidity), convergence palsies, and convergence spasms, as well as nuclear oculomotor pareses (causing diplopia), in addition to the vertical gaze palsy. Diplopia, however, may also be caused merely by a dissimilar involvement of the two eyes in their vertical conjugate movements (sometimes even visible in a sort of skew deviation, one eye being higher than the other). A vertical gaze palsy impairing downward gaze is particularly frequently associated with loss of convergence and accommodation. The symptoms just described, occasionally combined with retraction of the lids on an attempt to gaze upward, *convergence-retraction nystagmus* (attempt of gaze upward produces jerking bilateral movements of retraction or convergence or both), and displaced pupils (corectopia, after Wilson), form, in a variety of combinations, *Parinaud's syndrome* (also called the sylvian aqueduct syndrome). It is caused by tumors in the area of the sylvian aqueduct, the thalamus, the splenium of the corpus callosum, the quadrigeminal plate, the fourth ventricle, the vermis of the cerebellum, and in particular, the *pineal gland*. This may be a direct effect of the tumor on the lateral pretectal area of the midbrain, or it may be a remote influence. Among our patients, *pinealomas* accounted for 50% of the cases, thus being the major cause of Parinaud's syndrome (therefore also called the pineal syndrome). Of 10 patients with tumors manifesting a vertical gaze palsy (six with pinealomas), nine showed impairment of elevation, one showed impairment of elevation and depression, and none showed an isolated impairment of depression. We observed convergence palsy three times, convergence spasm twice, and nystagmus retractorius once. Pupillary disturbances of the light-near dissociation type were seen eight times in the bilateral form and once in the unilateral form.

*Convergence palsy* is the inability of the eyes to converge and to fix on a near object. There is crossed diplopia at close range, with the separation of the two images practically remaining constant for lateral and vertical movements of the eyes. Distant objects are seen single. In its pure form a convergence palsy shows no other limitations of ocular motility. (The internal rectus muscles manifest no weakness during simple adduction!) A pure convergence palsy is quite rare, but usually occurs in combination with other symptoms, for instance, a vertical gaze palsy (see discussion of Parinaud's syndrome in the section on vertical gaze palsies), a fact that is related to the location of a convergence center in the rostral midbrain. (Whether Perlia's nucleus is the midbrain center for convergence is still a controversial issue; also bilateral occipital lesions produce convergence paresis!) A convergence palsy, together with a vertical gaze palsy, occurs in patients with tumors of the midbrain and pinealomas, and it may be combined with a horizontal gaze palsy in patients with expansive tumors of the pons. It has been mentioned that smaller pontine lesions leave the convergence intact. Convergence palsy must be differentiated from *convergence insufficiency*, a functional disturbance. In convergence palsy, an adduction of the visual axes is all but impossible; a prism base out in front of one eye already causes diplopia for distance. In convergence insufficiency, some degree of adduction can always be demonstrated; up to a certain power a base-out prism can be overcome. Only if the impaired adduction is taxed too much will diplopia result.

*Divergence palsy* is the inability to bring the eyes to a parallel position in looking at a distant object. There is homonymous diplopia with a corresponding convergent position of the eyes for far, but not for near. There is no impairment of the function of the individual muscles, in particular the lateral rectus muscles, during abduction. The separation of the double images remains constant in all directions of gaze, but the greater the distance of the object is, the greater the separation. It is possible to confuse a divergence palsy with a convergence spasm. Autopsy findings have revealed tumors in the brain stem between the sixth nerve nuclei, the hypothetical divergence center (Savitsky and Madonick; Robbins;

Lippmann). Paralysis of divergence occurs with increased intracranial pressure from brain tumors or subdural hematomas.

*Internuclear ophthalmoplegia* is characterized by a failure of the medial rectus muscle on the side of the lesion to act in horizontal gaze to the opposite side and nystagmus of the abducting eye on lateral gaze to the side opposite the lesion. If, for instance, the patient is asked to look to the right, the right external rectus muscle works normally and brings the right eye into abduction (however, with the abducting nystagmus); in contrast, the left internal rectus muscle does not contract and the left eye remains immobile in a median position (thus producing exotropia with crossed diplopia). There is no real palsy of this left medial rectus muscle; it is able to function normally in convergence. The adduction paresis concerns either pursuit movements or voluntary saccades. Internuclear ophthalmoplegia can also occur bilaterally (Fig. 1-25); both medial rectus muscles fail to work when an attempt is made to look to the side, but they work normally in convergence. For detecting milder cases of internuclear ophthalmoplegia, two subtle signs, the "optokinetic sign" and the "ocular dysmetria sign," have been described (Cogan). If the patient is asked to move the eyes between two fixation objects, there will be a distinct difference between the slower saccades of the weak internal rectus muscle and the rapid saccades of the intact external rectus muscle, a phenomenon that can also be demonstrated in

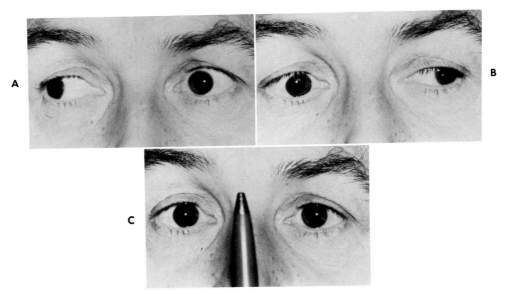

**Fig. 1-25.** Bilateral internuclear ophthalmoplegia. On gaze to right, **A**, and on gaze to left, **B**, both medial rectus muscles fail to work in presence of normal abduction (combined with nystagmus of abducting eye). Some degree of skew deviation is visible in **B** and retained ability to converge in **C**.

the fast phases of optokinetic or vestibular nystagmus. The ocular dysmetria sign is a result of the fact that the abducting eye in such fixation saccades over-shoots, whereas the adducting eye undershoots. Since unilateral internuclear ophthalmoplegia is vascular in origin in three fourths of the cases, and bilateral internuclear ophthalmoplegia is pathognomonic for multiple sclerosis, cerebral tumors rarely have to be considered. Internuclear ophthalmoplegia results from unilateral or bilateral lesions of the *medial longitudinal fasciculus* be-tween the nuclei of the third and sixth nerves. If an internuclear ophthalmo-plegia is associated with a horizontal gaze palsy, a facial palsy, or an abducens nerve paresis, there is a lesion of the pontine medial longitudinal fasciculus. If an internuclear ophthalmoplegia is combined with convergence paresis or a nuclear palsy of the internal rectus muscle (exotropia in primary position), the lesion is probably located in the mesencephalic area.

### Nystagmus

*Nystagmus is an involuntary rhythmic oscillating type of movement of one or both eyes in all or some fields of gaze.* There are two principal forms of nystag-mus (Fig. 1-26):
1. *Pendular* nystagmus, in which both phases of the movement are of equal speed
2. *Jerk* nystagmus, which shows a biphasic rhythm with an initial slow phase to one side and a following fast phase to the other side

Pendular nystagmus rarely remains pendular in all fields of gaze; outside the "neutral" zone, on lateral gaze, there is often a change from pendular to jerky movements. It is important to know that nystagmus involves one or more of the oculomotor gaze systems (saccadic, pursuit, vergence, nonoptic reflex, and fixa-tion). The fast phase of nystagmus is always mediated by the saccadic system, whereas the slow phase is mediated by one or more of the other systems.

According to the *plane,* horizontal, vertical, and rotary nystagmus (pendular or jerk) can be distinguished; there may also be combinations of these types (horizontal-rotary, oblique). *In jerk nystagmus, it is customary, by conven-*

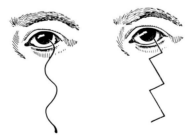

**Fig. 1-26.** Two general types of nystagmus. Left, Pendular nystagmus with undulating move-ment of eyes. Right, Jerk nystagmus with biphasic rhythm; quick phase is to nasal side and slow phase is to temporal side.

*tion, to designate its direction according to the direction of the fast phase.* At the same time, it is important to know that the direction may change in various fields of gaze. For clinical purposes, it is convenient to use the following classification based on *intensity* (Fig. 1-27):

*First degree*
No nystagmus with the eyes straight; nystagmus only when the eyes turn toward the side of the fast phase

*Second degree*
Slight nystagmus with the eyes straight; very active nystagmus if the eyes turn toward the side of the fast phase; no nystagmus if they turn to the opposite side

*Third degree*
Very active nystagmus with the eyes straight; extremely active nystagmus if the eyes turn toward the side of the fast phase; slight nystagmus if the eyes turn to the opposite side

Nystagmus can be also divided according to its *amplitude* into a fine type (excursions of less than 3 degrees), medium type (excursions between 5 and 15 degrees), and coarse type (excursions of more than 15 degrees). As a general rule, the amplitude of jerk nystagmus increases when the patient looks toward the side of the fast phase. The *frequency* of the nystagmus should also be considered. In general, the faster the rate, the smaller the amplitude, and vice versa. In some cases the amplitude may be so small that the existence of nystagmus is only noted by observing the optic nerve head with the direct ophthalmoscope (eventually only when occluding one of the patient's eyes). Jerk nystag-

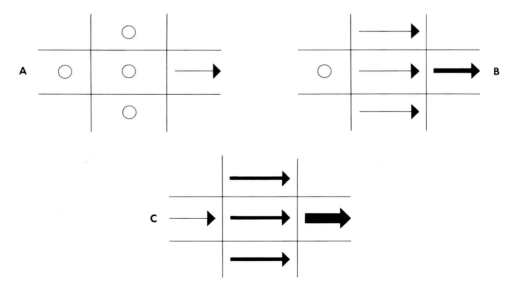

**Fig. 1-27.** Schematic representation of horizontal jerk nystagmus. **A,** First-degree horizontal jerk nystagmus. **B,** Second-degree horizontal jerk nystagmus. **C,** Third-degree horizontal jerk nystagmus.

mus usually shows the same amplitude in both eyes; unilateral or incongruent jerking nystagmus, however, may occur.

The *technique of examining* patients with nystagmus is simple and can be performed for clinical purposes without complicated instruments. First, the examiner notes whether or not there is nystagmus in the primary position of the eyes. Next, the examiner directs the patient to look to the sides, up, and down; these movements can be performed on command or by following a finger or a pencil. The examiner then notes whether nystagmus occurs that was not present in the primary position or in which direction of gaze an existing nystagmus increases. The type of nystagmus (pendular or jerk), its plane (horizontal, vertical, rotary), its degree (first, second, third), its amplitude (fine, medium, coarse), and its frequency are observed, if necessary with the aid of a loupe to magnify the ocular movements and at the same time to eliminate fixation. *Bartels'* spectacles with +20-diopter lenses or, even better, *Frenzel's* goggles are suitable for this purpose. The latter have, in addition, a built-in illumination that dazzles the patient to the extent that fixation is impossible if the examination is performed in an almost or completely darkened room. Visual fixation will increase the tonus of the extrinsic eye muscles to the extent that a slight nystagmus (for instance, first degree) may be suppressed, and thus not infrequently the eye may appear at complete rest although a nystagmus is actually present. Therefore *for an absolutely reliable observation, particularly if the nystagmus is of weak intensity* (either the spontaneous or induced type), *it is imperative to eliminate fixation.* Only the elimination of fixation will make it possible to determine the degree of the nystagmus accurately. Generally, nystagmus will increase by one class after fixation is eliminated. In other words, if there seems to be a first-degree nystagmus with the ordinary finger method, it will prove to be a second-degree nystagmus with the Frenzel goggles. The determination of the true class of the nystagmus, after fixation has been eliminated, is quite essential for its proper diagnosis. A first-degree nystagmus is in many cases of no pathologic significance. On the other hand, a *second-degree nystagmus always indicates a pathologic process.*

A correct analysis of nystagmus includes, in addition to examination in the erect position, testing with the head tilted to the left and to the right, forward and backward, if necessary with the patient in a supine position, and after shaking the head. It is frequently useful to repeat the examination several times with the Frenzel goggles in the position in which the patient reports vertigo. Induction of prerotatory and postrotatory nystagmus, caloric nystagmus, galvanic nystagmus, and compression nystagmus as methods of examination should, for technical reasons, be left to the otologist.

As already mentioned, the direction of the jerk nystagmus is determined by the direction of its fast phase. The direction of the slow phase as a rule corresponds to the side to which the patient has a tendency to fall if there are disturbances of gait or to the side of passpointing in the finger-nose test.

As a rule, there is some relationship between the direction of gaze and the direction of nystagmus: a nystagmus to the right occurs more readily when looking to the right, and a nystagmus to the left occurs more readily in gaze to the left. The most frequent combination is right nystagmus in gaze to the right together with left nystagmus in gaze to the left.

In recent years, *nystagmography* (Ohm; Coppez), especially *electronystagmography* (ENG), has come to play an increasingly important role in the examination of the eyes for spontaneous or induced nystagmus. It permits not only more exact observations of frequency, amplitude, and direction of the nystagmus, but also permanent objective recording of these ocular movements. In addition to its use in spontaneous nystagmus, ENG is gaining increasing practical value in the examination of induced nystagmus (caloric, rotational, optokinetic) and also in recording and analyzing various other types of eye movements such as saccades and pursuit mechanisms (Huber and Meyer).

The principle of ENG consists in picking up the corneoretinal potentials of both eyes by using four electrodes placed as near as is conveniently possible to the left and right outer and inner canthi. Direct current (DC) recording and amplification are definite needs in ENG. Special devices permit recording of the concomitant gaze positions of the eyes at the same time: in any ENG recording, this information is as essential as the information about the character and magnitude of the nystagmus. Apart from the facility to control the direction of gaze, there must be a means to measure it accurately when fixation is removed. Fixation can be eliminated either by closing the eyes or by testing the subject in total darkness. It is a well-known fact that removing optic fixation brings about a marked increase of vestibular nystagmus (either spontaneous or induced) of peripheral origin. In a spontaneous nystagmus caused by a lesion above the level of the vestibular nuclei (for example, cerebellar tumor), eye closure and darkness cause complete abolition of the nystagmus.

The reader is referred to special textbooks and papers for further information on the technical and clinical problems of ENG (Franceschetti; Cawthorne, Dix and Hood; Hallpike, Hood and Trinder; Jung and Kornhuber; Hart).

All spontaneous pathologic nystagmus can be related to four basic biologic mechanisms: the fixation mechanism, the mechanism of the vestibular apparatus, the mechanism of conjugate eye movements or gaze mechanism, and the convergence mechanism. Therefore it is customary to divide the numerous forms of pathologic nystagmus into four main groups:

1. *Fixation nystagmus*
2. *Vestibular nystagmus*
3. *Gaze nystagmus*
4. *Convergence nystagmus*

**Fixation nystagmus.** The fixation nystagmus group includes above all the so-called *ocular nystagmus* arising from disturbances of the retina and its connections with the visual cortex (sensory deprivation nystagmus): *pendular nystagmus* (Fig. 1-28), which begins during the first few months and persists throughout life, often being associated with severe refractive errors, media opacities, aniridia, macular defects, optic atrophy, albinism, or achromatopsia and sometimes hereditary, although occurring only in males; *spasmus nutans*, which is characterized by torticollis, head nodding, and horizontal pendular nystagmus beginning during the first 18 months and invariably disappearing by the third year of life; *latent nystagmus,* which is elicited by covering one eye and characterized by jerk nystagmus of both eyes away from the covered eye and is often associated with strabismus, especially esotropia and unilateral amblyopia; *miner's nystagmus,* which is a pendular, horizontal, or oblique form generally restricted to the upper field of gaze and improved when illumination is increased; and *congenital nystagmus,* which may be of the pendular or jerking type, with typical head turning of the patient so that he is looking toward the neutral position, thus giving himself maximum visual acuity.

Apart from the ocular forms, this group of fixation nystagmus syndromes also contains neurologic types caused by lesions in the posterior fossa, and these have neuro-ophthalmologic importance: *acquired pendular nystagmus,* which is usually horizontal, although becoming vertical on upward gaze, acquired later in life, characterized by a sensation of moving of the surroundings, and most frequently seen in multiple sclerosis; *ocular flutter* and *ocular dysmetria,* the former a periodic series of pendular, rapid horizontal movements while fixating on an object and the latter a series of dampening movements when the object of regard is shifted, both signs of cerebellar disease; *see-saw nystagmus,* which is a disjuncted pendular nystagmus characterized by one eye rising and assuming a position of intorsion and the other eye falling and assuming a position of extorsion and frequently associated with bitemporal defects caused by a chiasmal lesion; and *postural nystagmus* which occurs only with a shift of the head and is presumably caused by traction or pressure exerted on the brain stem by a neoplastic or vascular lesion in the posterior fossa.

**Vestibular nystagmus.** Evoked vestibular nystagmus such as prerotatory, postrotatory, caloric, galvanic, and compression nystagmus will not be discussed

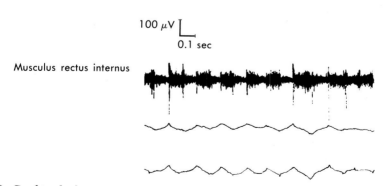

100 μV

0.1 sec

Musculus rectus internus

**Fig. 1-28.** Combined electromyogram and electronystagmogram (electro-oculogram) in congenital pendular nystagmus. Upper curve shows electromyogram of right internal rectus muscle, representing spindle-shaped rhythmic discharges. Two lower curves manifest rhythmic pendular movements of both eyes.

here. For details of these conditions, see textbooks on physiology and otolaryngology.

*Spontaneous* vestibular (or labyrinthine) nystagmus may appear as a *peripheral* nystagmus caused by lesions of the labyrinth or its nervous connection to the brain stem or as a *central* nystagmus resulting from a lesion of the vestibular nuclei or from a lesion of the central connections of the vestibular nuclei (such as the connections with the cerebellum or with the eye muscles via the reticular formation). *Vestibular nystagmus, the peripheral as well as the central type, is always jerky, usually horizontal rotary,* and may be first degree, second degree, or third degree.

*Peripheral* vestibular nystagmus remains in the same direction in all fields of gaze and is independent of the position of the body. An irritation of the labyrinth (for example, labyrinthitis) usually causes a horizontal-rotatory nystagmus in both directions (that is, in gaze to the right, nystagmus to the right; in gaze to the left, nystagmus to the left). Destruction of the labyrinth or an interruption of the vestibular nerve results in nystagmus to the other side, away from the lesion (fast phase away from the lesion). A prominent symptom is *vertigo,* usually associated with acoustic disturbances such as transient or permanent *deafness* and *tinnitus.* Peripheral vestibular nystagmus and the associated vertigo show a gradual decrease in intensity and disappear after a few weeks even if the underlying cause continues. ENG reveals the peripheral vestibular nystagmus to be enhanced (if present) or made manifest (if not present) by eliminating fixation by closing the eyes or testing in darkness.

*Central* vestibular nystagmus, also of the horizontal rotary type, may change its direction on right and left lateral gaze and may even become vertical on upward or downward gaze, a phenomenon never observed with a peripheral lesion. Therefore the determination of the direction of the nystagmus is not conclusive evidence of the side of the lesion. Changes in the position of the body frequently cause central nystagmus to change its direction. Vertigo may be present, but is not nearly so severe as in peripheral vestibular nystagmus. Tinnitus and deafness are not present. In contrast to peripheral vestibular nystagmus, the central type may persist for months and years if the underlying cause does not disappear. Often there is an associated oculomotor disturbance, such as abnormal pursuit movements of optokinetic nystagmus. ENG findings show central nystagmus (caused by a lesion above the level of the vestibular nuclei) to be abolished by eye closure or by testing in darkness.

From the clinical point of view, central vestibular nystagmus may be the result of a process in the brain stem or in the cerebellum.

In *tumors of the pons,* central vestibular nystagmus is an almost constant symptom. We found such a nystagmus in 12 of 13 patients with pontine tumors. Seven showed a horizontal type, four a combined horizontal-vertical type, and only one a vertical type. Most authors are of the opinion that a vertical component is the result of a long-distance effect on the midbrain tegmentum. The direction of the nystagmus in patients with lesions of the brain stem does not permit localization to a particular side unless there is an asymmetry (p. 59).

Long-distance effects of certain tumors on the brain stem are well known. Thus tumors of the occipital lobe may cause nystagmus of the central vestibular type (p. 197). A similar effect has been observed with tumors of the mesencephalon or the pineal body. Whether the nystagmus occasionally seen in frontal lobe tumors is caused by such long-distance effects is a matter of dispute.

Nystagmus occurs with extraordinary frequency in patients with *cerebellar tumors* (50% or more). This *cerebellar nystagmus* usually has the character of a central vestibular nystagmus and sometimes also of horizontal symmetric or vertical gaze nystagmus (p. 287). Cerebellar nystagmus is predominantly horizontal in nature. It may be spontaneous or only appear during lateral movements. It is distinguished by the fact that the fast phase occurs in the direction of the patient's gaze. In unilateral cerebellar lesions the amplitude varies with the direction of gaze: despite some exceptions, it can be generally stated that the *direction of gaze associated with the coarse form of nystagmus corresponds to the side of the lesion*. In the case of a median location of the tumor (for instance, in the vermis), there may be a purely vertical nystagmus (pressure effect on the tectal area?). According to Spiller, this also indicates a considerable anterior extension of the tumor from the posterior fossa anteriorly. It is still a controversial subject whether the nystagmus associated with cerebellar tumors truly represents a cerebellar sign or whether it is the result of a long-distance effect on the brain stem. In patients with tumors of the *cerebellopontine angle,* especially acoustic neurinomas, a horizontal nystagmus can be observed as an almost constant sign. This horizontal jerk nystagmus is usually coarser in its excursions toward the side of the tumor than toward the opposite side. In some instances, we have seen, in addition to the horizontal nystagmus, a rotary or, with eyes up, even a vertical component. The fact that nystagmus in association with cerebellopontine angle tumors is persistent and does not disappear suggests that it is less the result of a lesion of the vestibular nerve than a phenomenon of compression of the brain stem or the cerebellum. In other words, it is a central type of nystagmus similar to the one seen in association with cerebellar tumors. This is equally true for the very frequent occurrence of a vertical component (probably caused by a remote effect on the midbrain tegmentum), especially if it occurs as an isolated phenomenon and without a horizontal component.

**Gaze nystagmus.** One of the most common causes of nystagmus is a failure of the muscles involved in the gaze mechanism. *Muscle paretic nystagmus* is caused by a paresis of a single extraocular muscle. A progressive exhaustion (slow phase) alternates with a contraction (fast phase) induced by a renewed impulse. Since the repeated impulses are automatically sent equally to both eyes, the nystagmus occurs in both eyes. The movements in the normal eye are even greater than in the paretic eye. Its direction corresponds to the direction of action of the paretic muscle. This type of muscle paretic nystagmus does not occur with a completely paralytic muscle. The paresis may be of myopathic, synaptic, or peripheral neurogenic origin. Here it may be mentioned that myasthenic patients sometimes manifest peculiar jerky movements of the eyes following the administration of a cholinergic drug.

Related to muscle paretic nystagmus is *gaze nystagmus,* also called *gaze paretic nystagmus*. It is characterized by the *absence of nystagmus when looking straight ahead and the appearance of nystagmus in one or more fields of gaze with the fast component always in the direction of gaze*. In such an instance not a single muscle but a group of muscles executing a conjugate movement is involved.

The so-called physiologic *end-position nystagmus* represents a form of gaze nystagmus occurring in many healthy individuals (either with or without a latency period) as an expression of weakness or fatigue of gaze; instead of a steady position of the eyes in lateral gaze, repeated quick impulses to the side of gaze and slow deviations toward the midline alternate. This form of nystagmus has no clinical significance and is usually exhausted after a short time (maximally after 10 or 15 jerks). Tired and nervous individuals are especially subject to end-position nystagmus (fatigue nystagmus, neurasthenic nystagmus).

End-position nystagmus and fatigue nystagmus actually belong to the group of gaze nystagmus syndromes, but differ in that they are exhaustible. Nevertheless, it is possible to mistake an end-position nystagmus, which after extended observation changes to a fatigue nystagmus, for an inexhaustible gaze nystagmus. This mistake can be avoided if the test for gaze nystagmus is never performed in the extreme lateral position. In other words, pathologic gaze nystagmus always appears in lateral gaze before the end position is reached.

There are two types of pathologic gaze nystagmus: *horizontal symmetric gaze nystagmus* and *horizontal asymmetric gaze nystagmus* (Fig. 1-29). "Symmetric" means a nystagmus appears at the same distance from the primary position to the right and to the left, with an identical increase in its intensity in both directions. "Asymmetric" nystagmus appears earlier to one side, with a more pronounced increase in intensity to this side (a sort of gaze weakness to the same side). These forms of horizontal gaze nystagmus are characteristically jerking and almost purely horizontal, without a rotary component. The fast phase is toward the lateral side and the slow phase toward the midline. There is accentuation of nystagmus when the eyes are closed. In severe cases of symmetric gaze nystagmus, there may also be a vertical component, which is of no importance in itself. On the other hand, an isolated *vertical gaze nystagmus*,

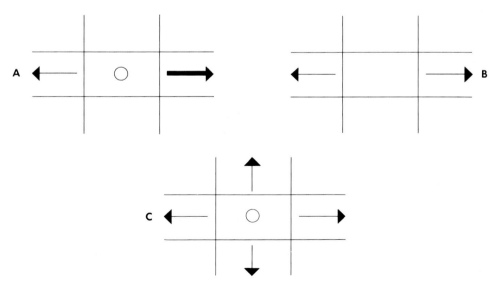

Fig. 1-29. Schematic representation of gaze nystagmus. **A**, Horizontal asymmetric gaze nystagmus. **B**, Horizontal symmetric gaze nystagmus. **C**, Horizontal and vertical gaze nystagmus.

when looking up or down, may be the prodromal stage of a vertical gaze palsy, suggesting a lesion in the midbrain tegmentum (p. 281). In symmetric or asymmetric gaze nystagmus the underlying lesion is located in the brain stem. According to Kestenbaum, asymmetric gaze nystagmus is a localizing sign indicating the site of the lesion to be within the pons. Also, cerebellar tumors may present with asymmetric gaze nystagmus when the head is turned to the side of the lesion. The causes of symmetric or asymmetric gaze nystagmus include various possibilities: vascular disease, tumor, multiple sclerosis, degenerative disease, intoxication (barbiturates), etc.

**Convergence nystagmus.** Convergence nystagmus is characterized by *intermittent convergence movements produced on horizontal gaze and often exaggerated on attempts at near vision or upward gaze.* In severe cases the convergence movements may be associated with more or less rhythmic jerking retraction movements of the eye: *retraction nystagmus,* or *nystagmus retractorius.* This convergence nystagmus is diagnostic for a lesion of the midbrain tegmentum. In its full form the so-called *Parinaud's* or *sylvian aqueduct syndrome* consists of vertical gaze palsy, pupillary disturbances, convergence retraction nystagmus, and paresis of one or more extrinsic eye muscles (p. 280).

In addition to the various pathologic types, one form of experimental nystagmus based on the normal fixation mechanism should be considered here: *optokinetic nystagmus,* which may play a significant role in the topical diagnosis in patients with homonymous hemianopia. This nystagmus was known for a long time as "railroad nystagmus." If the patient observes a revolving drum with a broad black stripe (a so-called optokinetic drum), a characteristic horizontal nystagmus is induced with its slow phase in the direction of the movement of the drum and its fast phase to the opposite side (Fig. 1-30). The drum should be about 13 cm high with a diameter of 25 cm; its surface should be painted with vertical black and white stripes 1.5 cm in width. If an optokinetic drum is

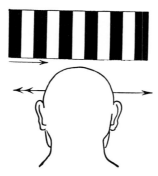

Fig. 1-30. Optokinetic nystagmus, or "train nystagmus." Patient fixes on drum that moves in direction of arrow. Drum is painted with broad black stripes. Resulting jerk nystagmus has slow phase in direction of movement of drum and quick phase in opposite direction. (After Duke-Elder.)

not available, a large newspaper can be used. It is slowly moved before the patient's eyes in a horizontal direction with the printed lines in a vertical position. If the patient is inattentive (for instance, in a slight stupor or in aphasia), the optomotor strength of the black stripes on the drum is insufficient. A better result may be obtained in such patients if pictures of persons or objects are substituted for the stripes, a method that is also more suitable for children. *Optokinetic nystagmus may be elicited horizontally or vertically.* Under normal conditions, it is equal in both horizontal and vertical directions, but it may be greater on downward than upward movement.

The *slow phase* of optokinetic nystagmus is identical to the pursuit movements and is mediated through the occipitoparietal lobe and the occipitomesencephalic pathways for the pursuit mechanism. The pathway for the *fast phase* of optokinetic nystagmus requires frontal lobe activity and is probably identical with the frontomesencephalic pathways for the saccadic mechanism.

*Horizontal optokinetic nystagmus disturbances can only be interpreted when there is a definite asymmetric response between the two sides.* If the optokinetic nystagmus is identical or approximately identical for both directions of the drum (tested according to the method just described), this is called a *negative optokinetic nystagmus sign.* In a patient with homonyous hemianopia, this indicates, with a certain degree of probability, that the lesion is in the optic tract, the external geniculate body, the anterior part of the optic radiation, or the cortex itself near the calcarine fissure (Kestenbaum; Stenvers; Cords). A *positive nystagmus sign* is present if no optokinetic nystagmus or only an attenuated nystagmus can be elicited toward the side of the hemianopia. (The optic radiations lie adjacent in the parietal lobe to the corticocortical connections between the occipital and frontal lobes.) In other words the nystagmus is absent or diminished when the drum moves out of the blind side. In patients with asymmetric optokinetic nystagmus the most significant abnormality is the loss of the fast phase of the optokinetic nystagmus to the opposite side (disconnection of occipitofrontal integration). According to different authors (Kestenbaum; Ling and Gay), *the positive nystagmus sign indicates quite reliably a lesion in the white matter of the parietotemporal or the parieto-occipital region, in other words a lesion in the middle or posterior part of the optic radiation.* Abnormal optokinetic nystagmus is therefore observed most frequently in lesions of the *parietal lobe* (interuption of the connections from both occipital lobes via pathways deep in the parietal lobe to the frontal lobe). Stadlin has described a patient with a parieto-occipital astrocytoma with homonymous hemianopia. Following surgical removal of the tumor, the optokinetic nystagmus, which was equal on both sides before the operation, disappeared toward the side of the hemianopia, only to return after an interval of almost 2 months, at first in an irregular and saccadic manner. This and many similar observations indicate a mechanism that compensates for such disturbances of the optokinetic nystagmus. Moreover, one must be aware of the fact that occasionally the optokinetic nystagmus may be missing or may be easily exhaustible in normal individuals.

In summary, the practical importance of the optokinetic nystagmus can be stated in the following manner: *In cases of homonymous hemianopia a missing or attenuated optokinetic nystagmus toward one side points toward a lesion in the medial or posterior part of the optic radiation, most frequently in the parietal lobe.* If, in the presence of hemianopia, the optokinetic nystagmus is more or less identical on both sides, no localizing value can be established.

In diffuse frontal lobe lesions (and lesions along the frontomesencephalic pathways), there may also be an impairment of the optokinetic nystagmus. The fast phase of the optokinetic nystagmus is impaired, but fixation and pursuit responses are intact. In addition, voluntary conjugate eye movement to the opposite side is defective or absent; also, the caloric response is impaired (especially the fast phase). Unilateral occipital lesions produce no abnormality of optokinetic nystagmus. Bilateral occipital lesions lead to complete loss of response to optokinetic stimulation only if there is complete cortical blindness.

*Asymmetry of optokinetic response in the vertical plane* may suggest a *disturbance in the brain stem,* but one must always be aware that a slight asymmetry may be normal. Symmetric disturbances in the horizontal and vertical plane have no localizing value. Only asymmetries between the horizontal and the vertical responses suggest a lesion in the brain stem. A vertical optokinetic nystagmus (fast phase up) producing convergence-retraction nystagmus is characteristic for Parinaud's syndrome.

The reader is referred to other publications for details of the theoretical and, to some extent, hypothetical principles of these empiric observations (Bárány; van Bogaert; Cords; Holmes; Ohm; Stenvers; Kestenbaum; Cawthorne, Dix, and Hood; Ling and Gay).

It should be of interest to examine briefly the relationship between disturbances of optokinetic nystagmus and those of pursuit movement (cogwheel movement, p. 48). Kestenbaum's studies on this subject are particularly penetrating. A disturbed pursuit movement to one side is always accompanied by an impaired optokinetic nystagmus to the other side. On the other hand, impairment of the optokinetic nystagmus is not always associated with a cogwheel movement. This may justify the assumption that the pathways of the occipitomesencephalic tracts for the conjugate movements, producing changes in either the optokinetic nystagmus or the pursuit movements, do not coincide completely. *Anomalies of either one of these phenomena* (optokinetic nystagmus or pursuit movement) *are of localizing value only if differences between the two sides can be demonstrated.* In such an event the lesion responsible for the hemianopia lies either in the middle or in the posterior part of the optic radiation (especially the parietal lobe). The absence of optokinetic nystagmus and the pursuit movement or symmetric changes of these phenomena to both sides are of no diagnostic importance. If the lesion involves the anterior part of the optic radiation or the area of the calcarine fissure, the optokinetic nystagmus and the pursuit movement are, as a rule, normal.

## Fundus

The external aspects of the eyes, the corneal sensitivity, the pupils, and the motility can easily be examined without major accessories. The pupils impose a formidable barrier to the examination of the eyegrounds. This barrier is created by the usually small size of the pupils or eventually by some opacities of the refracting media (lens and the vitreous). A special instrument, the ophthalmoscope, is necessary for the visualization of the eyeground. The examiner needs some dexterity and considerable personal experience in the use of this instrument to obtain reliable results.

We cannot always count on the pupils to remain in satisfactory mydriasis or perhaps even be rigid to light. In older persons, there is frequently a very annoying miosis that, in combination with a physiologic nuclear sclerosis of the lens, can render ophthalmoscopy all but impossible. Despite these obstacles, one should *attempt at all cost to examine the eyeground of a patient with a suspected brain tumor without instilling a mydriatic.* Any drug-induced mydriasis will mask the original state of the pupils for a varying length of time. During this time, complications might occur that would make evaluation of the pupils (for instance, a unilateral dilation in increased intracranial pressure) highly desirable. Ophthalmoscopy without artificial mydriasis is facilitated by *darkening the examining room,* which will tend to dilate the pupils. If that is impossible, the patient should turn the face from a bright window so that the eyes are shaded by the head. Occlusion of the other eye eliminates the consensual miotic impulse of the eye to be examined. To minimize the pupillomotor effect of the ophthalmoscope light, it is best to begin the examination with the disc, which, as a "blind spot," is insensitive to light. The light bundle of the ophthalmoscope entering the eye through a small pupil should be as narrow as possible to avoid scattering and reflection of the light at the pupillary area of the iris. The modern direct ophthalmoscopes are equipped with apertures of different sizes that permit the selection of a light bundle in accordance with the size of the pupil.

Only after these measures have failed is one justified in *dilating the pupil artificially* if a satisfactory view of the eyeground cannot be obtained because of a small pupil or because of opacities of the refracting media. The pupillary reaction to light and in convergence as well as the power of accommodation should be tested before drops are instilled. The mydriatic selected should be short lasting and should interfere as little as possible with accommodation.

In many cases, tropicamide (Mydriacyl) is suitable for this purpose. A dose of 2 to 4 drops, a few minutes apart, is instilled into the conjunctival sac. The maximal mydriatic effect is reached after 10 to 15 minutes. It disappears rapidly and is scarcely noticeable after an hour. Disturbances of accomodation are practically nonexistent or at the most quite insignificant and transitory. Cyclopentolate (Cyclogyl) should be used only if tropicamide does not cause a satisfactory mydriasis. It takes effect a little more slowly and lasts much longer (8 to 15 hours). It also immobilizes the accomodation almost completely for a considerable length of time. As a rule, the use of cyclopentolate cannot be avoided in patients with diabetes, in whom it is difficult to dilate the pupils. Atropine should never be used because its cycloplegia lasts for days (up to 1 week) and because of the danger of precipitating an acute glaucoma in older persons.

The artificial mydriasis not only eliminates the difficulty of performing ophthalmoscopy with small pupils, but also increases the visibility of the eyeground in the presence of slight *opacities of the media.* At the same time, such opacities of the lens or vitreous become visible, especially if a +10 lens is used, allowing some magnification. Any type of opacity manifests itself as a black moving (vitreous) or fixed (lens) shadow on a red background. If indicated (for instance, in pseudopapilledema seen in hyperopia), retinoscopy can be done with the pupil dilated. (The use of homatropine or cyclopentolate is essential for this purpose.)

It would seem almost superfluous to discuss the *ophthalmoscope* within the framework of this dissertation. Nevertheless, personal experience prompts us to make a few pertinent remarks. In our opinion, *direct ophthalmoscopy* (upright image) is best suited for neuro-ophthalmologic examinations, for it frequently has to be performed by nonophthalmologists. The modern ophthalmoscopes have a brilliant light source. They are provided with a number of apertures to adjust the width of the light bundle and the size of the pupil, with rheostats to regulate the light intensity, with a Recoss disc that will permit a sharply focused image of the fundus and compensation for refractive errors of the eyes of the patient or the examiner, and perhaps even with filters for red-free light. These qualities should make the direct ophthalmoscope an excellent tool for examination. Compared with indirect ophthalmoscopy, it has the advantages of greater simplicity and higher magnification (16×) of the fundus picture. Its disadvantage is that the total retinal area visible at one time is smaller than that seen with the indirect method. This is, however, of no great importance because, for the neuro-ophthalmologic examination, the central part of the retina (namely, the disc and the macula) is of primary interest. With adequate mydriasis, however, the peripheral parts of the fundus can be evaluated fairly completely with direct ophthalmoscopy. The instrument, supplied with a battery handle, makes the examiner completely independent of an external light source. Those who are trained to use the indirect "high plus" lens ophthalmoscopy will use the electric binocular instrument, with a 12-diopter lens held in front of the patient's eye and a distance of 40 to 50 cm between this lens and the ophthalmoscope. Only this method allows a full stereoscopic view of the fundus. This method is indispensible for quick screening of the ocular fundus, especially in children.

As the first landmark in examining the fundus, the disc should be visualized by asking the patient to turn the eye to be examined slightly nasally. The examiner should attempt to relax his accommodation as much as possible; this can be facilitated if he imagines himself looking into a spacious room through the ophthalmoscope. A refractive error of the patient's eye can be compensated by the lenses in the Recoss disc. After examining the papilla and the retinal vessels, one continues with the macula and its surroundings and finally with the periphery of the fundus in all meridians. Details of eyeground changes in brain tumors and the differential diagnosis of such conditions will be discussed in more detail in subsequent chapters. Essentially, these changes are papilledema and optic atrophy. The ophthalmoscopic aspects of these phenomena will be described and differentiated from similar affections (p. 94).

The ophthalmoscopic evaluation of the retinal vessels also affords the opportunity of measuring *arterial* and *venous blood pressures*. Under certain conditions such data can be of importance in the diagnosis of increased intracranial pressure and may help rule out complications such as carotid artery occlusion, vertebrobasilar artery occlusion, or carotid-venous communications. Bailliart's or H. K. Müller's ophthalmodynamometer (clock-dial type or straight model) is suitable for this purpose, especially for measuring the arterial pressure. There are similar instruments with a finer calibration and a lighter spring action for testing the venous pressure. For accuracy of results the pupils are dilated and the eyes anesthetized topically. The intraocular pressure is measured by Schiøtz or applanation tonometry. Direct or indirect ophthalmoscopy may be used. The advantages of indirect ophthalmoscopy, especially with a binocular indirect ophthalmoscope, are stressed by many ophthalmologists familiar with the difficulties of ophthalmodynamometry. Some authors (Rintelen; Weigelin and Lobstein; Smith; Gay) suggest that two observers perform the dynamometric examination: one places the instrument on the globe in the lateral canthal angle, taking care that the footplate is always tangential and that the plunger points at all times toward the center of the globe, gradually increasing the pressure inside the eye; the other looks through the ophthalmoscope and observes the behavior of the retinal vessels as they emerge from the disc. If the force is gradually increased, first there will be a venous pulsation. As soon as this occurs, the pressure of the spring is noted; it expresses the venous pressure in grams. The pressure on the plunger is continued until pulsation (more precisely an intermittent collapse) of the central artery at the site of its branching becomes visible; the spring tension measured is the equivalent of the *diastolic arterial pressure* in grams. The *systolic pressure* is reached with a spring pressure that causes the arterial pulsation to cease completely. To eliminate the errors of only one reading, it is advisable to perform several measurements of both the systolic and the diastolic pressure and to take an average of the spread of pressure values found. Since this blood pressure is naturally a function of the systemic blood pressure, immediately after measuring systolic and diastolic pressures in both eyes the brachial blood pressure is taken and recorded. Comparative measurements of the pressure in the ocular vessels should be performed with the patient either in a sitting or a supine position, but always in the same position.

The actual ophthalmodynamometric values read on the instrument (Bailliart or Müller) are in grams. They have to be converted to millimeters of mercury (mm Hg) and brought into relation with the intraocular pressure (Schiøtz, applanation). For this purpose the conversion tables of *Bedavanija* and *Niesel* are preferred to convert the pressure values in grams measured at a certain intraocular pressure level directly into the real pressure values of the ophthalmic artery in millimeters of mercury.

The ophthalmic artery pressures are of significance for the analysis of disorders of the cerebral circulation only when brought into relation with the brachial pressure. In this connection, one has to consider the *equation of Weigelin and Lobstein*, which is based on vast statistical material:

$$P_{m\ ophth} = 0.73\,(P_{m\ brach} - T) + T$$

where

$P_{m\ ophth}$ = Median ophthalmic artery pressure (diastolic pressure + 42% of the difference between systolic and diastolic pressures)

$P_{m\ brach}$ = Median brachial pressure (diastolic pressure + 42% of the difference between systolic and diastolic pressures)

$T$ = Intraocular pressure (Schiøtz, applanation)

There are special tables (Bedavanija) that replace the calculations according to this equation. They give the normal values of median ophthalmic artery pressures expected for a given intraocular and brachial pressure. To make a decision as to whether there exists a disorder of the intracranial circulation or not, these normal values have to be compared with those found in the patient.

An abnormal increase of the ophthalmic arterial pressure can be a sign of dilatation of the carotid artery or of obliteration or contraction of the cerebral arteries, whereas an abnormal decrease can point to a stenosis of the carotid or to a dilatation of the peripheral cerebral vessels. The behavior of the vascular pressure in cases of brain tumors will be discussed in the section on the choked disc (p. 117). Errors in interpretation of ophthalmodynamometric results are caused by the fact that there exist major anastomoses between internal and external carotid arteries via the orbit, so that the eye receives some, and sometimes all, of its blood supply from the external carotid artery. For a more specific consideration of the pathophysiologic principles involved in the pressure of the ophthalmic artery and its measurement, the reader should consult the monographs by Bailliart, Streiff and Monnier, and Weigelin and Lobstein as well as the contributions by Hollenhorst, Smith, Gay, Barut, and others.

A relatively new method of "objective" ophthalmodynamometry is represented by the *ophthalmodynamography* based on the instrument and technique devised by Hager. The ophthalmodynamograph is a tambourlike apparatus that, applied to the surface of the eye, transmits and records pulsations from the orbital vascular structures. The tracings obtained give information on the systolic and diastolic ophthalmic artery pressure, the pulse volume, and the pulse-wave speed within the internal carotid artery. Abnormal ophthalmodynamographic patterns are especially characteristic in carotid artery occlusive disease, low-tension glaucoma, ischemic papillitis, migraine disease, and temporal arteritis (Hager; Bettelheim; Salmon and Gay). Special ophthalmodynamographic data in cases of increased intracranial pressure have been collected by Finke. These findings will be discussed in the section on papilledema (p. 118).

A new method for detecting the presence of a stenosis in the internal carotid artery between the bifurcation and the branching of the ophthalmic artery is the percutaneous measurement of the blood flow by *Doppler ultrasound technique* over the supratrochlear and supraorbital arteries (both terminal branches of the ophthalmic artery). Besides the diagnosis of obstructions the technique may also help to evaluate the hemodynamic effect of an endarterectomy in the extracranial portion of the carotid artery (Keller, Bollinger, and Baumgartner).

*Fundus photographs,* black and white or color, easily performed today with a hand camera (Kowa, Olympus, etc.) as a bedside procedure, furnish important records that, by comparison at different time intervals, give valuable information on the development and morphologic changes of any fundus process (papilledema, optic atrophy, vascular affections, etc.). A new method to record function and structure in the living eye became available with the introduction of the serial photography of fluorescein in the circulating blood of the human ocular fundus (Novotny and Alvis).

*Fluorescein angiography* of the ocular fundus (Fig. 1-31) has not only become a popular method for studying the circulation and vascular changes of the eye, but also for visualizing some aspects of the appearance and function of the vasculature of the optic nerve head not revealed by ordinary ophthalmoscopy.

For fluorescein fundus photography, 10 ml of 5% fluorescein is injected into the antecubital vein. Any retinal camera can be modified for fluorescein fundus photography. All that is required is the insertion of two light filters: the first a blue filter (Kodak Wratten No. 47) over the aperture of the illumination diaphragm and the second a green-yellow filter (Kodak Wratten No. 15) in front of the film. This filter cuts out the blue exciting light and allows as much of the fluorescent light as possible to reach the film. The power supply for the electronic flash has to be strong enough to allow pictures to be taken at a time interval of 1 to 2

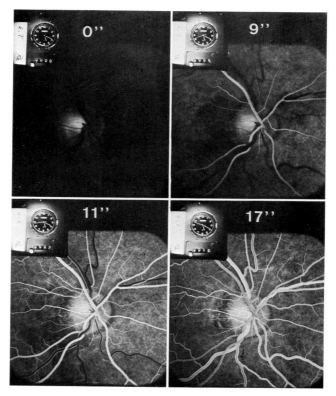

**Fig. 1-31.** Fluorescein angiogram of normal fundus and disc. At time mark 0, faint glow (incomplete filtering) of disc is visible. Nine seconds after intravenous injection of fluorescein, retinal arteries become stained with dye, and background of fundus shows mottling as a result of staining of large choroidal vessels. At time mark 11 seconds, retinal arteries are fully stained, disc manifests distinct fluorescence with numerous fine capillary vessels, and veins begin to show laminar inflow of fluorescein. At time mark 17 seconds, retinal veins are fully stained (laminar flow in some places still visible), arteries become less fluorescent, disc still reveals fine capillary vessels, and background fluorescence reaches maximum.

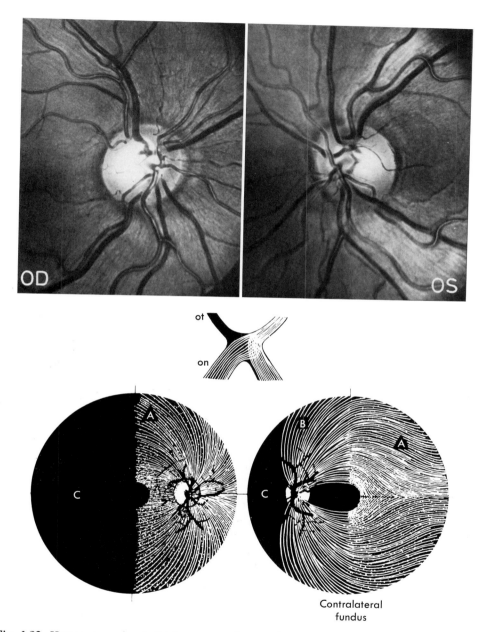

**Fig. 1-32.** Homonymous hemiretinal patterns of nerve fiber loss after transsynaptic degeneration from lesion in right occipital lobe (upper photograph). Nerve fiber patterns in two eyes can be compared with diagram of pattern of nerve fiber atrophy from right optic tract lesion (lower diagram). This is asymmetric atrophy of discs with left disc showing horizontal "band pallor" and right disc temporal pallor. *ot,* optic tract; *on,* optic nerve. (From Hoyt, W. F., and Kommerell, G.: Klin. Monatsbl. Augenheilkd. **162:**456-464, 1973.)

seconds or even more rapidly. Twenty-four serial pictures taken at an interval of 1.5 seconds are sufficient to demonstrate the characteristic arteriolar, arteriolar-venous, and venous filling phases, whereas demonstration of the arteriolar-venous recirculation phases requires further pictures for 5 to 20 minutes.

If a fundus camera is not available, the examination of the fundus and the observation of the passage of the fluorescein into the vessels and the tissues can also be observed with the ordinary direct or indirect ophthalmoscope using an additional blue filter (Kodak Wratten No. 47 or No. 47a) and an intensive light source. The personal observation of the patient's fundus during fluorescein passage may sometimes supply even better information than photography; it becomes equivalent in a certain way to *fluorescence cinematography* of the ocular fundus, which has the advantage of allowing visualization of all the circulatory phases without interruption.

Normal and pathologic patterns of fluorescein angiograms will be discussed in connection with papilledema (p. 107) and optic atrophy. For further information concerning the method and results of fluorescein fundus photography, the reader is referred to the monographs by Wessing and by Jütte and Lemke as well as to the numerous contributions by Amalric, Bessou, and Aubry; Charamis, Katsourakis, and Mandras; Ferrer; Matsui, Koh, and Tashiro; Norton; Smith; and Witmer.

In 1913 Vogt pioneered the direct ophthalmoscopic technique for observation of retinal nerve fibers using *red-free light* (selectively filtered from a carbon arc light). In 1972 and 1973 Hoyt adapted Vogt's method for the evaluation of retinal nerve fiber abnormalities in patients with optic nerve disease, optic tract affections, and glaucoma. For this purpose, he introduced *red-free fundus photography* using the Zeiss Oberkochen fundus camera with the 2× magnification attachment. The fundus is recorded directly on Kodak Plus-X black and white film, using a Wratten No. 65 (green) filter to enhance the contrast of gaps in the nerve fiber layer. The black and white negatives are printed on Kodak Ektamatic SC paper with a high-contrast filter. Final magnification ranges between 20× and 40×. Red-free fundus photography furnishes objective fundus findings, especially of the nerve fibers of the retina, which are of particular value when perimetric investigations fail to give reliable data (Fig. 1-32).

**Visual acuity**

In the course of a neuro-ophthalmologic examination, it is absolutely necessary to determine visual acuity as one of the functions of the retina and the visual pathways. The visual acuity and the visual fields, possibly with the addition of the color sense, are the principal criteria used in the evaluation of the functional state of the optic nerve and the higher visual pathways under normal and pathologic conditions. The examination of every patient with proved or suspected brain tumor must include the measurement of visual acuity.

*Distance* vision is tested with the aid of a chart to be used at 5 or 6 meters (Snellen or Birkhäuser type). These charts are arranged in rows of letters or numbers of certain sizes, the smallest of which should just be readable by the normal eye with a visual acuity of 1.0 (subtending an angle of 1 arc minute).*

---

*Actually, these characters subtend an angle of 25 arc minutes, with five squares in the horizontal and five squares in the vertical line. Each of these individual squares subtends an angle of 1 arc minute. It should stimulate an isolated retinal cone. If one cone lies between two cones thus stimulated by two black squares, these two squares are appreciated separately ("minimum separabile"); otherwise they are seen as just one black area.

The actual visual acuity of the patient results from the size of the line he is just able to read. It can be expressed in the form of a decimal (1.0; 0.1) or common fraction (6/6; 6/60). For the sake of uniformity, it would be desirable if the value of the visual acuity were always expressed in the form of a decimal fraction. If the patient is unable to read the largest characters on the chart (corresponding to a visual acuity of 0.1), he should be tested at half the distance (3 or 2.5 meters). The resulting values, accordingly, should be divided by 2. If the vision is still poorer, the reading distance can be further reduced. For a distance of 1 meter or less, it is better to have the patient count fingers and then express the visual acuity as "finger counting" (for instance, "fc at 50 cm"). If the vision is impaired very severely (for instance, secondary optic atrophy after papilledema), fingers may not be recognized—only the gross movement of the entire hand. The visual acuity is then recorded as recognition of hand movements (for instance, "HM at 50 cm"). If even the recognition of form is impossible, only the *light projection* can still give some idea of the visual faculty. A flashlight or the beam of an ophthalmoscope is brought in from the periphery in various meridians, and the patient is asked to indicate where he perceives the light. This type of examination also gives a rough idea of the visual field in patients with severely impaired visual acuity (p. 76).

*Near* vision is tested with suitable reading charts (Birkhäuser; Keeney), which consist of text matter printed in paragraphs of varying size corresponding to a visual acuity that ranges from 0.1 to 1.5. For this examination, one should maintain a normal reading distance of 30 cm. The near vision test is unreliable if there is a paresis of accommodation.

Whenever possible the *binocular visual acuity* should be determined after each eye has been tested individually; usually it is somewhat higher than the monocular vision. Proper illumination of the charts is essential for a reliable vision test. It should always be of the same intensity so that the results of the tests, if repeated, can readily be compared. Refractive errors are a factor that always has to be considered in the determination of the visual acuity. As a rule the physician who performs the neurologic examination has neither a trial case at his disposal nor the time to be concerned with the problem of refraction. Patients with high refractive errors (myopia, astigmatism) usually already have a correction. The glasses should be worn, of course, for the testing of the visual acuity. The hyperopia of younger patients is of little importance for the testing of distance vision because it can be compensated without difficulty by accommodation. Like presbyopia, hyperopia definitely has to be taken into consideration for the determination of the near vision; if necessary, it must be corrected with convex lenses. If no trial case is available, one may dispense with the determination of near vision in older persons (older than 45 years of age) and in persons with hyperopia because the results would not be of much value.

During the performance of a neuro-ophthalmologic examination in patients with suspected brain tumors, *malingering* probably will have to be considered only rarely in the determination of the visual acuity. This problem is of considerable greater importance for medicolegal evidence with regard to persons having suffered from brain injuries. A large number of "tricks" for the discovery of malingerers feigning poor vision has been suggested. They are described in detail in textbooks of ophthalmology. We want to mention here only the possibility of using *optokinetic nystagmus for an objective determination of visual acuity* (Ohm; Goldmann; Günther).

A pattern of minute black dots or squares is moved evenly either horizontally or vertically before the eyes of the patient to be examined. He is asked to observe this pattern without too much concentration. If his vision is keen enough to recognize this pattern and its movements, he will show an involuntary optokinetic nystagmus. The patient then is moved away from the instrument until the nystagmus is just barely noticeable or shows a tendency to disappear. The ratio between this distance and the actual visual acuity has been determined empirically for subjects with normal vision. This method permits a very reliable objective determination of the visual acuity. Since this form of examination is based on special instruments, it can be performed only in well-equipped eye departments. Those satisfied with less accurate results can easily improvise a similar arrangement with an optokinetic drum (p. 61).

In the discussion of symptomatology, it has been stressed that it is necessary for the patient to recognize and understand letters and words if visual acuity is to be tested. This may cause a great deal of difficulty for patients with *sensory-aphasic disturbances* of the *alexia* type (for instance, those with tumors near the angular gyrus and the adjacent areas of the parietal or occipital lobes). In most instances, such patients also will not understand gestures or pantomimes; hence attempts to test the vision in such a manner will also be unsuccessful. If the descending occipitomesencephalic pathways in the middle and posterior part of the optic radiation are intact, an attempt can be made to determine the visual acuity roughly with the aid of the optokinetic nystagmus (p. 61). The situation is far less complicated in patients with *motor aphasia* (tumors of the inferior posterior part of the left frontal lobe) because the patient understands quite well what he reads. Although unable to express what he has read, the patient can indicate distinctly to the examiner by signs or gestures, for instance, nodding, whether or not he is able to read a certain line on the visual acuity chart (Fig. 1-1).

Under certain conditions, discriminative and minute testing of the visual acuity may uncover other valuable details among the symptoms found in patients with brain tumors. The near vision test may disclose a *homonymous hemianopia*, especially if it is on the right side, because of the difficulty the patient has in reading a whole sentence fluently. *Concentric constrictions of the visual field* may become evident if it is difficult for the patient to locate the chart or if he sees only a few letters instead of a whole line. *Central scotomas* are particularly annoying to the patient while reading. If they are quite large, they prevent reading altogether. Smaller scotomas cause the fading of letters in a word or of complete words in a sentence. *Metamorphopsias* (micropsia, macropsia, irregular distortion) become quite obvious in reading. As a matter of fact, letters are an ideal test object for pathologic distortion, magnification, or diminution of an image. However, it should be emphasized that central metamorphopsias are rare; any lesion along the entire visual pathway may cause them (p. 6). Before such a diagnosis is made, retinal changes always have to be ruled out. A *paresis of accommodation* should be suspected if the patient's distance vision is satisfactory, but he is unable to read small print at a distance of 25 to 30 cm. Presbyopia and high hyperopia must be ruled out in such a case. Crossed diplopia on near vision without double vision for distance may be the result of a central *convergence palsy* (the result of tumors in the midbrain) (p. 51). This must be differentiated from the purely functional convergence insufficiency.

In special cases in which the determination of visual acuity is difficult or impossible (cataract, vitreous opacities, cortical blindness, malingering), *electroretinograms* (ERG's), eventually combined with *electroencephalograms* (EEG's) (evoked potentials, determination of retinocortical time), can be extremely helpful and provide important additional information on the functional state of the retina and the optical pathways, including the occipital cortex.

### Color sensation

Any damage to the optic nerve or optic tract by an intracranial neoplasm results in a more or less severe disturbance of conductivity; this can also modify or completely destroy the color sensation. According to experience, the *color sensation for red is most vulnerable and will be modified or destroyed before alterations of the sensation for white appear.* Sensations for green and blue will be involved only later. This rule applies to inflammatory and toxic disturbances of the conductivity of the optic nerve and tract as well as to those caused by a tumor. Traquair is of the opinion that this disturbance of conductivity for red, which is so important for an early diagnosis, is not caused by a selective vulnerability of the fibers conducting the red sensation. The test for red is generally considered a particularly suitable and refined clinical test for disturbances of conductivity, which actually could be demonstrated in the early stages just as well for white and blue if one would take the trouble to search for them with suitable test objects. Impairments of the color sensation in disturbances of conductivity caused by a tumor are usually concomitant with the appearance of a more or less advanced optic atrophy. This may take the form of a primary descending atrophy as the result of direct pressure of a tumor on the nerve, chiasm, or optic tract (pituitary tumors, meningiomas of the tuberculum sellae or the sphenoid ridge, craniopharyngiomas, tumors of the optic nerve or its sheaths), or it may be an atrophy secondary to a chronic papilledema associated with tumors in almost any location. *Disturbance of the color sensation frequently precedes the visible manifestation of the atrophy, thus assuming important diagnostic significance as an early sign of a retrobulbar disturbance of conductivity.* As a rule, this disturbance is not a general depression. In the early stages, it usually manifests itself as a more or less extensive *central scotoma for color*, especially for red; it will expand from the point of fixation toward the periphery. Such a scotoma for red may at first be only *relative* (that is, the red target will appear less saturated in a certain central area than in the remainder of the field). In a later stage the relative scotoma for red becomes *absolute*. In other words the form of the red target of a given size used for the test will be recognized, but its color cannot be perceived any longer. In even later stages, scotomas will develop for green, blue, and white (in that order) until the disturbance of conductivity and the resulting atrophy of the nerve fibers terminate in the complete extinction of all color sensations. This experience is encountered time and again in patients with severe chronic atrophic papilledema.

In every case of an acquired disturbance of the color sensation a *congenital form* (red-green deficiency, yellow-blue deficiency) must be excluded. This is customarily done with the standard *pseudoisochromatic plates by Ishihara or Hertel* or with the *Farnsworth-D-15 hue test*. These plates may also be used for color disturbances in nerve and tract lesions, but only in the relatively severe stages of general depression of the color sensation over wide areas of the visual field. In the early stages with only scotomatous defects the results are unsatisfactory. To demonstrate a color scotoma, one uses either a *perimeter* or *campimeter* (p. 79). This is the best and most reliable method. For a quick survey to determine the presence of a scotoma for color the so-called *scotometer* is suitable. A black wand is provided with colored dots of varying size and color. For the examination the patient is instructed to fix on a certain colored dot with one eye (it is important to make sure that the patient fixes properly!) and to indicate whether he perceives color and, if so, what color. Dots of the same color but of a different size are shown to the patient. In this simple manner, scotomas for red and other colors can be rapidly demonstrated and, to a certain extent, their size can be determined. Such a color scotometer can be improvised whenever the need arises without great technical resources. Even colored crayons can be used for this purpose; they are covered by black paper with holes of varying sizes.

For the more exact methods of testing the color vision (Farnsworth-Munsell 100-hue test), especially for a description of the use of the Nagel *anomaloscope* with regard to the Rayleigh equation, textbooks of ophthalmology should be consulted.

Although the peripheral disturbances of conductivity involving the visual pathways (namely, the optic nerve, the chiasm, and the optic tract) are the principal causes of a defective color sensation in connection with brain tumors, it should be remembered that there are also *central forms* associated with certain lesions of the visual cortex or the higher visual centers (Fig. 1-2).

In describing cortical blindness (p. 7), it has been stated that color sensation is last to return during the phase of recovery (that is, after light and form sensation). In partial lesions of the visual cortex the color sensation seems to be the most vulnerable part of the visual function and the one that is most easily impaired. In lesions of the calcarine area a homonymous hemianopia in a unilateral process or an extensive concentric constriction of the visual field in a bilateral process with sparing of the macula may be associated with a complete or partial disturbance of color sensation (achromatopsia or dyschromatopsia). Disturbances of space and form perception, which usually occur simultaneously, should make it possible to differentiate cortical blindness from the peripheral forms.

An entirely different type of disturbance of the color sensation is *amnestic color blindness* (Wilbrand) in patients with lesions in or near the angular gyrus of the dominant hemisphere. In this type of disorder the visual pathway, including the calcarine cortex, is intact. Only the associative interpretation of the color impression via the higher visual centers is impaired. The patient is unable to recognize the color he sees (color agnosia) or, in less severe forms, confuses colors and calls them by the wrong names (amnestic color aphasia). Again, associated symptoms such as simultaneous object agnosia, alexia, and apractic and sensory-aphasic symptoms (Fig. 1-2) will usually suggest central origin.

### Dark adaptation

Dark adaptation is the faculty of the eyes to adjust to varying intensities of light by an increased or decreased response of the light-sensitive retinal elements. This adaptation is primarily the function of the rods of the retina.

It should be recalled in this connection that the very *first sign of a disturbed conductivity of the optic nerves and tracts is an impairment (that is, a reduction or complete loss) of the dark adaptation* (Behr; Rutgers; Gasteiger). It can be determined before the appearance of changes in the visual acuity, the visual fields, the color sensation, or the fundus. A dark adaptation test therefore may be of considerable importance for the early diagnosis of a tumor causing disturbance of the conductivity of the optic nerve, the chiasm, or the optic tract. Unfortunately, the value of this test is limited because it requires relatively complicated instruments that are not always available. The determination of the visual field in the dark-adapted eye and its comparison with that of the light-adapted eye may, to a certain extent, serve as a suitable alternative (Goldmann).

The adaptometers of Nagel and Della Casa are useful for dark adaptation tests. Goldmann has constructed a self-registering adaptometer that is ideal for research purposes (manufactured by Haag-Streit, Bern).

### Visual field

Next to ophthalmoscopy and visual acuity estimation the examination of the visual field is one of the most important procedures in the neuro-ophthalmologic evaluation of brain tumors. It is so important because *visual field changes occur so frequently in association with brain tumors.* They occur in about 50% of the total number of patients with brain tumors and, according to Cushing and to Sanford and Bair, in 70% to 80% of patients with temporal lobe tumors. Furthermore, certain types of defects have a definite *localizing value* (in about 25% of the patients). This fact is important because the determination of the visual field is a procedure that can be performed relatively simply as part of a neurologic examination. A reliable field can be plotted by every physician without special training. We said intentionally "by every physician" because we are of the opinion that testing the visual field in a neuro-ophthalmologic examination is too important a task to be entrusted to a technician. Such a person is not familiar with the physiologic principles involved and does not possess the necessary basic training. The modern methods for exact tumor localization (such as computerized axial tomography, pneumoencephalography, arteriography, electroencephalography, and scintigraphy) should in no way lessen the localizing value of the visual field. By its use the patient eventually may be spared disagreeable and potentially harmful diagnostic procedures. It would be wrong for the neurosurgeon to take the attitude that examination of the visual field should be performed by the referring physician or by an ophthalmologist. On the contrary, he should insist on performing the test himself according to the principles of exact perimetry and campimetry so he can form his own opinion regarding the usefulness of the method and its results in a given patient. Naturally, this does not exclude cooperation with the ophthalmologist, especially in difficult and obscure cases.

During the past decades the methods of perimetry and campimetry have become incredibly refined and perfected. In particular, the instruments for perimetry (for instance, the ones designed by Goldmann or Harms) come equipped with all sorts of perfections that make examination of the visual fields quite valuable and furnish, in certain cases, data of the utmost importance. However, reliable *cooperation* on the part of the patient is an absolute necessity when such instruments are used. *Unfortunately, this is not always the case, especially in patients with brain tumors.* For one thing the patient may be drowsy because of increased intracranial pressure. Also, a tumor causing central disorders of visual integration may make it impossible for the patient to comprehend certain events in the surroundings (for instance, a visual field test). He may be unable to understand a task requested of him (sensory aphasia) or to express his thoughts in words (motor aphasia). The complicated instruments used in perimetry and campimetry therefore frequently fail with such patients because of their lethargic or impaired cooperation. The technical perfection of the instrument is out of proportion to the mental alertness of the patient. There is no advantage in using minute test objects with a variety of light intensities if a dull and indifferent patient is unable to follow and appreciate them! We ophthalmologists are the last to deprecate the value of the modern perimeter. *Yet in our contact with patients with brain tumor, we have come to recognize that, in certain cases, crude and seemingly simple methods of testing the visual field may be just as valuable, if not more so, as some such highly sophisticated instruments.* For this reason, we shall discuss "crude bedside methods" before discussing the methods of perimetry and campimetry.

### Qualitative testing of the visual fields without special instruments (crude methods)

For the so-called *confrontation test* the patient and physician face each other, with the light (daylight or artificial light) in back of the patient. The patient is instructed to cover one eye with his hand and to fix the eye to be examined on the examiner's opposite eye. The latter moves his entire hand or only the index finger in a frontal plane equidistant between the patient and himself in various (preferably eight) meridians from the periphery toward the center. As soon as the patient sees the hand or finger in his field, he should indicate this. With this method the examiner's own field serves as a control. Testing by confrontation can also be performed using a pencil or by asking the patient to count the examiner's fingers in the various quadrants of the visual field. Traquair has modified this test by using a white disk, 2 to 6 cm in diameter, mounted on a stick. As a further refinement of this method he has advised reducing the illumination of the room because a reduction in the brightness of the test object may render pathologic changes of the visual field more conspicuous. The *simultaneous binocular testing of the visual fields* is quite an important variant of the confrontation test. Both eyes of the patient are uncovered. The examiner moves both hands or extended index fingers symmetrically from the temporal sides (upper, lower, or middle) toward the center. It is important to have even illumination. The patient has to indicate whether he sees one or two hands and whether he recognizes one hand earlier or more distinctly. If there is a difference in perception of the two sides or perhaps no perception on one side, one speaks of a so-called *relative hemianopia* (p. 4). This is in contrast to the absolute hemianopia that becomes manifest in the separate examination of each individual eye. *The relative hemianopia must be considered an incomplete form of the absolute hemianopia.* In the former only partial functions of vision of a qualitative nature (recognition of form, perception of movement, spatial orientation, and others) are disturbed. Ordinary perimetry performed separately for each eye will not uncover a relative hemianopia, even with the most minute methods, unless a test object from the nasal side and one from the temporal side are moved simultaneously from the periphery toward the point of fixation (Dufour; Thiébaut, Guillaumat, and Brégeat). Since, as mentioned previously, only relatively primitive partial visual functions are disturbed, only a relatively crude method such as the one outlined will uncover such a relative hemianopia, also called *"unilateral visual inattention"* or *"visual extinction in homonymous fields."* An example such as this should emphasize how valuable and at times even indispensable such simple methods can be in the testing of the visual fields. In case one does not find field changes with the exact methods of perimetry in patients with tumors of the parietal or parieto-occipital area, he should always, by means of the confrontation tests, search for a relative hemianopia, this important form of "visual inattention," which is in the same class as other manifestations of the so-called *anosognosia* (for instance, the unawareness of a hemiplegia or a central deafness). Unilateral visual inattention may also be observed when there is regression or disappearance of homonymous hemianopia after any lesion (vascular, tumor trauma).

Kestenbaum describes another modification of the confrontation test that, in our opinion, is also valuable and that supposedly will furnish even more accurate results. He has observed that the *visual field in the plane of the face corresponds with a surprising exactness to the outline of the face when the eye looks straight ahead*. Whereas in the ordinary confrontation test the field of the examiner serves as a control, the outline of the patient's face serves this purpose in Kestenbaum's *"outline perimetry."*

The patient is instructed to look straight ahead. One eye is covered. The examiner brings a pencil or his finger from the periphery into the field of vision. This is done in a plane not more than 2 or 3 cm in front of the patient's face and repeated in 8 to 12 meridians. As soon as the test object appears in the periphery of the field, the patient should indicate this. If the visual field is normal, it will coincide with the outline of the face (nasally with the border of the nose, temporally with the lateral orbital rim). On the basis of this normal outline, a pathologic field can be recognized without difficulty. Kestenbaum is of the opinion that the margin of error with this method is less than 10 degrees in the hands of an experienced examiner. It would be expedient to include this outline perimetry in the general screening of every patient even if no field defects are suspected at first.

*As a bedside test, especially in patients who fatigue easily or who are slightly stuporous or in aphasic patients showing poor cooperation, outline perimetry may, except for the confrontation tests, be the only way to determine the visual field.* This also applies to patients whose visual acuity is reduced to finger counting or recognition of hand movements and in whom ordinary perimetry would fail.

Patients with a brain tumor may not even respond to outline perimetry. In such instances, even cruder methods may be called for. For the so-called *reflex lid closure test* the examiner uses the hand or fist and abruptly approaches the eye to be examined from both sides as well as from above and below. The presence or absence of the lid closure reflex will allow some conclusions as to whether the visual field is normal or abnormal. Other *optically induced reflex movements of the eyes* may be used instead of the lid closure reflex. An article that will attract the patient's attention, such as a pencil, cigarette, key, coin, or food (for instance, a piece of fruit), is moved toward the patient. If the field is intact, he will perceive the object already in the periphery of his field and will direct his gaze toward it (optically induced reflex movement, p. 45). The eight meridians should be tested for each eye, and the response should be recorded. The persistent absence of a reflex in a particular meridian should be considered as an indication of a field defect. In aphasic patients the small test objects mentioned are inadequate. Kestenbaum is right when he mentions that the strongest stimulus to gain the attention of such patients is the human face. The examiner stands behind the patient in a position that enables him to bring his own face into the patient's visual field from various directions. If the patient turns his eyes toward the physician's face, he probably has an intact field for that particular meridian, and vice versa. This *"face test"* is particularly useful for the determination of field defects not only in aphasic patients, but also in children.

If the visual field is reduced to light perception, *testing light projection* is the only means of gaining information concerning the visual field. A bright point source of light (for instance, an ophthalmoscope or flashlight) is moved toward the eye in various meridians. The patient has to indicate the direction from which the light comes and, if possible, the moment a light sensation is perceived. This test can be performed similar to Kestenbaum's outline perimetry test.

### Quantitative determination of visual fields

If during a neuro-ophthalmologic examination a field defect has been discovered with these crude methods, it should be investigated, if possible, with the *more refined methods of perimetry and campimetry.* If a superficial screening has shown no definite defect, a further and more subtle analysis is even more indispensable.

The customary *quantitative examination of the visual field* is based on the *principle of the determination of the differential threshold.* This can be accomplished in two ways.

The first way is to expose the target in a fixed position and to vary its size or its light intensity until the patient recognizes it. This determines the differential threshold for a given point of the retina (static perimetry). Point after point of the field is tested in this manner— an extremely cumbersome procedure but one that furnishes extremely reliable results, especially in neurologic patients (Harms; Ferree and Rand). The second way, and the one followed in most perimetric procedures (including those that will be described here), follows a procedure whereby a target of a certain size and luminosity is moved from the periphery toward the point of fixation (or in the opposite direction) until the patient recognizes it. This is the determination of retinal points with the same differential threshold (kinetic perimetry). All points thus determined are connected to form a curve, the so-called *isopter,* which represents a line formed of points with the same differential threshold for the chosen test. In the more common types of perimeter the illumination and the contrast between background and target are constant. The only variable is the size of the target (perimetry with one variable). Newer instruments have been designed that permit a variation of the size and luminosity of the target according to a definite ratio (perimetry with two variables; for instance, the Goldmann or Tübinger perimeter).

For an exact evaluation of the visual field in its entirety, it is in principle still advisable to use two instruments: a *perimeter* and a *campimeter* (tangent screen). *The former is used primarily for testing the peripheral field and the latter for the intermediate and particularly the central areas.* The need for two separate procedures is a consequence of the enormous difficulty of constructing targets sufficiently small for the exploration of the central area on the perimeter. (With the use of the Goldmann or Tübinger perimeter, however, the central areas can be examined so accurately that campimetry often may be omitted.) It is not the purpose of this book to describe the exact techniques used for perimetry (static and kinetic) and campimetry. We recommend the excellent and detailed monographs on this subject by Traquair; Lauber; Malbrán; Harrington; Hughes; and Dubois-Poulsen as well as the valuable articles by Goldmann; Harms; Aulhorn; Walsh and Hoyt; Schmidt; and others. Nevertheless, we want to stress a few points that are important in the neuro-ophthalmologic examination (especially in brain tumors) and that are, in part, based on personal experience.

**Examination of the visual field with the perimeter.** A large number of various instruments are available for this purpose. Essentially, they are modified and improved types of the classic *Foerster* perimeter. This instrument can still be recommended if it is equipped with a suitable illuminated arc. More up-to-date models have been designed by Ferree and Rand, Magitot, Harms, Maggiore, and Aimark. Next to the Goldmann perimeter, the two last-named instruments are still popular in our eye clinics. The Maggiore, Aimark, Tübinger, and Goldmann models are so-called projection perimeters because the test marks are replaced by projected light dots. The instruments employing test marks are for perimetry with one variable. Projection of a light target allows perimetry with two variables (that is, a variation in size and brightness of the light marks). As a rule, the radius of the perimeter arc is 33 cm. The test objects or light marks usually have a diameter of 10, 5, 3, 2, or 1 mm.

For the determination of the absolute outer limits of the visual field on the perimeter, one begins with a 10 mm target. It is moved slowly from the periphery toward the point of fixation at a steady rate of about 2 degrees/second. Next follows the exploration of the isopters. The differential threshold varies considerably in pathologic cases; thus no set rules can be stated for the determination of the isopters. Nevertheless, one should be guided by the following directions: the isopters determined should be rather evenly distributed from the periphery toward the point of fixation and, if possible, should include most zones of the peripheral visual field. The central zones are part of the examination on the tangent screen. In addition to the absolute outer limit, which is determined with a 10 mm target, it is desirable to have an isopter of the 60-degree zone (with a test object of 5 or 3 mm for the normal individual) and one in the 30-degree zone (with a test object of 2 or 1 mm for the normal individual). At least 12 meridians have to be tested in a routine examination. The use of targets smaller than 1 mm is unreliable and should be avoided in usual perimetry. Instead of moving the target from the "nonseeing" to the "seeing" part of the field, this method can be reversed. This will result in a somewhat greater sensitivity of some retinal areas (desirable in cases of poor cooperation); for instance, scotomas will appear smaller, and the peripheral limits of the field will extend farther out.

The isopters obtained in this fashion will be transferred to a visual field chart and identified in the form of a fraction (10/330, 5/330, 3/330, 2/330, 1/330). It is best to *use the same chart for perimetry and campimetry and to record the isopters found by the two different methods on the same chart* (Fig. 3-13).

With projection perimeters, the number of isopters can be increased by the use of each of the different-sized targets with varying degrees of brightness.

This is perhaps the appropriate time to describe the *Goldmann projection perimeter*, which, as a perimeter with two variables, can be considered one of the most modern, most complete, and most efficient instruments, apart from the Tübinger model. The two variables are the size of the object and its brightness or, more precisely, its contrast with the background of the perimeter bowl. The illumination of this bowl is such that an extended adaptation of the patient is superfluous. By means of a telescope-like arrangement the examiner can constantly check the patient's eye against a thread cross to assure central fixation, which is of the utmost importance for neuro-ophthalmologic field determinations. A pantograph permits the direct registration of the findings from the projection arm to the visual field chart. Six targets of different sizes and four different intensities of illumination make the determination of a large number of evenly distributed isopters possible. The relationship between the size of the objects and the intensity of illumination has been arranged according to the law of summation; therefore the same isopters can be determined either with a large but less luminous or with a small but bright target.

It has been observed that in patients with certain affections (papilledema, p. 94) it is indispensable to determine not only the isopters, but also the capacity for summation of various retinal areas (Dubois-Poulsen; Goldmann). This can be easily accomplished on the Goldmann or Tübinger perimeter by means of either the large, dimly illuminated or the small, brightly illuminated test marks that have been arranged according to the law of summation. A number of methods permit the determination of the sensitivity of any retinal area between the examined isopters: Goldmann's skiascotometry, Harms' method of static perimetry, and flicker fusion perimetry as elaborated by Hylkema, Weekers and Roussel, and Miles. Since it is possible to vary the brightness of the inner surface of the bowl of the Goldmann perimeter, the use of this instrument makes it possible to examine and compare visual fields for the light-adapted (photopic perimetry) and the dark-adapted (scotopic perimetry) eye.

For a detailed description of the technique used with the Goldmann perimeter, we recommend the original publications of Goldmann as well as the monograph by Dubois-Poulsen, whose material was mostly obtained with the aid of this perimeter. One of the chief advantages of this instrument, so extremely valuable for neuro-ophthalmologic examinations, is the ability to *control fixation*. Also, unlike the older perimeters, it furnishes reliable results *for the peripheral as well as the central areas of the field*. The same can be said for the Tübinger perimeter, where, especially for testing the central visual field, the accuracy of registration can be augmented three times. The use of the Goldmann perimeter is simple and rapid—in experienced hands more rapid than that of other perimeters. We regard it as the instrument of choice for a detailed and exact visual field test in patients with brain tumors, provided there is proper or at least halfway satisfactory cooperation. Examples of visual fields determined with the Goldmann perimeter can be found in later chapters (Figs. 3-37 and 3-42).

Goldmann and Schmidt briefly make the following suggestions for a proper and suitable technique with this perimeter—suggestions that prove to be satisfactory in our experience. The good eye or the eye with the better vision is examined first. The size of the pupil is recorded. For the examination of the central and intermediate field the patient should wear his spectacle correction (if indicated, a presbyopic correction!). There should be a preadaptation of the patient using the illuminated perimeter for 4 to 5 minutes. The examination begins with target size 1 and intensity 4 (the corresponding isopter is recorded as "1/4"). For healthy persons between the ages of 20 and 30 years, this isopter should extend to the normal peripheral limits of the field. If a constriction of the field is found, the size of the target should be increased, and the test should be repeated for 2/4 and, if necessary, 3/4 or even 4/4 and 5/4. The target should be brought from the periphery toward the center in the meridian examined with a steady speed of about 5 degrees/sec. This is performed every 30 degrees, but every 5 degrees or at even lesser intervals for the meridians of a field defect. After the peripheral limits of the field have been determined, one proceeds with the investigation of the intermediate and central isopters with the use of targets of less intense illumination or smaller size (for instance, 1/3, 1/2, 1/1, and 0/1). The outline of the blind spot should be determined with the target for the isopter that just includes the blind spot (usually 1/2). The target should be moved from the blind toward the seeing area. In the case of a scotoma the extent of the scotoma is first determined with the target corresponding to the isopters including the scotoma. The test is repeated first with a target of higher intensity and next with one of larger size. For instance, if the scotoma lies in the 1/2 isopter, the test is performed with the 1/2, 1/3, 1/4, 2/4, and 4/4 targets. Paracentral scotomas are tested by flashing the 1/1 and 0/1 targets. If malingering is suspected, the binocular field should be examined. Even the Goldmann perimeter does not furnish absolutely reliable findings in the area central to the blind spot, particularly around the point of fixation and its immediate surroundings. For the exact evaluation of this part of the field, one still cannot dispense with the time-proved method of campimetry.

**Examination of the visual field with the campimeter (tangent screen).** For the examination of the visual field with the campimeter, it is best to use the *Bjerrum screen* at a distance of either 1 or 2 meters. We definitely prefer the large screen at a distance of 2 meters for neurologic patients, especially those with brain tumors. A large number of the fields reproduced in this book have been obtained by this method. For the very smallest central defects, Krayenbühl recommends Vogt's method of testing at a distance of 6 meters (Wiesli). The tangent screen permits the use of objects that are very small as measured in degrees and yet large enough in actual extent to be easily handled. The examined dimensions being larger than at the perimeter, the examination can be performed with more accuracy.

The Bjerrum screen should be provided with concentric circles, if possible, in addition to the radial meridians. It should be evenly and intensely illuminated with floodlights. The patient is seated at a distance of 2 meters exactly opposite the fixation mark, with his eyes level with the latter. His head should be supported by a chin rest. The examiner should wear a black coat, black gloves, and, if possible, a black mask of the type used in the operating room.

First the target just inside the boundary of the screen for the eye examined is determined. With this target the most peripheral isopter is plotted. It is also used for a superficial survey of the size and position of the blind spot. This enables one to check the patient's fixation at the same time. Other isopters are determined by choosing the targets in such a manner that one isopter is outside the outer border and one inside the inner border of the blind spot. The most suitable targets are 3, 2, and 1 mm, the last one for the central and paracentral zone. After the preliminary test the blind spot should also be examined with the smaller 2 and 1 mm targets—a test that may be of particular help when demonstrating an increase in size of the blind spot resulting from a papilledema.

The isopters thus obtained are recorded on the blank and labeled as 3/2000, 2/2000, and 1/2000. If possible, perimetric and campimetric results should be plotted on the same blank (Fig. 3-60).

We use *color test objects* for the *visual field examination* only as a test for the central color sensation (that is, to demonstrate a scotoma for red in early disturbances of conductivity of the optic nerve and tract). As a rule, relatively larger objects should be used for color perimetry (for instance, 5/330) as well as for campimetry. In agreement with Dubois-Poulsen and Goldmann, we are of the opinion that *nothing can be accomplished with color perimetry that could not be accomplished with a carefully performed "white" perimetry,* particularly because the former is rendered less valuable by a number of disadvantages in the form of a large number of inconstant factors, most of them of a technical nature. Many authors are still of the opinion that the initial disturbance

in the conductivity of the optic nerve, the chiasm, or the optic tract is a disturbance in the central red field. A possible explanation for this misconcept is that
a detailed "white test" has been omitted or performed in a faulty manner in such
cases. An examination on the perimeter and tangent screen that has been carefully performed according to the previously described principles will eliminate
the need for color perimetry and campimetry in the neuro-ophthalmologic examination.

The *Amsler-Landolt grid* is quite useful in certain patients for testing the
very central part of the field (that is, the macula and its surroundings), especially for the demonstration of an absolute or relative central scotoma or of

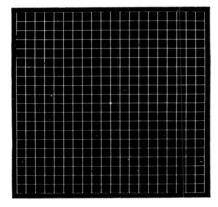

**Fig. 1-33.** Amsler-Landolt grid in reduced ( ½ ) reproduction. In original, length of each small
square measures 5 mm and corresponds to visual angle of 1 degree at a distance of 28 to 30
cm. Under such conditions, entire grid occupies central area of 10-degree radius around point
of fixation in visual field.

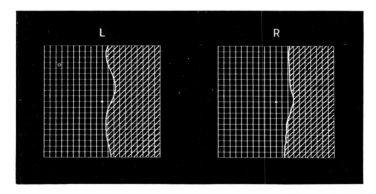

**Fig. 1-34.** Right homonymous hemianopia determined for central visual field on Amsler-
Landolt grid. Shaded squares mark field defect. Sparing of macula amounts to 2 degrees on
left side and 3 degrees on right side, measured from point of fixation. Patient had a tumor of
left occipital lobe.

metamorphopsia. Each individual square of this grid subtends a 1-degree angle if viewed at a distance of about 30 cm (Fig. 1-33). Even the central part of a hemianopic disturbance becomes manifest on this grid provided it extends to the point of fixation and provided the patient has no "unilateral visual inattention," as in a relative hemianopia. In such instances the patient himself may be able to indicate the distance that separates the fixation point from the line dividing the seeing from the blind area of the visual field. This method has been quite helpful in our field studies with patients after occipital lobectomies, especially in answering the question as to whether or not there was sparing of the macula (Fig. 1-34).

Cuendet and Dufour have suggested that the area enclosed by each isopter (especially the intermediate and central isopters found on the Goldmann perimeter) be determined with the help of a planimeter, using the simplified figures thus obtained for the magnitude of the visual field as a basis of comparison in repeat examinations.

The perimetric and campimetric methods are subjective methods of examination. They require full cooperation on the part of the patient. Naturally, they could be the source of numerous errors, which should always be considered judiciously. Fatigue of the patient should be taken into consideration. High refractive errors should be corrected by glasses. The response may be slow and the cooperation weary, especially with patients suffering from brain tumors. The result may be a spiral or, more rarely, a concentrically constricted field, although there is no organic defect of the visual pathways. Such an apparent contraction of the field caused by inattentiveness of the patient can be diminished if, during the perimetric or campimetric test, the examiner moves the targets away from the fixation point rather than toward it.

As has been mentioned previously, most methods of quantitative determination of visual fields (perimeter and campimeter) are based on the procedure of determination of retinal points with the same differential threshold and thus the principle of determination of isopters. *For neuro-ophthalmologic purposes, however, it is especially desirable to also know the retinal sensitivity of any retinal area between the isopters.* Two methods of perimetry making this possible deserve special consideration in this connection: flicker perimetry (Hylkema; Weekers and Roussel; Miles) and static perimetry (Harms).

*Flicker perimetry* consists of plotting visual fields by determining thresholds for a flickering light.

It is performed using an electronically driven glow modulator tube, presenting a target of about a 2-degree visual angle under the same conditions of illumination as in standard perimetry. Flicker thresholds are determined for 26 points in each eye at the 10-, 20-, and 30-degree circles.

Flicker perimetry appears to be more sensitive for central nervous system dysfunctions than standard field examination. Before it can be stated, on the basis of the standard examination, that central lesions (tumor, trauma, cerebrovascular accident) are present, extreme impairment of flicker discrimination must be demonstrable (Parsons, Chandler, Teed, and Haase).

In *static perimetry* a stationary target is used that can be placed in any part of the field and the differential threshold to light of the tested area measured.

For static perimetry, Harms has designed a special instrument (Tübinger perimeter, manufactured by Oculus) that at the same time can also be used for kinetic perimetry under different adaptations (photopic, scotopic, mesopic), for flicker fusion perimetry, and for adaptometry. With special additional devices, the Goldmann perimeter can also be used for static perimetry. The target used can be varied in diameter, enabling the exploration of the whole visual field. In the chosen retinal area, it remains absolutely immobile. Its luminosity decreases gradually, the time of presentation being less than 1 second and two different stimulations being separated at intervals of 2 to 3 seconds. The results obtained are points on the same meridian, which are plotted on a chart, the distance from the fixation point in degrees on the abscissa and the luminosity of the threshold stimulus in apostilb (asb) on the ordinate. Different meridians of the visual field are examined according to the defect.

The results of static perimetry can be compared with meridional sections through the "function mountain" of the retina (Harms) and thus represent on the whole a three-dimensional visual field where defects, especially of neurologic origin (scotomas, hemianopias), can be identified and mapped earlier and with more accuracy (especially very small defects) than by means of the two-dimensional kinetic perimetry. In static perimetry, meridians going through the center of the visual field are examined. The results obtained inform therefore only about the distribution of visual function in certain meridians. What meridians to choose can be decided beforehand by kinetic perimetry. *Especially for neuro-ophthalmologic examinations, the combination of kinetic and static perimetry is the ideal procedure of choice* (Fig. 1-35). Kinetic perimetry, giving a rough idea of the existing field defects, will instruct the perimetrist as to what meridians to use in static perimetry; static perimetry, on the other hand, will furnish important data for deciding what size and luminosity of target is necessary for successful kinetic perimetry.

A new method of fully automated *computer analysis of the visual field* is described by Fankhauser, Koch, and Roulier. The examination time with his program corresponds to that needed by a human perimetrist. The mathematic principles involved are valid for high degrees of pathologic field distortion. Each step of the computer analysis follows a rational strategy. The data may be displayed as isopters or as sections through the visual field, without time-consuming manual plotting.

**General pathology of the visual field in brain tumors**

The pathologic visual fields will be discussed in detail in connection with the various tumor sites. Nevertheless, we believe it is important to list first in a brief but systematic manner the field changes caused by disturbances in the conductivity of the visual pathways. This *brief general pathology of the visual field* is intentionally based on the *shape of the visual field* to provide the examiner with a guide that should enable him to localize a lesion from a given form of visual field change (Fig. 1-36).

The visual field changes observed in patients with brain tumors may be

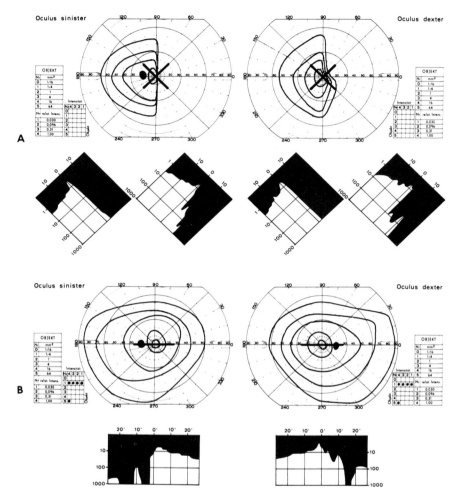

**Fig. 1-35. A,** Demonstration of kinetic and static perimetry in combination in patient with a tumor of left parietotemporal region. Above, Kinetic perimetry (Goldmann perimeter) shows right homonymous hemianopia with sparing of macula. Below, Static perimetry (Harms perimeter) performed in 45- and 135-degree meridians; "function mountain" of retina is cut away to right side with distinct sparing of macular area. Note striking congruity of field defects and its borderlines, which becomes manifest only in static fields (in contrast to kinetic fields, where by mistake not enough meridians have been examined in left field [right inferior area] and therefore apparent incongruity appears!). **B,** Kinetic and static perimetry in patient with suprasellar meningioma. Above, Kinetic visual fields (Goldmann perimeter), apart from slight temporal indentation of innermost isopters, show nothing pathologic (blind spots of normal size and site). Below, Static visual fields (Harms perimeter) manifest in 0-degree meridian bitemporal paracentral scotomas (extending from 3 to 10 degrees), which escaped kinetic perimetry because they are situated just between two isopters. (After Harms.)

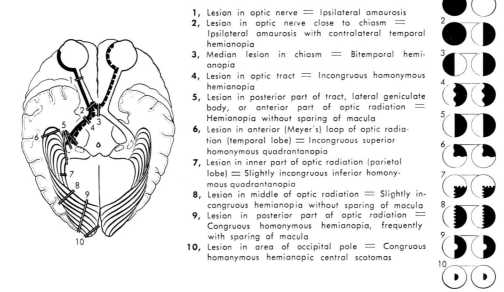

1, Lesion in optic nerve = Ipsilateral amaurosis
2, Lesion in optic nerve close to chiasm = Ipsilateral amaurosis with contralateral temporal hemianopia
3, Median lesion in chiasm = Bitemporal hemianopia
4, Lesion in optic tract = Incongruous homonymous hemianopia
5, Lesion in posterior part of tract, lateral geniculate body, or anterior part of optic radiation = Hemianopia without sparing of macula
6, Lesion in anterior (Meyer's) loop of optic radiation (temporal lobe) = Incongruous superior homonymous quadrantanopia
7, Lesion in inner part of optic radiation (parietal lobe) = Slightly incongruous inferior homonymous quadrantanopia
8, Lesion in middle of optic radiation = Slightly incongruous hemianopia without sparing of macula
9, Lesion in posterior part of optic radiation = Congruous homonymous hemianopia, frequently with sparing of macula
10, Lesion in area of occipital pole = Congruous homonymous hemianopic central scotomas

**Fig. 1-36.** Diagram of most important visual field defects for lesions in various parts of visual pathways. (After Duke-Elder.)

divided into five "morphologic" groups: general and concentric constriction (centric or eccentric), unilateral sector-shaped defects, scotomas (absolute or relative), bitemporal field defects, and homonymous field defects.

**General and concentric constriction (centric or eccentric).** A *bilateral* concentric constriction should always be evaluated with caution, especially in a patient with a brain tumor, because, as has just been mentioned, it could be merely the result of a general apathy in a lackadaisical subject rather than a manifestation of an actual organic interference with the visual pathways. We have had occasions to observe such concentrically contracted fields or spiral fields in patients with frontal lobe tumors (Fig. 3-8). A concentric contraction progressing to a typical "gun barrel" field in *chronic atrophic papilledema* is caused by progressive nerve fiber destruction (Fig. 2-19). A bilateral "gun barrel" field may also result from a bilateral homonymous hemianopia with macular sparing, an event suggesting a bilaterally expanding tumor process in the region of the calcarine fissure. A *unilateral* concentric constriction suggests a *lesion of the optic nerve between the globe and chiasm,* provided an even more peripheral etiology such as a diseased retina (heredodegenerative retinopathy, among others) or glaucoma can be ruled out; *usually there is an additional central or cecocentral scotoma* with quadrantal features (Fig. 3-4). The etiology for such a defect may be a tumor of the optic nerve itself or of its sheaths; a meningioma of the tuberculum sellae, the sphenoid ridge, or the olfactory groove; a craniopharyngioma; a pituitary adenoma with an extrasellar extension; a tumor at the inferior surface of the brain in the anterior or middle fossa (eventually with an accompanying cavernous sinus or superior orbital fissure syndrome); and occasionally a frontal lobe tumor (presenting itself in the form of a Foster Kennedy syndrome). Especially in a unilateral concentric contraction of the visual field, it is not always easy (or may even be impossible) to differentiate disturbances of conductivity caused by a tumor from those resulting from other etiologies, whether inflammatory, toxic, or degenerative. In the differential diagnosis, one should therefore always consider glaucoma, tapetoretinal degeneration of the retina, secondary atrophy after optic neuritis (multiple sclerosis), tabes, toxic amblyopia (tobacco, alcohol, quinine), and traumas.

Concentric contraction can also be the expression of generally diminished vision and must not be confused with real loss of the periphery of the visual field as the result of a local neurogenic process. True field defects and such "spurious" concentric contractions can be differentiated as follows: spurious contraction always parallels a corresponding decrease of the central vision; the outline of the field becomes normal again if a large enough object is used; and in a true defect of the periphery the bigger target will give the same or only a moderately larger field, but not a normal outline.

Tubular fields are generally contracted fields that become smaller as the patient moves away from the tangent screen. They are always a sign of malingering or hysteria (Goldmann).

**Unilateral sector-shaped defects.** Unilateral sector-shaped defects may occur *in combination with central scotomas* (quadrantal feature, extension to the blind spot) *resulting from tumor compression of the optic nerve* (see section on concentric constriction), an indication that only part of the optic nerve is damaged (Fig. 3-84). Sector-shaped defects in retrobulbar disturbances of the optic nerve are much rarer than concentric constrictions. Sector-shaped or wedge-shaped defects extending from the periphery of the field toward the blind spot are more *characteristic for an involvement of the disc,* for instance, secondary optic atrophy after choked disc (with a predilection for the nasal side) papillitis, glaucoma (in the early stages also predominantly on the nasal side), and juxtapapillary chorioretinitis. In the differential diagnosis, vascular changes of the retina must be considered, especially branch embolisms of the central retinal artery. The latter usually cause a sector-shaped defect involving an entire quadrant, with the apex characteristically touching the blind spot, in contrast to nerve fiber bundle disturbances of the disc or optic nerve where the apex of the sector defect points toward the point of fixation or actually coincides with it.

**Scotomas (absolute or relative).** Scotomas may be classified as central, paracentral, or cecocentral (extending from the blind spot to the point of fixation). A scotoma is relative if it exists only for color or small white targets; it is absolute if it exists for color and white targets of any size. The *blind spot* is a physiologic paracentral scotoma. Characteristically, it shows a symmetric enlargement in papilledema (Fig. 2-10). Many authors attribute some importance to this enlargement of the blind spot in the early differential diagnosis of choked disc (Chamlin and Davidoff; Davis; and others).

*Central, especially cecocentral, scotomas* suggest a *disturbance of conductivity of the nerve fibers of the papillomacular bundle within the homolateral optic nerve* and are sometimes associated with a concentric constriction of the visual field (see previous discussion). They are *negative* (that is, they are not appreciated by the patient) in slowly progressing lesions of the optic nerve or tract (for instance, tumors), but *positive* (causing the sensation of veils, gray spots, or shadows) in an acute embarrassment of the infrageniculate pathways (for instance, an inflammatory process or a hemorrhage). The papillomacular bundle, the anatomic structure involved in these scotomas, forms a separate entity not only in the optic nerve, but also in the chiasm. Thus a tumor causing a lesion in the chiasm may also be responsible for scotomas, which may occur unilaterally or bilaterally and which in their typical form, may assume a characteristic *temporal hemianopic* shape. Frequently, it is difficult to demonstrate them (Fig. 3-42). Color campimetry may be justified for this type of scotoma: scotomas for red may represent an early sign of an impaired conductivity of the papillomacular bundle. However, even in these early stages it should be possible to demonstrate similar defects if careful campimetry (or even perimetry, static and kinetic) is carried out with small white targets. *Homonymous hemianopic central scotomas* in principle may be caused by a lesion anywhere along the suprachiasmal visual pathway. It is known that they are rarely caused by tumors along the optic tracts. If they occur in connection with the optic radiation, they will almost always take the form of a negative scotoma. The corresponding *lesion* is most likely cortical or subcortical (in other words, in the *region of the occipital pole or the calcarine fissure*).

We have observed a typical case of such homonymous hemianopic scotomas in a patient with jacksonian epilepsy (Fig. 3-26). There was a visual aura (flashing, sparking, and blazing lights). This was the residue of an old meningitis. Surgical exploration revealed a circumscribed internal hemorrhagic pachymeningitis over one occipital pole.

**Unilateral temporal or nasal hemianopia.** If the optic nerve is compressed within the orbit or within the cranium, central field loss in the form of central scotomas is almost always the rule. Compression of the orbital optic nerve produces a central scotoma with quadrantal features and extension to the blind spot, forming an arcuate defect. Involvement of the *intracranial optic nerve,* especially in the region of the anterior angle of the chiasm, may give rise to *unilateral hemianopic defects,* either nasal (affection of the noncrossed fibers) or temporal (affection of the crossed fibers) with a midline separation of normal from blind areas. In cases of unilateral temporal hemianopia, one has to examine very carefully the visual field of the opposite eye in order not to overlook an upper temporal field defect that proves that the affection is no longer confined to one optic nerve, but has extended to the anterior angle of the chiasm, involving there the crossed fibers of the opposite side from a ventral direction. Unilateral hemianopic defects may occur in gliomas or meningiomas of the optic nerve, in meningiomas of the sphenoid ridge, in olfactory groove meningiomas, in meningiomas of the tuberculum sellae, and sometimes also in intracranial aneurysms of the ophthalmic artery (originating from the junction of the ophthalmic artery with the intracranial internal carotid artery).

**Bitemporal field defects.** Bitemporal field defects generally indicate a *lesion of the central part of the chiasm* (that is, a lesion of the crossing fibers). The involvement of the fibers may originate from above, below, in front, or behind the chiasm. The typical bitemporal hemianopia is usually caused by *pituitary tumors*. It may also occur in an incomplete or modified form, depending on the pressure effect on the chiasm and its surroundings from a different direction. A *bitemporal quadrantanopia* of the superior quadrants is usually produced in the initial stages of a pituitary tumor. A symmetric progress of the defect is characteristic for a pituitary tumor. An *asymmetric bitemporal hemianopia* or *quadrantanopia* with incongruous field defects progressing in an asymmetric manner is more characteristic for extrasellar (parasellar or suprasellar) neoplasms such as craniopharyngiomas, meningiomas of the tuberculum sellae, or meningiomas of the olfactory groove. The asymmetric growth of these tumors frequently causes a direct lesion of the optic nerve if the tumor is in an anterior location or a direct lesion of the optic tract if the tumor is in a posterior location, resulting in *amaurosis of one eye with temporal hemianopia of the other eye*. Occasionally, such a picture is also seen in association with a pituitary tumor, but here as a sign of a lesion involving the entire half of the chiasm (Figs. 3-41 and 3-68).

**Homonymous field defects.** Homonymous field defects indicate a *contralateral lesion in the region of the optic tract or the geniculocalcarine optic radiation*. A homonymous hemianopia is caused by a complete or almost complete interruption of the pathway, and a *homonymous quadrantanopia* is caused by an incomplete interruption of the corresponding upper or lower section of the optic tract or radiation. An incongruous onset and progress of the field defects, a limiting line through the point of fixation without sparing of the macula, and pallor of the discs (only the temporal half of the disc on the side of the lesion, but the entire disc on the contralateral side), which may develop after months, are indicative of a *lesion of the tract*. Such a lesion may be caused by a meningioma of the sphenoid ridge, a tumor of the temporal lobe, a tumor of the middle fossa, a tumor of the thalamus, or a tumor of the quadrigeminate plate (Fig. 3-30). According to Cushing, a *superior homonymous quandrantanopia* (damage to Meyer's loop) is almost pathognomonic for *tumors of the temporal lobe* (Fig. 3-13). An *inferior homonymous quadrantanopia* occurs with tumors of the parietal lobes. A *complete homonymous hemianopia* with a striking congruence of both defects is characteristic for a large number of *tumors of* *the occipital lobe* (Fig. 3-24). Sparing of the macula, which becomes most pronounced in tumors near the occipital pole, is seen much more frequently in such tumors than a vertical boundary line of the field through the point of fixation. In our opinion the absence of *sparing of the macula* does not necessarily rule out a suprageniculate site, but may indicate a very extensive involvement of the entire optic radiation, as visual field examinations in cases of occipital lobectomies (Huber) have demonstrated. Of course, an involvement of the entire optic radiation is much more likely to occur in its anterior part, where the fibers are close together, than in the posterior occipital section. Thus if there is sparing of the macula, the tumor probably is in the posterior part of the optic radiation. This is of some significance for purposes of localization. If there is no sparing of the macula, it is of no value in this respect. Other methods for the localization of a lesion causing homonymous field defects have already been discussed (optokinetic nystagmus, saccadic pursuit movement, p. 61).

# TWO

## General signs and symptoms of increased intracranial pressure in patients with brain tumors

The signs and symptoms of a brain tumor can be divided into two different groups of symptoms: *general signs and symptoms,* mostly the result of increased intracranial pressure and of no localizing value, being more or less independent of the site of the tumor, and *focal signs and symptoms,* which are of decided localizing importance and are the result of irritation of or damage to a specific part of the brain and its immediate surrounding area. It is always important to keep in mind the chronologic sequence of these signs and symptoms. As a rule, the focal signs are the first to occur and depend strictly on a lesion of a specific part of the brain (jacksonian epileptic seizures, pareses, sensory disturbances, ataxia, agnosias, anosmia, etc.). As the growth increases in size, there may be remote effects. Finally, there will be the general signs and symptoms of increased intracranial pressure caused by a space-consuming lesion. This *sequence of focal and general signs and symptoms* is significant for a large number of brain tumors, especially those that develop in a highly differentiated part of the brain: here even a minute circumscribed focus may lead to manifestations of neurologic disturbances. In the diagnosis of brain tumors this *steady and more or less rapid progression of focal signs and symptoms,* which are *complicated by the general signs and symptoms of increased intracranial pressure only in the later stages,* is an important and pathognomonic feature. However, the chronologic development does not always follow this pattern. It may not be observed with tumors of silent parts of the brain (for instance, in the frontal or occipital lobes), with tumors that tend to cause an early internal hydrocephalus (for instance, tumors of the third or fourth ventricles), or with tumors producing intensive concomitant brain edema. In such instances the general signs and symptoms of increased intracranial pressure may be the first indications of a tumor (in 34% of all intracranial tumors, according to Tönnis). They may remain the only signs and symptoms, or the *sequence may be reversed* and the general signs and symptoms may precede the focal ones.

This discussion already clearly indicates a general *classification of the ocular signs and symptoms* in brain tumors. Analogous to other neurologic signs, we distinguish between *general signs and symptoms* that are independent of the site of the tumor and that primarily indicate an increased intracranial pressure and *signs and symptoms of localizing significance* that represent the direct result of damage to a specific part of the visual system caused by the brain tumor.

Such a classification is justified for a number of reasons. There are actually ocular signs and symptoms associated with a brain tumor that are only general ones, but that are so typical that they alone frequently enable one to make a general diagnosis of increased intracranial pressure caused by a space-consuming lesion. *Papilledema* is such a sign. These signs and symptoms do not depend on the site of the tumor and develop regardless of whether the tumor is in direct contact with the visual apparatus or not. On the other hand, intracranial neoplasms may produce quite specific ocular focal signs and symptoms if there is a direct interference with the visual apparatus. Such signs and symptoms frequently permit the localization of the tumor in an amazingly exact manner. This fact must be attributed in no small way to the highly differentiated structure of the visual sensory and oculomotor apparatus and its close topographic and functional relationship to the brain. As the sensory organ trusted with visual perception, the eye is particularly well equipped to register the minutest disturbances and to make the patient conscious of functional disorders that may not always be so obvious in other sensory organs and nervous elements.

*The nonocular general symptoms of increased intracranial pressure are headaches, vomiting, circulatory and respiratory disturbances, and psychic changes.* We purposely want to stress these symptoms briefly in order to put the ocular general signs and symptoms into the proper perspective and to clarify their relationship to the nonocular symptoms.

There is no question that *headache* is one of the most frequent symptoms of increased intracranial pressure and thus of a brain tumor. The headache is rather diffuse in character ("the head is ready to burst"; "there is a band of iron around the head") and its intensity typically increases with an additional rise in the ventricular pressure, which may be caused by coughing, sneezing, or defecating. If the headache is localized, it may occasionally indicate the site of a superficial tumor, but more often not. According to present opinion, the headache caused by a brain tumor is caused by the effect of traction on sensitive intracranial structures (large venous sinuses, meningeal blood vessels, arteries on the base of the brain, dura of anterior and posterior fossa). This may be either a local effect of the tumor or a remote effect resulting from displacement of brain substance.

*Vomiting* is usually associated with the morning headache. It affords relief from the steady or paroxysmally aggravated headache. Vomiting that occurs without nausea and without relationship to the intake of food should always arouse suspicion of increased intracranial pressure.

*Circulatory disturbances* associated with increased intracranial pressure are

tachycardia, arrhythmia, and, in later stages, bradycardia (vagus effect). Together with *respiratory disturbances* (increased rate, Cheyne-Stokes breathing),
they are, from the prognostic point of view, unfavorable signs that, as a rule,
occur in the late stages of acute increased intracranial pressure.

*Psychic disturbances* are usually a manifestation of diffuse damage to the
brain. Clouding of the consciousness ranging from slight somnolence to severe
coma is one such disturbance (lesion of the midbrain). Delirium is a form of
disturbance of consciousness in which the patients exhibit a pronounced motor
unrest because of hallucinations and delusions. An increase of the intracranial
pressure may also produce an *organic brain syndrome* (Bleuler), with disturbances of apprehension, memory, and power of association, a tendency for per-
severance and confabulation, and increased emotional lability, yet a general lack
of impulse and dullness of emotional activity.

The *ocular general signs of increased intracranial pressure consist of papilledema, nonspecific extraocular muscle pareses (especially of the abducens
nerve), the transtentorial herniation syndrome (pupillary disturbances and abnormalities of the oculomotor system), and occasionally a bilateral exophthalmos.*
They will be discussed in the order of their importance. Without doubt, the
chocked disc has to be named first because its occurrence alone frequently permits one to make a diagnosis—not only as an ocular general sign but also as the
one most important general sign of increased intracranial pressure.

The *local signs and symptoms* will be discussed in a separate chapter. In
certain tumor localizations the ocular signs are prominent, that is, in patients
with tumors that directly involve the structures of the visual apparatus (visual
pathways, nerves and nuclei of the extrinsic muscles). In patients with tumors in
other sites the ocular local signs are of equal importance to the other neurologic
signs. Again, there are other types of tumors that cause the ocular signs to take
a somewhat subordinate place of importance in the total clinical picture. It is
just for such reasons that it will be necessary to consider the ocular local signs
and symptoms not as isolated phenomena but in their proper relation to the entire neurologic status of a given patient. Thus we want to *appeal to the ophthalmologist* to never evaluate either the ocular general or the ocular local signs and
symptoms in patients with suspected brain tumors as isolated from the total
clinical picture but to always *consider them with the entire neurologic symptomatology.*

## PAPILLEDEMA

Krayenbühl in his contribution on neurosurgery in *Lehrbuch der Chirurgie*
states: "*Among the signs of increased intracranial pressure, papilledema should
be considered the most important one.*" This statement of a well-known neurosurgeon points out the prominent position papilledema occupies as a general
sign in the diagnosis of increased intracranial pressure. The significance of this
fact for the general practitioner, for the neurologist, and in particular, for the

ophthalmologist is obvious. The recognition of increased intracranial pressure and thus of a brain tumor may depend on the familiarity of the examiner with this fundus picture. Its recognition could be of absolutely vital importance for the patient in view of the chances of successful outcome with modern neurosurgical procedures.

First, a few terms should be defined. The German term *"Stauungspapille"* indicates a *passive edema of the optic disc that is caused by increased intracranial pressure but is not associated with primary inflammatory changes and frequently not with functional disturbances.* Thus the term "Stauungspapille" is, to a large extent, identical to the English term "papilledema." The German term "Papillenödem," however, is in no way identical to the English term. It is, so to speak, a neutral expression for an edematous swelling of the disc that may be caused by stasis, inflammation, or toxic agents. In our opinion, it is a mistake to reserve the term "Stauungspapille" for the more extensive forms of swelling of the disc (Uhthoff) and to call lesser forms "Papillenödem." One should limit the term "Stauungspapille" to cases with proved or at least probable increased intracranial pressure. Minor stages of "Stauungspapille" can be simply designated as incipient "Stauungspapille." However, if there is uncertainty as to the etiology of the swelling of the disc and if, on the basis of the ophthalmoscopic findings and the clinical picture in its entirety, other etiologies (for instance, a malignant hypertensive retinopathy) must be considered, the neutral terms "Papillenödem" or "Papillenschwellung" are permitted without any compulsion to use a term implying a specific interpretation of the underlying etiologic factors. *"Papillitis"* ("optic neuritis" in the English nomenclature) indicates an *inflammatory swelling of the nerve head with functional loss.* It must be differentiated from papilledema, which it resembles quite closely from the standpoint of appearance. The terms "pseudopapilledema" and "pseudoneuritis" refer to ophthalmoscopic pictures, which will be treated in greater detail in the discussion of the differential diagnosis of papilledema.* For a functional classification of optic disc edema syndromes based on pathogenesis, Lubow suggests the following: papilledema (increased intracranial pressure); papillitis (inflammation of optic nerve head); ischemic, hypoxic, and static optic neuropathy; compression optic neuropathy; and pseudodisc edemas.

---

*This entire dissertation may be of little interest to the English-speaking reader. There is no similar ambiguity in the terms used in the English literature. Nevertheless, this paragraph has been retained in the English translation to guard the English reader in his perusal of the German literature against any misunderstanding that might arise from this inconsistency in the German terminology (Stefan Van Wien). In modern French literature (Brégeat; Bonamour, Brégeat, Bonnet, and Juge) the corresponding terms are clearly differentiated: "oedème papillaire pure" means an interstitial edema of the disc without primary affection of the nerve fibers (= papilledema, *Stauungspapille*), whereas "oedème papillaire accompagnée" refers to edema of the disc with primary affection of the nerve fibers (= papillitis, optic neuritis, ischemic papillitis, toxic and traumatic syndromes of the optic nerve) (Frederick C. Blodi).

The *presence of papilledema,* especially in bilateral form, is now considered *pathognomonic for increased intracranial pressure* provided an ocular or orbital etiology can be ruled out. A number of etiologic factors can produce such an increase in the intracranial pressure (for instance, displacement of brain substance by a tumor or a hemorrhage, increase in the volume of the cerebrospinal fluid, diffuse or circumscribed edema of the brain, or disproportion between the cranium and the volume of its contents). By far the greatest number of cases are caused by tumors of the brain (about 75% according to Uhthoff's figures), perhaps because here the etiologic factors just mentioned are frequently superimposed (volume of tumor + edema of the brain + hydrocephalus). In consideration of these facts, one may state that papilledema indicates the *presence of a brain tumor* (in the broad sense of the word) *with a very high degree of probability.* Its absence, on the other hand, does not exclude the possibility of a brain tumor. As a matter of experience, papilledema usually is not an early general sign of increased pressure, or it may even be missing in patients with slowly growing tumors (for instance, a benign meningioma) despite a marked increase of the intracranial pressure. The infratentorial tumors, especially those of the cerebellum, are known to cause a relatively early papilledema quite frequently (obviously as a result of their tendency to interfere with the circulation of the cerebrospinal fluid at an early stage), whereas supratentorial tumors cause a choked disc less frequently (if papilledema is present, it occurs in the later stages and progresses slowly).

Papilledema is much more frequently observed in children than in older persons (81% in the age group between 1 and 5 years and 43% in the age group between 60 and 70 years, according to Bonamour, Brégeat, Bonnet, and Juge and to Brégeat). The relative frequency of choked discs and the presence of extreme degrees of papilledema in children can be explained by the special character of infantile cerebral tumors (infratentorial site, early blockage of cerebrospinal fluid circulation, rapid growth) and by the soft nature of the disc tissue and its vessels. In elderly men, papilledema is rarely found or even completely absent (rarity of cerebral tumors at this age, sclerosis of disc tissue).

Although papilledema frequently does not develop simultaneously and symmetrically in both eyes, a *bilateral form is the rule.* The unilateral form (for instance, a Foster Kennedy syndrome) is rare (8% according to Bonamour's statistics). A *unilateral papilledema is usually ocular or orbital in nature,* or if this is not the case, there must be a local cause (unilateral optic atrophy, unilateral disc anomaly, unilateral glaucoma, unilateral congenital anomaly of the sheaths of the optic nerve) that prevents the increased intracranial pressure from producing swelling of the disc on the corresponding side. There will be a fuller discussion of unilateral papilledema in a separate section. Formerly, it was frequently maintained that the more advanced papilledema corresponded to the side of the tumor location (Gibbs). However, modern neurosurgical experience has taught us that certain tumors, especially those of the temporal and parietal lobes, may cause a unilateral internal hydrocephalus of the opposite side as a result of displacement of brain substance and a partial obstruction of the interventricular foramina of Monro; in other words, the more advanced papilledema in such cases corresponds to the side opposite the tumor. *Differences in the two sides regarding the rate of development as well as the appearance of the fully developed choked discs are therefore of no value for diagnosing the laterality of the tumor.*

Our statement that not every brain tumor causes papilledema needs some elaboration by examining the ratio of tumors with and without papilledema as well as the influence of the localization and type of tumor on this ratio. Our own statistical material includes 1166 patients with brain tumors: 698 (59%) showed papilledema, whereas in 468 (41%) the ophthalmoscopic findings were *negative in this respect.* In other words, *a little more than half of all patients showed a papilledema.* Compared with older statistics (Paton; Uhthoff) in which papilledema was reported in up to 80% of patients with brain tumor, our figure of 59% may appear somewhat low. However, it is in striking agreement

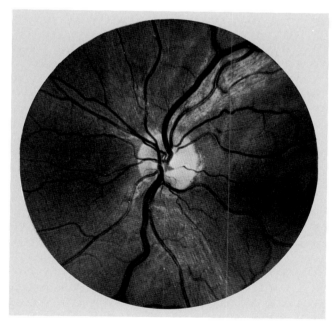

**Fig. 2-1.** Photograph of normal fundus (left eye). (Enlargement ×10.) Papilla is contrasted with surrounding eyeground as a pale red disc with sharply outlined margins except for slight blurring of the nasal border caused by larger number of nerve fibers crossing it. Level of papilla is in plane with surrounding area. Because of papillomacular bundle, temporal half of disc normally is lighter in color than nasal half. Bright red arteries and dark red veins are of normal structure and caliber. Caliber ratio of veins to arteries is 3:2. Normal diameter of disc is 1.5 to 1.7 mm.

with a newer publication by Petrohelos and Henderson, who analyzed 358 cases and reported an incidence of 59% and with a statistic of Tönnis, who, among 3000 cases of intracranial tumors, found papilledema in 60%. One may wonder what could cause such a discrepancy between the more recent and the older figures. We believe that we are justified in assuming that *these figures unmistakably reflect the progress made in the diagnosis and treatment of brain tumors during the past few decades.* In other words, thanks to our modern diagnostic methods (electroencephalography, arteriography, pneumoencephalography, ventriculography, echography, scintigraphy, computerized axial tomography, and others), we are able to make an earlier diagnosis of a brain tumor in the average case. Thus fewer patients reach the state of increased intracranial pressure showing papilledema. In a scrutiny of the total number of our own cases (Table 3) with regard to the occurrence of papilledema in patients with supratentorial and infratentorial tumors, we find confirmation of the familiar and well-established fact that there is a *distinct prevalence of choked disc in patients with infratentorial tumors (70%) as compared with those with the supratentorial type (60%).* These figures are also in close agreement with those of other authors. Petrohelos and Henderson report an incidence of 53% in patients with supratentorial tumors and 75% in those with infratentorial tumors. *Bilateral papilledema occurred in practically all our patients.*

Apart from the localization of the tumor, the presence of a papilledema also depends on the type and particularly the rate of growth of the tumor. Papilledema is seen in 50% of our patients with rapidly growing and malignant glioblastomas. In patients with the rather slowly progressing and benign group of astrocytomas and meningiomas, there is an incidence of 65%. The figure in patients with cerebral metastases is 61%. Even though these numerical differences are not very large or significant, there seems to be a slightly greater tendency for the development of papilledema in patients with slowly progressing tumors than in those with the rapidly expanding malignant forms. There are cases of increased intracranial pressure in which papilledema is absent. This occurs commonly in congenital hydrocephalus, in which the patient develops optic atrophy instead. When the disc is atrophic from any cause, papilledema does not develop. For further details, see Table 3.

**Ophthalmoscopic appearance of papilledema**

The clinical picture of *fully developed papilledema* (Figs. 2-2 and 2-3) is relatively distinct and can be summarized as follows:
1. Increase of the disc diameter
2. Nasal, temporal, upper and lower pole indistinctness and blurring of the disc margins
3. Elevation of the disc and mushrooming of the nerve head into the vitreous ("doughnut" or "champagne cork" shape)
4. Reddish discoloration of the disc (capillary stasis), later visible network of dilated capillaries all over the nerve head

**Table 3.** Manifestation and frequency of papilledema in 1166 patients with brain tumor*

| Location / Papilledema | Glioblastomas + | Glioblastomas − | Astrocytomas and astroblastomas + | Astrocytomas and astroblastomas − | Meningiomas + | Meningiomas − | Metastases + | Metastases − | Medulloblastomas + | Medulloblastomas − | Hemangiomas + | Hemangiomas − | Craniopharyngiomas + | Craniopharyngiomas − | Others + | Others − | Totals + | Totals − |
|---|---|---|---|---|---|---|---|---|---|---|---|---|---|---|---|---|---|---|
| Frontal | 60 | 50 | 37 | 25 | 38 | 16 | 14 | 11 | 2 | 0 | 0 | 1 | — | — | 18 | 16 | 169 | 119 |
| Temporal | 23 | 23 | 22 | 6 | 14 | 2 | 8 | 4 | 1 | 0 | 1 | 1 | — | — | 13 | 6 | 82 | 42 |
| Parietal | 4 | 12 | 4 | 6 | 7 | 6 | 2 | 4 | 1 | 0 | 0 | 1 | — | — | 5 | 7 | 23 | 36 |
| Occipital | 19 | 13 | 11 | 2 | 1 | 2 | 10 | 3 | — | — | 0 | 1 | — | — | 6 | 2 | 47 | 23 |
| Sagittal, parasagittal | — | — | — | — | 15 | 9 | — | — | — | — | — | — | — | — | — | — | 15 | 9 |
| Third ventricle | 3 | 0 | 2 | 0 | — | — | 3 | 0 | 2 | 0 | — | — | 11 | 2 | 7 | 2 | 28 | 4 |
| Fourth ventricle | 4 | 1 | 12 | 0 | — | — | — | — | 7 | 0 | — | — | — | — | 6 | 0 | 29 | 1 |
| Base of brain | — | — | — | — | — | — | 1 | 1 | — | — | — | — | — | — | 5 | 2 | 6 | 3 |
| Lateral ventricle | 0 | 2 | — | — | 1 | 0 | — | — | — | — | — | — | — | — | 0 | 2 | 1 | 4 |
| Cerebellum | 0 | 6 | 24 | 6 | 6 | 4 | 10 | 4 | 15 | 8 | 11 | 9 | — | — | 9 | 5 | 75 | 42 |
| Cerebellopontine angle | 4 | 2 | 2 | 0 | 2 | 3 | 1 | 0 | 3 | 0 | 4 | 2 | — | — | 0 | 3 | 16 | 10 |
| Not localized | 60 | 62 | 40 | 33 | 26 | 19 | 19 | 16 | 11 | 1 | 5 | 3 | 11 | 2 | 46 | 41 | 207 | 175 |
| Totals | 177 50% | 171 | 154 66% | 78 | 110 64% | 61 | 68 61% | 43 | 42 | 9 | 21 | 18 | 11 | 2 | 115 | 86 | 698 59% | 468 41% |

*Of the total 1166 patients with brain tumors, 698 (59%) had papilledema and 468 (41%) did not have papilledema.

5. Venous congestion and tortuosity of the veins, with relatively normal arteries (increase of ratio in caliber of veins and arteries)
6. Deflection of the vessels over the disc margin
7. Hemorrhages at the disc margin and within the disc
8. White "exudates" over the surface and at the margin of the disc
9. No primary disturbances of the sensory functions

Anyone who has seen fully developed papilledema a few times should thereafter recognize its ophthalmoscopic picture without difficulty. The reddish discoloration of the disc that abolishes the contrast with the surrounding retina may render its recognition quite difficult, especially in ophthalmoscopy through a small pupil. However, the retinal vessels converging toward the disc will assist the examiner in finding the optic nerve head.

Fully developed papilledema is truly indicative of an increase in the intra-

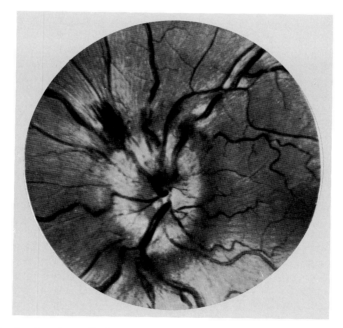

**Fig. 2-2.** Fully developed papilledema (left eye) in 20-year-old patient with hemangioma of right tonsil and hemisphere of cerebellum. Enormous enlargement of diameter of disc, in areas up to twice normal diameter. Blurring of nasal and temporal disc margins. Mushroom-like swelling and prominence of about 2.5 diopters of nerve head. Loosening and veiling of texture of disc, with capillary congestion. Preservation of vascular funnel. Congestion, dilation, and tortuosity of retinal veins, with ratio of veins to arteries of 4:2 to 5:2. Deflection of vessels at disc margin, with partial concealment of vessels by edema of papilla. Peripapillary retinal edema with markedly increased display of nerve fiber pattern. "Flame-shaped" radial hemorrhages in the nerve fiber layer at 11 o'clock position of disc margin. Intraocular arterial pressure, O.U. 40 grams diastolic (Bailliart). Visual fields, except for enlarged spot on both sides, normal. Visual acuity, O.U. 1.0, distance and near.

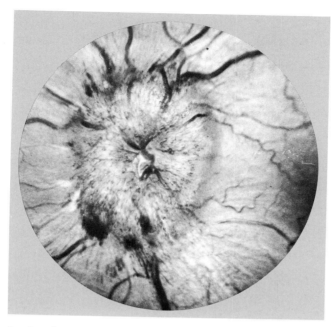

**Fig. 2-3.** Fully developed papilledema in 46-year-old patient with hemangioma of cerebellum. "Champagne cork" protrusion of enlarged edematous papilla (prominence of about 3 diopters), intensive congestion of venules and capillaries, obscuration of major vessels, nerve fiber layer hemorrhages at upper and lower margins of disc, and two white "exudates" within retina at nasal border. Visual acuity, O.U. 1.0, distance and near.

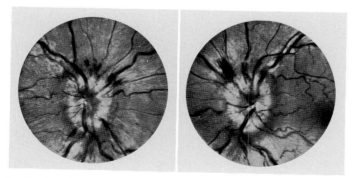

**Fig. 2-4.** Fully developed papilledema in patient with hemangioma of right tonsil and hemisphere of cerebellum (same patient as in Fig. 2-2). (Enlargement ×6.) Left illustration corresponds to right eye and right illustration to left eye.

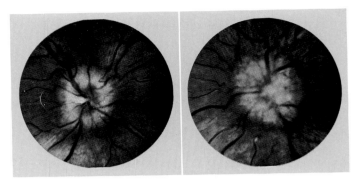

**Fig. 2-5.** Advanced stage of bilateral papilledema in 27-year-old patient with neurinoma of choroidal plexus in area of left lateral ventricle. Papillae show mushroomlike prominence of approximately 3 diopters. Conspicuous edematous veiling of tissues of disc with complete filling of left cup. Slight radial folding of retina near disc, especially toward left fovea. Visual acuity, O.U. 1.0. Both visual fields intact. Left illustration corresponds to right eye and right illustration to left eye.

cranial pressure. The force of this pressure has caused the "mushrooming" of the nerve head into the vitreous, drawing the tortuous and dilated veins with it—a picture that could be called the *grotesque other extreme of increased intraocular pressure,* that is, *a glaucoma, with its excavation of the disc into the opposite direction,* in other words, an "inverse glaucoma." Despite the round shape of the disc, which is usually retained, the disc *diameter* is usually more or less *increased* in papilledema. This enlargement is caused by the swelling of the nerve head itself and the spreading of the edema into the surrounding retina. The functional equivalent of this extension of the disc with a consecutive *lateral displacement of the adjacent retina* (which can occasionally be seen ophthalmoscopically as *concentric peripapillary* curvilinear reflexes) is an enlargement of the blind spot, which will be discussed subsequently (Fig. 2-10).

A parallel development of the enlargement is an indistinctness and *blurring of the disc margins* caused by the edema, which, especially in the early stages, may be less pronounced on the temporal side than on the nasal side, but most noticeable at the upper and lower poles. This diffuse indistinctness of the disc margin, however, is caused not only by the edema, but also by scattering of the light reflexes by the edematous tissues of the nerve head and the surrounding retina. This edema also changes the aspect of the nerve fiber bundle pattern. Even with normal light, but more so with red-free light (especially with magnified red-free photography according to the method of Hoyt), the pattern of the peripapillary *nerve fibers* appears erased, with disappearance of all surface details from the nerve fiber layer and with a deep red and lusterless retina around the disc. This is in distinct contrast to the normal peripapillary retina with the fine, radially oriented striations from the surface of the nerve fiber layer and the glistening reflexes on the vessels. The serous infiltration of the disc, however, is not limited to the margin, but involves the disc in its entirety. The central funnel is usually filled, and a previously existing physiologic cup has been completely smoothed out and can no longer be recognized. As a result of the serous infiltration, the *entire tissue of the disc is loosened,* less compact than under normal conditions, and of a *finely striated* or *reticular structure,* which is in distinct contrast to the rather uniform and smooth appearance of the normal optic papilla (Fig. 2-1).

The *mushroomlike prominence of the choked disc* is one of its most conspicuous signs. In the end stage of this development the prominence usually is approximately equal on the nasal and temporal sides. In the incipient stages a difference is possible, with the upper, lower, and nasal margins progressing more rapidly and more strikingly than the temporal rim. Even with the monocular ophthalmoscope, the elevation of the papilledema is obvious at once, provided this elevation is of a fairly marked degree. Naturally, the stereoscopic picture obtained with a binocular ophthalmoscope makes this situation even more conspicuous; thus this instrument is a favorite in the early diagnosis of a beginning prominence. One point that should aid in recognizing an early mushrooming is the *deflection of the vessels at the disc margin* that, so to speak, underscores and accentuates this particular contour.

The difference in the planes of the retina and of the nerve head in which the retinal vessels course leads to the phenomenon of the *parallax;* its magnitude can be used to express the degree of prominence of the papilla.

In order to determine the parallax the examiner has to move his head, together with the ophthalmoscope, a little up and down as well as to the right and to the left without, of course, losing sight of the fundus. He should compare the behavior of one and the same vessel first in the plane of the nerve head and then in the plane of the retina. The section of the vessel that is closer (that is, on the disc) will seem to move in a direction opposite to the movement of the head of the examiner, whereas the more distant section will move in the same direction. The more pronounced this relative movement of the two sections of the vessel is, the greater should be the prominence of the disc (Fig. 2-6).

The *prominence of the disc* can be quantitatively measured with the ophthalmoscope. Although this is a relatively crude method, it is quite adequate for our clinical needs provided it is performed properly.

*The prominence is measured in diopters* because the lenses in the Recoss disc of the ophthalmoscope are used with this method. For a more conventional expression of this magnitude, it should be mentioned that *3 diopters correspond approximately to 1 mm of prominence.* The elevation of the disc is determined in the following manner: the ophthalmoscope is first focused on the most prominent vessel on the nerve head, and the strongest plus or weakest minus lens giving a clear picture of this vessel is noted. It should be understood that the examiner must be emmetropic or wear a correction. The next step is to select a vessel, parallel to the first observed vessel, near the disc margin in the retinal plane and again to find the strongest plus or weakest minus lens allowing a clear image of this vessel. The difference in the strength of these two lenses expresses the prominence of the disc in diopters. This can be easily converted into millimeters.

A more exact method for the determination of the prominence of the disc has been described by Heinz. He retinoscopes the fundus, beginning at a point temporal to the macula,

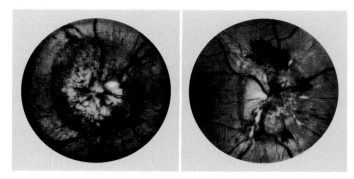

**Fig. 2-6.** Advanced bilateral papilledema in 52-year-old patient with meningioma of left sphenoid ridge. Enormous enlargement of disc diameter, especially on right side (up to three times normal size). Pronounced venous congestion with intense congestive hyperemia of fine vessels of disc and conspicuous capillary loops at summit of discs (especially right one). Numerous streaklike and punctate hemorrhages on and near disc. Retinal arteries obscured by edematous tissues of disc. White and grayish white dots (cytoid bodies) on discs and disc margins. Distinct parallax between vessels in plane of retina and those on disc. Visual acuity, O.D. 1.0; O.S. 0.6. Left illustration corresponds to right eye and right illustration to left eye.

and using successive points, he progresses over the disc into the nasal part of the horizontal meridian. In this manner, he obtains a sort of profile of the papilla and the surrounding parts of the retina. He uses the Maddox cross for fixation and progresses from degree to degree in the horizontal or vertical meridian.

The *prominence of the choked disc* parallels the progress of its development. Prominence and enlargement of the papilla, however, need not always be parallel. The prominence may reach values as high as 8 or 9 diopters. Based mostly on our material, the *average is between 2 and 4 diopters.* There are a number of references in the literature (Uhthoff; Kestenbaum; and others) to the effect that the diagnosis of a papilledema less than 2 diopters in prominence is quite difficult and unreliable. According to our own experience, we cannot agree with such an opinion, but would rather lower this value to about 1 diopter of prominence before it actually becomes difficult to decide whether or not there is a choked disc. In our opinion, a prominence of more than 1 diopter can be definitely interpreted as favoring a diagnosis of papilledema if other symptoms are taken into consideration. In reviewing our cases of brain tumors, we were able to observe a fairly close correspondence between the increase in the intracranial pressure found on the operating table (tension of the dura, force of escape of the cerebrospinal fluid after ventricle puncture) and the degree of prominence of the disc. In the absence of increased intracranial pressure, there was no choked disc. If the pressure was high, we usually found a choked disc. (Supposedly there were no preexisting alterations of the optic nerve that made the swelling of the nerve head impossible, for example, optic atrophy.) *Regression* of the papilledema and of the elevation of the disc usually occurs either after successful neurosurgical intervention (Fig. 2-7) or together with the onset

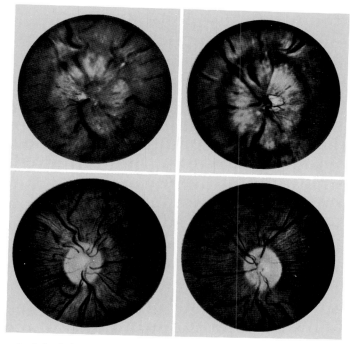

**Fig. 2-7.** Bilateral choked discs showing all characteristic signs of advanced stage in 33-year-old patient with astrocytoma of left temporal lobe. Lower photographs taken 7 months after extirpation of tumor. They demonstrate capacity of edema of disc to regress almost completely. Only slight atrophy of discs and circumpapillary radial folding of retina, evidenced by reflex lines, are visible. Left illustrations correspond to right eye and right illustrations to left eye.

of a secondary optic atrophy (p. 123). Spontaneous regression can be observed in cases of serous meningitis, pseudotumoral encephalitis, or pseudotumor cerebri. Sometimes resolution of the papilledema seems incomplete. This is the result of a more or less pronounced proliferation of glial tissue that may obscure the disc margins and thus sometimes give the "postpapilledema" optic atrophy a special aspect. A *recurrence* of the elevation and of the swelling of the disc is possible if there is a recurrence of the increase of the intracranial pressure. However, this recurrence cannot occur if the nerve fibers have degenerated and glial cicatricial tissue has invaded the papilla.

The *reddish discoloration of the disc* is a result of *venous congestion* extending into the smallest capillaries and rendering them frequently visible as an arborizing network of very small telangiectatic vessels in the edematous tissue of the disc (Fig. 2-3). This hyperemia of the disc is also an important early sign and one that is conspicuous by its absence in other conditions that might be mistaken for papilledema. As a result of this reddish discoloration, the color of the disc is almost identical with that of the surrounding retina. This factor, together with the blurring of the disc margins, makes it even more difficult to differentiate the disc from the remaining fundus. The direction of the large vessels converging toward the disc will always make it possible to identify the latter. Whereas the arteries maintain their normal caliber or actually become somewhat attenuated, the *retinal veins show a characteristic engorgement in the case of a choked disc, which can be recognized as a broadening of their lumens* (the ratio of veins to arteries, which is normally 3:2, increases to 4:2 or even 5:2) and a distinctive *increased tortuosity.* The deflection of the vessels at the disc margin caused by the prominence of the papilla has already been mentioned. The sloping or almost vertical direction of the vessels at the neck of the papilla usually causes them to lose their wall reflex in this area. They may actually become invisible if they are buried in the edematous tissues of the disc. In such cases, they seem to be interrupted in their course (Fig. 2-3).

A direct result of the venous and capillary congestion is the occurrence of *hemorrhages* (either on the disc itself or in its immediate surrounding area) near the large branches of the retinal veins. If the hemorrhages are in the nerve fiber layer, they are flame shaped, have a radial arrangement, and occupy the outer slopes of the edematous nerve head (Fig. 2-4). Occasionally they are in the outer nuclear layer of the retina, in which case they appear punctate. Sometimes these may also be subhyaloid hemorrhages extending into the vitreous. Only rarely are the hemorrhages far from the disc. This is an important point against the diagnosis of a central retinal vein thrombosis, in which the hemorrhages reach far out into the periphery. Hemorrhages do not occur with any great regularity in papilledema. They may appear as an important early sign (for instance, in a rapidly developing choked disc, Fig. 2-12), or they may be missing completely, even in some advanced stages. It should be emphasized that the *presence of hemorrhages on the disc itself or in the area surrounding it is not absolutely pathognomonic for papilledema.* Similar hemorrhages are seen, for instance, in an inflammatory papillitis (Fig. 2-26).

The soft, *white patches* seen occasionally on the disc or at its margin, especially in the later stages, are definitely not exudates. They consist of varicosities and so-called cytoid bodies resulting from terminal nerve fiber swellings of Cajal, identical with those of "cotton-wool exudates" in the retina. Some of the white or grayish white spots in the retina surrounding the disc are remnants of absorbed hemorrhages. In reviewing our material, we found hemorrhages and white dots on the disc in patients with tumors of the occipital lobe (Fig. 3-28) and the cerebellum with striking frequency.

If the edema increases in intensity, it may extend into the adjacent retina to reach the macular area. There is a turbid milky appearance of the retina with blurring or loss of all light reflexes from the surface of the nerve fiber layer and blood vessels, especially well visualized in the red-free light (Hoyt). *As a result of the edema,* droplets of fluid occasionally accumulate underneath the internal limiting membrane between the *disc* and the *macula* and become visible as *minute brilliant white dots in a radial arrangement* and assume the *shape of a fan*. This picture contrasts with the macular fan seen in malignant hypertensive retinopathy, which is composed of lipids and lipid-laden macrophages. Such a fan-shaped macular structure may recede completely with the resolution of the papilledema (Fig. 2-8), and the related impairment of central vision disappears.

In the *fluorescein angiogram* of the fundus the papilledema shows characteristic signs (Fig. 2-9). The first one occurs during the arterial and the early venous phase. During this phase a net of dilated, tortuous capillaries is visible on the disc. They come from the depth of the physiologic cup and show great irregularities of caliber and occasionally aneurysmatic dilatations. The margins between the vascular net on the elevated disc and the surrounding retina seem to be remarkably sharp. The second sign is a diffuse fluorescence of the entire

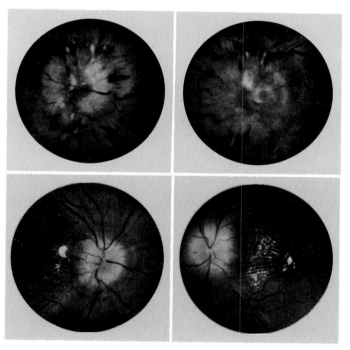

**Fig. 2-8.** Chronic atrophic papilledema with beginning star figure in fovea in 26-year-old patient with astroblastoma of frontal lobe. Above, Already transition to atrophy of papilledema measuring 4 diopters before surgical intervention. Below, Fundus after craniotomy (7 weeks later). Edema of papilla is considerably less distinct. Prominence is only 1.5 diopters. There is conspicuous pallor, a sign of atrophy. Right fundus shows incomplete and left fundus shows almost complete macular star consisting of brilliant white dots in radial arrangement. Suggestion of these changes can already be recognized in preoperative stage. Left visual field shows marked nasal constriction. Left illustrations correspond to right eye and right illustrations to left eye.

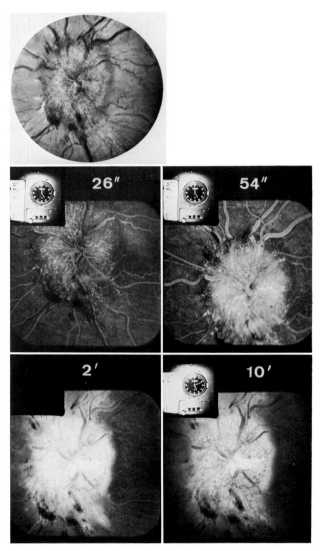

**Fig. 2-9.** Fluorescein angiogram of fully developed papilledema in 46-year-old patient with hemangioma of cerebellum (same patient as in Fig. 2-3). Typical for arterial and early venous phase (26 seconds) in papilledema is net of dilated congested capillary vessels with irregularities of caliber and sometimes microaneurysms. Fluorescence of disc increases gradually to reach maximum in late venous phase of angiogram (2 and 10 minutes), at which time capillary stasis on fluorescent background of disc is distinctly visible. Diffuse staining of papilla, limited to disc and its immediate surroundings, may last for several hours and reflects uptake of dye by edema itself.

edematous disc tissue. This begins in the late venous phase and may last several hours; it is also generally well demarcated and confined to the disc itself. (Sometimes the abnormal fluorescence of the disc fades away into the adjacent retina with extensions along the retinal vessels.) In other types of elevation and edema of the disc, such as papillitis, pseudopapilledema, and drusen (p. 150), the fluorescein angiogram looks entirely different.

In this connection the *angiogram of a normal disc* should be mentioned. The optic nerve head has a weak bluish green autofluorescence. Immediately after the dye reaches the ocular fundus, the disc begins to fluoresce. This occurs a fraction of a second before the retinal vessels are filled and is caused by the circulation of the dye in the opticociliary capillary net deriving from Zinn's anastomoses, respectively from the posterior ciliary arteries. A little later the capillary branches of the central retinal artery are filled, together with the main artery. The disc is overlaid by a net of fine fluorescing vessels densely covering the nerve head. For this reason the expected optic illusion that usually occurs in areas of autofluorescence does not appear. This illusion appears a little later, approximately 5 seconds later, when the dye has disappeared from the ciliary capillary network. The background of the disc now appears dark. The fluorescing capillary branches of the central retinal artery are still yellowish green and contrast vividly with the dark, nearly black, background. This darkness remains for 30 seconds. With decreasing fluorescence of the entire fundus, in the late stages the disc regains its original autofluorescence (Fig. 1-31).

## Symptomatology

The *symptoms* in fully developed papilledema usually are insignificant. Despite a considerable prominence, even one of long standing, visual acuity and visual fields may be completely intact. *This very preservation of the visual functions is characteristic of the papilledema* and may become quite important in the differentiation of choked disc from similar ophthalmoscopic pictures. However, we should be aware that patients with severe papilledemas occasionally have subjective symptoms that will bring them to the ophthalmologist, such as fleeting "attacks" of obscuration lasting only seconds or minutes, blurred vision, or even transient amaurosis, so-called *amblyopic attacks.*

An intelligent patient who had an acoustic neurinoma with bilateral papilledema of about 2.5 diopters described his attack as follows: Especially at night under artificial light, there was a more or less dense but always transparent fog that started at times from the right side, at other times from the left side, but always from the side. There was no headache or any other discomfort. The sensation of this fog lasted from 3 to 5 seconds. No obvious cause (such as, for instance, some strain) could be observed to provoke an attack. Rather the sensation of the fog occurred during a period of quiescence. For a few days, four or five times daily, a peculiar luminous ring was seen in the upper left field and lasted 20 to 30 seconds.

If one searches for these amblyopic attacks in a large series of patients with papilledema—they occur in about one-fourth of all patients with brain tumor (Ethelberg and Jensen)—one will be able to differentiate *three degrees of intensity of these obscurations:*

1. Sudden appearance of blurred vision as if a heavy fog, smoke, or a veil obscured the surroundings. There is a simultaneous impairment of color sensation.

2. Sudden appearance of a bluish or bluish green cloud; daylight changes to twilight, or the patient has the sensation of a momentary night blindness. There is a striking shift of color sensation toward blue-green.

3. Sudden appearance of complete darkness or actual blindness.

The average duration of such obscurations and amblyopic attacks is spectacularly short and lasts, as a rule, not more than 30 seconds—mostly a few seconds up to 10 seconds. Attacks lasting for minutes are quite rare. This observation is important for the differential diagnosis of migraine, with its obscurations lasting much longer (that is, minutes, a quarter of an hour, or more). Another characteristic sign is the complete restoration of the visual function after the obscuration. This occurs just as abruptly as the onset of the attack itself. In the majority of patients the obscuration involves the entire visual field uniformly. Occasionally, it is limited to a central scotoma or to one half of the field, similar to a homonymous hemianopia. Attacks may occur simultaneously in both eyes or may alternate between them. At times, patients report peculiar uncharacteristic and *unformed photopsias,* which they describe as flashes, sparks, stars, lightning, or luminous spheres or rings and which occur during, before, or after the amblyopic attacks (occasionally even independent of such attacks). The patient who described his attacks as quoted previously also had photopsias. If one probes the conditions that are likely to trigger these obscurations, one frequently may find that they are prone to occur when the patient arises (a change from the horizontal to the vertical position of the body) or when the head is turned abruptly. They may also occur after bodily exertion. *Occasionally the onset of the amblyopic attacks is accompanied by a fit of violent headache,* or an already existing headache may become more intense. There seems to be a direct relationship between the frequency of the attacks and the state of development of the papilledema (Ethelberg and Jensen), respectively, the severity of increased intracranial pressure.

The pathogenesis of these obscurations and amblyopic attacks is still quite controversial. A number of theories have been proposed, such as cortical origin as an equivalent to epileptic amaurosis, sudden pressure of the dilated third ventricle on the chiasm (Leber; Paton; Holmes), transient spasms of the retinal arteries, or compression of the optic nerves in the optic canals (Behr). Ethelberg and Jensen relate the amblyopic attacks (which they have seen frequently in association with changes of the muscular tone, that is, hypertonia and hypotonia, or an impaired sensorium, ranging from numbness to coma) to a transient strangulation of the mesial part of the temporal lobe in the tentorial notch (transtentorial herniation), which causes a temporary vascular disturbance as the result of the compression of the posterior cerebral arteries, or rather their branches, especially the calcarine artery, supplying the visual cortex.

*The amblyopic attacks, just like the papilledema itself, occur relatively late in the course of a brain tumor.* With tumors in silent zones of the brain, they may be the first symptom that brings the patient to the physician. Considering the typical and unmistakable ophthalmoscopic picture of papilledema, the diagnosis of amblyoptic attacks, as a rule, causes no great difficulty. *Migrainelike ob-*

*scurations* last from several minutes to quarter hours and are often accompanied by typical scintillating scotomas. Unilateral blackouts from carotid insufficiency are different and last a few minutes. The fogginess of *acute and subacute angle-closure glaucoma* lasts longer. The sensation of rainbow colors (a result of the edema of the corneal epithelium!) as well as an increased intraocular pressure, eventually a glaucomatous excavation of the disc, and visual field changes (starting with sector-shaped nasal defects) usually help in confirming such a diagnosis. The situation becomes somewhat more complicated if the *obscurations occur as the premonitory signs of impending epileptic attacks.* The latter may be the well-known accompanying signs of a growing brain tumor, but yet there may be a different etiology, such as a cicatricial or an idiopathic epilepsy. Careful ophthalmoscopic examinations in such cases should also aid in differentiating amblyopic attacks associated with increased intracranial pressure and papilledema from other types.

*Despite the occasional occurrence of obscurations, the visual acuity and peripheral fields in a patient with papilledema remain intact for a long time.* The patient is not conscious of the *concentric enlargement of the blind spot* caused by the edematous enlargement of the disc and the resulting lateral displacement and compression of the adjacent retina (Fig. 2-10). The normal blind spot lies in an area between 13 and 18.5 degrees temporal to the point of fixation. Its medium width in emmetropes is 5.5 degrees and its height 7.5 degrees, with a 5 or 10 mm target used on the tangent screen at a distance of 2 meters. According to Chamlin and Davidoff, an additional relative blind zone of 1 degree surrounding the blind spot can be demonstrated with smaller targets (for instance, a 2 mm object at the same distance of 2 meters). This zone corresponds to retinal elements of lesser sensitivity. Thus it can be stated that the *normal blind spot tested with a 2 mm white target at a distance of 2000 mm has a width of 7.5 degrees and a height of 9.5 degrees on the tangent screen.* An increase of these figures, if it amounts to 1 degree or more, has to be considered

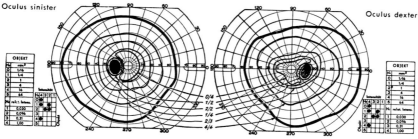

**Fig. 2-10.** Visual field changes (Goldmann perimeter) in bilateral papilledema: (1) marked enlargement of blind spot (up to three times normal size) and (2) disturbance of law of summation of isopters surrounding blind spot. The 2/2 isopters with larger sized targets include Mariotte's spot, whereas the 0/4 isopters with smaller targets bare it. (After Dubois-Poulsen.)

as enlargement of the blind spot. Enlargement in the horizontal direction is more important because the mapping of the upper and lower poles is rendered somewhat unreliable by angioscotomas. The enlargement is generally as much as three to four times, although enlargement of as much as eight times can be observed. These figures naturally apply only if there are no circumpapillary or parapapillary changes such as a scleral crescent, peripapillar choroidal atrophy, or medullated nerve fibers. We agree with numerous other authors that *in practically every case of papilledema there is an enlargement of the blind spot.* This empiric fact is easily explained by the pathologic-anatomic findings. There is such a striking correlation between the enlargement of the blind spot and the extent of the papilledema that some authors prefer the size of the blind spot as a criterion of the status of the edema to its prominence as determined using the ophthalmoscope (Davis; Chamlin and Davidoff).

A further perimetric symptom of papilledema may be seen in the relatively *smooth slopes of the borders of the blind spot,* which contrast with the abrupt limits of the normal disc. Dubois-Poulsen and Brégeat rightly call attention to a *sign typical for papilledema* that can be determined on the Goldmann perimeter. This sign indicates an *anomaly of the law of summation of the isopter surrounding the blind spot* (photometric disharmony); the shape of some isopters determined by targets with the same additive qualities do not correspond any longer. In other words, isopters that should coincide recede from each other in such a manner that the isopters for the larger targets surround the blind spot, whereas those for the smaller ones bare it and are situated centrally to it (Fig. 2-10). However, this phenomenon is only the result of the edema of the nerve head and thus not absolutely pathognomonic for papilledema caused by increased intracranial pressure. For this reason, we believe we cannot agree with Dubois-Poulsen and consider this sign as an early indication of a choked disc. Also, we can hardly agree with the opinion expressed by some researchers (de Schweinitz; Chamlin and Davidoff; Brégeat) that an enlargement of the blind spot can be demonstrated before the choked disc manifests itself ophthalmoscopically. *On the basis of our personal experience, we believe it is neither possible nor reliable to depend solely on the size of the blind spot for the early diagnosis of a papilledema.* There is some justification in using an enlargement of the blind spot for such purpose if combined with other early signs; it should never serve as the basis for a diagnosis if it is the only sign. In our opinion, the real importance of an enlarged blind spot lies in the fact that it permits us to differentiate papilledema from conditions with a similar ophthalmoscopic appearance (p. 131). If the edema of the nerve head expands toward the macula, the enlargement of the blind spot will extend toward the point of fixation. A macular edema will produce metamorphopsia and a *relative central scotoma* with a slightly reduced central visual acuity. According to Traquair, such a scotoma shows a relative blue-blindness, which he considers characteristic for a disturbance of the outer retinal layers. In the even more severe and advanced stages of papilledema the enlarged blind spot and the central scotoma may merge to form a relative cecocentral scotoma. Edema of the nerve head extending into the macular region generally causes only a minor loss of central vision —an important criterion in favor of papilledema. A more extensive impairment of the visual acuity (possibly in combination with small or even large absolute scotomas) is caused by secondary changes in the macula, such as hemorrhages, horizontal ridging of the retina, or the fan-shaped accumulations of white retinal dots in the macular region described previously.

The *perimetric syndrome of papilledema,* characterized by enlargement of the blind spot, smooth slopes of its borders, and an anomaly of the law of summation of the isopters surrounding it, can be easily demonstrated by photopic and scotopic perimetry and campimetry. Scotopic perimetry and campimetry show proportionally more pronounced pericecal defects around the blind spot than photopic methods. In the fully developed stage (without any signs of atrophy) the papilledema manifests normal electrophysiologic signs (ERG, objective and subjective frequency of fusion, occipital evoked response in the EEG, retinocortical time).

### Incipient papilledema

Although fully developed papilledema should not offer any diagnostic problems, its early stages may present a much more delicate and complex situation. Yet it is in these early stages that we as ophthalmologists are called in consultation by the neurologist and the neurosurgeon to make such a weighty and grave decision. Occasionally, it depends on this very decision whether or not the patient will be subjected to all the diagnostic procedures of modern neurosurgery and neuroradiology, procedures that are not only disagreeable to the patient but are potentially dangerous, even with all possible precautions.

Indeed, early papilledema (Fig. 2-11) is frequently mistaken for similar conditions with the same ophthalmoscopic picture, but with a different etiology and significance. Which are the more or less reliable signs of incipient papilledema? In agreement with numerous authors, we believe they are as follows: *hyperemia and redness of the papilla* (caused by dilation of the capillaries within the tissue of the optic disc), together with *blurring of its margins* at the superior and inferior poles, later on the nasal side and finally on the temporal side; a slight *elevation* of the papillary margin with a corresponding deflection of the vessels at first on the nasal side and then on the temporal side; and *widening of the veins and increased visibility of the capillaries of the disc* (Fig. 2-12). Venous distention is a sign of incipient papilledema, but is significant only if accompanied by progressing hyperemia and blurring of the disc margins. The early stages of papilledema are characterized by minimal prominence of the disc margins. More pronounced or even measurable elevation of the optic disc is not an early sign of papilledema. (Elevation of the disc may also be congenital and absolutely unrelated to increased intracranial pressure!) In the pres-

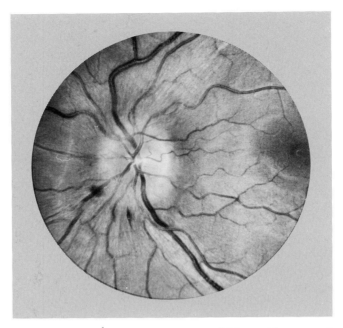

**Fig. 2-11.** Incipient papilledema of left eye in 9-year-old boy with tumor of posterior fossa. Slight enlargement of diameter of disc. Blurring of entire disc margin. Beginning flat prominence of papillary margin (about 0.5 diopter) with slight deflection of retinal vessels. Preserved vessel cup. Moderate dilation and tortuosity of retinal veins. Discrete peripapillary edema with two splinter hemorrhages in nerve fiber layer. Visual acuity, O.U. 1.0. Diastolic pressure of arteries, 40 to 50 gm (Bailliart).

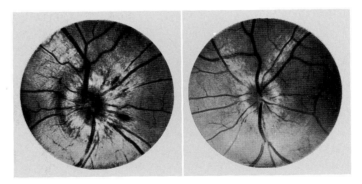

**Fig. 2-12.** Incipient papilledema in 35-year-old patient with meningioma in area of right temporal region. There is a distinct difference between the two eyes in development of choking. Right papilledema is already fully developed and shows pronounced venous congestion and hemorrhages at nasal disc margin. Left disc shows discrete bulging of about 0.5 diopter of its margin, with slight deflection of vessels, blurring of entire disc margin, and slight venous congestion—all signs of incipient papilledema. Visual acuity, O.U. 1.0. Diastolic pressure of arteries, O.U. 50 gm (Bailliart). Left illustration corresponds to right eye and right illustration to left eye.

ence of disc hyperemia and disc blurring, *small hemorrhages* in the nerve fiber layer at the border of the disc represent, especially if they multiply in serial examinations, a definite and reliable sign of incipient papilledema. In this connection, even a single splinter bleeding may be significant.

Other authors also mention filling of the physiologic cup and grayish sheathing of the vessels in the funnel of the disc (widening of the perivascular lymph spaces) as important early symptoms. In other words, we have all the characteristic signs that have already been mentioned in the description of the fully developed choked disc here in an attenuated form. The correct diagnosis is rendered more difficult because these signs in the early stages do not involve the entire nerve head, but are frequently confined to only part of it, especially the nasal part. Even the experienced ophthalmologist will hesitate to consider these early signs of absolute and unequivocal evidence, because they may occur in a very similar form (either singly or in combination) in various physiologic (for example, hyperopia with pseudoneuritis and congenital tortuosity of the retinal vessels) and pathologic (for example, incipient hypertensive malignant retinopathy, papillitis) conditions (p. 131). It is absolutely essential to caution against a rash evaluation of these signs!

For further evaluation of early papilledema the *examination of the optic disc with the slit lamp using the contact glass* may furnish important data. In this connection, Goldmann mentions two important symptoms of incipient papilledema: hyperrefringency of the papillary border and elevation of the prepapillary internal limiting membrane. A further biomicroscopic sign is the enlargement of the perivascular lymphatic spaces.

There is no doubt that *fluorescein angiography of the fundus* can contribute to the early diagnosis of papilledema. In favor of such a diagnosis are a rapid diffuse coloration of the disc tissue and the increased visibility of dilated capillary vessels (p. 107). Especially important in this connection is the exact timing of the observed phenomena, which is different from other pathologic conditions of the disc.

*Magnified red-free photography* in early papilledema reveals a deep red and lusterless peripapillary retina with blurring or loss of all light reflexes from the surface of the nerve fiber layer and blood vessels. This aspect differs completely from the normal peripapillary retina (and also from the retina in eyes with congenitally blurred disc margins!) with the normal striated nerve fiber bundle patterns, the glistening reflexes on the vessels, and the scattered point highlights (Gunn's dots). According to Hoyt, red-free ophthalmoscopy and photography permits accurate clinical differentiation between incipient papilledema and pseudopapilledema-like congenital disc blurring (Fig. 2-13).

In the opinion of some authors (de Schweinitz; Chamlin and Davidoff; Dubois-Poulsen; Brégeat), the enlargement of the blind spot (p. 112) is considered a reliable early sign that may even precede the ophthalmoscopic manifestation of swelling of the papilla. We tend to follow Traquair and cannot agree

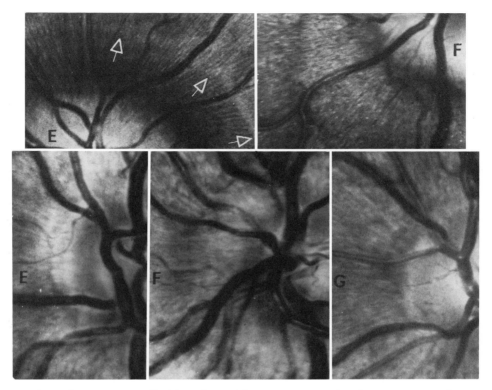

**Fig. 2-13.** Above, *Congenitally blurred optic disc margins* with fine linear striations of nerve fiber bundles approaching disc margins, superficial retinal reflexes such as Weiss' line (open arrows in **E**) and Gunn's dots (**F**), and distinct light reflexes from surface of arterial and venous vessels. Below, *Incipient papilledema* with blurring of disc margins, loss of all light reflexes from surface of nerve fiber layer and blood vessels, and no Weiss' line or Gunn's dots. All fine striations are obliterated; most major vessels without light reflexes appear dark and dull. (From Hoyt, W. F., and Knight, C. L.: Invest. Ophthalmol. **12:**241-247, 1973.)

with this opinion. After all, the enlargement of the blind spot is merely the non-specific evidence of an edema of the disc that, in addition to increased intra-cranial pressure, may be caused by other factors, such as an inflammation or a toxic agent. For early papilledema, we are tempted to accept Dubois-Poulsen's *observation on the Goldmann perimeter that indicates an anomaly of the law of summation for the isopters surrounding the blind spot.* However, again we have to make the reservation that this phenomenon is merely a nonspecific sign of damage to the retina surrounding the disc as a result of the edema (Fig. 2-10).

There is a loathsome uncertainty regarding the early signs of papilledema. If papilledema is a direct consequence of increased intracranial pressure, proof of the latter should assist in arriving at a diagnosis. A spinal or occipital puncture could establish the existence of such an increase. However, it is a well-founded fact that such a puncture in patients with increased intracranial pressure harbors the immense danger of incarceration of the brain stem into the foramen magnum, an event that would lead to a grave aggravation of the existing condition, requiring immediate neurosurgical intervention. *A lumbar or occipital puncture for the verification of an incipient or an already fully developed choked disc is strictly contraindicated and would betray extremely poor judgment on the part of the physician.*

The *pressure in the ophthalmic artery* is not only related to the systemic blood pressure, but also to the intracranial pressure. This is obvious if one is mindful of the origin of these ocular vessels from the large cerebral vessels and of their partly intracranial course. Thanks to the fundamental investigations of Bailliart, it is possible to determine the arterial as well as the venous pressure of the ocular vessels with the aid of the ophthalmodynamometer (p. 118) with some accuracy. Bailliart and, with him, the majority of investigators, especially of the French school (Coppez, Rasvan, Magitot, Pereyra, Spinelli, Gallois, Bauwens, Winther, Ascher), originally were of the opinion that there is always an increased pressure in the ophthalmic arteries in patients with brain tumors. De Morsier, Monnier, and Streiff were able to prove that this belief is not always correct. They made the observation on 21 patients with brain tumors (verified either during operation or postmortem) that *tumors of the anterior or middle fossa were usually associated with normal or decreased pressure of the ophthalmic arteries,* whereas *those of the posterior fossa were, as a rule, associated with increased pressure.* Streiff was able to confirm this observation in an additional series of ten patients. He concluded that the variations of the pressure in the arteries were not a direct result of the space-consuming process, but an indirect effect on the central mechanism governing the circulation of the cerebral vessels. Bailliart later arrived at the conclusion, confirmed by numerous authors (Rossano; Gauddisart; Suvina; Streiff and Monnier; Redslob; Toyama), that in *brain tumors an increase in pressure in the ophthalmic arteries precedes the appearance of the papilledema,* and that once the latter develops, this pressure becomes normalized or even gives way to a decrease in pressure. This increase of the pressure in the arteries is an *isolated discordance,* since the pressure in the brachial artery in patients with space-consuming lesions is usually normal.

Bailliart calls this drop of pressure in the arteries at the onset of papilledema "asystoly." The ophthalmic artery seems to resist the increased intracranial pressure for a while (initial increase in pressure) only to give up in the end; the drop in pressure is quasi a sign of an insufficiency of the arterial wall. Bailliart believes that the fall in pressure of the arteries, together with the resulting insufficiency of the venous return flow, is the true basis for the pathogenesis of the choked disc.

According to Weigelin, the ophthalmodynamometric results in patients with brain tumors (with or without papilledema) do not give any concordant results from which one could draw practical conclusions.

In 31 patients having cerebral tumors with papilledema, Weigelin registered the median ophthalmic arterial pressure in relation to the median arterial brachial pressure; in four patients the pressure was elevated, in nine it was lowered, and in 18 it was normal. In 34 patients with cerebral tumors without papilledema the median ophthalmic arterial pressure in relation to the median brachial pressure was found to be elevated in eight, lowered in four, and normal in 22.

*Therefore Weigelin came to the conclusion that there is no characteristic alteration of the ophthalmic arterial pressure resulting from increased intracranial pressure.* An increase of intracranial pressure no doubt causes an increase of the resistance of flow within the intracranial vessels, which at the same time, however, may be compensated by a dilatation of the terminal vessels. This is just the phenomenon that explains so many normal values of intraocular arterial pressure in patients with papilledema. As this compensation varies greatly from subject to subject, the measurement of the intraocular arterial pressure, according to Weigelin, cannot be used for evaluation of the intracranial pressure.

Important data gained with the method of *ophthalmodynamography* are reported by Finke, who examined 20 patients with intracranial tumors using the method of Hager (p. 67).

Fourteen patients with no or only minimal signs of increased intracranial pressure revealed normal conditions in the ophthalmodynamogram. In seven patients with distinct signs of increased intracranial pressure, ophthalmodynamography revealed a normal general pressure with relative cranial hypertonia in two, a general hypertonia with ophthalmobrachial isotonia in one, and a general hypertonia with relative cranial hypotonia in four. The five patients with general hypertonia had never before had any signs of hypertonia of an essential nature. In these cases the increased pressure in the brachial artery is an expression of the tendency to overcome the increased intracranial pressure, as mentioned by Cushing in 1902. Of special interest in this series are the patients with general hypertonia and relative cranial hypotonia. Finke calls this the *decompensated intracranial pressure:* despite an increase of the brachial artery pressure, a further decrease of the ophthalmic artery pressure occurs because the increased intracranial pressure can be overcome incompletely or not at all.

With regard to ophthalmodynamography, Finke comes to the conclusion that this method gives information as to whether and how far a compensatory increase of the brachial artery pressure is accompanied by an increase of the cranial blood pressure. It may also give information in certain cases of increased intracranial pressure as to whether, despite an increase of the arterial brachial pressure, there is a decrease of the ophthalmic artery pressure (decompensated intracranial pressure). Furthermore, the ophthalmodynamogram is able to control the effect of dehydration of the brain on the ophthalmic artery pressure. If a relatively low ophthalmic artery pressure does increase despite an unaltered brachial artery pressure, this is a sign of improvement of the so-called decompensated intracranial pressure.

In summary, the following rule is suggested for practical purposes: the determination of the pressure in the ophthalmic artery (ophthalmodynamometry) for the early diagnosis of a papilledema as well as of a brain tumor must be regarded with caution and should never be the single fact on which such a diagnosis is based. *In a patient with suspected incipient papilledema an increase in the pressure of the ophthalmic artery may be interpreted as an indication of increased intracranial pressure*. Its absence or even a decrease, however, never rules out increased intracranial pressure. One always has to keep in mind that in cases of pronounced increased intracranial pressure there might be a general arterial hypertension with relative intracranial hypotonia manifested by a relatively low ophthalmic artery pressure, a phenomenon that can be registered especially well by ophthalmodynamography. The relation between the pressures within the brachial artery and the ophthalmic artery gives valuable information as to whether the increased intracranial pressure still permits an increase of the cranial blood pressure or leads to a decompensation of the arterial cerebral blood flow.

Since a beginning venous congestion is an early sign of papilledema, the determination of the *pressure of the veins* should be of special interest. The intraocular venous pressure depends on the intracranial venous pressure, which, on the other hand, is a function of the pressure of the cerebral spinal fluid. Even in recent publications, we frequently find the opinion expressed that an increased intracranial pressure can be excluded if a spontaneous venous pulsation is present or occurs after exerting slight pressure on the eye (Lauber; Sobanski; Duke-Elder; Redslob; and others). We are in agreement with Streiff, Serr, and Williamson-Noble that the disappearance of spontaneous venous pulsation is of no significance for the diagnosis of increased intracranial pressure, especially not for the early diagnosis of choked disc. In numerous patients with brain tumors with an incipient papilledema as well as a fully developed choked disc, we have seen a positive venous pulse or at least an immediate collapse of the retinal veins when slight pressure is applied to the eye, an observation confirmed also by Toyama and by Primrose. Actual measurement of the retinal venous pressure with a special dynamometer likewise does not supply additional information, although various authors (Baurmann; Lauber; Sobanski; Marchesani; Redslob) regard an increased venous pressure pathognomonic for increased intracranial pressure. There is a considerable division of opinion concerning the significance of the venous pressure. Other authors (Riser, Calmettes, Garipuy, Pigassou, and Pigassou) are convinced that they found a pronounced lowering of the venous pressure in the majority of their verified cases of brain tumor. Such discrepancies demand a cautious interpretation. Perhaps these discrepancies are related to the technical difficulty of the method. Streiff is so right when he states in his monograph on the retinal blood pressure: *"The exact determination of the pressure of the retinal veins is, however, very difficult and subject to many sources of errors; for that reason one should not attach too much significance to it, neither to the indirect evaluation of the intracranial pressure—an attempt that is made time and again."* Our own experience in the evaluation of the pressure of the retinal veins for the early diagnosis of a papilledema is in full agreement with Streiff's opinion.

This discourse should make it quite plain how difficult the diagnosis of an incipient papilledema is. Often it cannot be made merely on the basis of the ophthalmoscopic examination and some of the ophthalmologic ancillary methods. We maintain that *we, as ophthalmologists, should not evaluate the ophthalmologic findings as data detached from the complete clinical picture, but that we should consider the entire neurologic picture and the results of appropriate tests in our interpretation of changes of a disc if papilledema is suspected*. If it is impossible to arrive at a definite decision as to whether or not there is an early papilledema, there are, in our opinion, two avenues of approach. If the general condition of the patient permits it, the ophthalmoscopic examination can be repeated at a later date (perhaps 1 or 2 weeks later); a definite progress of the signs of edema of the disc may be observed at that time. We would like to stress in this connection the enormous importance of having a complete record of the previous findings for the sake of comparison; color and red-free *photographs* of the fundus (also fluorescein angiograms) taken on different occasions in the sense of a serial documentation are particularly valuable. If the situation in a suspected papilledema is more urgent, especially in view of the general condition of the patient, one should not hesitate to refer the patient to the neurologist or the neurosurgeon. With the advanced modern diagnostic facilities, it is preferable to make such a referral once too often!

### Unilateral papilledema

As mentioned previously, the swelling of the disc resulting from increased intracranial pressure usually occurs bilaterally (in 20% of the cases there is a predominance on one side); a unilateral form is rare (8%). This bilateral manifestation of a choked disc is sometimes forestalled by local factors. One of these factors is a *previous unilateral atrophy of the optic nerve*. An atrophic optic nerve is incapable of developing edema. This is one reason why pituitary tumors that produce a descending optic atrophy do not cause papilledema, even though there might be a fairly large space-consuming lesion. Another possible mechanism is the *blockage of the communication between the vaginal spaces of the sheaths of the optic nerve and the subarachnoidal space* as a result of some inflammation, compression, or congenital anomaly. The *Foster Kennedy syndrome* is cited as a typical example. Its characteristics are an optic atrophy on the side of the tumor (caused by direct pressure on the intracranial part of the optic nerve) and a choked disc on the opposite side. In addition to this fully developed picture of the Foster Kennedy syndrome, there are a number of incomplete forms that belong to the same group: there may be a preponderance of signs of atrophy on the side of the tumor, with a preponderance of swelling of the disc on the opposite side, but definitely a bilateral papilledema with a distinct difference on the two sides; there may be a normal disc with central scotoma on the tumor side and a papilledema on the opposite side; or there may be an atrophic papilledema (secondary optic atrophy) on the side of the tumor and an ordinary papilledema on the opposite side. We shall consider the Foster Kennedy syndrome in the discussion of the ocular symptoms found in patients with frontal lobe tumors and in those with meningiomas of the olfactory groove and the sphenoid ridge (p. 242). Apart from tumors (68%), the Foster Kennedy syndrome may also be caused by nontumoral conditions (32%), such as arteriosclerosis, optochiasmatic arachnoiditis, and carotid aneurysms. In some cases the unilateral optic atrophy may be explained by some pressure on the optic nerve, but the contralateral papilledema is not explained by an increased intracranial pressure. Here the swelling of the disc must have some relation to circulatory disorders of the optic nerve itself (for instance, as in ischemic papillitis).

A much less known and recognized cause of unilateral papilledema associated with increased intracranial pressure is *unilateral myopia* of medium or higher degree. A medium myopia measures 5 to 10 diopters; high myopia measures 10 to 15 diopters or more. The anatomic peculiarities of the myopic disc and the area surrounding it (myopic crescent) either prevent the development of a papilledema or cause its development at a later stage and in an atypical form (Marchesani; Bietti; Morone). In bilateral myopia a papilledema may never become manifest despite existing increased intracranial pressure.

If increased intracranial pressure can be ruled out as the cause of a unilateral chocked disc, an *orbital process* should be considered next. As a rule, it will produce a more or less distinct *exophthalmos,* which is of considerable importance for diagnostic purposes. Usually the closer such a process is to the globe, the more pronounced is the edema of the disc. The etiologic factor of such a unilateral papilledema may be tumors, aneurysms, inflammatory conditions, abscesses, or an edema of the orbit. It should be mentioned that occasionally tumors of the middle and anterior fossa (for instance, meningiomas of the sphenoid ridge) may extend into the orbit and cause a unilateral papilledema in such a manner. However, such a condition will mostly cause a Foster Kennedy syndrome with papilledema on the side opposite the tumor.

*In reviewing our material, we have observed a unilateral papilledema only rarely as the result of increased intracranial pressure* (8%). This may occasionally be the case in cerebral abscesses or in temporal lobe tumors. The Foster Kennedy syndrome, likewise, is not so frequent as is generally assumed. Orbital and purely *ocular conditions* can be recognized with relative ease. Such ocular conditions are hypotension of the globe (for instance, after a fistulating operation for glaucoma), swelling of the papilla in the case of a unilateral iridocylitis, or an edema of the disc caused by central retinal vein thrombosis. One should also keep in mind the possibility of *unilateral drusen of the disc* and, in the presence of hyperopia, a *hyperopic pseudoneuritis* (p. 152 and Figs. 2-14 and 2-42).

Unfortunately, on the basis of our observations, a fairly large number of so-called unilateral papilledemas ·cannot be accounted for despite the benefit of all kinds of diagnostic procedures. A certain number of cases that cannot be explained properly must be listed under the unsatisfactory category of unilateral *pseudopapilledema* or *pseudopapillitis,* since they are accompanied neither by increased intracranial pressure nor by orbital or ocular conditions. We have no less than eight cases of so-called unilateral "choked disc" on record, cases that were referred because of a suspected brain tumor and that did not yield a satisfactory explanation for the unilateral fundus changes. One cannot help but consider these pseudoforms (for the ophthalmoscopic appearance, see Fig. 2-15) of a unilateral choked disc as insignificant morphologic deviations of a normal disc, provided they do not change their original picture during an extended period of observation (p. 156).

There are also transient forms of *unilateral papilledema*. We have examined a 25-year-old man with an unquestionable unilateral papilledema of a 1-diopter prominence, hemor-

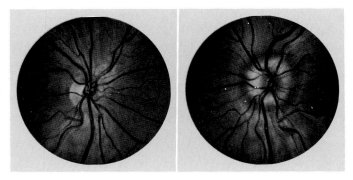

**Fig. 2-14.** Unilateral apparent choked disc (left side) with intrapapillary drusen of papilla in 18-year-old patient. Left disc enlarged, with indistinct margin and slight prominence over level of retina. No venous congestion. Drusen hidden in depth of papilla just manifest themselves by slightly protuberant outline of left disc margin. They could be visualized by means of posterior slit-lamp microscopy (Goldmann's or Hruby's method). Left illustration corresponds to right eye and right illustration to left eye.

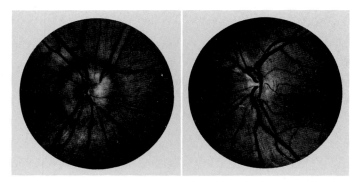

**Fig. 2-15.** Unilateral pseudopapilledema in 20-year-old patient. Enlarged disc diameter. Blurred disc margin. Slight bulging of right disc margin. Insignificant deflection of vessels but no venous congestion of either large veins or capillaries of disc. Left disc appears blurred on nasal side but not prominent. Left illustration corresponds to right eye and right illustration to left eye.

rhages, white dots, and a distinct engorgement of the retinal veins. The neurologic and neuroradiologic findings were negative. There was no increased intracranial pressure. The visual acuity and fields were not remarkable. A year later the choked disc had disappeared completely without leaving any residual or functional disturbances! An etiologic explanation for this transient choked disc was pseudotumor cerebri with an abnormality of the optic nerve sheaths on the side without papilledema ( ? ) (Wagener).

These rather gloomy statements regarding the chances of interpreting a unilateral papilledema (including pseudopapilledema) should not allay the zeal of the examiner. On the contrary, because of the very difficulties just described, every attempt should be made at least to rule out the possibility of increased intracranial pressure. In most instances, this will hardly be possible without the assistance of the neurosurgeon and neuroradiologist.

### Chronic atrophic papilledema

Sooner or later any persistent papilledema will lead to a *secondary optic atrophy,* provided there is no intervention to relieve or at least to decrease the increased intracranial pressure. As a rule, this atrophy appears only a few months after the onset of the papilledema. The time required for the involution or collapse of a severe, fully developed papilledema to complete atrophy is 6 to 9 months, occasionally even up to more than 1 year.

The degenerative changes of the nerve fibers caused by the chronic edema produce a glial proliferation—the typical reaction in every kind of secondary optic atrophy. Ophthalmoscopically, it manifests itself as a *grayish white discoloration involving the peripheral parts of the disc initially, but, in the more advanced stages, also its center.* As the atrophy progresses, the prominence and the width of the disc decreases despite the persistent intracranial pressure. The disc becomes distinctly paler; the original reddish color gives way to the unmistakable grayish white gliosis as the end result. There is narrowing of the retinal arteries. The veins are less congested and may even approach a normal caliber, actually an indication of constriction of the vessels caused by glial proliferation. In certain stages a fine network of dilated superficial capillaries resembling telangiectasias can be observed overlying the white atrophic nerve head. Arteries and veins sometimes may be completely obscured by the glial proliferation in their course across the disc. Occasionally the picture of the chronic atrophic papilledema results in a whitish sheathing of the vessels that creates blurring and narrowing of the red blood column within them (Figs. 2-16, 2-17, and 2-20). In very chronic papilledema, yellow shiny exudates near the margins of the disc may simulate drusen of the optic nerve (p. 150). Even in the later stages after the prominence of the disc has receded considerably, the original aspect of the choked disc can be surmised from the increased size of the nerve head, from its blurred and slightly prominent border, from remnants of hemorrhages and white dots on or near the papilla (Fig. 2-8), and from an irregular arrangement of the retinal pigment in the surrounding retina. It still may be difficult to rule out a secondary optic atrophy after a papillitis if one depends only on the

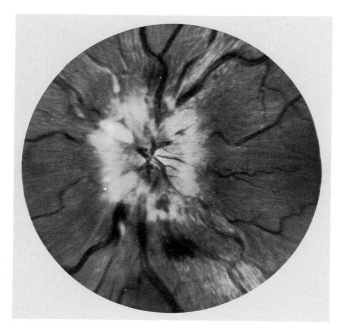

**Fig. 2-16.** Chronic papilledema of left eye showing beginning atrophy in 29-year-old patient with hemangioma of right cerebellar hemisphere with internal hydrocephalus. Papilla markedly enlarged with blurred outline and elevation of 4 diopters. Grayish white discoloration of peripheral as well as central parts of disc, indicating beginning atrophy of nerve fibers and secondary glial proliferation. Numerous white dots ("cytoid bodies") on disc. Dilation and tortuosity of veins that, in areas, are buried in disc. White accompanying stripes of vessels (dilation of perivascular lymph spaces). Hemorrhages at disc margin within nerve fiber layer. Visual acuity, 1.0. Slight concentric contraction of visual field.

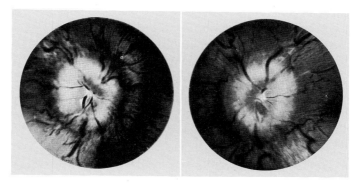

**Fig. 2-17.** Chronic atrophic papilledema in 36-year-old patient with syphilis of central nervous system and syphilitic meningitis. Conspicuous pallor of edematous discs showing prominence of 4 to 5 diopters. Veins are barely dilated and arteries rather narrowed. White perivascular sheaths. Visual acuity, O.D. 1.0; O.S. 0.7. Both visual fields intact. Left illustration corresponds to right eye and right illustration to left eye.

ophthalmoscopic findings. The presence of grayish arcuate lines (Paton's concentric lines) surrounding the disc and white perivascular sheathing is more suggestive of an atrophic papilledema. The final decision will usually depend on the functional examination, especially the determination of the central and peripheral visual fields (p. 4).

The visual functions will be preserved for a relatively long time during the acute stages of the papilledema. In contrast, the chronic atrophic papilledema is marked by significant disturbances of the visual function. It is imperative to detect these disturbances as early as possible and not to take chances with a grave, irreversible impairment. *A decompression for a papilledema should be performed before optic atrophy sets in or at least during its very early stages.* Otherwise a restitution of the visual function is no longer possible. In the later stages of a progressing atrophy, which occasionally develops quite rapidly, a decompression for the relief of the increased intracranial pressure may have catastrophic results for the visual function; we have had occasion to observe a reduction of the central vision and the visual fields amounting to complete bilateral amaurosis, especially in patients with tumors of the posterior fossa with chronic atrophic papilledema. Thus the importance of the *early signs of a beginning atrophy in papilledema* cannot be stressed enough. One should make it a rule to search for them carefully in serial examinations, especially in those patients with papilledema in whom, for some reason, neurosurgical intervention has to be postponed or is not indicated.

One of the first symptoms of beginning atrophy of a papilledema is a *concentric constriction* of the peripheral and middle isopters, which may be associated with peripheral sector-shaped defects or similar defects extending close to the center (Figs. 2-18 and 2-19). Unless the intracranial space-occupying lesion interferes directly with the visual pathways, thus causing specific field changes, these early symptoms are enormously valuable and reliable. It is essential to

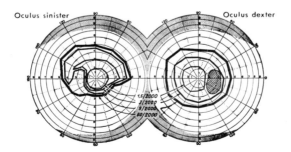

**Fig. 2-18.** Visual field changes in 19-year-old patient with chronic atrophic choked discs resulting from astrocytoma of fourth ventricle (see Fig. 3-122, p. 295). Concentric constriction of right field, particularly of peripheral isopters, and marked enlargement of blind spot. Contraction of inferior nasal and inferior temporal quadrants of left peripheral field, with formation of sector-shaped defects protruding toward center, as determined on tangent screen. There is a history of numerous amblyopic attacks. Visual acuity, O.U. 0.6.

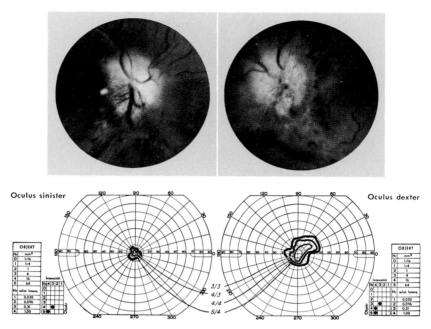

**Fig. 2-19.** Chronic atrophic papilledemas in 18-year-old patient with tumor of corpus callosum and septum lucidum in late stages. Bilateral prominence of discs of 4 to 5 diopters. Marked pallor and gliosis of discs. Superficial network of dilated capillaries; arteries partially obscured by glial proliferation. Left illustration corresponds to right eye and right illustration to left eye. Below, Corresponding visual fields taken on Goldmann perimeter. Extensive concentric contraction of peripheral isopters, especially of left field. Right field shows predominantly a loss of nasal parts. Central visual acuity is reduced to finger counting at 1 meter O.S. and at 0.8 meter O.D.

search for them with the most minute perimetric targets. Here again, the Goldmann perimeter is particularly well suited. It will indicate a *contraction of the peripheral visual field,* which may occur at a time when the more central isopters still appear relatively normal except for disturbances of the law of summation mentioned previously. Parallel with the increasing concentric contraction of the visual field is a *decrease of the central visual acuity.* As mentioned before, it may have been impaired already by the edema extending into the macular region (resulting in a cecocentral relative scotoma) and further impaired by hemorrhages or by a fan-shaped arrangement of droplets of fluid. As a rule, the concentric contraction of the visual fields progresses more rapidly in the nasal, especially inferonasal, halves of the field, thus stimulating some sort of a *binasal hemianopia* during certain stages. In the end, there remains a more or less centrally located island of the field that may or may not include the blind spot and that may barely enable the patient to find his way around. In these advanced stages, it may be impossible to determine a field defect caused directly by the pressure of the tumor (for instance, a homonymous hemianopia). Unfortunately, even this small island may be lost, giving way to a complete amaurosis with wide, fixed pupils. (This is in contrast to cortical blindness with intact pupillary reactions!)

In the presence of a chronic atrophic papilledema the size of the peripheral visual field, not the ophthalmoscopic aspect, is of prognostic importance with regard to postoperative loss of vision. When the cause of a persistent increased intracranial pressure cannot be eliminated for some reason or other, the visual field has to be examined repeatedly to detect any progression of the peripheral contraction. This could necessitate an orbital or temporal decompression and eventually a shunting procedure. In the atrophic stage of papilledema the *electrophysiologic responses* are also altered: decrease of the subjective frequency of fusion, increase of the retinocortical time, and delay or even absence of the specific evoked occipital response. Thus the electrophysiologic examinations may help to confirm an otherwise suspected tendency of a papilledema toward atrophy.

Not without reason did we give such a detailed description of the picture of chronic atrophic papilledema. *We know of numerous instances in which the patient initially consulted an ophthalmologist because of rapidly deteriorating vision and the ophthalmologist diagnosed a chronic atrophic papilledema and was the first to suspect a brain tumor.* Such tumors are mostly in a relatively silent part of the brain and have an early tendency to cause an internal hydrocephalus (cerebellum, third, or fourth ventricle). As mentioned previously, surgical removal generally was not followed by any functional improvement. On the contrary, in some of the patients there was a catastrophic drop of vision, even resulting in total bilateral blindness. Anybody who has experienced such complications once will appreciate the importance of recognizing a choked disc in its early stages, not only in view of the brain tumor, but also in consideration of the possible functional impairment of the optic nerve. From this point of view, one should almost regret that the papilledema remains asymptomatic for such a long time and that it becomes noticeable only when the dreadful signs of atrophy have already developed, indicating a condition that generally will not improve with active neurosurgical interference but frequently will even become worse. Fortunately, with the progress of modern neurologic and neuroradiologic diagnosis, such extreme evolutions of chronic atrophic papilledema become still rarer. The most common cause today is pseudotumor cerebri (p. 310).

Under certain circumstances (for instance, meningioma of the olfactory groove), papilledema and optic atrophy may develop at the same time. The optic atrophy (either unilateral or bilateral) depends on the compression of the optic nerves or the chiasm by the tumor. The papilledema is a function of the increased intracranial pressure, but may be handicapped in its evolution by the degree of the preceding optic atrophy. In such cases, it may become extremely difficult to decide whether one has to deal with a chronic atrophic papilledema or with a combination of simultaneous papilledema and optic

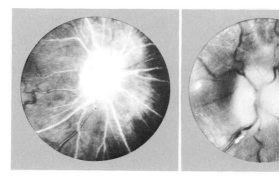

**Fig. 2-20.** Optic atrophy and gliosis following chronic untreated papilledema in 28-year-old patient with bilateral acoustic neuroma in neurofibromatosis. Amaurosis of both eyes. Right disc is flat, enlarged, and shows permanent gliosis with folds in peripapillary retina. Note perivascular sheathing extending from disc far out on periphery. Optic cup completely obscured by glial proliferation. Left disc is still prominent, but also atrophic, with gliosis and distinct perivascular sheathing. Arteries practically invisible within area of atrophic disc. Optic cup begins to be obscured by gliosis.

atrophy (Fig. 2-20). The functional disturbances and their character can help in making the differential diagnosis; if loss of central vision (including scotomas) and defects of the peripheral visual field occur early, one has to think of a primary optic compression; if headaches or other manifestations of increased intracranial pressure precede the visual disturbances, there is a great probability that papilledema has developed into secondary optic atrophy.

### Pathologic anatomy of the disc in papilledema

It may be of interest to touch briefly on the pathologic-anatomic changes of the disc in papilledema and their relationship with the clinical phenomena just discussed. In principle, there is a *simple edema of the nerve head with an edematous swelling of the glial cells surrounding the nerve fibers and a corresponding exudative infiltration of the rest of the tissues.* This edema is usually limited to a relatively small area and extends from the disc surface to the region in the trunk of the nerve where the retinal vessels leave the nerve. The edematous infiltration and swelling involve also the perivascular spaces within the nerve and close to the eyeball. There is an anterior convex displacement of the glial fibers of the lamina cribrosa, and the physiologic excavation appears to be filled. The entire disc mushrooms into the vitreous, displaces the adjacent retina laterally, and causes it to form fine folds. These folds can be recognized ophthalmoscopically as arcuate stripes concentric with the disc (Paton's concentric lines). The retina adjacent to the disc also shows a slight edema with blurring or loss of the light reflexes from the surface of the nerve fiber layer (as seen in red-free light ophthalmoscopy) and accumulation of exudate between the sensory retina and the pigment epithelium (also contributing to the enlargement of the blind spot in the visual field). The veins and capillaries in the area of the disc are markedly dilated. There may be aneurysmal dilatations, microaneurysms, or a resemblance to new vessel formation. Hemorrhages on the disc or at the margin appear predominantly in the nerve fiber layer. Ophthalmoscopically, they appear as "flame-shaped" hemorrhages. The subarachnoid spaces of the sheath of the optic nerve are filled by albuminous fluid, are markedly broadened, and show some ballooning at their scleral end (Fig. 2-21).

The nerve fibers show characteristic changes as a result of the edematous infiltration only in later stages. The edema first involves the periphery of the optic nerve and gradually pro-

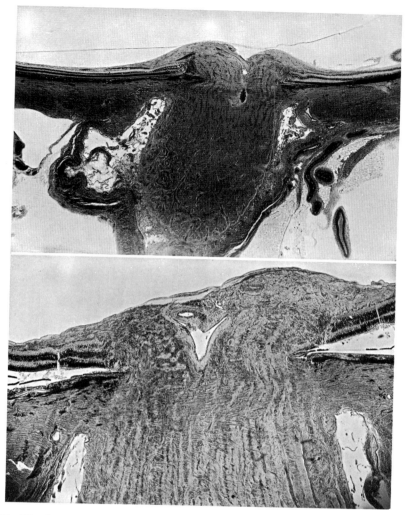

**Fig. 2-21.** Histologic section of papilledema (above, low power, about ×14; below, higher power, about ×30). Edema of nerve head with edematous swelling of nerve fibers and interstitial tissue. Cup in lower illustration is filled. Lateral displacement and folding of retina. Dilation of veins and capillaries. Dilation of perivascular lymph sheaths. Ballooning of intervaginal spaces by transudate.

gresses toward the axial area. This process has its functional equivalent in the progressive concentric constriction of the visual field. In the early stages, there is swelling of the non-medullated fibers of the disc, especially those near its margin. They show typical varicose dilations. Within these varicosities the fine neurofibrils, separated by the edematous fluid, can be recognized distinctly. As the papilledema progresses, these varicosities multiply and eventually fill the entire disc. After some time, *degenerative changes develop*—the equivalents of the chronic atrophic papilledema! The neurofibrils within the varicosities disappear by ischemic destruction and are replaced by fine granules. In the end these granules change to a homogeneous mass. The varicosities lose their connection with the nerve fibers. They are now called "cytoid bodies." These cytoid bodies undergo a lipoid degeneration and finally disappear altogether. In the final stages of chronic papilledema, there is an ascending and descending degeneration of the nerve fibers and at the same time a neuroglial proliferation. Ophthalmoscopically, this corresponds to the grayish white "milky" discoloration of the disc. The degenerated neural elements are phagocytosed by microglial cells and replaced by proliferating fibrous astrocytes. Inflammatory alterations play an insignificant and subordinate role during all of these processes.

## Pathogenesis of papilledema

From the multiplicity of theories proposing an explanation for the pathogenesis of papilledema, one can draw the conclusion that the mechanism is still controversial and by no means settled. A variable combination of anatomic, mechanical, vascular, and metabolic factors is responsible for the development and progression of papilledema. With regard to anatomic considerations, one has to realize that the *blood supply to the optic disc is from the short posterior ciliary arteries,* which end in the circle of Zinn and Haller, and that the venous return goes primarily through the central retinal vein with collaterals to the choroid. Probably in connection with the intense capillary vascularization and the special structure of the tissue, the optic nerve head, much more readily than other parts of the optic nerve, has a special tendency to swell and to manifest edema. *Forward transmission of the increased cerebrospinal fluid pressure into the sheaths of the optic nerve is an essential factor and element in the production of papilledema* (Hayreh). This is in agreement with the recently presented clinical work showing that established papilledema can be relieved by surgical fistulization of the optic nerve in the orbit (Davidson; Hayreh). The exact mechanism by which this increase of pressure in the intravaginal space around the optic nerve produces prelaminar edema is not yet clear. It could be a function of *interference with a centripetal flow of tissue fluids or of axoplasm* in the anterior part of the optic nerve, creating a flow of such fluid or axoplasm into the extracellular space of the papilla and producing the choked disc. Once edema has developed in the prelaminar region, it compresses the venous channels in this area, producing dilatation of the prelaminar vessels, more edema, and thus a vicious cycle, leading to more marked edema of the disc. It is further an experimentally proved fact that a chronic increase of intracranial pressure does not increase the pressure in the ophthalmic veins (Hedges) and that compression of the central vein in the sheath of the optic nerve by the increased cerebrospinal fluid pressure plays no role in the pathogenesis of papilledema (Hayreh). This is also in agreement with the clinical findings that papilledema has a different ophthalmoscopic aspect than occlusion of the central retinal vein. Arterial changes seem to be of more importance in the pathogenesis of choked disc. In early papilledema, there is a distinct increase in ophthalmic artery pressure, and this movement disappears when papilledema is fully developed (Baillart; Toyama). *Elevation of ophthalmic artery pressure and increase in orbital blood flow occur with increasing intracranial pressure* (reaching systolic levels), as could be shown experimentally (Hedges). An increase in arterial blood flow, combined with an impaired venous outflow, could account for the vascular congestion seen in papilledema. It is improbable that a direct extension of cerebral edema along the optic nerve could lead to edematous swelling of the disc. However, it has been possible to demonstrate that the tissue pressure in the orbital optic nerve increases with an increase of intracranial pressure (Hedges). Such an increased interstitial pressure within the optic nerve might extend to the prelaminar portion of the nerve, the specific area able to swell and to protrude anteriorly in the direction of the vitreous. Finally, one must consider the *importance of the pressure gradient between the optic nerve and the intraocular pressure* in the development of papilledema. Glaucoma tends to prevent papilledema; in eyes with lowered intraocular pressure, there is a tendency to optic disc swelling. These statements are the basis for the *concept of a hydrostatic mechanism underlying the pathogenesis of papilledema* (Hedges); in the presence of increased intracranial pressure, there may develop at the level of the optic nerve head varying degrees of vasodilatation as a result of microcirculatory congestion, stasis, and hyperemia; the degree of edema of the nerve head is determined by the degree of the disproportion between the capillary pressure or tissue pressure and the intraocular pressure at the nerve head. The hydrostatic concept combines all the anatomic, clinical, and pathologic facts known to date and serves as a good model for considering various causes and degrees of papilledema.

For more details concerning theories on the pathogenesis of papilledema, the reader is referred to special monographs and specific publications (Brégeat; Bonamour, Brégeat, Bonnet, and Juge; Walsh and Hoyt; Hayreh; Hedges; Sanders; Weigelin).

### Differential diagnosis of papilledema

The differential diagnosis is important considering the fact that a *papilledema does not indicate a brain tumor in all patients*. Seventy-five percent of all cases of papilledema are caused by brain tumors. For the remaining 25%, other possible factors must be considered in evaluating a papilledema. It is these 25% that occasionally make a definite diagnosis of a papilledema so difficult, especially in its early stages. These difficulties exist not only as a statistical fiction, but also in everyday practice. This is clearly demonstrated by the personal communication of a British ophthalmologist who is the consultant for a large neurologic and neurosurgical clinic. During the past 12 years, not less than 110 patients were referred with the diagnosis of bilateral "papilledema" in whom neither a brain tumor nor increased intracranial pressure could be proved with all the up-to-date methods of examination. In addition to the choked disc caused by increased intracranial pressure not related to a brain tumor, papilledemas resulting from a variety of noncerebral conditions with a striking resemblance to a true choked disc have to be considered. Finally, some congenital anomalies of the disc have certain ophthalmoscopic aspects that may easily lead to confusion with a choked disc. Thus in the differential diagnosis, three groups have to be considered: (1) papilledema caused by increased intracranial pressure other than that resulting from brain tumor, (2) optic disc edema of noncerebral origin, and (3) congenital anomalies of the disc resembling choked disc.

### Papilledema caused by increased intracranial pressure other than that resulting from brain tumor

In discussing this first group the term "brain tumor" must be defined more precisely. We limit it to true neoplasms; the percentage of 75% cited previously is based on this premise. As "brain tumor" in the broader sense of the term, the following conditions may naturally cause an increased intracranial pressure and thus a choked disc: *brain abscesses*, occasionally with ony an ipsilateral choked disc that would be of localizing value; *tuberculous* or *syphilitic granulomas*; *epidural* and *subdural hematomas*, perhaps also *subarachnoidal* or *intracerebral hematomas* if they assume large enough proportions (Fig. 5-2); and quite rarely, *aneurysms, cysticercus cysts,* and *cerebral phakomas*.

In addition to an increase in the volume of the brain tissue, an increased intracranial pressure may also be the result of an increase in the volume of the cerebrospinal fluid. Thus occasionally, we find a choked disc in patients with *internal hydrocephalus, epidemic encephalitis, epidemic purulent meningitis, nonpurulent meningitis-like syndrome, syphilitic meningitis, tuberculous meningitis, viral meningitis, infectious meningitis secondary to trauma,* further infectious polyneuritis (Guillain-Barré syndrome), poliomyelitis, and infectious mononucleosis (Figs. 2-22 and 2-23).

The rather frequently seen choked discs in patients with septic or aseptic *thromboses of the dural sinuses* are caused by cerebral edema, hemorrhage, and an increase in pressure of the cerebrospinal fluid resulting from an impairment

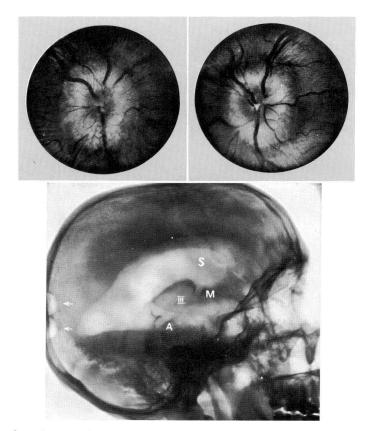

**Fig. 2-22.** Bilateral papilledema showing beginning atrophy in 34-year-old patient with internal hydrocephalus secondary to serous meningitis complicating an attack of flu. Enormous dilation of disc diameter. Prominence of right disc measured 4 diopters and of left disc, 3 diopters. Grayish pallor of discs as a sign of beginning atrophy. Peripapillary retinal edema with radial folding. Veins dilated and tortuous. Hyperemic congestion of small vessels of disc, especially on right side. Visual acuity, O.D. 1.0; O.S. 0.1 (atrophy!). Diastolic pressure of arteries, O.U. 70 to 80 gm (Bailliart). Left illustration corresponds to right eye and right illustration to left eye. Below, Ventriculogram of patient with internal hydrocephalus caused by occlusion of sylvian aqueduct (arrows mark burr holes). S, Lateral ventricle; *III,* third ventricle; *M,* interventricular foramina (Monro); *A,* sylvian aqueduct.

of the circulation through the main effluent channels of the intracranial circulation (Walsh; Wohlwill; Dill and Crowe; Weber).

Attention should be called here to those somewhat obscure cases in which the patients have bilateral papilledema and increased intracranial pressure, but negative neurologic and general physical findings. Characteristic is the finding of normal-sized ventricles on ventriculography (therefore no signs of obstructing hydrocephalus). A multitude of names has been used for this syndrome, among which are *"pseudotumor cerebri,"* "benign intracranial hypertension," "serous meningitis," *"meningeal hydrops,"* and "otitic hydrocephalus." This dis-

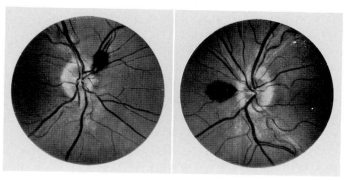

**Fig. 2-23.** Incipient papilledemas in 53-year-old patient with internal hydrocephalus as a result of cerebral arteriosclerosis. Disc margins are blurred throughout. Slight enlargement of disc diameters. Discrete elevation, especially of nasal disc margin, with minimal deflection of vessels. Minute venous congestion. Large blotches of retinal hemorrhages in nerve fiber layer on both nasal borders of discs. Diastolic pressure of ophthalmic arteries, O.U. 80 gm (Bailliart). Left illustration corresponds to right eye and right illustration to left eye.

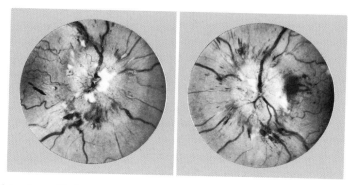

**Fig. 2-24.** Bilateral papilledema in 49-year-old patient with reticulum cell sarcoma of spinal cord (cauda equina) and concomitant increase of intracranial pressure. Both discs show distinct prominence, enlargement, blurring of margins, capillary venous stasis, and nerve fiber layer hemorrhages at disc margins. White "exudates" can be observed among nerve fibers of disc and within retina at disc margins.

ease occurs in young to middle-aged adults and is characterized by headaches, sixth nerve palsy, papilledema, occasionally field defects, and rarely blindness (caused by chronic atrophic papilledema). The affection lasts for weeks, sometimes for months, and generally has a good prognosis as long as damage does not result in optic atrophy. The pathogenesis of the syndrome is either a hypersecretion or an obstruction of resorption of cerebrospinal fluid. There are indications, at least in some of the patients, that thrombosis of the sagittal and lateral sinuses is involved. Otitis media, especially in children, may precede such a thrombosis (Chapter 5).

*Tumors of the spinal cord* may be the cause of a bilateral papilledema after blockage of the circulation of the cerebrospinal fluid and formation of a secondary hydrocephalus (Fig. 2-24). (Whether increased protein content of the spinal fluid here plays an additional etiologic role is still controversial.) Such instances have been described in neoplasms of the cervical portion of the spinal cord near the foramen magnum. However, the tumor may also be situated in the thoracic or lumbar spinal cord (Love, Wagner, and Woltmann). Choked discs have been observed even with *herniated intervertebral discs of the cervical spine;* they disappeared, together with the paresthesias of the hands, when traction was applied to the cervical spine (Girard, Devic, and de Gevigney) or surgical intervention performed.

An increase in the intracranial pressure may also result from a disproportion between the cranial vault and its contents. We have seen a few cases of unquestionable bilateral papilledema in infants with *craniosynostosis* (that is, a premature closure of the cranial suture and fusion of the skull bones). Papilledema and eventually simultaneous atrophic changes of the optic disc (either in unilateral or bilateral form) may be observed with other *malformations of the*

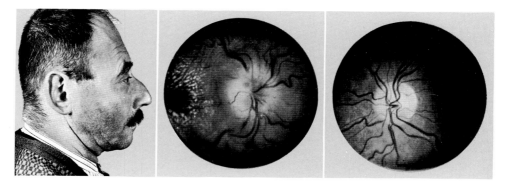

**Fig. 2-25.** Unilateral papilledema in 53-year-old patient with tower skull (oxycephaly). Right disc shows pronounced swelling and prominence with signs of beginning atrophy, venous congestion, macular star, and circumpapillary retinal edema. Left disc shows only slight blurring of nasal disc margin. It is slightly prominent and somewhat pale. Middle illustration corresponds to right eye and right illustration to left eye.

*skull,* especially *tower skull* (oxycephaly), craniofacial dysostosis (Crouzon's disease), basilar impression, and Paget's disease (Fig. 2-25).

The differential diagnosis of cases in the group just discussed is made purely on an etiologic basis. The common mechanism for all of them is increased intracranial pressure. The resulting ophthalmoscopic picture is more or less identical with that of a choked disc caused by a brain tumor and need not be described further. The same principles described for the incipient, the fully developed, and the chronic atrophic papilledema can be applied to these cases.

### Optic disc edemas of noncerebral origin

When increased intracranial pressure has been ruled out as an etiologic factor, we no longer apply the term "papilledema," but use the noncommittal terms "edema of the papilla" or "optic disc edema" in accordance with the terminology outlined previously. A first group includes *inflammatory* edemas and a second group includes *vascular* edemas of the papilla.

**Inflammatory optic neuropathy.** The inflammatory edemas include papillitis, juxtapapillary chorioretinitis, and isolated tuberculosis of the nerve head.

*Papillitis (intraocular optic neuritis).* In the differential diagnosis of every case of papilledema a *papillitis* (that is, an inflammation of the nerve head or the immediate area surrounding it) must be considered first of all. First, it should be emphasized that *it is impossible to differentiate a papillitis from a papilledema only with the aid of the ophthalmoscope.* In both instances an edema of the papilla manifests itself by blurred margins, an increased disc diameter, and a prominent nerve head. Common to both also are hemorrhages and white dots on the papilla or its margin (Fig. 2-26). Dense opaque intraretinal punctate exudates deposited around the disc and in the macula (where they may aggregate into a macular star figure) characterize a particular type of papillitis (neuroretinitis) common in children with signs of acute monocular visual loss (Hoyt and Beeston).

Of great importance in the differential diagnosis is the examination of the disc and the posterior pole of the eye using the *slit lamp,* preferably with the aid of the fundus contact glass. There are prepapillary vitreous changes that undoubtedly speak in favor of papillitis: vitreous haze (increased prepapillary Tyndall phenomenon) and prepapillary and preretinal inflammatory cells, eventually aggregating as precipitates at the posterior surface of a detached vitreous. In certain cases of papillitis the anterior uvea may participate and manifest a positive Tyndall phenomenon or even pathologic cells in the aqueous.

In the fluorescein angiogram, papillitis shows a characteristic vascular pattern of the disc (Fig. 2-27). This can be of great importance in the differential diagnosis, since it differs from the angiographic picture of papilledema and pseudopapilledema. In papillitis, we see a regular meshwork of radial capillaries connected by anastomoses covering the disc. This network extends beyond the disc margin and goes far into the retina, especially in the area of the large vessels. The capillary stasis, which is so conspicuous in papilledema (Fig. 2-9), is absent or only minimal in papillitis, perhaps confined to only one segment. In the venous phase the disc tissue will also fluoresce. This fluorescence, however, is never as intensive as in papilledema. At the same time, it lacks the conspicuously visible capillaries and microaneurysms so typical of choked disc.

True, the prominence of the edema of the papilla, as a rule, is less distinct in papillitis than in papilledema. Also, the dilation of the veins (including the

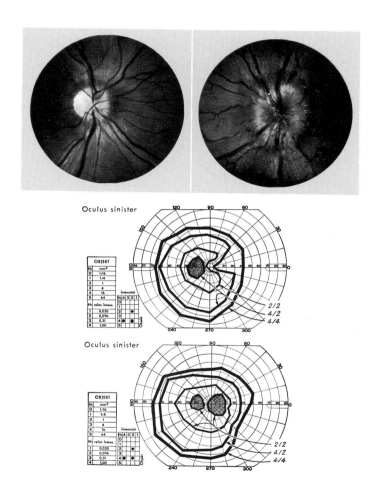

**Fig. 2-26.** Left acute papillitis (intraocular optic neuritis). Increased diameter of disc. Blurred disc margin. Grayish yellow edema of disc. Pronounced prominence of about 2.5 diopters. Deflection of vessels at disc margin. Slight venous congestion. Hemorrhages at 1 o'clock position of disc margin. This picture is very similar to that of choked disc! Left central visual acuity is reduced to 0.06. Left illustration corresponds to right eye and right illustration to left eye. Originally visual field showed nasal sector-shaped defect in addition to enlargement of blind spot (upper field). One week later (lower field) massive central scotoma had developed.

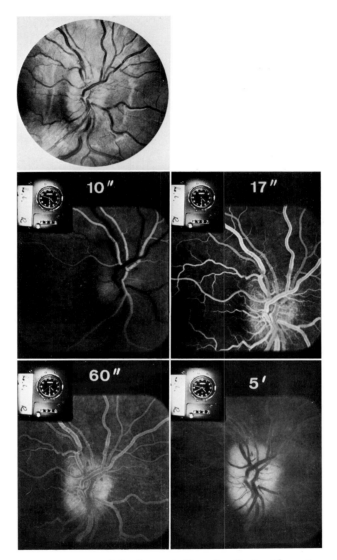

**Fig. 2-27.** Fluorescein angiogram of fundus and disc of patient with acute papillitis. In arterial phase (10 seconds), no capillary stasis is visible. There is diffuse fluorescence of papilla in venous phase (17 seconds). In late venous phase (60 seconds), there is still fluorescence of disc, but no capillaries can be detected. This angiographic pattern is in distinct contrast to that of papilledema (Fig. 2-9), in which capillary stasis, together with aneurysmatic dilatations of capillaries, represents one of the most pathognomonic signs.

capillaries), their tortuosity, and the degree of their deflection at the disc margin are more pronounced in a choked disc than in an inflammation of the nerve head. However, such ophthalmoscopic details are deceptive, especially in the early stages, where such distinctions are missing altogether. *Unilaterality,* in many instances, will weigh in favor of a papillitis. Yet we personally observed several cases of bilateral papillitis (which occurred simultaneously) whose appearance was indistinguishable from a choked disc. Nevertheless, a simultaneous bilateral papillitis is a rare event. In our experience the onset of the inflammation in the second eye is observed much more frequently after an interval of several weeks or even months. The ophthalmoscopic examination may reveal a receding stage in one eye and an incipient stage in the other eye. However, it is relatively easy to differentiate a papillitis from a papilledema by testing the visual functions. In most instances, one can follow the rule that there are *no disturbances of the visual function in papilledema in contrast to papillitis.*

The disturbances of visual function found in association with papillitis involve the central visual acuity as well as the visual fields. It has already been mentioned that, apart from the attacks of obscuration and the enlargement of the blind spot, the visual acuity and the visual field remain intact for weeks and even months in papilledema. The patient is unaware of the papilledema! The situation is entirely different with a papillitis. Perhaps even before fundus changes can be recognized ophthalmoscopically, the patient complains of a sudden foggy, blurred, or veiled vision that, in contrast to the transient obscuration of papilledema, is permanent. Within hours or a few days, it may lead to a *progressive loss of vision* and possibly to a *complete amaurosis.* Actually, this rapid deterioration of the visual function is pathognomonic for a papillitis, which, because of its inflammatory nature, causes an early disturbance in the conductivity of the nerve fibers. Only in rare cases does papillitis develop without impairment of central vision (leaving the macular bundle of the optic nerve intact). In the early stages, *pain in or behind the eye, especially on lateral movements, is characteristic for a papillitis.* The disturbance in the conductivity of the optic nerve may also be demonstrated by means of the so-called *Marcus Gunn pupillary phenomenon.* As a result of the impaired pupillomotor stimuli, the pupil on the involved side will be distinctly wider if the other eye is occluded than the pupil on the opposite side if the involved eye is occluded (p. 26). Such a sign can never be demonstrated in a papilledema—unless there is already evidence of a beginning atrophy.

*Visual field defects* are of cardinal importance in the differential diagnosis. The edema of the papilla and the immediate retinal area surrounding it frequently causes enlargement of the blind spot and a disturbance of the law of summation for the surrounding isopters (as in papilledema). Important and decisive, however, is the *demonstration of the early occurrence of central and paracentral scotomas.* Their form is not typical and is quite variable. Resulting from an early impairment of the papillomacular bundle, these scotomas usually are of the *cecocentral* type (in about 50% of the cases); they originate from the point of fixation and tend to merge with the blind spot. A number of authors still stress the importance of a *scotoma for red* for the early diagnosis of such disturbances of conductivity. With the more refined methods of perimetry, but also on the tangent screen, a carefully performed examination should demonstrate similar defects for small white targets even during these stages. The scotomas may also show an arcuate shape and originate from the upper or lower pole of the blind spot, expanding toward the periphery to merge with sector-shaped or quadrantal peripheral defects. This phenomenon is the so-called "breaking through" of a central scotoma. We have also seen central and even cecocentral scotomas in cases of papilledemas; they are the result of an edema extending into the macular area and occur only in the more advanced stages. They are relative scotomas, according to Traquair, especially for blue.

In addition to the central scotomas, the early occurrence of a *peripheral sector-shaped* or *quadrant-shaped field defect,* indicating damage to the peripheral nerve fiber bundles, is typical for a papillitis and may precede the loss of central visual acuity. These defects may even break through toward the central field and merge with central or paracentral scotomas to form one large defect. In order to give a complete description of these characteristic disturbances of the visual function, it should be added that there may be a *complete or almost complete recovery of the central vision and the field defects* within a few days or weeks. This is in contrast with the defects found in chronic atrophic papilledema. This is not the place to go into detail concerning the numerous etiologic factors that may be responsible for a papillitis, except for a reminder that a great percentage of all cases are caused by disseminated sclerosis. We do want to stress that an acute or chronic *iridocyclitis* is occasionally accompanied by a secondary papillitis, which may resemble a choked disc. We have personally observed such cases that had been referred as a suspected brain tumor—primarily because of an alarming unilateral loss of vision with disc swelling.

Electrophysiologic examinations are an additional aid in the differential diagnosis of papilledema and papillitis. In papillitis, there is a distinct decrease of frequency of subjective fusion, an increase of the retinocortical time, an absent or delayed specific evoked cortical response on illumination of the affected eye, and sometimes a supernormal ERG.

*In summary, it can be stated that every case of optic disc edema—regardless of how much the ophthalmoscopic appearance resembles a papilledema—must be interpreted as a papillitis if there are early disturbances of the central vision, central scotomas, or sector-shaped or quadrant-shaped visual field defects or both.*

*Juxtapapillary chorioretinitis (Jensen).* Juxtapapillary chorioretinitis is a *peculiar type of chorioretinitis,* a simultaneous inflammation of the choroid and retina, that does not involve the entire fundus, but shows a predilection for the immediate surroundings of the disc and may come in actual contact with it and the nerve fibers. There is an *edematous swelling of the papilla* and its immediate surroundings that could be mistaken for a papilledema or a papillitis. The similarity with the latter can be even more striking because damage to nerve fiber bundles may produce either a central scotoma or a sector-shaped field defect. The parapapillary lesion has a moldly grayish green color in its early stages that changes to a bright yellow and finally becomes white with vicarious heaping of black pigment. This typical picture of a choroidal atrophy, together with its location, should help to clarify the situation. There may be other similar foci, either in the acute or in more advanced stages (the latter pigmented!), scattered over the fundus that will also reveal the true nature of this lesion. More specific diagnostic signs such as posterior vitreous opacities and keratic precipitates, cells, and an aqueous flare in the anterior chamber are of interest only to the ophthalmologist. They may aid greatly in establishing the diagnosis. Toxoplasmosis seems to be a frequent cause of this type of chorioretinitis. We know from personal experience that juxtapapillary chorioretinitis is not only of theoretical interest in the differential diagnosis of the papilledema. We have seen a patient who had been referred because of a suspected unilateral papilledema. The ophthalmoscopic findings of a subsequently developing atrophic parapapillary choroidal scar that showed an extensive marginal accumulation of pigment enabled us to make the proper diagnosis (Fig. 2-28). Sometimes juxtapapillary chorioretinitis, even after healing, may lead to a residual chronic disc swelling (reactive glial tissue growth) that resembles congenital pseudoneuritis or pseudopapillitis (Hoyt and Beeston).

Juxtapapillary chorioretinitis has a typical fluorescein angiogram. Corresponding to the clinically visible edema, the disc and the focus close to the disc fluoresce even before the dye enters the retinal vessels. The retinal vasculature fills and empties the dye in a normal fashion. The fluorescein in the disc and the peripapillary area increases, and the peak of fluorescence occurs in the center of the inflammatory focus. This results in an irregular area of fluorescence lasting for a considerable period of time. This area shows a peculiar feathery, blurred margin and encompasses the entire clinically visible edema, including the disc.

*Isolated tuberculosis of the nerve head.* Isolated tuberculosis of the nerve head is a rare condition that, however, may be easily mistaken for a papilledema. There is a more or less pronounced edema of the papilla. In contrast to a true papilledema, it is of a striking whitish, spotty appearance. Furthermore, the swelling is quite uneven, with nodular prominences of different sizes. The papillary border is conspicuous by its uneven outline. There may be tonguelike projections of the edema into the retina. The disc is covered by a veillike membrane with several perforations that allow visualization of more or less indistinct parts of the nerve head in addition to sharply outlined areas. The veins are dilated. There are numerous hemorrhages on the disc and in the retina. Characteristic is a rapid breakdown

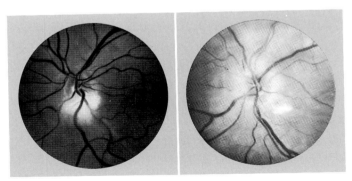

**Fig. 2-28.** Juxtapapillary chorioretinitis (Jensen) with disc edema. Left photograph shows small chorioretinitic patch that extends to lower part of disc. Right photograph shows diffuse edema of disc with venous engorgement, small linear hemorrhages in nerve fiber layer between 5 and 6 o'clock, and as a probable cause, chorioretinitic patch at inferior temporal margin (marked loss of vision, sectorlike defect in visual field).

of the visual functions. Duke-Elder considers the diagnosis of a tubercle of the nerve head very difficult, even in the presence of a simultaneous granulomatous iridocyclitis or an active tuberculosis elsewhere in the body. He observed several cases where enucleation became necessary. Only the histologic examination of the globe revealed the true nature of the condition.

We have the record of a patient with Boeck's sarcoid who showed abnormalities of the disc very similar to papilledema. Boeck's nodules buried in the depth of the disc may have been responsible for this misleading ophthalmoscopic picture. Sometimes the disc forms one yellowish white mass with an irregular surface, pronounced neovascularization, and a prominence of 5 diopters or more. The differential diagnosis of a real tumor or a tuberculoma of the nerve head may be extremely difficult (positive Kveim test in sarcoidosis!).

**Vascular optic neuropathy.** The vascular edemas include malignant hypertensive retinopathy, occlusion of the central vein, ischemic papillitis, edema of the disc in emphysema, and edema of the disc in anemias and leukemias.

*Malignant hypertensive retinopathy.* Aside from papillitis, edema of the papilla in patients with malignant systemic hypertension is probably the most important and most common entity to be considered in the differential diagnosis of choked disc (Fig. 2-29). One of the most important reasons is that the *edema of the disc in patients with hypertensive retinopathy practically always occurs bilaterally.* A number of systemic symptoms common to both conditions (for instance, headache, vomiting, vertigo, and cerebral vascular accidents causing hemiplegias, aphasias, and other neurologic complications) are responsible for optic disc edema in patients with malignant hypertensive retinopathy too frequently being diagnosed as a choked disc. Quite frequently, patients suffering from malignant hypertension with bilateral edema of the papillae are referred to the department of neurosurgery as having suspected brain tumors. Reasons for these referrals are based either on the ophthalmoscopic findings alone or on additional cerebral complications.

Disc swelling in malignant hypertensive retinopathy may closely resemble acute or chronic papilledema in brain tumor; under both circumstances, increased diameter of the papilla, blurring of the disc margins, prominence of the nerve head, deflection of the vessels at the disc margin, exudates, and hemorrhages within the papilla or the adjacent retina may occur. In contrast to papilledema in brain tumors, the disc swelling in malignant hypertension manifests a lighter, even anemic color, but no capillary dilatation and no telangiectasias. The retinal veins seldom appear significantly dilated in disc edema caused by malignant hypertension. Narrowing of the arteries and arterioles occurs only in late atrophic stages of papilledema, but is a constant and important sign in all stages of hypertensive edema of the papilla. The elevation of the optic disc is not a criterion of diagnostic value; it can go as far as 6 diopters in hypertensive retinopathy! Like papilledema, hypertensive disc swelling after appropriate treatment may disappear completely and may, if left untreated for long periods, also lead to severe optic atrophy with functional disturbances. In contrast to papillitis, hypertensive disc swelling and papilledema can be differentiated with the ophthalmoscope.

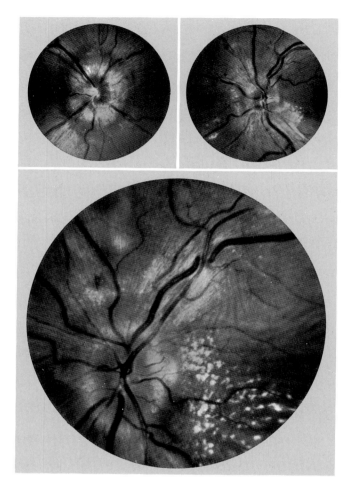

**Fig. 2-29.** Edema of papilla in patient with malignant hypertensive retinopathy (severe systemic hypertension). Disc swelling similar to chronic papilledema. Prominence and edematous imbibition of discs with enlargement of their diameter. Blurring of disc margins and deflection of retinal vessels at disc margins. Slight congestion and tortuosity of veins. Arteries show extensive attenuation with irregularities in their caliber; in places they are threadlike with silvery reflex stripes (silver wire arteries). Distinct Gunn's signs at arteriovenous crossings. Peripapillary retinal edema, with patches of ischemic cloudiness of retina. Soft, fluffy, white cotton-wool exudates, in addition to yellowish white foci of lipoid and fatty nature, especially in macular region. Isolated streaklike and punctate hemorrhages. Diastolic pressure of ophthalmic arteries, O.U. 120 gm (Bailliart)! Left illustration corresponds to right eye and right illustration to left eye.

The diagnosis should be based on the *unmistakable vascular changes* resulting from hypertension and the renal damage as well as the secondary retinal lesions representing the *retinopathy* proper. These pathologic signs are missing in patients with papilledema, but are absolutely pathognomonic in those with malignant hypertension. The vascular changes apply primarily to the *arteries* and consist of generalized *narrowing* of caliber with considerable localized irregularities. The angiospasm may become so severe that the arteries can scarcely be recognized. The increasing sclerosis of the intima and the proliferation and hypertrophy of the media cause marked thickening of the vessel wall, with narrowing and obscuring of the blood column. The wall reflexes increase in brightness until the stage of *silver wire arteries* or even segmental obliteration is reached. Because of the rigidity and the increased tension of the arteries, *Gunn's sign* will appear at the arteriovenous crossings: the vein appears indented at the point of the crossing, with a tapering of both the distal and proximal adjacent sections; there may even be some arching (Salus' sign). In even more advanced stages the angiospasm may extend to the veins (which are seldom significantly dilated), with caliber variations if they are only partially involved. The retinal changes proper, which are only rarely missing (if so, perhaps only in the initial stages) in patients with malignant hypertension, are just as important in making the diagnosis. The increased arterial pressure leads to extravasations of varying sizes and forms, mostly near the vessels. In contrast to the choked disc, the *hemorrhages* are not only on or near the disc margin, but quite characteristically extend far into the fundus periphery. Some of the retinal changes are soft, grayish white, fluffy *cotton-wool* exudates in the superficial retina that, in contrast to the white spots of the papilledema, do not appear on the disc but in the surrounding retina. There are also hard yellowish white punctate *exudates* deep within the retina that have a fatty and lipid nature, that show a predilection for the macular area, and that appear as sharply outlined, pointed, brilliant dots. Frequently, they form a macular star or show a wreathlike arrangement around the macula (circinate retinopathy). If such a macular star is incomplete, it may quite closely resemble the fan-shaped arrangement of the intraretinal droplets seen in papilledema (Fig. 2-8).

Ophthalmodynamometry is quite helpful for differentiating papilledema and edema of the papilla in hypertensive retinopathy. It has been stressed already that the blood pressure of the ophthalmic arteries in fully developed papilledema shows either a normal or even an abnormally low value (p. 117). *In malignant hypertension an abnormally and even discordantly high diastolic pressure in the ophthalmic arteries is a constant sign.*

In summary, it can be stated that *edema of the papilla in hypertensive retinopathy* (although it closely resembles a choked disc) *can be differentiated with some degree of certainty from papilledema on the basis of the characteristic vascular and retinal changes.* Sometimes the retinal changes and hemorrhages may be minimal or even absent despite pronounced disc swelling.

In these cases the presence of the characteristic hypertensive arteriolar changes will help to distinguish optic disc edema in malignant hypertension from papilledema caused by brain tumor. One still has to consider the *possibility of the co-existence of malignant hypertension and brain tumor!* If the ophthalmoscopic findings leave any doubt, the findings of a general physical examination, including blood pressure, urinalysis, nonprotein nitrogen determination, and tests for kidney function, should confirm the diagnosis. We recall a number of hemiplegic patients in whom the question of whether or not there was a papilledema caused by cerebral tumor or malignant hypertension had to be considered quite seriously. In every patient the exact evaluation of the ophthalmoscopic findings, especially proof of arterial and retinal changes, clarified the situation and eliminated the need for unnecessary neuroradiologic examination or even neurosurgical intervention.

Together with hypertensive malignant retinopathy, some quite similar ophthalmoscopic pictures should be mentioned, for instance, in *Kimmelstiel-Wilson syndrome* in patients with diabetes, *Fahr's malignant sclerosis, retinopathy of pregnancy*, and *secondary renal hypertension after chronic glomerulonephritis, pyelonephritis, amyloidosis*, and *periarteritis nodosa*. Frequently in such patients, we find pronounced optic disc edema resembling a choked disc. In the differential diagnosis the same considerations as in malignant hypertensive retinopathy are valid.

*Occlusion of the central vein.* The process of occlusion of the central vein is usually unilateral. A blockage of the venous drainage may at times cause quite a severe edema of the disc, with prominence of the latter and numerous other signs that are common in papilledema. The diagnosis is not difficult, if one is cognizant of the *enormous venous congestion* and the distinct corkscrewlike tortuosity of the veins, but most of all the *massive extravasations extending far into the periphery of the fundus.* The dominant factor in the ophthalmoscopic picture of an occlusion of the central retinal vein is the hemorrhages over the swollen disc and the surrounding retina, which mostly show a radial arrangement. Also typical and unmistakable are the immediate disturbances of the visual function caused by macular hemorrhages and interference with the arteriolar circulation (Figs. 2-30 and 2-31). A chronic disc swelling resembling unilateral papilledema and sometimes persisting for months may result from primary inflammation of retinal veins, leading to central vein occlusion *(papillophlebitis* or *optic disc vasculitis)* that occurs in young adults and manifests only minimal loss of vision. Characteristic is the enormous dilation and tortuosity of the veins and the presence of retinal hemorrhages in and around the disc and especially along the veins. The affection leaves discrete partial sheathing of the veins (sign of resolved phlebitis) and sometimes newly formed venules on the surface of the disc, which may resolve the edema completely (Hoyt and Beeston). Venous pressures are close to or equal the arterial diastolic pressure when measured by ophthalmodynamometry (Lubow).

*Edema of the disc seen in hemorrhages into the sheaths of the optic nerve* after fractures of the base of the skull (especially if the optic canal is involved) should also be mentioned. Its probable cause is an impediment of the venous circulation. We have observed one case. The appearance of the disc differs little from that of a choked disc (Fig. 2-32). There are, however, early disturbances of the conductivity of the involved optic nerve. In some patients, there is an immediate or early amaurosis following the trauma. After a few weeks, there is invariably an optic atrophy with partial or complete loss of vision, unless such an event has been prevented by neurosurgical interference. In most cases, however, a hemorrhage into

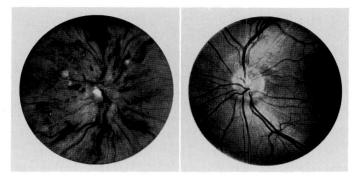

**Fig. 2-30.** Right central vein occlusion in 41-year-old patient. Right papilla shows edematous cloudiness, swelling, and blurring of entire disc margin with insignificant prominence of 0.5 diopter. Edema of surrounding retina. Veins markedly dilated and engorged with enormous tortuosity, in some areas protruding over level of retina. Massive hemorrhages on disc extending into fundus periphery. Isolated white exudates on disc and in retina. Left illustration corresponds to right eye and right illustration to left eye.

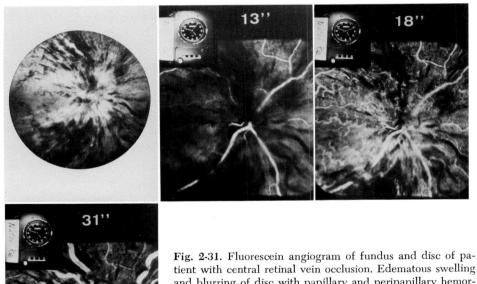

**Fig. 2-31.** Fluorescein angiogram of fundus and disc of patient with central retinal vein occlusion. Edematous swelling and blurring of disc with papillary and peripapillary hemorrhages, veins engorged with tortuosity. Distinctly delayed fluorescein filling of retinal arteries. In late venous phase, staining of veins and permeation of dye into surrounding disc tissue. Capillary stasis, although present, should not be confused with congested capillary vessels (including microaneurysms) of fully developed papilledema (see Fig. 2-9).

the sheaths of the optic nerve does not produce an edema of the disc, but merely functional disturbances of the optic nerve with no primary changes of the disc. Only after weeks is there a primary optic atrophy with a sharp outline of the disc margin. Papilledema with possible hemorrhage in the optic nerve sheaths in intracranial hemorrhage is late in its development and of relatively low degree.

*Ischemic papillitis.* To the vascular group of disc swellings of noncerebral origin also belongs *ischemic papillitis* (apoplexia papillae, vascular pseudopapillitis, ischemic edema of the disc), which occurs especially in elderly patients with arteriosclerosis and hypertension, but sometimes also in younger individuals with collagen vascular diease (polyarteritis), temporal arteritis, carotid occlusion, or diabetes. The disc swelling resembles that of ordinary inflammatory papillitis, but there are some characteristics that cannot be overlooked and help to confirm the diagnosis: the pale color of the disc from the beginning that changes within a few days to a whitish, nearly avascular pallor; feathery hemorrhages between the nerve fiber

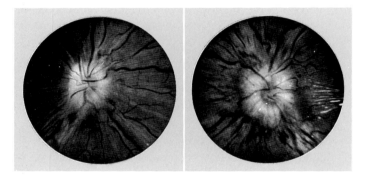

Fig. 2-32. Bilateral papilledema with beginning atrophy in 19-year-old patient with hemorrhage into sheaths of optic nerve caused by a fall on a concrete floor. Contusion of brain. Conspicuous pallor of edematous, swollen discs. Radial folding of surrounding retina. Beginning left "macular star." Severe impairment of sensory functions. Reduced visual acuity to 0.1 O.U. Bilateral concentric contraction of visual fields. Left illustration corresponds to right eye and right illustration to left eye.

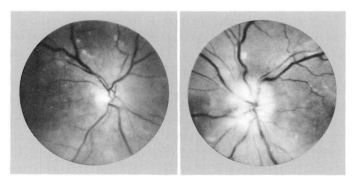

Fig. 2-33. Left ischemic "papillitis" in 85-year-old patient with general arteriosclerosis. Pale avascular swelling of disc with no capillary stasis, narrowed sclerotic arteries, slight prominence, and completely blurred margins (infarction of nerve head). After a few weeks, edema disappeared, leaving snow-white disc. Visual acuity remained at original level of 0.1.

bundles; no capillaries visible on the disc; distinct narrowing of the arterioles at their exit from the disc; and moderate dilation of the major veins (Fig. 2-33). Ischemic papillitis, the result of total or segmental infarction of the optic nerve head (the result of occlusion of one or more of the posterior ciliary arteries), usually produces rapid impairment of central vision and fascicular visual field defects (especially inferior quadrantanopia or inferior altitudinal hemianopia), which shows a poor or no chance of recovery. Fluorescein angiography reveals the absence of filling of the posterior ciliary circulation in the optic disc and peripapillary choroid (Hayreh). Bilateral forms of ischemic papillitis may occur, most often in the sense that the second eye becomes involved after an interval of some weeks or months or even later. The disc swelling on the one side and the optic atrophy on the other side (as a product of the earlier attack, when the edema of the nerve head has subsided) may produce a *pseudo-Foster Kennedy syndrome*. The leading symptoms, described previously (narrowed arterioles in both fundi, visual loss in both eyes, the field defects indicating bilateral optic nerve involvement, and also the history of the affection), speak against a brain tumor genesis. Thus by careful ophthalmologic examination, further neuroradiologic examination or even neurosurgical intervention can be avoided (Bonamour, Brégeat, Bonnet, and Juge; Rintelen).

*Edema of the disc in emphysema.* There have been reports of cases of emphysema in patients with chronic bronchitis (usually during the stages of cardiac insufficiency) that show a bilateral edema of the disc, together with an increased pressure of the cerebrospinal fluid (Simpson; Cameron). The appearance of such cases is similar to that of choked discs. We observed such a picture in one of our patients with a similar condition (Fig. 2-34). The cause

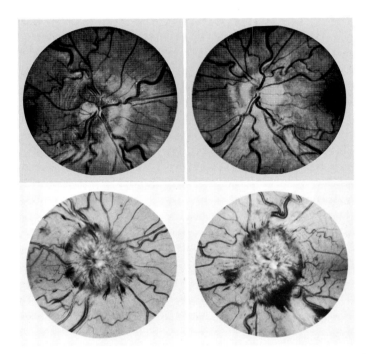

**Fig. 2-34.** Above, Edema of discs in 40-year-old patient with bronchiectasis and cardiac insufficiency (marked cyanosis and polycythemia). Below, Massive disc swelling in 32-year-old patient with chronic pulmonary heart disease caused by bronchial asthma. Note striking resemblance to papilledema as a result of increased intracranial pressure (capillary stasis, venous engorgement, hemorrhages, white "exudates," etc.).

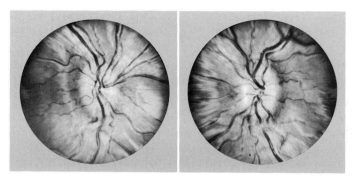

**Fig. 2-35.** Papilledema (bilateral) in 12-year-old boy suffering from leukemia (leukemic meningitis with increase of intracranial pressure). Prominence, blurring, venous engorgement of both discs, but no signs of leukemic retinopathy. Latter finding favors a diagnosis of true papilledema caused by increased intracranial pressure and not local infiltration of disc tissue by leukemic cells. Left illustration corresponds to right eye and right illustration to left eye.

of the elevated pressure of the cerebrospinal fluid supposedly is a decreased concentration of oxygen and an increased concentration of carbon dioxide in the blood (hypercapnia), which may cause dilation of the cerebral veins. For these optic disc edemas the term "hypoxic optic neuropathy" has recently been introduced (Lubow).

Based on a similar mechanism are the edemas of the disc (usually not very pronounced) seen occasionally in patients with congenital or acquired *valvular defects of the heart* with a severe venous congestion. The enormous dilation of the veins as well as the unmistakable cyanosis of the retina should make the diagnosis easy (Fig. 2-34).

*Edema of the disc in anemias and leukemias.* We have seen a case of bilateral edema of the papilla resembling choked discs in a patient with acute anemia following a hemorrhage. This hemorrhage resulted from anticoagulant therapy. No signs of increased intracranial pressure could be demonstrated. Similar edemas of the disc have been described in leukemias, chlorosis (Jaensch; Huber; and others), macroglobulinemias, and polycythemias. In anemias the probable mechanism for papilledema is a combination of hypoxic optic neuropathy and optic disc edema resulting from increased intracranial pressure caused by cerebral edema (Lubow).

The disc swelling with *leukemias* manifests three different forms that, with regard to the ophthalmoscopic appearance, have no special characteristics. All types and grades of swelling may be observed. The first form represents the disc swelling accompanying leukemic retinopathy; it is characterized by scattered retinal and preretinal hemorrhages, an edematous retina, and typical venous engorgement. The second form represents local infiltration of disc tissue by leukemic cells and is accompanied by more or less pronounced visual defects as a sign of affection of the nerve fibers. The third form is a real papilledema caused by increased intracranial pressure in connection with a "meningoneuroleukosis" that develops after treatment with antimetabolites, even in the phase of clinical and hematologic remission of the disease (Huber; Hamard) (Fig. 2-35).

## Congenital anomalies of the disc resembling papilledema (pseudodisc edemas)

Neither the ophthalmoscopic appearance nor the pathologic-anatomic findings indicate an edema of the disc or papilledema. There are only certain similarities in the morphologic appearance of the optic disc, which anybody acquainted with these anomalies should recognize as being different from

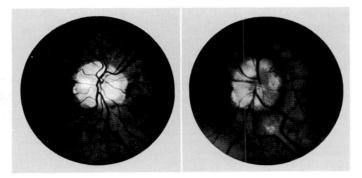

**Fig. 2-36.** Combination of drusen of discs with papilledema in case of giant tumor of right frontal lobe in 37-year-old patient. Right disc shows a few exposed drusen in lobulated surface of atrophic disc. Left disc is edematous, prominent, and enlarged, with isolated hemorrhages at disc margin. Absence of edema on right side and choked disc on left side represent type of Foster Kennedy syndrome! Left illustration corresponds to right eye and right illustration to left eye.

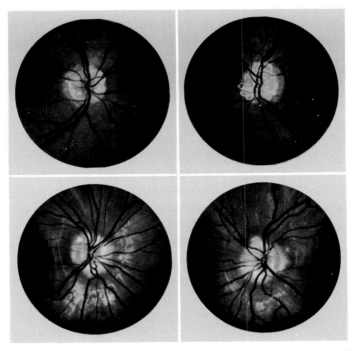

**Fig. 2-37.** Bilateral drusen of discs. Above, Exposed drusen that appear as yellowish white, sagolike granules and cause lobulated surface of disc. Below, Drusen are buried in depth of discs except for a few superficial ones. Swelling, enlargement, and slight prominence of discs. Absence of venous congestion! (See Fig. 2-15.) Left illustrations correspond to right eye and right illustrations to left eye.

papilledema. Unfortunately, *these elevated disc anomalies are sometimes confused with real papilledema, and thus the suspicion of a brain tumor may lead to unnecessary and unjustified diagnostic procedures or even neurosurgical interventions.* On the other hand, one must not forget that there is always the possibility of the coexistence of such congenital elevated disc anomalies and a brain tumor (Fig. 2-36); however, in such cases the general nonocular symptomatology will most often help make the right diagnosis. In doubtful cases in which a neurosurgical investigation is not yet indicated because of lack of neurologic signs, examining the patient at regular time intervals and, if possible, taking fundus photographs (colored, red-free, etc.), possibly combined with fluorescein angiography of the retina, are recommended.

**Drusen of the optic disc ("hyaline bodies").** The deposition of granular hyaline-like substances in the disc may lead to a swelling, enlargement, and prominence of the papilla that could be mistaken for a papilledema. This is especially true in those cases in which the hyaline drusen are situated in the depth of the disc and cannot be recognized with the ophthalmoscope (Fig. 2-37), which is mostly the case in children. An occasional enlargement of the blind spot, arcuate scotomas, or peripheral, mostly nasal field defects (occurring first only in early adult life) or obscurations may contribute to the possibility of such a mistake. Also, these drusen of the optic disc usually involve both sides (Fig. 2-38). The following observations should help to overcome some of the diagnostic difficulties.

In distinct contrast to the reddish discoloration of papilledema, drusen give the disc a yellowish color. There is a complete absence of venous and capillary dilation, exudates, and hemorrhages (only exceptionally will papillary or peripapillary bleeding occur)—an important and absolutely reliable sign. As a result of the deposition of the granular hyaline substances, the surface of the disc frequently assumes an irregular, nodular appearance that is especially pronounced if isolated drusen extend to the disc margin and lie exposed on the *surface* of the disc. *In such a case the disc margin shows nodular excrescences, with the drusen being visible as glassy, yellowish white, sagolike grains—findings usually sufficient to make the correct diagnosis.* With multiple drusen at the disc margin, the nodular appearance of the surface is characteristically described as "mulberry-like." The peripapillary retinal pigment in some areas is eroded and looks "moth-eaten." Premature branching and other anomalies of retinal arteries are common. If one suspects drusen, a search should always be made for these superficial translucent hyaline grains, which are usually at the disc margin. Both fundi should always be examined, for the drusen may be completely hidden on one side but quite superficial on the other side. By means of posterior slit-lamp microscopy and with the use of a contact lens, it is occasionally possible to visualize hidden drusen of the disc. These drusen of the optic disc are frequently hereditary (irregular dominance).

The hyaline bodies of the optic disc can usually be recognized with fluores-

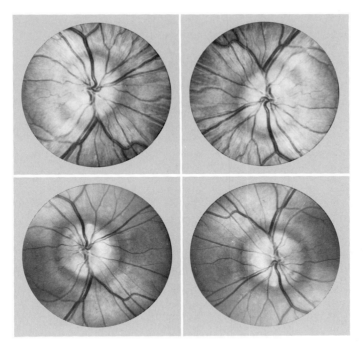

**Fig. 2-38.** Bilateral drusen of optic disc. Above, Buried intrapapillary drusen producing anomalous disc elevation ("pseudopapilledema") in 4-year-old boy with hypermetropia of 7 diopters. Below, Optic discs of same patient 10 years (!) later, indicating exposed intrapapillary drusen, especially on nasal side of disc and in some places "moth eaten" appearance of pigment epithelium surrounding disc. Good demonstration of gradual exposure of buried drusen over period of 10 years. Left illustrations correspond to right eye and right illustrations to left eye.

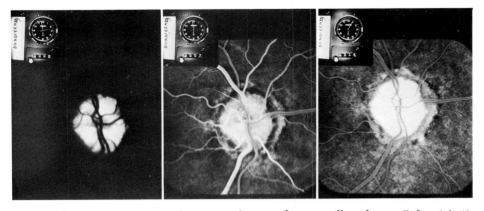

**Fig. 2-39.** Fluorescein angiogram of patient with exposed intrapapillary drusen. Before injection of fluorescein, there is intensive apparent "spontaneous" fluorescence of drusen (left). In arterial and venous phases (middle and right), no capillary stasis is visible; rather a lack of small vessels in disc tissue. Moderate staining of disc tissue. Characteristic polycyclic margins of slightly enlarged disc.

cein angiography. The primary fluorescence of these drusen, which can be seen in the preliminary photographs taken before the injection of the dye, is important (Fig. 2-39). Drusen do not take the dye, but show their sharp polygonal outlines during the entire angiogram. The hypoplastic glial tissue of the disc may take the dye to a moderate degree, usually with irregular intensity. This, however, is never as intensive or as long lasting as the fluorescence that occurs in papilledema or papillitis. There is absolutely no capillary stasis. Deep-lying drusen are often better visualized with fluorescein angiography than with the usual ophthalmoscopy.

Drusen of the optic disc are also seen in tuberous sclerosis (hyaline bodies also in the retina!), optic atrophy, pigment degeneration of the retina, angioid streaks (associated with pseudoxanthoma elasticum), or high hyperopia. According to the investigations of Chalmers and Walsh, a brain tumor in the presence of drusen is very unlikely. Among several hundred cases of brain tumors, they found only one patient with drusen of the optic disc. Our own observations are in agreement with the findings of these authors (Fig. 2-36). It is interesting that intrapapillary drusen occur especially in children (Fig. 2-39). With increasing age, the hyaline bodies seem to expose themselves first near the border and later on the whole surface of the disc as well, although some drusen remain deeply situated and invisible with the ophthalmoscope throughout life. These remarks explain the frequent occurrence of manifest exposed drusen in the parents and of anomalous disc elevations (often first interpreted as pseudoneuritis or pseudopapilledema) caused by submerged intrapapillary drusen in their children (Hoyt and Beeston).

A 22-year-old girl had a pronounced swelling of one optic papilla, although without venous congestion or hemorrhages. The suspected drusen of the optic disc (hidden drusen) could be confirmed by the finding of manifest bilateral drusen in the mother (upper photographs in Fig. 2-37).

In summarizing, we can state that *hidden intrapapillary drusen of the optic disc could be mistaken for papilledema.* The absence of dilation of the veins or of hemorrhages as well as the yellowish color of the disc are valuable criteria in the differential diagnosis. Frequently, drusen manifest themselves by the nodular appearance of the surface of the disc. Their typical appearance corroborates the diagnosis. Examination of other members of the same family may furnish valuable diagnostic data. In the discussion of *chronic papilledema* (p. 123), yellow, hyalinized exudates simulating congenital drusen were mentioned. These *drusenlike bodies* near the margins of the elevated, pale, atrophic disc are easily differentiated from real drusen if one considers the typical aspect of chronic atrophic papilledema with capillary telangiectasias, pallor and gliosis of the disc, narrowing of the arterioles, perivascular sheathing, and finally concentric contraction of the visual fields.

**Pseudoneuritis and pseudopapilledema (with or without tortuosity of the retinal vessels).** The terms "pseudoneuritis" and "pseudopapilledema" are used for anomalies of the disc that may resemble either a papillitis or a papilledema. Since our previous discussion should have made it clear that there is great similarity between the morphologic picture of papillitis and papilledema, we would like, for simplicity's sake, to dispense with a distinction between these pseudoforms and to discuss pseudoneuritis and pseudopapilledema as one entity. Practical experience has taught us that *such a distinction* is artificial unless one reserves the term "pseudoneuritis" for the description of elevated anomalies of the optic disc combined with mildly defective visual functions and anomalous retinal vessels and the term "pseudopapilledema" for anomalous elevation of the disc without any visual field defects and signs of visual impairment.

The terms "pseudoneuritis" and "pseudopapilledema" indicate a congenital anomalous elevation of the disc consisting of hyperplastic glial tissue interlacing among the nerve fibers. As a consequence, the nerve fibers appear raised, and the ensuing picture is that of a blurred, enlarged, and occasionally elevated disc. Sometimes hyperplastic glial tissue overhanging the edge on one side is found with *tilting of the optic disc* ("supertraction" papilla). *Two forms* can be distinguished: *one without and one with vascular anomalies.* If the vessels appear normal, the pseudopapilledema (or pseudoneuritis), in contrast to the genuine papilledema, shows a more grayish white opaque discoloration. Edema of the optic nerve head and congestion of the capillary network are characteristically missing. The disc is usually only slightly or not at all prominent and appears to be rather firm and compact. In the other form, the one with the vascular changes, in addition to the characteristic findings just described, there are a marked *tortuosity and anomalous early branching of the vessels,* the arteries as well as the veins. Sometimes an excess number of vessels is also present. The veins, however, are of normal caliber or only moderately dilated (Fig. 2-40). Despite this

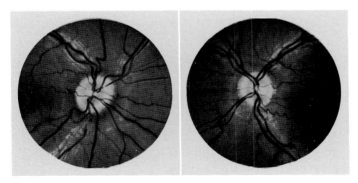

**Fig. 2-40.** Pseudopapilledema (pseudoneuritis) of right eye with tortuosity of vessels. Right disc is barely enlarged, compact, and not edematous and has relatively distinct margins. Veins, like arteries, are tortuous but not congested. Premature branching of arteries and veins. No hemorrhages. Size of blind spot is normal! Left illustration corresponds to right eye and right illustration to left eye.

tortuosity, their course remains in the same layer of the retina. This is the reason why the hue of their color does not change, in contrast to the choked disc, in which bright sections of the vessels alternate with dark ones. Hemorrhages and white spots are missing entirely. Papilledemas show a certain relationship between the degree of elevation and blurring of the disc on the one hand and the tortuosity of the vessels on the other hand. In the pseudoforms,

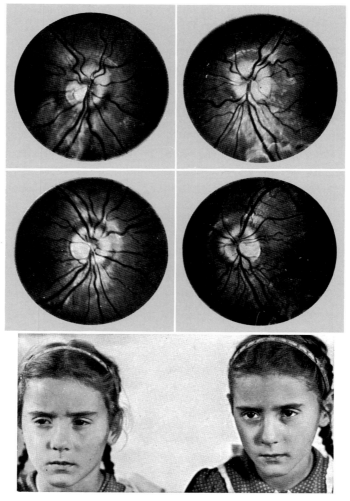

**Fig. 2-41.** Pseudoneuritis or pseudopapilledema (congenital blurring of disc margins; "supertraction" of papilla) in both eyes of identical twins. Upper photographs belong to twin on left and lower ones to twin on right. Blurring and elevation, especially of nasal halves of discs. Tortuosity of vessels. There is an amazing similarity of twins to smallest morphologic details of fundus! Upper left illustrations correspond to right eye and upper right illustrations to left eye.

there is always a more pronounced tortuosity in comparison with the elevation of the disc. *The size of the blind spot is completely normal, a characteristic sign that differentiates it from a true choked disc!* The visual functions are usually intact, although pseudoneuritis is sometimes accompanied by mild amblyopia. Pseudopapilledema is a congenital anomaly that may frequently involve several members of a family or that may even occur as a hereditary trait (Fischer). We have observed pseudoneuritic changes in both eyes of *identical twins;* both had a bilateral myopia of 4 to 5 diopters. Ophthalmoscopic examination revealed a distinct blurring and elevation of the discs (especially on the nasal side) with tortuosity of the vessels (Fig. 2-41). The myopia has been mentioned purposely; frequently one hears the opinion expressed that pseudopapilledema or pseudoneuritis occurs only in persons with high hyperopia. This is only a conditional truism. We have records of 11 cases of pseudoneuritis in which nine of the patients show a *hyperopia* between 2 and 15 diopters. The hyperopia is not necessarily one of a high degree; it may be quite moderate. In two patients, we found a unilateral pseudoneuritis (Fig. 2-42). In one patient with pseudoneuritis, we found a pronounced brachycephaly and an arched palate. Here we would like to call attention to a certain relationship between pseudoneuritis and *malformations* of the skull. Also, Uhthoff's observation that pseudoneuritis occurs twice as often in patients with mental disease as in normal individuals should be mentioned. The occasional unilateral occurrence of a pseudoneuritis plays an important part in the differential diagnosis of unilateral choked disc (p. 120).

Pseudoneuritis and pseudopapilledema in general show no pathologic change on fluorescein angiograms (Fig. 2-43). This differentiates them unequivocally from papilledema or papillitis. The fluorescein picture is that of a normal fundus. There are only a few vessels visible on the disc and these are of normal caliber.

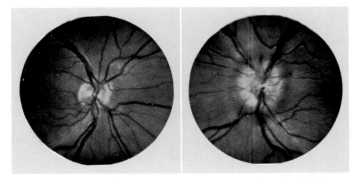

**Fig. 2-42.** Hyperopic pseudoneuritis ("congenital glial hyperplasia") of left eye. Right eye is emmetropic and left shows hyperopia of 5 diopters. Picture is similar to that of papilledema; however, there is no venous congestion! Left illustration corresponds to right eye and right illustration to left eye.

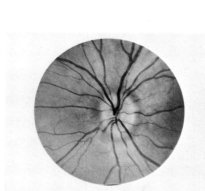
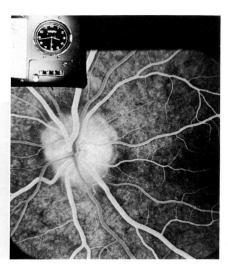

**Fig. 2-43.** Fluorescein angiogram of patient with pseudoneuritis ("pseudopapilledema") of papilla. Left, Appearance of pseudoneuritic disc with slightly blurred margins, discrete prominence, but no capillary stasis and no venous engorgement. Right, Fluorescein angiogram of same disc; it behaves like normal disc and manifests no capillary stasis and no signs of increased permeability of vessels as does real papilledema.

The late fluorescence is minimal and lasts only a short time after the vessels have emptied. It is advisable to repeat the fluorescein angiogram (including color and red-free photographs) at regular intervals when beginning papilledema has to be differentiated from a pseudopapilledema.

*The diagnosis of pseudoneuritis or pseudopapilledema is not always easy.* It is no coincidence that there are so many cases of this anomaly in our series. The patients were referred to the neurosurgical clinic as suspected of having choked discs and brain tumors. A thorough examination revealed completely negative results. These cases of pseudoneuritis have to be *carefully observed for some time* before the correct diagnosis can be made. One should not forget that most of the cases of pseudoneuritis or pseudopapilledema in children represent *intrapapillary drusen* that only later in adult life become exposed and can be diagnosed as such. Repeated perimetric examinations of the blind spot and photographs of the eyeground at certain intervals aid enormously in making the correct diagnosis. *One should always take heed of the principle that every patient with pseudoneuritis or pseudopapilledema should be suspected of having papilledema until proved otherwise—that is, when there is no increase in the intracranial pressure.*

**Medullated nerve fibers.** Normally the medullary sheaths of the fibers of the optic nerve begin immediately behind the lamina cribrosa. Occasionally they may extend distally to the papilla and the adjacent retina. They can be recognized as snow-white, flame-shaped stripes that seem to originate from the upper or lower disc border. Thus the disc may appear enlarged

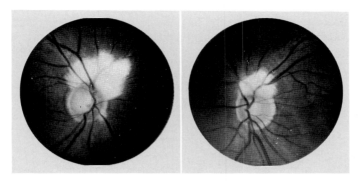

**Fig. 2-44.** Medullated nerve fibers of both eyes of same patient. Feathered edges of myelinated patches are especially obvious on right side. Left illustration corresponds to right eye and right illustration to left eye.

and its outline blurred. This picture conceivably could be mistaken for a papilledema. However, anybody who has seen the extraordinarily characteristic appearance of medullated nerve fibers even once is not likely to make such a mistake (Fig. 2-44). It is well known that medullated nerve fibers are often associated with ocular malformations such as epipapillary membranes, persistent prepapillary glial tissue, congenital tortuosity of the vessels, and prepapillary vessel loops. Enlargement of the blind spot or localized relative scotomas may be registered in the visual fields. Of course, a real papilledema caused by increased intracranial pressure may be superimposed on medullated nerve fibers, and the primary condition of the altered disc manifests itself only after corresponding treatment.

Anomalies of the retinal vessels. Although *tortuosity and anomalous early branching of the retinal vessels* have been mentioned previously in connection with pseudoneuritis and pseudopapilledema, they actually should be included as congenital anomalies in this discussion.

There are congenital vascular anomalies of such extraordinary morphologic variety that some of them might simulate a papilledema, especially if they are localized very close to or directly on the disc. Most of all, we should mention the *arteriovenous aneurysms (racemose angiomas* or *cirsoid aneurysms) of the retina,* which show an incredible variety in their ophthalmoscopic aspects, as pointed out by Wyburn-Mason. *The finding of a visible connection between an artery and a vein* (either a direct connection or via a distinct, markedly dilated capillary network) is important and decisive for the diagnosis. Such an arteriovenous shunt causes widening and tortuosity of the veins in one form or another, which contrasts distinctly with the caliber of the arteries. If such an arteriovenous rete mirabile is located near the disc or directly on it, it may cause an edematous blurring, an indistinction of the disc margin, and some prominence of the papilla—signs that may be similar to a papilledema. The protrusion of such a disc usually is minor. The venous congestion and, last but not least, the dilated capillary network in the area of the disc are very closely related to the changes that occur in papilledema. The arteriovenous communication, however, can always be found with careful ophthalmoscopic examination. This should confirm the diagnosis of an arteriovenous aneurysm (Figs. 2-45 and 2-46). Sometimes some larger vessels are sheathed by white tissue neoformation, and in some cases the periphery of the fundus may be covered by grapelike aneurysms surrounded by hard, white exudates (Hoyt and Beeston).

We personally observed an instructive case of a 24-year-old girl who had been referred by a neurologic clinic because of a suspected meningioma of the olfactory groove and a unilateral "choked disc." All neurologic findings were negative. An EEG revealed nothing unusual. After careful ophthalmoscopic examination, the changes of the disc that had been interpreted as "choked disc" turned out to be a typical arteriovenous aneurysm of the retina, or rather the papilla (Fig. 2-46), with a distinctly dilated capillary network interpolated between an artery and a vein, in addition to several arteriovenous shunts.

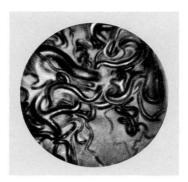

**Fig. 2-45.** Arteriovenous aneurysm of retina in left eye of 12-year-old girl. Enormous dilation of veins and arteries form convolution covering disc. There was also an arteriovenous plexus within orbit (Wyburn-Mason syndrome).

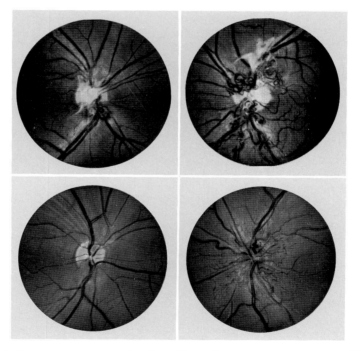

**Fig. 2-46.** Arteriovenous aneurysms of retina. Above, Racemose aneurysm at papillary margin with distinctly visible arteriovenous shunts in 43-year-old patient. Below, Racemose aneurysm with very fine vessels immediately above left disc of 24-year-old patient; it resembles a low degree of papilledema. Left illustrations correspond to right eye and right illustrations to left eye.

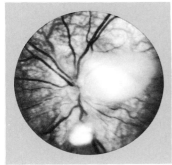 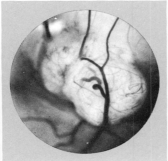 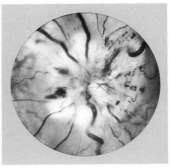

**Fig. 2-47.** Tumors of disc simulating papilledema. Left, Congenital tumorlike malformation of disc (not verified histologically). Middle, Malignant melanoma involving disc. Right, Bronchogenic carcinoma metastatic to optic disc and nerve (first diagnosed as acute papillitis because of sudden functional loss, unilateral disc swelling, and edema; only association with other intraocular and extraocular metastases led to correct diagnosis!).

It may be of interest to mention that such *arteriovenous aneurysms of the retina are occasionally associated with similar lesions of the optic nerve, the orbit, the maxilla, and mandible, or the brain* (basifrontal area, sylvian fissure, posterior fossa, or midbrain). This may explain the occurrence of supranuclear conjugate gaze palsies and bilateral ptosis that has been described in cases of arteriovenous aneurysms of the retina (Wyburn-Mason syndrome).

**Tumors of the disc.** In rare cases, it can happen that tumors of the disc (gliomas, meningiomas, neurinomas, neurofibromas, metastatic tumors) are misinterpreted as papilledema. The predominantly unilateral occurrence should caution against such a diagnosis. The same is true for malignant melanomas of the choroid near the disc, with secondary invasion of the latter. We have observed a few such malignant melanomas of the disc. The conspicuous pigmentation of such a prominent structure, its size, and its eccentric position with regard to the vessel trunk usually lead to the correct diagnosis (Fig. 2-47). In rare instances of *von Hippel–Lindau disease* an angiomatous hamartoma (hemangioma) may be located directly in the center of the disc and thus simulate papilledema. One should always search for other angiomas far peripherally in the retina and not forget the possibility of the coexistence of similar angiomatous hamartomas in the cerebellum and other organs (kidney, pancreas, etc.).

## PARESES OF EXTRAOCULAR MUSCLES

In addition to papilledema, increased intracranial pressure caused by a brain tumor may cause a few other ocular signs and symptoms that, likewise, are of no localizing significance. One should be cautious not to use them as a basis for a hasty conclusion regarding the site of the space-consuming cerebral process. Cushing actually called a *unilateral paresis or the more rarely occurring bilateral pareses of the sixth nerve a "false localizing sign,"* a statement repeated by Collier and Gassel. It seems that the sixth nerve, because of its long intracranial course, is particularly vulnerable. Displacement of the brain stem by the tumor may easily cause it to be tugged in exposed areas. Cushing has called attention to an important anatomic deviation. Normally, the sixth nerve lies between the dura and the branches of the basilar artery after it emerges from the pons. In a certain number of cases, however, it lies for a short stretch between these vessels and the pons. An increased intracranial pressure may cause a compression of the sixth nerve between the pons and branches of the basilar artery, especially the inferior anterior cerebellar artery. The result is a partial disturbance of the conductivity of the nerve with a corresponding *weakening in the action of the lateral rectus muscle of the ipsilateral eye.*

If the paresis is severe, diplopia will occur even in the primary position, but will be noticeable only on lateral rotation of the involved eye in the case of a mild paresis. The diplopia is horizontal and homonymous. (For details about diagnosis and symptomatology of sixth nerve paresis, see p. 38.) If the intracranial pressure decreases, the nerve may recover its function and the paresis may recede. These variations in the intracranial pressure explain the daily or even hourly "fluctuations" of a sixth nerve paresis as occasionally observed in patients with brain tumors. Pathologic-anatomic investigations have demonstrated conclusively that the compression of the sixth nerve between the pons and the branches of the basilar artery causes some damage to the nerve (Fig. 2-48).

In addition to the point at which the sixth nerve leaves the pons, there is another vulnerable area during its extended course along the base of the skull.

1, Superior orbital fissure
2, Trigeminal nerve (first and second branches)
3, Oculomotor nerve
4, Trochlear nerve
5, Posterior cerebral artery
6, Cerebellum
7, Vertebral artery
8, Upper ridge of petrous portion of temporal bone
9, Sixth nerve

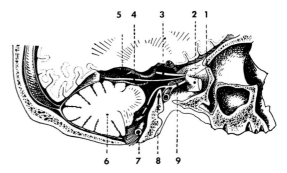

Fig. 2-48. Vertical section through base of brain and skull to demonstrate intracranial course of sixth nerve. Bend over sharp upper ridge of petrous bone is marked by arrow.

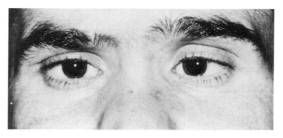

Fig. 2-49. Left sixth nerve paresis caused by increased intracranial pressure in a case of sagittal sinus thrombosis.

If a tumor displaces the brain stem inferiorly, superiorly, or posteriorly, it may tug on the nerve at the sharp superior ridge of the petrous bone. The displacement of the brain stem can be caused by supratentorial as well as by infratentorial tumors and has no relation to the side where the space-consuming lesion is located. Therefore a paresis of the sixth nerve (which usually is unilateral) will not permit any conclusions regarding the site of the tumor causing the increased intracranial pressure (Fig. 2-49).

In summary, it can be stated that *a unilateral sixth nerve paresis occurring during the development of a brain tumor is without value whatsoever for purposes of localization* (except when it is a component of a topically important syndrome, as, for instance, the superior orbital fissure or the cavernous sinus syndrome) (Fig. 2-49); *it is merely a general sign of increased intracranial pressure*. However, a bilateral sixth nerve paresis and one that occurs during the early stages of a space-consuming lesion is of decisive value and is highly suggestive of an intrapontine focus.

A paresis of the trochlear nerve does not occur merely as a nonspecific general sign of increased intracranial pressure. Also, nonspecific pareses of the extrinsic muscles supplied by the oculomotor nerve are rare. They may occur only in the terminal stages of a severely increased intracranial pressure (p. 39). There are, however, *nonspecific pupillary disturbances* caused by increased intracranial pressure. They are most likely to occur if the oculomotor nerve is pressed against the clivus ridge of the tentorial notch or the medial petroclinoid ligament. They will be discussed in the following section in connection with the transtentorial herniation syndrome.

## TRANSTENTORIAL HERNIATION

Similar to a sixth nerve paresis resulting from increased intracranial pressure is a *unilateral lesion of the oculomotor nerve that is manifested by a fixed mydriatic pupil*. It is part of the transtentorial herniation syndrome—another general sign of increased intracranial pressure, especially of a high or an acute degree. Actually, the basic lesions of the sixth and oculomotor nerves are quite similar in nature, with only a gradational difference in the resulting pictures. In the case of the sixth nerve, there is only a paresis of the corresponding lateral rectus muscle, since there are no other fibers. In the case of the oculomotor nerve, on the other hand, the pupillomotor fibers are impaired first as a result of their particular vulnerability. Occasionally, this is actually the only sign of the impairment. At least in the early stages, there is no paresis of any of the extrinsic muscles, but only a unilateral fixed mydriasis. However, in contrast to unilateral sixth nerve paresis, which has no localizing significance, the *unilateral fixed mydriatic pupil is highly suggestive of an ipsilateral or a predominantly unilateral space-consuming supratentorial process*.

The ipsilateral mydriatic fixed pupil is only one sign of a broader and more comprehensive clinical picture, namely, progressing *brain stem dysfunction associated with transtentorial herniation;* in addition to the somatic components (that is, the oculomotor paresis, cardiorespiratory signs, pyramidal tract symptoms), there is a *psychic component* in the form of varying degrees of *disturbances of consciousness.* Thus we have a combination of ocular and systemic signs of increased intracranial pressure in the transtentorial herniation syndrome. The disturbances of consciousness are brought about by pressure damage and circulatory disturbances in the diencephalon and mesencephalon.

An increase in intracranial pressure may be compensated under certain conditions by various mechanisms (Fig. 2-50). Expulsion of cerebrospinal fluid from the internal and external cerebrospinal fluid spaces is the most important one. If the space available in the supratentorial area is no longer capable of containing the expanding process, *herniation of the soft brain occurs through the only possible passage between the supra- and infratentorial spaces, that is, through the tentorial incisura.* In this *transtentorial herniation* first the midbrain, then the temporal lobes, especially the hippocampal gyrus and uncus, participate. As most supratentorial space-occupying processes (tumors, epidural or subdural hematomas) are predominantly or exclusively unilateral, such a herniation is more pronounced on one side than on the other and leads to *lateral displacement of the brain stem* with compression (ischemic and hemorrhagic lesion of the brain stem), to *compression of the posterior cerebral artery,* and to *oculomotor nerve damage.* The latter will be discussed in detail subsequently.

Compression of the brain stem as a consequence of transtentorial herniation results in hemorrhages, especially in the midbrain and upper pons. The clinical signs of *midbrain–upper*

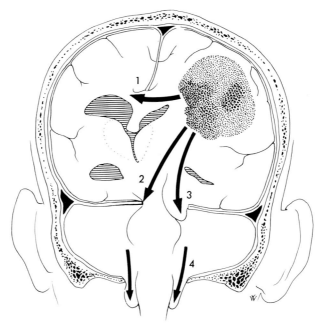

**Fig. 2-50.** Diagrammatic representation of distortion of brain caused by growth of brain tumor (parietotemporal area). *1,* Sideward displacement of falx and ventricles; *2,* caudal displacement of brain stem (including midbrain) through tentorial incisura and pressure against clivus ridge; *3,* transtentorial herniation of hippocampal gyrus through tentorial aperture; *4,* downward displacement of brain stem and herniation of cerebellar tonsils into foramen magnum.

*pons impairment* are temperature fluctuations, respiratory disorders (Cheyne-Stokes respiration or central hyperventilation), dilatation and rigidity of the pupils, dissociated ocular movements with signs of internuclear ophthalmoplegia, and deterioration of motor functions (bilateral decerebrate rigidity). In the syndrome of uncal transtentorial herniation the early stages are characterized by oculomotor nerve damage (unilateral dilatation and sluggish reactions of the ipsilateral pupil), whereas midbrain damage occurs only in the late stages and progresses quickly to the disastrous symptoms mentioned above.

Compression of the posterior cerebral arteries or branches as a result of transtentorial herniation may lead to *occipital cortical hemorrhagic infarctions* with homonymous field defects. Such homonymous hemianopias secondary to transtentorial herniation can be observed in patients with acute supratentorial pressure increases (Hoyt). In epidural or subdural hematomas, such homonymous hemianopias have a distinct localizing value (similar to the homolateral pupil dilatation), although they must also be considered false localizing signs.

In 1867 Hutchinson was among the first to describe unilateral fixed mydriasis in connection with cerebral traumas. Since the original observations, a number of investigators have become interested in the origin and mechanism of this clinical sign and its importance in the recognition of the site of an acute intracranial space-consuming lesion (McKenzie; McNealy and Plum; Plum and Posner; Zülch). There is almost unanimous agreement among the various authors that the ipsilateral fixed mydriasis is caused by *pressure on the peripheral oculomotor nerve* (particularly the smaller, more vulnerable pupillomotor fibers) and not by stimulation of the sympathetic fibers (Scharfetter).

How can increased intracranial pressure cause a specific lesion of the oculomotor nerve? There are two possibilities that may occur in a number of com-

**U,** Uncus of hippocampal gyrus (**Hip.**) of temporal lobe (**Tp.**)
**R,** Gyrus rectus of frontal lobe with orbital sulcus (**F. orb.**)
**H,** Oblique position of pituitary stalk (displaced from left to right side)
**Car.,** Internal carotid artery
**Co. post.,** Posterior communicating artery
**Cb. sup.,** Superior cerebellar artery
**Impr. T.,** Tentorial notch
**B,** Pons
**Bas.,** Basilar artery
**C.P.,** Posterior cerebral artery

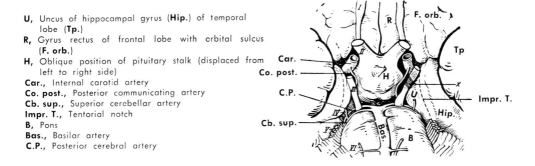

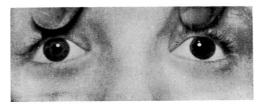

**Fig. 2-51.** Transtentorial herniation syndrome of left oculomotor nerve in 25-year-old patient with petechial hemorrhages distal to area of pressure. Abscess of left side of frontal lobe with breakthrough into ventricle. Below, Clinical picture of syndrome. Fixed mydriatic pupil of left eye, with slight outward deviation of left eye, a sign of paresis of left medial rectus muscle.

binations (Zülch; Fischer-Brügge): (1) *the third cranial nerve may be pushed against the ipsilateral clivus ridge of the tentorial notch by increased intracranial pressure to one side or strangulated at the medial petroclinoid ligament* and (2) *the oculomotor nerve may be compressed immediately after its emergence from the inner surface of the cerebral peduncle between the posterior cerebral artery and the superior cerebellar artery.* The anatomic-pathologic manifestation of such a compression of the nerve consists of a pressure groove (Fig. 2-51) on the caudal surface of the nerve or, more rarely, of a vessel groove (cranial surface of the nerve). Just as important as the groove formations are circulatory disturbances. Frequently, there are patches of extravasation in the area of the oculomotor nerve distal to the point of compression, manifest signs of interference with the blood supply. *It is just this interference with the intraneural and perineural blood circulation that explains satisfactorily* the frequently only transitory nature of *the pupillary signs of the transtentorial herniation syndrome.* They are known to recede completely, for instance, immediately following a decompression or even subsequent to an intravenous injection of a hypertonic saline, glucose, mannitol, or urea solution in the treatment of a cerebral edema, together with a simultaneous clearing of the consciousness.

In the clinical picture of the transtentorial herniation syndrome, four stages can be distinguished.

The *first stage* shows a *narrowing of the ipsilateral pupil,* which might be considered an irritation of the oculomotor nerve preceding the lesion (Tönnis). This miosis on the side of the lesion is, however, quite transient and for that reason quite easily overlooked.

The *second stage* is by far the most frequent and the one phase that can be observed longest during the course of progressively increasing intracranial pressure. *The pupil is dilated but will still react to light and in convergence.* Occasionally, a slight ptosis can be seen. The patient's sensorium is either completely free or already shows a suggestion of somnolence.

The transition to the *third stage* manifests itself by an increasingly *sluggish reaction of the dilated pupil* and a beginning loss of the pupil's regular shape. With the increase in the intracranial pressure, the somnolence and apathy of the patient become more severe and terminate in complete *coma* (impairment of diencephalon and midbrain). The *pupil* becomes *mydriatic, irregular,* and *completely fixed to light.* During this stage, not only the oculomotor fibers supplying the pupil, but also those supplying the extrinsic muscles may be impaired. There may be *pareses of the extraocular muscles supplied by the third cranial nerve.* The eye shows a mydriatic fixed pupil, sometimes ptosis, and assumes a divergent position (Fig. 2-51).

During the *fourth* (terminal) *stage* the contralateral pupil becomes mydriatic and fixed to light, obviously on the basis of midbrain damage in connection with uncal herniation.

*In general the unilateral fixed mydriatic pupil is a nonspecific sign of gen-*

*erally increased intracranial pressure of higher degree or acute nature.* For this reason, it has been discussed with the general symptoms. The cause may be a space-consuming process (tumor, abscess, or hemorrhage, especially a subdural or epidural hematoma) in the supratentorial region or an edema accompanying a hemispheric tumor. This is definitely a remote effect of a space-consuming process on the oculomotor nerve. The expansion of the supratentorial content causes downward displacement of the brain stem and the compression of the third cranial nerve previously described.

In *tumors of the temporal lobe,* there is a *local effect* in addition to the remote effect. Frequently, the hippocampal gyrus and uncus on the tumor side are forced into the tentorial notch. The result is a so-called *herniation of the temporal lobe into the tentorial notch,* which may cause a compression of the oculomotor nerve by direct pressure. We were able to observe unilateral fixed pupils particularly frequently in our patients with temporal lobe tumors. We can assume a direct pressure effect on the oculomotor nerve in tumors close to the diencephalon, especially craniopharyngiomas.

Although the transtentorial herniation syndrome, with its striking sign of a unilateral fixed mydriatic pupil should be primarily considered a general sign of increased intracranial pressure, it may be of localizing value for certain tumor sites (for instance, tumors of the temporal lobe, p. 185). Thus the discussion of this syndrome leads to a discussion of focal symptoms in the next chapter.

*In conclusion, we can state that a unilateral mydriatic fixed pupil is usually a general sign of increased intracranial pressure caused by pressure damage to the oculomotor nerve.* This pupillary sign is seen on the ipsilateral side with unilateral supratentorial space-consuming lesions. With temporal lobe tumors, it may be either a general sign of increased intracranial pressure or a local sign (herniation of the temporal lobe into the tentorial notch). The pupillary disturbances are part of a more extensive picture, the transtentorial herniation syndrome, which includes, apart from cardiorespiratory signs and pyramidal tract symptoms, also disturbances of consciousness.

## EXOPHTHALMOS

In Chapter 1, it was stated that a *bilateral exophthalmos* (more rarely, a unilateral exophthalmos) may be a general sign of increased intracranial pressure (p. 16). This is less a simple protrusion of the globes than an "extrusion" of the entire orbital contents—obviously the result of the transmission of the increased intracranial pressure through the orbital fissures into the orbits or the result of pressure effects on the cavernous sinus (Skydsgaard). Among our cases, bilateral exophthalmos as a general sign of increased intracranial pressure has been observed especially in patients with expansive parasagittal meningiomas, meningiomas of the falx, and tumors with a tendency to early hydrocephalus formation (for instance, cerebellar tumors and tumors of the third and fourth ventricles). This exophthalmos is usually quite inconspicuous and can be easily overlooked in certain cases, perhaps because it is of no diagnostic and particularly no localizing value. A bilateral exophthalmos also cannot be evaluated properly with the customary instruments intended for relative exophthalmometry.

A *unilateral exophthalmos* may result from the remote effect of an intracranial growth (Elsberg, Hare, and Dyke), *but should be primarily considered a local orbital sign.* One should consider here primarily orbital processes, but also brain tumors of the anterior and middle fossas, which may cause an exophthalmos by direct invasion of the orbit or indirectly by interference with the drainage of the ophthalmic vein or the cavernous sinus (Figs. 1-4, 1-5, 3-81, 3-88, and 3-96).

*In conclusion, it can be stated that a bilateral exophthalmos occurs occasionally as a general sign of increased intracranial pressure, but that it is irrelevant for clinical diagnostic purposes.*

# THREE

## Local signs and symptoms of brain tumors

The classification of the signs and symptoms of brain tumors into general ones caused by increased intracranial pressure and local or focal signs and symptoms was suggested in the introductory remarks to Chapter 2 (p. 92). *The local signs and symptoms are those that originate from localized damage to a definite brain area and thus assume definite significance for purposes of localization.* It has been stressed that, as a rule, the chronologic sequence of the two groups of signs and symptoms is as follows: the focal signs and symptoms, according to the lesion of a certain part of the brain, appear first, to be followed by the general signs and symptoms of increased intracranial pressure caused by the remote effect of a growth gradually increasing in size and the reactive edema and swelling of adjacent structures. This chronologic development is true for the majority of brain tumors. Thus the local signs and symptoms assume exceptional diagnostic importance. If they per se are not absolute proof of a neoplasm of the brain, *their steady progressiveness (with possible periods of quiescence, but seldom remissions or improvements) is, in fact, among the principal signs and symptoms of an intracranial tumor.* In 1904 Collier postulated that *local signs and symptoms occurring in the late stages of a brain tumor are unreliable.* Thus one should make an assiduous search for early signs and symptoms in patients with progressive cerebral deficits and, if possible, elicit them by taking a careful case history. In a certain number of patients with brain tumors the local signs and symptoms are so conspicuous and alarming that they may motivate an examination or even surgical interference before general signs or symptoms develop. It has also been mentioned that there are some tumors in silent zones of the brain and others with a tendency to cause an early internal hydrocephalus with general signs and symptoms of increased intracranial pressure as the first, or perhaps even the only, symptom.

What has been said in a general way with regard to the local signs and symptoms of brain tumors is also true in a stricter sense for the ocular local signs and symptoms in brain tumors. The nature of the visual sensory organ may cause even small circumscribed lesions of the visual pathway to develop distinct disturbances of vision. Early ocular local signs and symptoms in patients with brain tumors are therefore of decided significance for purposes of localization. The importance of some of these signs and symptoms, however, varies and depends on the site of the tumor, that is, its relation to the visual apparatus. Thus pareses of the extrinsic muscles supplied by the oculomotor nerve are usually quite significant, whereas pareses of the lateral rectus muscle (especially if they are unilateral) are generally of no value for purposes of localization but have to be considered as a general sign of increased intracranial pressure. Visual field disturbances in patients with brain tumors usually represent defects that are valuable for the localization of the lesion. It is rare for remote effects of brain tumors to cause visual field changes (occipital lobe infarction as a consequence of transtentorial herniation!) that could be mistaken for those of a focal nature. If at all, this usually occurs in the late stages. It should be clear that the ocular local signs and symptoms in patients with brain tumors assume diagnostic significance only in their relationship with other neurologic local signs and symptoms. *We ophthalmologists should therefore appraise ocular local signs and symptoms only as part of the entire clinical picture.* The importance of the ocular local signs and symptoms in the overall picture varies a great deal with the location of the tumor. The ocular signs and symptoms may be the outstanding feature, may be of equal significance with other signs and symptoms, or may be a subordinate accompanying sign or symptom of other neurologic symptoms. It certainly would be a mistake to discuss only ocular local signs or symptoms in this presentation. *We consider it our duty to assign the ocular local signs or symptoms in brain tumors to their proper place within the framework of the entire clinical picture.* For this reason, we plan to give a brief summary of the other neurologic signs and symptoms for each symptom complex according to its topographic basis and to point out their proper relationship with the ocular signs and symptoms.

The ocular local signs and symptoms and their diagnostic significance will be discussed from the topographic point of view (Fig. 3-1). The brain tumors will be classified into supratentorial and infratentorial groups. The *supratentorial* group consists of the hemispheres with their frontal, temporal, parietal, and occipital lobes, the pituitary gland and its surrounding area, the anterior and middle fossa, the diencephalon, including the third ventricle, the thalamus, the basal ganglia, and the midbrain. The *infratentorial* group includes tumors of the cerebellopontine angle, the cerebellar hemispheres, the cerebellar vermis, the pons, and the medulla oblongata. Tumors in the mesencephalon may expand in a supratentorial or infratentorial direction. They will be discussed in the concluding discussion of the supratentorial group.

The classification of the tumors into supratentorial and infratentorial groups is used for didactic reasons. It is also based on the symptomatologic difference between tumors of these two groups and, last but not least, on the difference of their surgical accessibility. Also, the so-called tentorium cerebelli forms a definite natural barrier between the supratentorial and infratentorial spaces of the cranium. In its middle section the cerebellar tentorium shows an opening of the

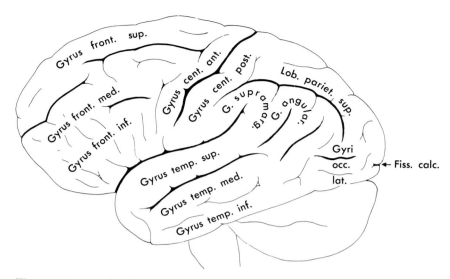

**Fig. 3-1.** Topography of cerebral lobes, gyri, and sulci: convexity of left hemisphere.

dura, the so-called tentorial notch. The stalklike brain stem passes through this opening. Even though the tentorial notch causes a certain discontinuity of the tentorium, the latter presents a mechanically effective barrier that creates a fairly sharp separation between the supratentorial and infratentorial contents of the cranium. A growth in the infratentorial area is not likely to extend into the supratentorial space. The membrane of the tentorium protects the occipital lobe against direct invasion by a tumor as well as, to some extent, against the pressure effect from cerebellar or paracerebellar tumors. The tentorium especially forms the lateral dividing line between the infratentorial and supratentorial region. It lies between the cerebellar hemispheres and the poles of the occipital lobes. In the region of the brain stem the separation line coincides with the isthmus, that is, approximately the area where the mesencephalon passes into the rhombencephalon. This area roughly corresponds to the anterior cranial part of the fourth ventricle.

*A topographic discussion of the ocular local signs and symptoms of brain tumors is essential because in numerous patients the ocular signs and symptoms suggest a definite site for the tumor. In other words, they are of localizing value.*

In the diagnosis of brain tumors, it is equally important to determine the *nature* of the tumor, especially in view of possible surgical intervention. Certain histologic types of intracranial tumors show a specific and characteristic symptomatology. Some of them (for instance, pituitary adenomas, craniopharyngiomas, and some meningiomas, for example, meningiomas of the tuberculum sellae and the sphenoid ridge) also cause specific ocular local signs and symptoms. In the majority of patients with brain tumors, however, ocular signs and symptoms, if present at all, do not depend on the type of tumor. Following the topographic discussion of the ocular signs and symptoms, we propose to touch briefly on the relationship between the histologic structure of the tumors and their ocular local signs and symptoms. This chapter should aid in the initial and differential diagnosis of the various types of tumors.

## SUPRATENTORIAL TUMORS
### Tumors of the frontal lobe

In patients with tumors of the frontal lobe the mental changes dominate the picture. Such changes may manifest themselves either in the form of a more or less characteristic psycho-organic syndrome or occasionally as local signs of a frontal lobe syndrome. The latter may be described as lack of impulse (for movement, speech, and thinking), apathy, striking changes in social behavior, euphoria, and occasionally a peculiar silly jocularity (moria). In frontal lobe tumors, with their pronounced tendency to relatively early increase of intracranial pressure, the mental changes may be mixed with disturbances of consciousness in such a way that their differentiation is sometimes almost impossible. Obviously as a result of loss of inhibitory action on the frontopontine tracts, a motor phenomenon appears that is known as forced grasping or groping—a sign that is almost pathognomonic for frontal lobe lesions, especially those of large size with extension into the corpus callosum or the basal ganglia. It consists of a violent grasping movement of the hand and the fingers if an object is placed into the hand. This sign can also be produced by stroking the palm at the proximal end of the fingers. Frontal lobe ataxia is characterized by a tendency to fall forward or toward one side. A lesion in the left lower frontal lobe gyrus (Broca's center) in a right-handed patient causes motor aphasia that is often associated with agraphia. One of the most frequent signs of a frontal lobe tumor is a central paresis of the facial nerve that occurs on the side opposite the tumor. If the damage caused by the tumor extends to the motor cortex of the anterior central region, there may be either signs of irritation in the form of local (jacksonian) or generalized seizures, or there may be signs of paresis or paralysis in the form of a contralateral spastic monoplegia that, depending on the site of the process, are more prominent in the face, the arm, or the leg. The focal motor epilepsy (with turning of the head and the eyes to the side opposite the tumor) as well as the paralyses actually belong to the *syndrome of the anterior central gyrus* but have been mentioned intentionally because we include the anterior central gyrus in the discussion of the frontal lobe. Of interest to the ophthalmologist is the fact that in frontal lobe epilepsy there is a specific motor discharge from the frontocortical adversive field that consists of a spasmodic horizontal conjugate deviation of both eyes to the side opposite the lesion (possibly with turning of the head in the same direction). The corresponding signs in damage of the frontal lobe are a horizontal gaze paresis or palsy to the side opposite the tumor, frequently resulting in a conjugate deviation of the eyes and turning of the head to the side of the lesion (Fig. 1-12). Frontal lobe tumors, especially glioblastomas, and metastatic processes, with their exquisite tendency to increased intracranial pressure, produce acute, chronic, or intermittent transtentorial herniation syndromes characterized by unilateral or bilateral pyramidal tract signs, anisocoria, and sixth nerve and hypoglossal nerve pareses. As just mentioned, these are all signs of a general increase of intracranial pressure, but may in certain cases occur so early or be so prevalent as to lead to severe diagnostic errors (Fig. 3-2).

Because of the relatively distant position of the frontal lobe from the visual pathways, ocular localizing signs or symptoms are rather rare in patients with tumors of this region. They actually appear only if the tumor lies at the base of the frontal lobe and extends into the area of the chiasm. Accordingly, ocular symptoms in patients with frontal lobe tumors are usually uncharacteristic and are frequently manifestations of a generally increased intracranial pressure. Pa-

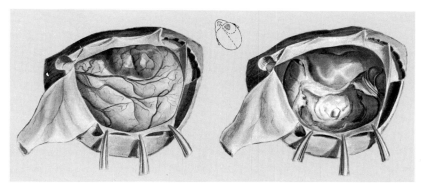

**Fig. 3-2.** Malignant astroblastoma of right frontal lobe in 47-year-old patient before and after extirpation (frontal lobectomy).

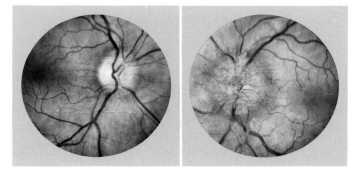

**Fig. 3-3.** Foster Kennedy syndrome in 32-year-old patient with frontobasal astrocytoma on right side. Fully developed papilledema with blurring and mushrooming of disc (note distinct capillary stasis) on left side, and slight nasal blurring and slight temporal atrophy of disc on right side. Visual acuity, O.D. finger counting; O.S. 1.0. Marked concentric contraction of right visual field, and normal visual field on left side.

tients occasionally complain of double or foggy vision, glittering before the eyes, dark spots suddenly occurring on one side, or formed figures in a certain part of the visual field. The topical symptoms, however, are considerably more important! These are complaints ranging from *unilateral loss of visual acuity to amaurosis.* We have seen this in a number of patients whose conditions assumed various forms of the Foster Kennedy syndrome (Fig. 3-3). However, it should be stressed that in a little more than one half of the patients with frontal lobe tumors, no ocular symptoms were present.

To draw a true picture of the ocular signs and symptoms, we want to emphasize that numerous tumors, even if they reach considerable size, may show no signs whatsoever that would implicate the visual apparatus. We have 46 verified cases of frontal lobe tumors on record (glioblastomas, astrocytomas, oligodendrogliomas, meningiomas, metastases). In two thirds of the patients (31), there are absolutely no visual changes—an observation that is in agreement with the statistics of Guillaumat and Robin. In about one third (17) the fundi of both eyes were completely negative (that is, not even a papilledema could be found as a general sign of increased intracranial pressure). Such figures speak for themselves. We should be aware *that the ocular symptomatology of frontal lobe tumors is frequently disappointing.*

In the literature the localizing value of the *Foster Kennedy syndrome* is often stressed. It consists of a primary optic atrophy with a central scotoma on the side of the tumor and a papilledema on the opposite side (Fridenberg; Glees). It must be assumed that the unilateral optic atrophy results from direct pressure on one optic nerve between the optic foramen and the chiasm by a tumor situated at the base of the lobe with a backward extension. It is a well-known fact that an atrophic optic nerve will not develop edema. Hence an increased intracranial pressure will manifest itself only on the side of the intact nerve. *Such a textbook case of a fully developed Foster Kennedy syndrome did not occur in any of our cases.* In the discussion on unilateral papilledema (p.

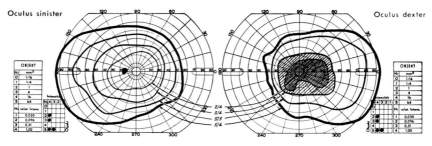

**Fig. 3-4.** Hemangioblastoma of right frontal lobe with compression of right optic nerve (optic atrophy!). Visual field on side of tumor shows slight constriction of peripheral isopters as well as large relative central scotoma. (Case of Dr. Guillaumat; from Dubois-Poulsen.)

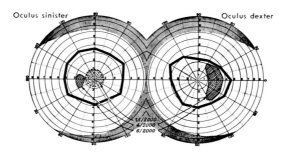

**Fig. 3-5.** Glioblastoma multiforme of left frontal lobe. Slight concentric constriction of peripheral visual fields. Enormous enlargement of right blind spot (choked discs). Left relative central scotoma.

120), it was stated that there are numerous incomplete forms of this syndrome that occur more frequently than the typical picture. Thus we found a unilateral primary optic atrophy with sharp borders of the disc, concentric constriction of the peripheral visual field, and a central or cecocentral scotoma in four of 46 patients with tumors (Figs. 3-4 to 3-5). The atrophic papilla was always on the side of tumor. On the opposite side, there was either a completely normal or only slightly blurred nerve head but never a pronounced choked disc. The tumor causing these incomplete forms of the Foster Kennedy syndrome was always situated on the side with the optic atrophy—more precisely at the base of the lobe, with a deep basal expansive growth. In one instance a meningioma originating from the roof of the orbit was seen to surround and compress the ipsilateral optic nerve. *The optic atrophy is the pathologic basis for the subjective sensation of a unilateral loss of vision,* which usually does not escape the patient's attention. In the case of a frontal suprasellar cholesteatoma causing such an incomplete Foster Kennedy syndrome, loss of vision was noted first in the ipsilateral eye 5 years prior to surgical intervention! Originally, a retrobulbar optic neuritis had been suspected. In the discussion of the basal tumors, especially those of the chiasm and its surroundings, we shall meet frequently with instances in which damage to the optic nerve caused by tumor pressure in the initial stage cannot be differentiated from an ordinary retrobulbar neuritis. *Every case of retrobulbar neuritis should be suspected as being caused by tumor compression of the optic nerve if recovery of the visual function is only temporary or does not take place at all and if there is further deterioration of the visual acuity as well as of the visual field.* By the way, it is interesting to note that Foster Kennedy himself talked about a retrobulbar neuritis and a central scotoma with a subsequent primary optic atrophy on the side of the lesion and a papilledema on the other side when he described his syndrome in 1911! We are in agreement with various other authors (David and Sourdille; Dubois-Poulsen; Walsh and Hoyt; Tönnis; François and Neetens) that the value and the topographic significance of the Foster Kennedy syndrome generally is somewhat overrated. We want to state quite emphatically that this syndrome is not pathognomonic for frontal lobe tumors. It is found, for instance, with meningiomas of the olfactory groove (p. 242), meningiomas of the sphenoid ridge (p. 248), and other basal tumors (for instance, suprasellar meningiomas)—all of them tumors that may involve the optic nerve. The value of the Foster Kennedy syndrome is lessened by the fact that even tumors of the third ventricle or the cerebellum can cause similar symptoms by remote effect (for instance, via an internal hydrocephalus and dilation of the third ventricle) and that there are also nontumoral causes (arteriosclerosis, optochiasmatic arachnoiditis). In the very early stages, it is actually not always easy to differentiate a unilateral retrobulbar neuritis from a beginning Foster Kennedy syndrome, particularly since signs of papilledema are usually missing on the opposite side at this stage. Only the bilaterality of the visual field changes will give actual proof of an intracranial lesion. One has to search for the first minute signs of visual field changes in the other eye. Such signs usually consist of minimal losses in the superior temporal quadrant. Dubois-Poulsen is right in pointing out how important it is to search for such field defects of the better eye by repeated tests. In addition to the central scotoma in the eye with the reduced vision, there usually occur during this stage bitemporal superior or perhaps inferior quadrant defects as signs of damage to the crossing fibers of the optic nerves in the area of the median parts of both optic nerves or the anterior angle of the chiasm (Fig. 3-6).

Thus an extension of the tumor into the chiasmal region (eventually also herniation of the gyrus rectus into the anterior chiasmal angle) may cause the development of a *bitemporal hemianopia*. We have observed a tumor of the base of the frontal lobe with extension into the suprasellar region that caused a bitemporal superior quadrantanopia (Fig. 3-6).

An actual *homonymous hemianopia* or homonymous quadrantanopia with distinctly incongruous field defects occurred in our series only twice. The tumor causing these defects expanded from the frontal area into the temporal direction. Guillaumat and Robin recorded such defects in 8% of their patients with frontal lobe tumors. We are convinced that in such cases tumor pressure from above causes a tract hemianopia (Fig. 3-7).

Tumors located in the frontal region may also cause a homonymous hemi-

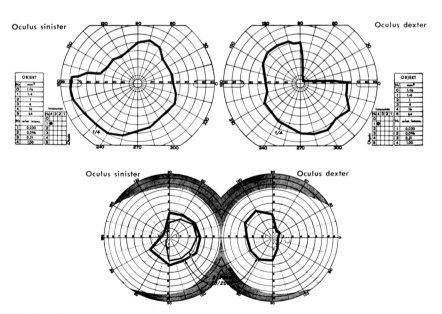

**Fig. 3-6.** Glioblastoma multiforme at base of left frontal lobe with expansion into suprasellar region. Above, Bitemporal asymmetric superior quadrantanopia on Goldmann perimeter. Below, Almost complete asymmetric bitemporal hemianopia on tangent screen. These signs indicate interference of tumor with anterior chiasmal angle.

anopia by remote rather than by direct effect. This is clearly demonstrated by two patients in our series (one with a falx meningioma of the middle third and the other with a parasagittal meningioma of the anteror third of the sinus), both with a distinct homonymous hemianopia. The field defect must be interpreted as a propagation of the pressure caused by the tumor on the optic tract. The mechanism of this propagation is still quite obscure. Possibly, compression against an artery at the base of the skull may lead to such a lesion of the optic tract (Fig. 3-30).

Despite normal fields on the perimeter and tangent screen, one may be able to demonstrate a so-called *pseudohemianopia* (Silberpfennig) in frontal lobe tumors. As a rule, it is associated with a gaze palsy toward the side opposite the tumor or a conjugate deviation toward the side of the tumor. This pseudohemianopia consists of a loss of the visual attention toward the side of the gaze palsy. It is assumed that objects in the missing "field of gaze" do not attract attention despite an intact "visual field" on this side. The asymmetry of this phenomenon alone indicates that it does not result only from a general lack of attention, as frequently seen in patients with frontal lobe tumors. In such patients the fact that, in addition to the voluntary saccadic movements, the optically induced movements (including the optokinetic nystagmus) are impaired in the field of the gaze palsy suggests the following mechanism: the occipital optomotor centers probably function properly only if they are

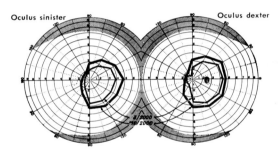

**Fig. 3-7.** Malignant glioma of right frontal lobe with expansion into temporal region. Left homonymous hemianopia with sparing of macula (tract hemianopia?).

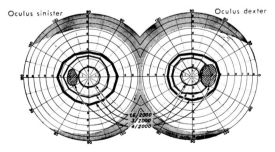

**Fig. 3-8.** Astrocytoma of frontal lobe (edge of pallium) with expansion through falx and corpus callosum toward right side. Enormous bilateral enlargement of blind spot (bilateral choked discs of 5 diopters prominence; amblyopic attacks!). Insignificant concentric constriction of peripheral fields (patient became exhausted rapidly).

adequately coordinated with the frontal oculomotor centers. An object must stimulate some interest before the eyes will fix on it. This interest originates in the frontal centers. It is note-worthy that a gaze palsy as well as a pseudohemianopia can be temporarily improved by an increase in the general attention, by stimulation of the visual attention, and by stimulation of the vestibular apparatus. We have observed a patient with an astrocytoma of the frontal lobe in whom the visual fields for very small white and red targets were normal. However, a crude simultaneous test of both visual fields with the hand demonstrated a distinct visual in-attention on the side opposite the tumor, although without an accompanying disturbance of the conjugate eye movements.

The *scotomas* are on the side of the optic atrophy and may be central, para-central, or cecocentral (either relative or absolute), as previously mentioned. Especially in the early stages, they can be the very first signs of a unilateral lesion of the optic nerve (Fig. 3-4).

A markedly *concentric constriction* or *spiral visual fields* in frontal lobe tumors should be interpreted with caution. Usually, they are the consequence of the general apathy and lack of impulse on the part of the patient (Ecker) (Figs. 3-5 and 3-8).

A unilateral exophthalmos occurred three times in our series. It should be considered a sign of the direct transmission of tumor pressure into the ipsilateral orbit.

It is known that optomotor centers for the horizontal voluntary saccadic gaze movements are located in the posterior part of the second frontal convolution (area 8 of Brodmann). Nevertheless, we were unable to observe gaze palsies, with or without conjugate deviation, in our patients with frontal lobe tumors. However, during epileptic attacks we found two instances of *turning of the eyes toward the side opposite the tumor,* together with a corresponding torsion of the head into the same direction (frontal adversive attack). It is striking that gaze palsies in patients with frontal lobe tumors are so rare and of such short duration. It is possible that the missing conjugate functions are vicariously taken over by the opposite hemisphere after a brief interval.

There are reports in the literature (Silberpfennig) of cases of gaze palsies accompanied by conjugate deviations toward the side of the tumor. Some of the patients show an isolated impairment of voluntary saccadic movements, with intact optically induced pursuit and vestibular movements. Others show impairment of the saccadic (frontal) and pursuit (occip-ital) movements associated with pseudohemianopia. (See previous discussion.) Since a lesion in the occipital area is not likely with a tumor in the frontal region, one must assume in such a case that the occipital gaze mechanism does not function properly because the connection with the frontal oculomotor centers (whose function, among others, is to stimulate interest for objects in the field of fixation) is missing.

*Gaze palsies resulting from frontal lobe lesions are practically always horizontal; ex-tensive bilateral lesions, however, lead to a total absence of saccades (global saccadic paralysis).*

In diffuse frontal lobe lesions, in addition to a horizontal gaze palsy, there may also be an *impairment of optokinetic response.* The fast phase of the optokinetic nystagmus is im-paired, whereas the slow phase (identical to a sort of pursuit movement) remains intact (p. 62).

A true gaze palsy must be differentiated from a motility disturbance caused by *lack of attention* as seen frequently in patients with frontal lobe tumors. The latter, as a rule, is equal on both sides. In addition to an impairment of the saccadic voluntary movements, in lack of attention the pursuit movements characteristically may be more disturbed and in-volved earlier than optically induced movements (Kestenbaum).

Nystagmus in frontal lobe tumors is rare. We have observed it in only four patients (central vestibular, respectively, of cerebellar type). The amplitude was fine, medium, and even coarse. The direction in one patient was toward the side of the tumor and in another toward the opposite side. It should be kept in mind that minor gaze pareses occasionally manifest themselves in the form of nystagmoid movements (gaze paretic nystagmus).

*The general symptoms of increased intracranial pressure in patients with frontal lobe tumors are quite pronounced.* We found bilateral papilledema in one half of the patients, mostly with a prominence of from 1 to 3 diopters and frequently with numerous hemorrhages. More developed papilledema on the side of the tumor occurred in about 20% of the cases, especially in association with meningiomas. A unilateral papilledema without optic atrophy or central scotoma on the opposite side (in other words, without a Foster Kennedy syndrome) occurred twice, both times on the tumor side. There is not an absolute but a considerable correlation between increased intracranial pressure found during surgery and an existing papilledema. Nevertheless, it should be stressed that there are frontal lobe tumors with markedly increased intracranial pressure that will not produce papilledema. Of 27 patients in whom increased intracranial pressure was demonstrated, 10 did not show papilledema. Interestingly, almost none of the meningiomas caused papilledema. *Unilateral sixth nerve paresis* with a corresponding subjective diplopia has been noted only in one tenth of the patients. Bilateral paresis occurred only twice. A *unilateral mydriasis* as part of the transtentorial herniation syndrome previously described was always on the side of the tumor. However, it is a relatively rare sign and occurred only eight times among a total of 46 patients.

*In summary, it can be stated that the ocular symptoms as well as the ocular signs are frequently missing in patients with frontal lobe tumors. Further, the Foster Kennedy syndrome, which is frequently considered almost pathognomonic for an involvement of the frontal lobe, is practically never found in its typical form. It occurs occasionally in an incomplete form, with a unilateral optic atrophy and a contralateral normal or blurred disc if the tumor lies at the base of the lobe and expands toward an optic nerve. Bitemporal field defects result if a tumor expands toward the chiasmal region. Homonymous defects are the direct result of pressure by a tumor on the optic tract from above, or they must be interpreted as a remote effect of a frontal lobe tumor on the tract. Unilateral or bilateral scotomas in frontal lobe tumors are the first signs of a pressure lesion of one or both optic nerves. Frequently, they precede the Foster Kennedy syndrome. The rather rare gaze palsies, with or without conjugate deviation, are occasionally accompanied by a pseudohemianopia (that is, a lack of visual attention in the missing "field of gaze"). General signs of increased intracranial pressure are frequent and pronounced, especially papilledema. Nevertheless, it happens that very large tumors remain completely "silent" as far as ocular general signs and symptoms of an increased intracranial pressure are concerned. Concentric contractions of the visual fields should be evaluated with caution. Usually they are an indication of a general lack of attention on the part of the patient.*

### Tumors of the temporal lobe

The so-called uncinate fits are important as an indication of an irritation of the temporal lobe. These are paroxysmal, usually unpleasant olfactory or gustatory hallucinations of brief duration, which occasionally are accompanied by peculiar sniffing movements or smacking of the lips. These uncinate fits may occur as isolated symptoms or occasionally in association with strange dreamy states. They may even present themselves as the aura of epileptic attacks. These epileptic convulsions dominate the initial clinical picture of temporal lobe tumors and manifest an aura (olfactory, gustatory, optic, acoustic) in about 40% of the cases. Other symptoms of temporal lobe epilepsy are the "déjà vu" or "déjà raconté" phenomena, psychomotor attacks (periods of confusion and abnormal behavior), and paroxysmal optic hallucinations in the form of entire scenes and episodes, which will be described in more detail subsequently. If the tumor is localized in the dominant hemisphere, there may be a sensory aphasia in the form of a disturbed comprehension of speech and word blindness and word deafness, or, if the anterior part of the temporal lobe is involved, a difficulty in finding the proper words in the sense of jargon motor aphasia (Fig. 1-2). However, it must be stressed that also in temporal lobe tumors these local symptoms may often be partially or totally masked by the general signs of increased intracranial pressure, producing not only headache, vomiting, and vertigo but also transtentorial herniation syndromes with consequent compression of the brain stem, characterized by unilateral mydriasis, ptosis, oculomotor or sixth nerve pareses, and pyramidal tract signs. Sometimes, especially in lesions of the right temporal lobe, the signs of increased intracranial pressure represent the whole neurologic symptomatology. The temporal lobe is affected by the same tumor types (glioblastomas, astrocytomas, oligodendrogliomas, and meningiomas) as the frontal lobe (Figs. 3-9 and 3-10).

The number of localizing ocular signs and symptoms associated with frontal lobe tumors is disappointingly small; this situation, however, is quite different in temporal lobe tumors. Even the symptoms alone, if present, may furnish important localizing cues. The major or minor epileptic fits or dreamy states so typical in patients with temporal lobe tumors may be accompanied by *visual hallucinations* in addition to olfactory and gustatory hallucinations. The patient has sensations (usually on the side of the field defect, provided such a defect is present) of objects, scenery, people, animals, or plants—hallucinations of a definite, formed, and highly organized nature, often reenacting scenes of past life, with little relation to the immediate surroundings. Their duration is limited to a few seconds. There are also disturbances of the sensorium of varying, but usually slight, degree. Sometimes the visual hallucinations represent an aura of generalized or jacksonian epileptic attacks. It is assumed that these hallucinations are the result of an irritation of the optic radiation, which is spread out largely in the temporal lobe.

In our own series of 30 patients with temporal lobe tumors, we found olfactory hallucinations relatively frequently (30%). Visual hallucinations were quite rare. Actually, they occurred only twice. In both instances, there were undifferentiated, unformed, and primitive hallucinations in the form of glowing rings,

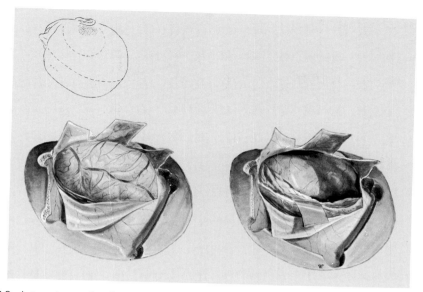

**Fig. 3-9.** Astrocytoma of right temporal lobe in 37-year-old patient before and after extirpation (total right temporal lobectomy).

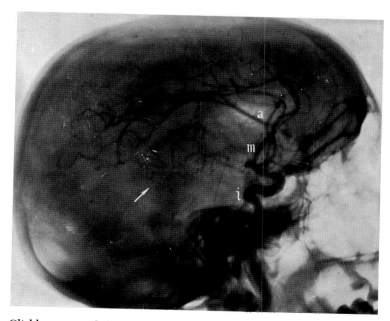

**Fig. 3-10.** Glioblastoma multiforme of left temporal lobe. Arteriogram of left carotid artery. Abnormal vessels in tumor area (arrow). Upward displacement of middle *(m)* and anterior *(a)* cerebral and internal carotid *(i)* arteries.

bright stars, multicolored circles, or snowflakes. In the literature, it is emphasized time and again that undiffierentiated visual hallucinations are characteristic for lesions of the occipital lobe, whereas complex and differentiated visual sensations suggest a temporal site. Actually, both of our patients showed a distinct expansion of the temporal tumor toward the occipital lobe. *It is correct that temporal lobe tumors are more frequently the cause of differentiated and complex visual hallucinations* (Horrax). On the other hand, this type of hallucination is not exclusively found in association with temporal lobe tumors and is not absolutely pathognomonic for such a location. There may be unformed primitive photopsias in patients with tumors limited entirely to the temporal lobe without occipital expansion. According to a number of publications (Paillas, Boudouresques, and Tamalet; Weinberger and Grant), complex visual hallucinations may also originate from a parietal or occipital location. Nevertheless, in the presence of highly differentiated visual hallucinations, one should consider primarily the temporal lobe. However, in making a topical diagnosis, and especially in differentiating between the temporal and occipital lobes, one should not depend entirely on these symptoms but should consider the entire neurologic status of the patient. It certainly would be a mistake to base conclusions regarding the site of the tumor on the nature of the hallucinations. Visual hallucinations generally occur in the blind half of the visual fields, and if there is no hemianopia, they occur in the fields opposite the side of the tumor. There are, however, records of visual hallucinations in the seeing half of the fields.

Ocular symptoms are found in about one half of the patients with temporal lobe tumors. Since visual hallucinations occur quite rarely, these symptoms are mainly limited to manifestations of a generally increased intracranial pressure in the form of flickering or fog before the eyes, temporary blackouts, or unilateral or bilateral decrease of vision. Occasionally, there is photophobia or diplopia.

The *visual field changes* must be counted among the most important *visual symptoms* in temporal lobe tumors. They could be demonstrated in two thirds of the patients in our series. Of course, the reduced general condition or somnolence of some patients will sometimes not permit an exact determination of the visual fields. Actually, this was the case only in one tenth of our patients. If an exact testing of the fields on the perimeter or tangent screen is impossible, the confrontation method or the determination of a relative hemianopia (Thiébaut) may still furnish important clues.

The visual field changes in patients with tumors of the temporal lobe may be labeled with the password *homonymous hemianopia*. We must differentiate between a complete homonymous hemianopia involving both the superior and inferior quadrants and a quadrantanopia. Our own series as well as a number of reports (for instance, Guillaumat and Robin) indicate that a *complete homonymous hemianopia is considerably more frequent than a quadrantanopia*. The former occurs in about one third and the latter in about one sixth of all cases. This greater frequency of complete homonymous hemianopias (Fig. 3-11), in our opinion, is caused by the expansive growth of the tumors, especially in a posterior direction. We found the macula spared in all types of complete homonymous hemianopias. There were no instances of division of the halves of the visual fields through the point of fixation in patients with tumors of the temporal lobe (described by Penfield as the result of excision of the posterior portion of the temporal lobe), as is seen so frequently in those with occipital lobe tumors. In contrast to hemianopias caused by occipital lobe tumors, those resulting from tumors of the temporal lobe (especially those situated anteriorly)

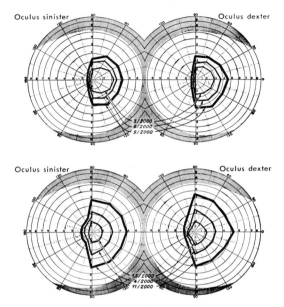

**Fig. 3-11.** Above, Astrocytoma of right temporal lobe. Below, Granuloma in posterior part of right third temporal gyrus. In both cases, there was complete homonymous left hemianopia with sparing of macula and slight incongruence of visual field defects.

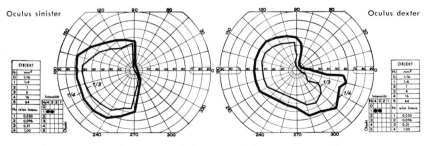

**Fig. 3-12.** Glioblastoma multiforme of left temporal lobe. Pronounced incongruence of field defects: left eye with subtotal hemianopia of right part of field; right eye with quadrant defect of right superior part of field. Patient reported differentiated visual hallucinations!

are characteristic in our series because of a striking *incongruence of the two field defects* or the remaining islands of vision. Time and again, this incongruence is stressed by numerous authors (Harrington; Traquair) as typical for the temporal location (especially on the anterior part). *This incongruity of the visual fields can go so far that occasionally there is a complete hemianopia on one side with only a quadrantanopia on the other side* (Fig. 3-12). There is a difference of opinion as to whether the larger defect is on the side of the lesion or on the opposite side. Our own opinion is that this sign does not permit any conclusions as to the site of the tumor. It should be stressed emphatically that the complete homonymous hemianopia associated with temporal lobe tumors does not differ in principle from that associated with occipital lobe tumors. Even an incongruence of the visual fields is no definite proof for a temporal location, if for no other reason than that tract hemianopias must be considered in the differential diagnosis. However, it is a fact that the congruence of the field defects becomes increasingly more complete the farther posterior the tumor is located in the radiation (Harrington; Hoyt).

In summarizing his experience, Kestenbaum states that a pronounced incongruity of homonymous hemianopic field defects (a positive "incongruity sign") for all practical purposes rules out a lesion in the parietal or occipital part of the visual radiation. On the other hand, congruence may be found in any location (that is, the optic tract as well as the optic radiation). A homonymous hemianopia merely indicates an interruption of the visual pathways above the chiasm. Incongruence of the visual fields is useless for the differentiation of lesions in the infrageniculate or suprageniculate tracts. Traquair even suggests that the incongruity of the field defects, as seen in association with temporal lobe tumors, is indicative of damage to the optic tract below the temporal lobe. The fact that temporal lobe hemianopias usually leave the macular function intact seems to refute this opinion, because optic tract hemianopias result relatively early in the formation of central scotomas (isolated or splitting of the macula by a complete homonymous hemianopia). This opinion has been generally abandoned since Meyer published his fundamental investigations on the course of the optic radiation in the temporal lobe. His anatomic findings demonstrated that the incongruity of the visual fields, especially in processes of the anterior part of the temporal lobe, can be explained by the evidence of a dissociation of the fibers of corresponding retinal points in this region (Fig. 3-15).

*A superior homonymous quadrantanopia or sector-shaped defect is typical and almost pathognomonic for tumors of the temporal lobe* (Figs. 3-13 and 3-14). We have observed them in one sixth of our patients. In the majority the defect was rather congruous and in a smaller number incongruous. This defect is the *result of damage to Meyer's loop,* the ventral bundle of the optic radiation from the external geniculate body, which swings forward in the temporal lobe to form a loop around the apex of the lower horn and to run from there ventrally into the anterior part of the calcarine cortex (Fig. 3-15). Cushing was the first to investigate the superior homonymous quadrant defects in temporal lobe tumors and to point out their localizing value. The incongruity of these quadrant defects can also easily be explained as damage to the optic radiation, particularly if it involves the anterior part of the optic radiation where the crossed fibers still have an anterolateral and the uncrossed fibers a posteromedian course.

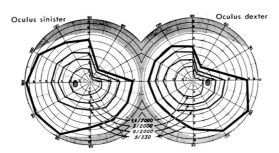

**Fig. 3-13.** Protoplasmic astrocytoma of left temporal lobe the size of a walnut. Tumor situated in depth of third left temporal, fusiform, and hippocampal gyri. Typical right superior homonymous quadrantanopia, a sign of tumor interference with Meyer's loop. Congruence of field defects.

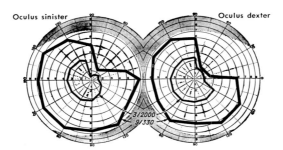

**Fig. 3-14.** Astrocytoma of left temporal lobe. Right superior homonymous quadrantanopia. Incongruence of quadrant defects.

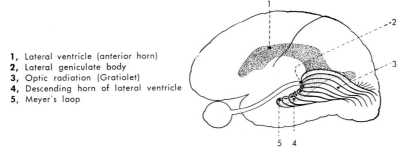

1, Lateral ventricle (anterior horn)
2, Lateral geniculate body
3, Optic radiation (Gratiolet)
4, Descending horn of lateral ventricle
5, Meyer's loop

**Fig. 3-15.** Diagram of Meyer's loop. Ventral fibers of optic radiation pass from lateral geniculate body anteriorly into temporal lobe to form loop around tip of descending horn.

If one remembers that only tumors of the posterior part of the temporal lobe area interfere with the optic radiation, one will understand the relatively rare event of this type of field defect. *But if present, a superior homonymous quadrantanopia definitely has localizing value.* The importance of the most careful perimetry, the use of very small targets, and the plotting of a number of isopters is urgently stressed. Otherwise, such field defects may go unnoticed (Krayenbühl). Frequently, they start merely with a slight indentation of the outer isopters in the superior quadrants and are likely to escape detection (Fig. 3-16).

In agreement with the experience of other authors, we have also observed an *inferior quadrantanopia* (involvement of the superior part of the temporal lobe) in addition to a superior quadrantanopia (involvement of the inferior part of the temporal lobe). This defect occurs much less frequently (one-fifteenth). If a superior quadrantanopia or sector-shaped defect increases in size, the incongruity becomes less distinct, and the defect changes to a com-

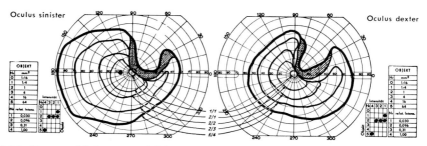

**Fig. 3-16.** Tumor of left temporal lobe. Typical right superior homonymous quadrantanopia. This is initial stage, with involvement of only part of right superior quadrants. Shaded areas indicate progressive deterioration of visual field during time of observation and before surgical intervention. (Case of Dr. Guillaumat; from Dubois-Poulsen.)

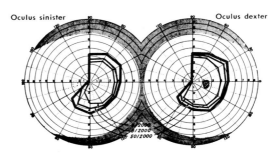

**Fig. 3-17.** Glioblastoma multiforme of right temporal lobe (second and third basal temporal gyri). Left partial homonymous hemianopia. Left superior quadrants are missing completely. Central parts of left inferior quadrants are still preserved. This is intermediate form between superior homonymous quadrantanopia and complete homonymous hemianopia. Neoplasm expanded from front and below in posterosuperior direction.

plete homonymous hemianopia. This is always a sign that the tumor process expands into a superior and particularly a posterior direction (Fig. 3-17).

In addition to these homonymous field changes, we have also observed concentric constrictions of an unspecific nature that had to be interpreted as signs of a beginning optic atrophy secondary to a chronic papilledema. Of course, they have no localizing value.

Other specific ocular signs of an involvement of the temporal lobe may be particularly helpful in a complicated diagnostic situation when complete homonymous hemianopias are difficult to differentiate from those caused by occipital lobe tumors. Such a sign is the *homolateral mydriatic fixed pupil described in the section on general signs of increased intracranial pressure as a component of the transtentorial herniation syndrome.* It has been stated (p. 165) that a unilateral mydriatic fixed pupil in patients with temporal lobe tumors may be caused by direct pressure of the neoplasm on the oculomotor nerve as well as by such pressure of the temporal lobe (hippocampus) herniating through the tentorial notch. Among 30 patients with temporal lobe tumors, we have observed this phenomenon of a unilateral mydriasis six times on the side of the tumor and three times on the opposite side. Once there was miosis in place of mydriasis, which, according to Fischer-Brügge and Tönnis, we took as an early sign of irritation on the oculomotor nerve (p. 164). However, as the transtentorial herniation syndrome is a general sign of increased intracranial pressure, unilateral mydriasis should be interpreted with caution as a localizing sign in temporal lobe tumors.

*Pareses of the oculomotor nerve, especially in the late stages* of tumor growth, may form part of the transtentorial herniation syndrome. We have seen such oculomotor pareses in one sixth of our patients. Usually such pareses can be recognized by the divergent position of the eyes (caused by a paresis of the medial rectus muscles) and by unilateral ptosis. We regard the pareses of the oculomotor nerves as components of the transtentorial herniation syndrome, although in the case of temporal lobe tumors, there is also the possibility of a direct pressure effect on the nerve, as described previously.

A *contralateral central facial palsy* in patients with temporal lobe tumors has been seen more frequently than pareses of the extrinsic ocular muscles—in approximately two tenths of our patients. In a central facial palsy the frontal branch of the nerve is not involved; thus no lagophthalmos occurs. In contrast to the ordinary supranuclear paralysis of the facial nerve, the emotional motility of the mimic muscles, according to Foster Kennedy, is impaired in addition to the spontaneous motility (pressure on the thalamus).

Occasionally, an *ipsilateral disturbance in the area of distribution of the trigeminal nerve with hyporeflexia or areflexia of the corresponding cornea* (Krayenbühl) is found in patients with temporal lobe neoplasms.

At times a unilateral *exophthalmos* is observed in patients with temporal lobe tumors. We have seen three such cases among 30 patients. It occurred twice in bilateral form as a general sign of increased intracranial pressure. A unilateral exophthalmos in the temporal lobe syndrome is mostly the manifestation of an extracerebral growth in this region (for instance, a meningioma).

Disturbances of motility have already been discussed in connection with the transtentorial herniation syndrome. They are oculomotor pareses as the result of a direct pressure effect of the temporal lobe herniating through the tentorial notch. We have never observed supranuclear gaze disturbances, although there are reports of disturbances of convergence and conjugate vertical movements (remote effect on the brain stem, especially the pretectal area) in the literature (Walsh and Hoyt; Bing). Not seldom, motility restrictions are only caused by lack of attention or poor cooperation on the part of the patient! Relatively often (in about one third of our patients), we found a horizontal *fine* or *medium,* easily exhaustible *nystagmus* of the gaze nystagmus type. This also must be a remote effect of the tumor on the brain stem.

The *general signs of increased intracranial pressure* are usually quite distinct. Bilateral papilledema, frequently with hemorrhages and a prominence of 1 to 4 diopters, was found in about one half of all patients. (Tönnis found them in 82% of his cases.) Among 30 patients, unilateral papilledema occurred three times: twice on the side of the tumor and once on the opposite side. There was considerable correlation between increased intracranial pressure determined during surgery and the presence of papilledemas. Nevertheless, in one sixth of the patients with increased intracranial pressure, no papilledema was seen. In our series of 30 patients with temporal lobe tumors, a sixth nerve paresis as a general sign of increased intracranial pressure was observed only once.

*The significance of the ocular signs and symptoms in patients with temporal lobe tumors can be summarized as follows: highly differentiated, formed hallucinations suggest a temporal location, whereas primitive, unformed photopsias are more typical for an occipital site. This differentiation is only conditionally, not absolutely, correct; differentiated as well as undifferentiated hallucinations may be triggered both by occipital and temporal lobe tumors. Superior homonymous quadrantanopia must be considered pathognomonic for a temporal site of the tumor. However, it is rare compared with the complete incongruous homonymous hemianopia. Practically, however, the latter cannot be differentiated from a similar lesion caused by an occipital tumor. Of localizing importance are an ipsilateral mydriatic fixed pupil and oculomotor pareses as components of the transtentorial herniation syndrome, as well as the frequent contralateral central facial palsy. There are no specific general signs of an increased intracranial pressure typical for the temporal lobe.*

### Tumors of the parietal lobe

The posterior central gyrus, by definition, is part of the parietal lobe. Lesions of this anterior part of the parietal lobe produce a characteristic syndrome known as the *syndrome of the postcentral gyrus.* An irritation of the postcentral convolution manifests itself in the form of sensory jacksonian fits. The region of the initial sensory sensation points out the localization of the focus. The destructive loss of this specific cortical area results in a disturbance of the epicritic sensibility; according to the site of the lesion, the arm or leg on the contralateral side is involved. Kinesthesia, position sense, vibration sense, and two-point discrimination are decreased or abolished. Recognition of objects by touch is limited or impossible (astereognosis). Lesions of the medulla of the supramarginal gyrus cause apraxia in the form of bilateral motor apraxia (ideokinetic apraxia or Liepmann's apraxia), that is, inability to carry out purposeful movements in the absence of motor paralyses or sensory disturbances. Affections of the various areas of the *angular gyrus* and its adjacent regions in the temporal or occipital lobe on the dominant hemisphere result in loss of comprehension of the written word and consequent inability to read (alexia), often associated with loss of ability to write (agraphia); in inability of calculation (acalculia); in disturbances of the body scheme; and in right-left disorientation. *Gerstmann's angularis syndrome* consists of finger agnosia, right-left disturbance, agraphia, acalculia, and right homonymous hemianopia (affection of dominant side). Lesions in the region of the angular gyrus of the nondominant hemisphere cause disturbances in spatial orientation (topographic agnosia), neglect of the contralateral side, and a left homonymous

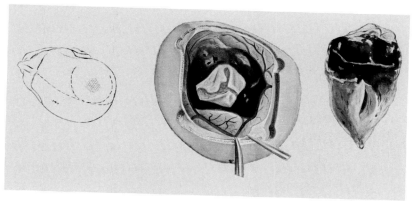

**Fig. 3-18.** Malignant glioma of right parietal lobe in 41-year-old patient before and after surgical extirpation (right parietal osteoplastic craniotomy).

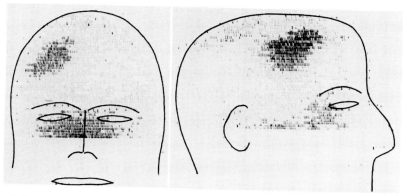

**Fig. 3-19.** Color scintigram of glioblastoma in frontoparietal region. Contrast medium is $^{197}$Hg-neohydrine.

field defect. Biparietal lesions may produce global visual object agnosia (inability to identify objects and to recognize persons), eventually associated with lack of voluntary control of eye movements (Balint's syndrome) (see Fig. 1-2). The distribution of the types of parietal tumors is as follows: meningiomas, 30%; glioblastomas, 20%; astrocytomas, 10%; oligodendrogliomas, 10%; and metastases, 5% (Zülch; Tönnis) (Figs. 3-18 and 3-19).

Parietal lobe tumors may produce ocular signs and symptoms of localizing significance that should not escape the ophthalmologist during the examination. Some of the most important sensory cortical centers are situated in the parietal lobe. As mentioned previously, defects caused by a parietal tumor involve important functions such as writing, reading, calculation, stereognosis, and others, in addition to sensory disturbances. A tumor in the region of the angular gyrus of the dominant hemisphere may cause *alexia,* or *word blindness; the patient is unable to read (in other words, he does not comprehend the significance of written words, musical notes, or figures).* In our series of 27 proved cases of parietal lobe tumors, we found complete alexia three times and an incomplete form (dyslexia) once. Alexia is usually combined with *agraphia,* the inability to write spontaneously or on dictation. Alexia without agraphia (a disconnection syndrome, p. 8) occurs in patients who have a unilateral occipital lobe lesion of the dominant side and a lesion of the splenium of the corpus callosum, but an intact angular gyrus (mostly the result of vascular infarction, seldom tumors). Alexia can be observed with or without hemianopia (usually right-sided homonymous hemianopia); it can occur independent of any lesion of the optic radiation. In our own patients the alexia and agraphia usually were combined with other sensory-aphasic and with apractic disturbances. We found no cases of visual object agnosia (that is, *mind blindness,* an inability to recognize and identify objects although they are seen). Visual object agnosia is also considered a result of damage to the angular gyrus or its association pathways. Even though we have not seen a typical case of visual object agnosia in our series of patients with tumors of the parietal lobe, we have observed one patient with findings suggestive of such a condition. This patient stated that he recognized his physician visually, but that he was unable to comprehend the entire significance of the situation he visualized. We were of the opinion that this was an incomplete form of visual object agnosia. So much for the subjective ocular symptoms concerning the higher visual centers in the parietal lobe (p. 8 and Fig. 1-1).

In two patients in our series, we were able to observe an aura before jacksonian fits, which always occurred in the form of *undifferentiated primitive visual hallucinations* such as stars, flickering, or dots before the eyes. Such visual sensations occur infrequently with parietal lobe tumors. They suggest an expansion of the tumor toward the optic radiation. As can be expected from the proximity of the occipital lobe, these hallucinations usually are unformed and undifferentiated in character.

Parietal lobe tumors will interfere with the optic radiation only in the case of a relatively extensive downgrowth. This is the reason for the *rather infrequent occurrence of visual field changes.* We observed them in only one third of our patients; Guillaumat and Robin reported them in only one fourth of their series. Some reports (Traquair; Dubois-Poulsen) indicate that *inferior homonymous quadrant defects* are characteristic for parietal lobe tumors (Figs. 3-20 and 3-21). This type of defect occurred in our series only once. In another patient, there was a bilateral superior homonymous quadrant defect. We observed a *complete homonymous hemianopia* much more frequently (especially in gliomas, most seldom in meningiomas). It occurred in seven of 27 patients with parietal lobe tumors. A *relative hemianopia* in the form of "visual inattention" that could not be demonstrated on the perimeter or tangent screen was found twice. Our own experience leads us to conclude that inferior homonymous quadrantanopia, which supposedly is characteristic for parietal lobe lesions, actually occurs quite rarely. Other visual field changes (especially complete hemianopias, mostly with sparing of the macula and with rather congruous defects) are difficult to differentiate from those caused by occipital lobe tumors. This differentiation actually is quite irrelevant because numerous parietal lobe tumors extend into the occipital lobe, and vice versa. *It is impossible to distinguish a "parietal" from an "occipital" homonymous hemianopia on the basis of the visual field.* Lack of awareness of the homonymous field defects (anosognosia) and a strange sensation of per-

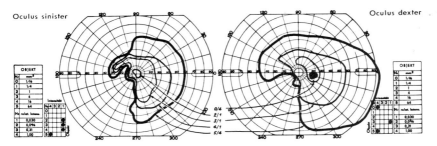

**Fig. 3-20.** Tumor of right parietal lobe. Left inferior homonymous quadrantanopia with distinctly incongruous field defects. Enlargement of right blind spot caused by papilledema. (After Dubois-Poulsen.)

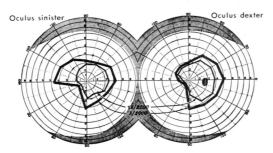

**Fig. 3-21.** Cortical and subcortical sarcoma of right parietal lobe. Rather congruous left inferior quadrantanopia.

sistence or recurrence of an afterimage in the blind half of the field (visual perseveration or paliopsia) accompany many parietal lobe lesions.

We have never observed the disturbances of the conjugate lateral movements reported by David and Hecaen in patients with parietal lobe tumors. *A rotation of both eyes toward one side* (usually opposite the tumor) *during an epileptic seizure* must be considered as a parietal adversive phenomenon—the "associated adversive looking" of Penfield. We have seen two such cases in our series. In view of the cortifugal occipitomesencephalic pathways in the middle and posterior thirds of the optic radiation, one should always search for asymmetric disturbances of optically induced movements, pursuit movements (cogwheeling!), and optokinetic nystagmus (p. 61) in patients with suspected parietal lobe tumors. Kestenbaum, by the way, emphasizes the strikingly constant manifestation of a positive optokinetic nystagmus sign (optokinetic nystagmus to the side of the hemianopia or to the side opposite the lesion strikingly less than to the other side) in deep or massive parietal lobe lesions. Lesions of the parietal lobe are by far the most common lesions seen in association with abnormal optokinetic responses. The most important feature is a decrease or *loss of the fast phase of the response to the opposite side* with retention of the pursuit response, that is, the slow phase of optokinetic nystagmus. Voluntary saccadic movements and the fast phase of nystagmus induced by caloric stimulation are normal, proving preservation of the frontomesencephalic pathways. The abnormal optokinetic response does not necessarily depend on the hemianopia; it may be positive with dorsal parietal lesions even when there is no affection of the visual radiation (disconnection of the corticocortical paths from the occipital lobes to the frontal lobes).

*Pursuit movements also are frequently disturbed in parietal lesions.* They may show a cogwheel phenomenon, interruption of smooth pursuit movements by saccades, (to the side contralateral to the hemianopia, or toward the side of the lesion). However, patients with a tumor of the parietal lobe in whom this sign is missing completely are seen time and again. Stadlin made some interesting investigations bearing on this subject in a case of a parieto-occipital astrocytoma; these are referred to in the section on occipital lobe tumors (p. 191). A gaze palsy of the upward movement was seen once; since there was simultaneously a diminished pupillary reaction to light, we interpreted this vertical conjugate impairment as a remote effect of the tumor on the midbrain. A fine or medium, easily exhaustible *horizontal gaze nystagmus* was noted in about one fourth of the patients.

In addition to a relatively *frequent contralateral central facial palsy,* we found *hypesthesia of the contralateral cornea* with diminution of the corneal reflex in one fourth of our patients with parietal lobe tumors, usually associated with a corresponding disturbance of the other trigeminal branches. This phenomenon is an analogue to other sensibility disturbances in patients with parietal lobe lesions.

*General signs of increased intracranial pressure* occur in about one half of the patients in the form of bilateral papilledema. It is noteworthy that increased intracranial pressure is frequently found during the operation (in about one fourth of the patients) despite the absence of papilledema. Generally, the prominence of the choked disc is rather minor (that is, between 1 and 2 diopters). Signs of optic atrophy secondary to papilledema occur rarely (3% of cases). Other ocular signs of increased intracranial pressure were surprisingly rare. In three of our patients the nonspecific sixth nerve paresis and a unilateral mydriasis were both on the side opposite the tumor!

*In summarizing, the localizing signs and symptoms in patients with parietal lobe tumors are the subjective phenomena of disturbances of the higher visual centers that occur in the form of the visual agnosias, especially alexia or dyslexia. An inferior homonymous quadrantanopia, which is somewhat pathognomonic for parietal lobe lesions, is rare. Much more frequent are complete homonymous hemianopias. The latter type, however, can hardly be distinguished from similar defects caused by occipital lobe tumors. Noteworthy are contralateral disturbances of the corneal sensitivity, usually associated with disturbances in the area of distribution of other branches of the trigeminal nerve. The general sign of increased intracranial pressure in the form of choked discs is rather rare or frequently completely absent despite a proved increased intracranial pressure.*

### Tumors of the occipital lobe

Except for the ocular symptoms, the occipital lobe is actually a neurologically silent zone. Manifestations of tumor-induced irritation in this area are epileptic seizures (generalized or focal), occasionally preceded by unformed visual hallucinations or ocular involuntary deviations. Defects involve primarily the visual field in the form of complete or incomplete homonymous hemianopia. (However, we know today that small lesions of the striate cortex may occur without a defect in the visual field.) If an occipital tumor extends forward and involves the peristriate and neighboring parietotemporal areas, there may result aphasia (motor, sensory, or mixed), alexia with or without agraphia (dominant hemisphere), topographic agnosia (nondominant hemisphere), visual object agnosia, achromatopsia (inability to recognize colors), and visual irreminiscence (inability to call up visual images from the past). Bilateral lesions of the occipital lobes may lead to cortical blindness, occasionally accompanied by a denial of the blindness (Anton's syndrome). In reality, about 70% of the occipital lobe tumors start with symptoms of increased intracranial pressure (Tönnis) and, because of disturbing neighborhood symptoms (parietal, temporal) and early herniation syndromes (tentorium notch, foramen magnum), occasionally lead to a false diagnosis. Pressure atrophy and enlargement of the sella, especially pronounced in occipital lobe tumors, may, in connection with visual disturbances, even simulate a lesion of the sellar region. Thus the *results of a proper ophthalmologic diagnosis will assume utmost importance* and supply the neurosurgeon with valuable data for a tumor localization. Glioblastomas and meningiomas are the preponderant types (25% each) of occipital lobe tumors; astrocytomas, oligodendrogliomas, and metastases occasionally involve the occipital lobe (7% each) (Fig. 3-22).

Occipital lobe tumors occur relatively infrequently. Nevertheless, we are able to report on more than 20 cases limited more or less exclusively to the occipital lobe.

To state the most important fact, *the ocular symptoms are related primarily*

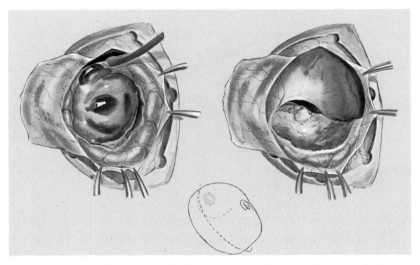

Fig. 3-22. Astrocytoma of left occipital lobe in 37-year-old patient before and after extirpation (left total occipital lobectomy).

*to the homonymous hemianopia.* However, it must be emphasized that quite a few patients are not aware of their hemianopia and will not mention it spontaneously (p. 4). Less intelligent patients, for instance, complain of a vaguely defined loss of vision, especially toward the side of the hemianopia. Much more frequently, patients will make *statements that imply a hemianopia:* the patient strikes a door post; the motorist misses a pedestrian or cyclist on one side; the cyclist cannot see the curb correctly; when reading, the patient sees only half a word; or when writing, he always writes past the margin of the paper (especially disturbing with hemianopias on the right side; with hemianopia on the left side there is difficulty in finding the next line of print). Occasionally a patient will only state that he cannot see very well with one eye. Another will say that "there is no depth" toward the side of the hemianopia. Much rarer are peculiar deformations of objects; they appear reduced in size (micropsia) or change their size. One patient with an extensive glioblastoma multiforme of the occipital lobe experienced attacks of micropsia associated with visual hallucinations. Similarly, another patient complained of undefined "deformed vision" (metamorphopsia).

*Visual hallucinations of an unformed primitive pattern, mostly in the blind half of the visual fields,* are surprisingly rare in patients with occipital lobe tumors. Such hallucinations may assume the form of fiery globes, stripes, discs, rings, zigzag lines, or flashing lights of purple, golden, or other bright colors and occur as transient attacks, even with the eyes closed. We observed visual hallucinations only three times in 20 proved cases of occipital lobe tumors. (According to Parkinson, Rucker, and McCraig and Hoyt, they are more frequent, occurring in about one fourth of the cases.) All of them were of the primitive type. Although there are occasional reports that more highly organized, refined forms of visual hallucinations can originate not only in the temporal but also in the occipital lobe (Weinberger and Grant), it can be stated on the basis of reports by numerous authors (Parkinson, Rucker, and McCraig; Penfield and Rasmussen) as well as our own experience that *occipital lobe tumors usually produce simple primitive visual hallucinations*. If, during the course of the disease, the latter give place to more complex visual sensations, this may be an indication of an expansion of the tumor into the temporal region. Although visual hallucinations are important localizing symptoms in the diagnosis of occipital lobe tumors, their importance unfortunately is diminished by their rare occurrence.

The subjective complaints of reading difficulties may make it difficult at times to decide whether they are caused by only the hemianopic field defect or by an additional alexia or dyslexia. In addition to field defects, twice we observed an unquestionable *alexia* and twice *agraphia* manifested by disturbances of writing. *Alexia without agraphia* occurs in patients with unilateral left occipital lobe lesions and associated lesions of the splenium. Such patients are able to write but are unable to read what they have written. If the tumor of the occipital lobe responsible for such symptomatology involves also the angular gyrus of the adjacent parietal lobe, it will produce the better known and more frequent syndrome of alexia with agraphia (p. 8).

In our series of patients with occipital lobe tumors, there were no instances of associated disturbances of the higher visual centers such as visual object agnosia or mind blindness, that is, the inability to recognize and identify objects although they are seen (Fig. 1-1).

Nor have we observed *cortical blindness* as the functional equivalent of bilateral tumor damage to the occipital cortex, especially the calcarine fissure. There was, however, one case of necrosis of both occipital lobes caused by x-ray treatment after an operation to remove a temporal lobe tumor. Another case occurred after a bilateral ventriculography performed through the occipital lobes. Obviously, this caused a localized edema, which proved to be reversible. The characteristic signs of cortical blindness were discussed in detail in Chapter 1 (p. 7). Briefly, cortical blindness is characterized by complete loss of all visual sensations, by loss of reflex lid closure, by intact pupillary reactions on light and convergence, and by intact motility of the eyes. Cortical blindness may occur as an indirect consequence of any supratentorial cerebral tumor causing herniation of the brain and brain stem through the tentorial notch and thus producing compression of the posterior cerebral arteries and their branches supplying the occipital cortices (Chapter 2, p. 163). Sometimes patients with cortical blindness deny their defect, using the most extravagant confabulations (Anton's syndrome). Cortical blindness must not be confused with *cerebral blindness* or *double homonymous hemianopia*. In such a case, there is complete loss of vision at the onset, but generally only for a relatively short, transient interval, and vision reappears in a small central field around the point of fixation (corresponding to both areas of the spared maculas!). Cerebral blindness is usually of vascular origin (arteriosclerosis, hypertension) and not related to cerebral tumors.

Some of the most typical and important symptoms of occipital lobe tumors are the visual field changes, which may be summarized with the phrase *complete or incomplete homonymous hemianopia on the opposite side. Visual field changes*

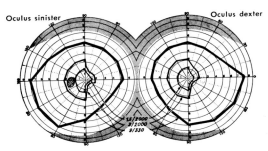

Fig. 3-23. Cherry-sized parasagittal metastatic hypernephroma of left occipital lobe. Right homonymous hemianopia of central isopters with distinct sparing of macula. The 9/330 isopters determined on perimeter do not reveal homonymous hemianopia at all!

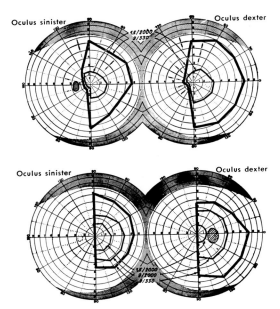

Fig. 3-24. Above, Glioblastoma multiforme of right occipital lobe. History revealed unformed visual hallucinations! Below, Oligodendroglioma of right occipital lobe. In both cases, there is complete homonymous hemianopia that is characteristic for occipital lesions. Upper fields reveal sparing of macula. This is missing in lower fields—splitting of macula is sign of total interruption of optic radiation. Field defects and remaining parts of fields are congruous. Hemianopia could be demonstrated on perimeter (peripheral isopters) as well as on tangent screen (central isopters).

*were not missing once among our 20 patients with occipital lobe tumors.* Ten (that is, one half) of the patients showed complete homonymous hemianopia with distinct sparing of the macula. In six (approximately one third) the complete homonymous hemianopia occurred with splitting of the macula (that is, with the dividing line between the seeing and the blind part of the field running directly through the macula). *There is a conspicuous congruence of the field defects and the remaining parts of the fields of these patients with complete hemianopia, both those with and those without sparing of the macula* (Figs. 3-23 and 3-24).

Incomplete hemianopia was seen only once in the form of an inferior homonymous incongruous quadrantanopia (Fig. 3-25). In two instances, we observed a concentric constriction on one side in the presence of an incongruous hemianopic field defect on the other side. In agreement with numerous authors (Dubois-Poulsen; Guillaumat and Robin; Walsh and Hoyt; Horrax and Putnam; and others), we feel that complete homonymous hemianopia is characteristic for tumor lesions of the occipital lobe. There is always a lively discussion concerning sparing of the macula. We examined the visual fields after occipital lobectomy in 15 patients operated on for occipital lobe tumors (Huber). We demonstrated that the *removal of the occipital lobe (that is, the complete interruption of the optic radiation) results in complete homonymous hemianopia without sparing of the macula* in the real sense of the word (that is, less than 3 degrees). However, there exists in most cases a definite sparing of the central fovea, which is rather difficult to explain and raises the problem of a possible bilateral representation of the fovea. On the basis of these findings, we have come to the conclusion that the absence of sparing of the macula is suggestive of a complete or nearly complete interruption of the fibers of the optic radiation or of the visual cortex. Sparing of the macula (that is, more than 3 degrees) occurs in homonymous hemianopia if the fibers of the optic radiation, particularly those of the macula, are not interrupted in their entirety. Since the optic radiation spreads out in its posterior part toward the calcarine fissure (Fig. 1-36), one can draw the con-

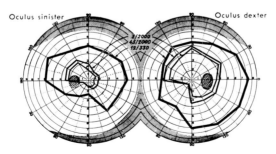

**Fig. 3-25.** Astrocytoma of right occipital lobe. Left asymmetric inferior quadrantanopia. This picture is similar to one seen in parietal lobe tumors. Enormous bilateral enlargement of blind spot caused by bilateral choked discs of 4 diopters' elevation.

clusion that very extensive tumors or those situated in a rather anterior part of the occipital lobe are more likely to produce homonymous hemianopia without sparing of the macula. And thus we are in agreement with Kestenbaum, who also considers *macular sparing as a sign that points to a lesion in the most posterior part of the optic pathway, that is, the hindmost part of the optic radiation or the calcarine cortex itself.*

Occasionally, the temporal part of one peripheral visual field (the one opposite the lesion), the so-called *"temporal crescent or half-moon,"* may be spared in cases of occipital lobe tumors producing homonymous hemianopia. In other instances a unilateral temporal crescent defect may be the only visual field sign in a cerebral tumor affecting the optic radiations (Bender and Strauss). We agree with Walsh and Hoyt that sparing of the temporal crescent in homonymous hemianopia indicates an occipital localization, whereas an isolated temporal crescent defect is of no value in the topical diagnosis.

We agree with Dubois-Poulsen that it is not possible to differentiate lesions of the optic radiation from those of the cortex on the basis of the visual fields. Furthermore, such a differentiation is irrelevant because many tumors involve the cortex as well as the gray matter. *Central or paracentral homonymous scotomas (with apices at the points of fixation) are generally regarded as signs of affection of the occipital cortex, especially in the area of the occipital pole.* They are also a characteristic finding in some early cases of occipital lobe tumors (Bender and Battersby). One of our own observations concerns a case of hemorrhagic pachymeningitis over the right occipital pole with paracentral homonymous scotomas in the left side of the fields (Fig. 3-26). It is noteworthy that the patient had epileptic seizures with a decided visual aura during which he experienced flashing concentric circles and sparks of light synchronous with the pulse in addition to certain noises. In case a tumor develops in the space between the two occipital poles, it may press on the upper or lower calcarine lips, thus creating a *vertical hemianopia.* Such cases have been described in the literature. We personally have never observed one.

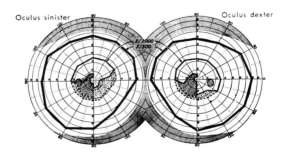

**Fig. 3-26.** Hemorrhagic pachymeningitis in region of right occipital pole after pneumococcal meningitis. Jacksonian epilepsy with visual and acoustic aura. Left paracentral homonymous hemianoptic scotomas with sparing of macula in left inferior quadrants. Vision, O.U. 1.0 Scotomas are absolute in shaded area. Dotted areas indicate relative scotomas (also involvement of left occipital pole?).

Next to visual field changes, ocular signs play a lesser role. In a little more than one fifth of our patients, we noticed a fine or medium horizontal *gaze nystagmus*. It is probably caused by a remote effect on the cerebellum or the brain stem. *Gaze palsies are extremely rare.* We observed only one patient with a gaze paresis up and toward the side opposite the tumor.

Let us add some remarks regarding the usefulness of *pursuit movement* and its change to cogwheel movement as well as *optokinetic nystagmus* for the differential diagnosis of a tract hemianopia and an optic radiation hemianopia (p. 62). In a patient with a parieto-occipital astrocytoma with homonymous hemianopia, Stadlin was able to demonstrate that following the extirpation of the tumor the optokinetic nystagmus toward the side opposite the tumor was missing. Before surgery, it had been symmetric to both sides. In the case of a homonymous hemianopia with an absent or weakened optokinetic nystagmus toward the side of the hemianopia, or an impaired pursuit movement toward the opposite side, one must assume a lesion in the middle or posterior part of the optic radiation (in other words, the parietal or parieto-occipital region). It is important, however, that the optokinetic nystagmus as well as the pursuit movement remains normal in patients with lesions of the cortex of the calcarine fissure.

Unilateral or bilateral *sixth nerve pareses* resulting from an increased intracranial pressure manifest themselves a little more often in occipital lobe tumors than in those of the parietal lobe (one fourth of the patients). A unilateral fixed *mydriasis* also occurred in one fourth of the patients. Usually it is homolateral, occasionally associated with a ptosis. Sometimes there is also homolateral miosis (sign of irritation of the oculomotor nerve).

There was a *conspicuous frequency in the occurrence of choked discs* (that is, in 17 of our 20 patients with occipital lobe tumors). We always found a *pronounced prominence of the disc of up to 5 diopters as well as excessive retinal hemorrhages and exudates*—findings that are in agreement with those of Walsh and Hoyt; Bailey; and Parkinson and McCraig (Fig. 3-27). The frequency and pronounced character of these choked discs may be related to the location of the neoplasms near the posterior fossa. Tumors here lead to a relatively early impairment of the circulation of the cerebrospinal fluid and formation of an internal hydrocephalus. Consequently, there is an almost complete parallelism between the development of a choked disc and the finding of increased intracranial pressure during surgery (Fig. 3-28).

Finally, it should be mentioned that a brain tumor, regardless of its location (that is, in the frontal or temporal lobe), may occasionally simulate an "occipital picture." Evidently, a compression of the posterior cerebral arteries during a transtentorial herniation process in relation with increased intracranial pressure may cause an *ischemic or hemorrhagic infarction of one or both occipital lobes.* (See discussion of cortical blindness, p. 7, and transtentorial herniation, p. 161.)

*The following is a summary of the important ocular signs and symptoms of occipital tumors. Frequently, either clear or disguised statements in the patient's history suggest homonymous hemianopia. Signs of irritation in the form of primitive undifferentiated visual hallucinations are relatively rare. An expansion of the tumor toward the parietal region leads to disturbances of the higher visual centers in the form of visual object agnosia, alexia, agraphia, and perhaps also micropsia or metamorphopsia. The most frequent visual field change is a complete homonymous hemianopia, with or without sparing of the macula, the former perhaps*

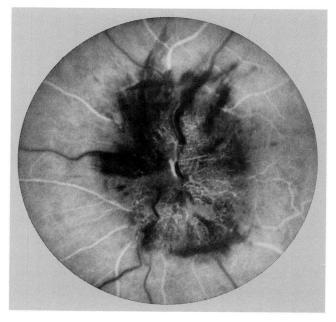

**Fig. 3-27.** Papilledema in patient with occipital lobe tumor. Fluorescein angiogram taken during early arterial phase.

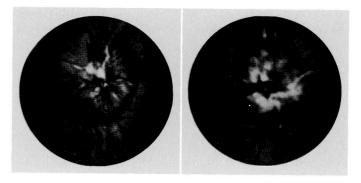

**Fig. 3-28.** Bilateral choked discs. Advanced chronic stage in glioblastoma multiforme of right occipital lobe. Pronounced elevation of 3.5 to 4 diopters. Numerous hemorrhages and white exudates (cytoid bodies) on disc and in adjacent retina. Left illustration corresponds to right eye and right illustration to left eye.

*being the more frequent one. Another typical sign is a striking congruence of the remaining halves of the visual fields. Quadrantanopia and a concentric constriction are both quite rare. A differentiation between cortical and subcortical lesions cannot be based on the visual fields. Signs of an increased intracranial pressure in the form of choked discs are remarkably pronounced and practically always present. Characteristically, the choked discs are relatively prominent and present numerous hemorrhages and exudates. In the presence of alexia and other central disorders of visual integration, it may be quite difficult to differentiate occipital lobe tumors from those of the parietal lobe. It may be irrelevant in cases of expansive growth of an originally occipital tumor. Generally, temporal lobe tumors can be differentiated from those of the occipital lobe on the basis of other neurologic symptoms. Superior homonymous quadrant defects and highly organized visual hallucinations suggest a temporal site. Complete homonymous defects and primitive hallucinations signify an occipital focus.*

### Tumors of the corpus callosum

A *unilateral apraxia* of the left hand generally is considered as the only, although rare, characteristic neurologic symptom of a tumor of the corpus callosum (disconnection syndrome). In addition, such tumors usually cause grave psycho-organic disturbances accompanied by marked hypokinesia or akinesia, lack of initiative, indifference, and urinary and fecal incontinence (symptomatology similar to frontal lobe tumors!). The clinical diagnosis of such tumors often is quite difficult, mostly because general signs of increased intracranial pressure may appear at an early stage and dominate the whole symptomatology (including signs of herniation through the tentorium and the foramen magnum). Tumors of the callosal region are most frequently glioblastomas ("butterfly gliomas"), astrocytomas, and lipomas.

The general ophthalmologic signs and symptoms of increased intracranial pressure, especially choked disc, may be seen in patients with tumors of the corpus callosum as the first symptoms. We found a papilledema, although lacking characteristic details, in every one of our patients. The tendency to secondary optic atrophy with loss of vision and concentric contraction of the visual fields is pronounced. Sixth nerve pareses and central facial palsies are rather common signs (Tönnis). Pupillary disturbances such as anisocoria and fixed pupils have been described (Bailey). We have not observed them in any of the patients in our series. Occasional field defects must be considered as a pressure effect on the neighboring structures, for example, the temporal lobes.

*In summary, it can be stated that the ocular signs and symptoms associated with tumors of the corpus callosum have no localizing value. They are merely manifestations of a general increase in the intracranial pressure, especially in the form of papilledema. With the tumor situated in the posterior part of the corpus callosum, the splenium, there may occur alexia of the left half of the visual field (in right-handed subjects), sometimes combined with difficulty in naming colors (posterior disconnection syndrome).*

### Parasagittal meningiomas and meningiomas of the falx

Meningiomas of the falx originate in the falx itself. The parasagittal meningiomas develop in the recess between the superior longitudinal sinus and the falx. One differentiates between meningiomas of the anterior, middle, and posterior thirds of the sinus according to their location and symptomatology. The neurologic signs depend on the effect on the adjacent part of the cerebral hemispheres. In meningiomas of the anterior third of the sinus, compression signs of the frontal lobe will predominate; those of the middle third of the sinus will show signs typical for the central region. Tumors of the posterior third of the sinus are associated with compression signs of the parietal and occipital lobes. Meningiomas of the falx and bilateral parasagittal meningiomas will result in signs involving both hemispheres (Fig. 3-29).

The ocular signs and symptoms of parasagittal meningiomas and meningiomas of the falx depend on the part of the brain compressed by the tumor. For this reason, we merely refer to the detailed discussion of the appropriate regions of the cerebral hemispheres. In our series of patients, parasagittal meningiomas and meningiomas of the falx *almost invariably caused papilledemas of 2 to 3 diopters' prominence, although without any peculiarities characteristic for this type of tumor.* The ocular symptoms usually are related to the general increase in intracranial pressure and occur in the later stages of the tumor growth. They manifest themselves as flickering before the eyes, blackouts, photophobia, and double vision. Visual field changes are relatively rare. If present, they must be interpreted as remote effects of the tumor, with the exception of homonymous hemianopias caused by meningiomas of the posterior part of the falx or the sinus with direct involvement of the occipital lobes. A tumor in the falx between the occipital lobes may cause *bilateral homonymous hemianopia,* for instance, in the form of a bilateral inferior homonymous quadrantanopia, which looks like an

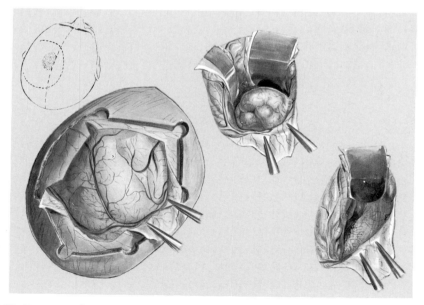

**Fig. 3-29.** Deep-seated meningioma of falx in left parietal region of 31-year-old patient before and after extirpation.

altitudinal hemianopia with a line separating the seeing and the blind half of the field in the horizontal meridian (Rucker and Kearns). Klingler and Condrau have called attention to the *misleading localizing signs of the visual field changes caused especially by meningiomas of this type.* For instance, a deep-seated parietal meningioma of the falx on the left side caused a central scotoma of the left eye, with concentric contraction of the peripheral field. In such a case, one must assume a remote effect of the tumor on the optic nerve; the exact mechanism cannot be explained (Custodis). We have observed a homonymous hemianopia of an incongruous type in a patient with meningioma of the middle third of the sinus as well as in a patient with a parasagittal meningioma of the frontal third of the sinus (Fig. 3-30). These homonymous hemianopias also must be interpreted as a remote effect on the optic radiations or possibly on the optic tract. A satisfactory explanation is difficult. In one patient with meningioma of the middle third of the falx, we even observed a defect resembling bitemporal hemianopia. We cite this case as an illustration of how complex the task of interpreting these visual fields may become in such meningiomas and how misleading the field changes may be.

Finally, it should be mentioned that meningiomas may directly invade the dural sinus and produce by their occlusion the misleading picture of pseudotumor cerebri (Marr and Chambers).

*In summary, it can be stated that parasagittal meningiomas and meningiomas of the falx are generally associated with distinct general signs of increased intracranial pressure in the form of choked discs. It is of importance that they may cause visual field changes, mostly in the form of a homonymous hemianopia. Since these tumors are quite distant from the optic radiation and the optic tract, they must have a remote effect (except for those in direct contact with the occipital lobes). This type of tumor seems to be disposed to produce visual fields with misleading features for an exact localization because of their slow growth and their relatively large size.*

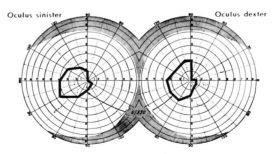

**Fig. 3-30.** Meningioma of falx in middle third of sinus (left frontoparietal region). Right incongruous homonymous hemianopia, possibly remote effect of tumor on optic tract. This visual field is of misleading localizing value.

## Intrasellar, suprasellar, and parasellar tumors

After the discussion of tumors of the cerebral hemispheres, we must consider the space-consuming lesions of the anterior fossa, especially those of the *region of the chiasm*. We proceed, so to speak, from the hub of this area, the sella and its contents, in radial directions to the suprasellar structures situated anterosuperiorly as well as to the parasellar area on both sides. Thus we plan to set forth a logical method to differentiate the various types of space-consuming sellar lesions (Fig. 3-31).

*Pituitary adenoma* is considered the prototype of an intrasellar neoplasm because it originates within the sella despite its frequent extrasellar expansion during later stages. *Craniopharyngioma* shows intrasellar and extrasellar growth, with the extrasellar expansion usually proceeding in a suprasellar direction. *Meningiomas of the tuberculum sellae* and *olfactory groove meningiomas* represent decidedly suprasellar types of growths. Finally, *meningiomas of the sphenoid ridge* will be discussed as typical examples of parasellar tumors. In the broadest sense of the word, tumors of the middle fossa and the cavernous sinus should be considered as growths of the parasellar space. The latter will be discussed in a special section because of the characteristic cavernous sinus syndrome they produce.

Statistics tell us that *one in four of all intracranial tumors arise in the region of the chiasm. In the majority, visual symptoms represent their initial manifestations.* As most of these sellar and parasellar tumors are of a benign nature, their early recognition is of utmost importance. Successful treatment therefore depends largely on the correct and well-timed diagnosis by the ophthalmologist!

### Pituitary adenomas (intrasellar and suprasellar tumor type)

The neuro-ophthalmologic examination reaches a maximum of importance with tumors of the pituitary gland, not so much because it permits exact localization, but because the symptoms produced by these tumors, in the initial as well as the fully developed stage, are *ocular symptoms* (Fig. 3-32). Sooner or later these symptoms will bring the patient to the ophthalmologist (Table 4). It is entirely the responsibility of the general practitioner or the ophthalmologist to detect pituitary tumors and arrange for early treatment. The neurologist and especially the neurosurgeon usually see these patients at a later date.

**Table 4.** Frequency of eye symptoms in different types of pituitary adenomas

| Adenoma type | With eye symptoms | Without eye symptoms |
|---|---|---|
| Endocrine-inactive | 20 | 7 |
| Acromegaly | 0 | 17 |
| Forbes-Albright | 0 | 4 |
| Nelson | 1 | 1 |

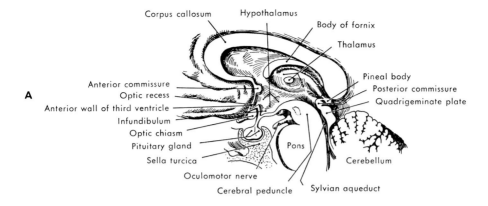

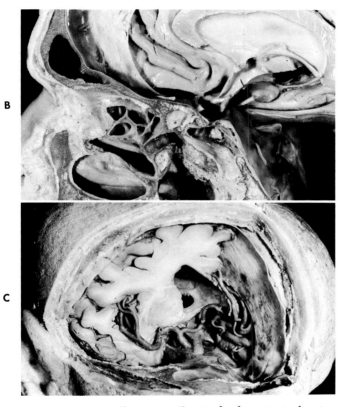

**Fig. 3-31. A,** Semidiagrammatic illustration (longitudinal section) showing pituitary gland, sella, optic chiasm, third ventricle, thalamus, hypothalamus, and brain stem. **B,** Median section through skull showing sella, pituitary gland, optic chiasm, third ventricle, thalamus, hypothalamus, and bony structures of forehead, nose, and epipharynx. **C,** Transverse section of right anterior part of skull and brain showing optic chiasm with its anterior rim and its relation to internal carotid artery, arterial circle of Willis, and adjacent brain areas (especially third ventricle). (**B** and **C** specimens of Prof. Kubic, Anatomic Institute of the University of Zurich.)

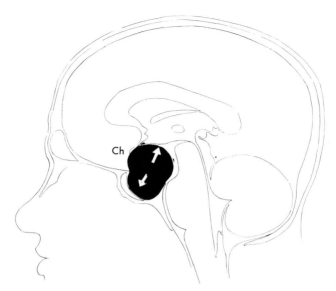

**Fig. 3-32.** Median section through skull showing pituitary adenoma growing out of sellar region. Note compression and upward displacement of optic chiasm, *Ch*, as well as narrowing of third ventricle in comparison with those structures shown in Fig. 3-31.

Pituitary adenomas have usually been divided into three or four groups according to their tinctorial behavior of the pathologic specimen in hematoxylin-eosin staining. The *eosinophilic* adenomas were usually related to acromegaly, the *basophilic* adenomas to Cushing's syndrome, and the *chromophobe* adenomas to space-occupying lesions with endocrine deficiency without signs of hormone production. The mixed-type adenomas containing both eosinophilic and chromophobe cells were found in different endocrinologic syndromes. A closer clinical and anatomic examination of the pituitary adenomas shows that this view is not correct, since conditions such as acromegaly and Cushing's syndrome are known to be caused in a number of cases by chromophobe adenomas and since the eosinophilic oncocytomas do not show any signs of endocrine secretion at all. The type of staining seen in routine pathologic specimens characterizes the amount of hormone secreted rather than its biologic type (Young, Bahn, and Randall; Robert; Landolt and Hosbach; Landolt). *A clinically oriented classification has to be based on the type of hormone secreted.* The largest group of adenomas with clinical signs of hormone secretion secrete growth hormone (10% to 33% of all adenomas in different series). They are more frequent in females than in males and produce *gigantism* in young individuals during the growth period and *acromegaly* in adults. The patients show enlargement of the hands and feet, prominence of the jaw and supraorbital ridges, thickening of tongue, hyperhydrosis, hypertrichosis, deepening of voice, headaches, arthralgias, insulin-resistant diabetes mellitus, amenorrhea, impotence, and loss of libido.

In this connection, we want to stress also that the hormone-secreting adenomas involve the chiasm far less commonly than the nonsecreting type. In our series of 23 patients with acromegaly a chiasmal syndrome was observed only five times (a frequency that is still lower than that found by others, for example, Mundinger, Riechert, and Reisert reported 30%; Tönnis, 36%; and Bakay, 41%). Furthermore, the compression of the chiasm caused by an acidophil adenoma is always minor. Surgical intervention is usually not necessary; radiotherapy will suffice in most cases. Apart from visual field defects and optic atrophy (described in the discussion of chromophobe adenomas), proptosis and, infrequently, palsies of the ocular muscles (resulting from a hemorrhage into the adenoma) may occur with acromegaly.

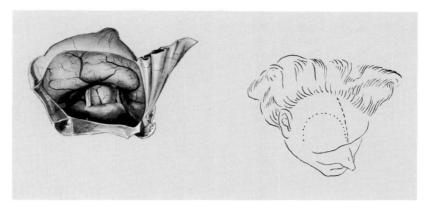

**Fig. 3-33.** Solid chromophobe pituitary adenoma (mostly intrasellar) with beginning suprasellar extension in 29-year-old patient. Tumor was approached via right frontal osteoplastic craniotomy. Note separation and compression of optic nerves caused by neoplasm growing upward from sella.

The *amenorrhea-galactorrhea syndrome* (Forbes, Henneman, Griswald, and Albright) is caused by a prolactin-secreting adenoma. The syndrome is rare (about 3% of the pituitary adenomas). *Cushing's syndrome* is usually caused by an adrenocorticotropin-secreting adenoma. The patients show adiposity, moon facies, hypertension, osteoporosis, steroid diabetes mellitus, and hypogonadism. Visual symptoms are extremely rare in uncomplicated cases, because the disease is usually caused by pituitary microadenomas. Patients with Cushing's syndrome caused by such a microadenoma who have been treated by extirpation of the hyperplastic adrenal glands develop visual disturbances and hyperpigmentation in about one third of the cases after some years. This is called *Nelson's syndrome* (Nelson). The increased growth of the primarily unrecognized pituitary microadenoma is a result of the loss of the negative feedback that was originally caused by the increased blood steroid levels. Adenomas causing Cushing's or Nelson's syndromes are also rare (2% to 3% of the pituitary adenomas). Pituitary adenomas with thyrotropin and gonadotropin secretion have been described, but are extremely rare and therefore of no practical importance.

The majority of pituitary adenomas (55% to 80%) present clinical signs of a space-occupying lesion with various degrees of pituitary insufficiency and no clinical signs of secretory activity. They are usually designated as *"chromophobe adenomas."* They are characterized by sexual disturbances (amenorrhea, impotence, loss of libido), decreased basal metabolic rate, weight gain, skin changes (straw color, wrinkling, scanty growth of beard in males), tiredness, loss of resistance in stress situations, tendency toward hypoglycemia, and decreased steroid excretion. Hypothalmic disturbances (diabetes insipidus, disorders of thermoregulation) are seen only in extremely rare cases (Fig. 3-33).

Ultrastructural and histoimmunologic examinations demonstrate that this group of pituitary adenomas showing only signs of hyposecretion is really a collection of different tumor types. The *oncocytomas* (Kovacs and Horvath; Landolt and Oswald) exhibit a fine eosinophilic granulation in routine sections. These patients seem to suffer from a defective metabolism and show an abnormal accumulation of altered mitochondria on electron microscopic examination. The ultrastructure of other adenomas demonstrates an ongoing secretory activity despite the absence of clinical signs of hormone production. Four possible explanations can be offered (Peillon; Zimmermann, Defendini, and Frautz; Landolt and Hosbach; Landolt): (1) The adenomas produce large amounts of prolactin, which does not cause galactorrhea because of the absence of other hormones necessary for lactogenesis. (2) The adenomas produce normal hormones (for example, growth hormone, prolactin) in low quantities that still fall within or only slightly above the normal limits. (3) The hormone proteins secreted show slight molecular changes that still allow their determination as "normal hormones" by radioimmunoassay, but that result in their no longer being recognized by the biologic receptor site and therefore being ineffective. (4) Grossly abnormal substances might be produced.°

Apart from the genuine pituitary tumors, there are numerous other tumors that may invade the hypophysis and thus produce pituitary dysfunction and eventually a chiasmal syndrome: tumors of the frontal lobe, tumors of the third ventricle, tumors of the chiasm, tumors extending from the sphenoidal sinus, and tumors from the nasopharynx. *Metastatic tumors* within the sella (for example, carcinoma of the breast, adrenal carcinoma) also occur. Other tumors that are not primary intrasellar are *intrasellar epithelial cysts, arachnoid cysts, mucoceles of the sphenoid sinus*, chordomas, osteochondromas, ectopic pinealomas, meningiomas, teratomas, and *aneurysms*. (See discussion of differential diagnosis of tumors of the sella, p. 227.)

Malignant tumors of the pituitary gland are mainly *primary carcinomas of the pituitary*, characterized by extension above the sella, invasion of the cavernous and sphenoidal sinuses, and sometimes dural or even extracranial metastases.

The cardinal ocular signs and symptoms of pituitary tumors can be expressed in two words: *chiasmal syndrome*. This syndrome consists primarily of *disturbances of the visual field, loss of vision,* and *fundus changes* (in other words, the consequences of an impaired conductivity of the chiasm, the optic nerves, or the optic tracts caused by the tumor). The functional endocrine changes of the pituitary gland previously mentioned produce secondary or accompanying signs and symptoms that may assume some importance for differentiation from other tumors in the sellar area.

*The subjective complaints of the patient* are strikingly similar and may in themselves lead to the right diagnosis. Time and again the complaints are a *decrease of vision* (in 70% according to Tönnis), *often at first on one side, but occasionally on both sides.* This decrease of vision is described as a veil, fog before the eyes, vision through a dirty or dull spectacle lens, a cloud, or vision through a tinted lens. Frequently, patients ask for new glasses. With the appearance of the visual disturbances, headache that may have been present for years and that was localized in the frontal region, in the temporal region, or in the eyes themselves may cease. Unfortunately, we have seen numerous patients who sought medical aid only after one eye had already become amaurotic and the other eye had begun to lose sight (24% of cases, according to Tönnis). It is characteristic and valuable that some patients assert that they notice a decrease of vision only at dusk or after physical exertion, in some cases also during pregnancy, with a transient improvement of vision post partum! Among the 33 patients with adenomas of the pituitary gland in our series, the more or less sudden onset of a unilateral loss of vision in three caused the consulting ophthalmologist to make *the misdiagnosis of a retrobulbar neuritis*. The retrobulbar injections were credited with a temporary improvement, which actually seemed to confirm the wrong diagnosis in these cases. This improvement, however, was only short-lived and was followed by final deterioration of

---

°We wish to thank Dr. Landolt, Neurosurgical Unit, University of Zurich, for contributing these general considerations on pituitary tumors.

vision. In the end the diagnosis of a pituitary tumor was made, although after considerable delay. Usually the onset of visual symptoms is insidious and their course slowly progressive, most patients having had complaints for up to 2 years.

Although the loss of vision in pituitary tumors is usually gradual, extremely rapid (within minutes or hours) loss of vision or onset of amaurosis in one or both eyes may occur. (See discussion of pituitary apoplexy and differential diagnosis of aneurysms of the sellar region, p. 258.) Patients complain only occasionally of attacks of transient amaurosis lasting from a few seconds to an hour or more.

*Hallucinations* among patients with adenomas of the pituitary are unusual, but according to Weinberger, Adler, and Grant, do occur either in the form of flashes of light or in the form of complex figures and complicated geometric patterns. They are explained on the basis of a secondary involvement either of the cerebral peduncles (peduncular hallucinosis) or of the temporal lobes. One extraordinary, interesting observation concerns a patient who noticed rapid bilateral deterioration of his visual acuity following a stellate ganglion block for trophic disturbances in one arm. A permanent impairment on the side of the injection caused annoying clouding and fogging of vision. Subsequently, an acidophil pituitary adenoma was discovered.

Although patients with pituitary tumors practically always complain of loss of vision, *they will less frequently mention disturbances of the visual field.* To some extent, this results from the fact that they are not conscious of the superior temporal field defects in the early stages of the development of a pituitary tumor—defects that, because of their peripheral situation, are not disturbing. In the later stages, however, complaints relating to visual field changes are quite characteristic. The patient states that he collides with people approaching from the side; that he drives his car over the sidewalk because he does not see the curb; that when reading he sees only part or perhaps only one half of the line; that he cannot see out of the corners of his eyes and must turn his head too much; that he feels as if he has *blinders* on both sides of his eyes (a motorist noticed these blinders for the first time after a strenuous drive); that at times he sees only the middle of people's faces; and that either one or both of the outer sides of his field appear in the shade. Such more or less spontaneous descriptions of field defects so characteristic for pituitary adenomas were recorded in more than one fourth of the patients in our series (28% according to Mundinger, Riechert, and Reisert). Occasionally, patients complain of transient or permanent diplopia, which usually can be traced to a corresponding extraocular muscle paresis.

The *ocular signs and symptoms of the chiasmal syndrome* consist of changes of the *visual field* and the *fundus.*

The characteristic field change is *bitemporal hemianopia.* We have seen such a characteristic field in a large number of cases (about one half of our patients, 60% according to Tönnis, 63% according to Bakay) during the first examination.

There has always been a more or less vertical line of separation either through the point of fixation or more frequently just sparing it. In such patients the subjective visual disturbances, especially symptoms of a hemianopia, have been pronounced. *Symmetry of the bitemporal field defects is characteristic for pituitary tumors. It is important for their differentiation from extrasellar conditions.* This symmetric bitemporal hemianopia usually involves the peripheral as well as the central field (Fig. 3-34). In some of our patients, peripheral isopters indicated perfectly normal limits and only the central isopters demonstrated the bitemporal defect (Fig. 3-35); in others only the peripheral field was defective.

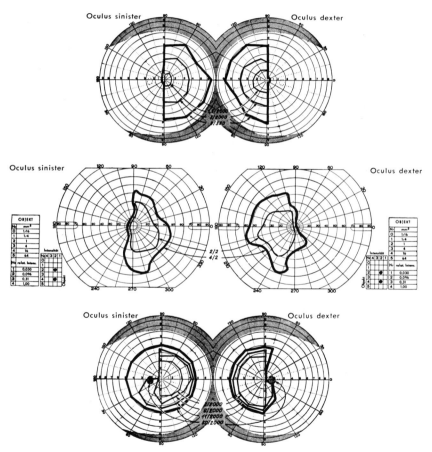

**Fig. 3-34.** Three cases of intrasellar and suprasellar chromophobe pituitary adenomas with typical chiasmal syndrome: bitemporal hemianopia, loss of vision, and optic atrophy. Above, Symmetric bitemporal hemianopia with vertical line of separation and only slight sparing of macula. Peripheral and central isopters are involved. Middle, Bitemporal hemianopia with slight asymmetry of missing and remaining parts of visual fields. Below, Symmetric, slightly incomplete bitemporal hemianopia with preservation of islands of vision in both inferior temporal quadrants. Left peripheral isopter (50/2000) does not reveal hemianopia!

The presenting visual field changes in patients with pituitary tumors are not always so typical. The classic fully developed bitemporal hemianopia actually is only an advanced stage in the gradual development of the field changes. *The very first defects in a pituitary tumor start in the superior temporal quadrants* (Cushing and Walker; Traquair). Frequently, these defects are bilateral and symmetric, indicating an impairment of the inferior surface of the body of the chiasm by the tumor protruding from the sella, in other words, an involvement of the crossing fibers originating from the inferior nasal quadrants of both retinas. Frequently, however, the field defect in a temporal upper quadrant is limited to one eye in the early stages (Figs. 3-36 and 3-37). Only at a later date will the other eye show a similar change. It is often necessary to search for such peripheral superior temporal field defects with the most painstaking methods of perimetry and campimetry (Chamlin and Davidoff). Again, we want to call attention to the signal value of kinetic perimetry performed with targets of

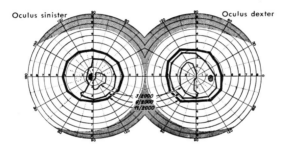

**Fig. 3-35.** Macrocystic chromophobe pituitary adenoma with marked compression of chiasm and optic nerves. Beginning bilateral optic atrophy. Corrected visual acuity, O.D. 0.6; O.S. 0.2. Slightly asymmetric bitemporal hemianopia of central isopters with normal peripheral (11/2000) isopters. Left paracentral hemianopic absolute scotoma temporally to vertical meridian ("junction" scotoma of Traquair).

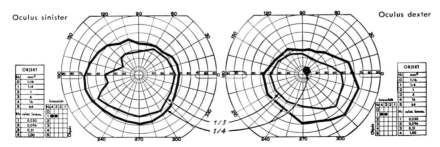

**Fig. 3-36.** Chromophobe pituitary adenoma with beginning extrasellar extension up to right optic nerve. Temporal pallor of right disc with visual acuity of 0.3. Normal left disc with visual acuity of 1.0. Very early beginning bitemporal indentation of superior fields, left somewhat more than right. Absolute paracentral scotoma of right eye temporally and superiorly to point of fixation.

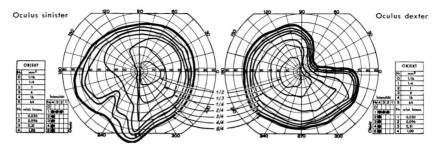

**Fig. 3-37.** Intrasellar chromophobe pituitary adenoma. Slight atrophy of left disc. Temporal pallor of right disc. Visual acuity, O.S. 0.9; O.D. 1.0. Subjective complaint of veil before eyes. Beginning loss of field in right superior temporal quadrant (peripheral and central isopters). At least central isopters of left field already show complete temporal hemianopic defect. (Case of Prof. Brückner.)

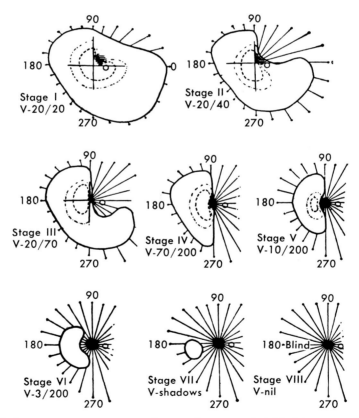

**Fig. 3-38.** Eight stages in progression of primarily temporal field defect in right eye with progressive growth of pituitary tumor. (After Cushing and Walker.)

varying light intensity and size on the Goldmann instrument, preferably combined with static perimetry performed on the Harms-Tübinger perimeter (p. 85).

It is imperative to determine a fairly large number of peripheral and central isopters because experience shows that the peripheral isopters show either no change or merely a superior temporal indentation, whereas the central isopters already indicate a distinct bitemporal hemianopia. In one sixth of the patients in our series, there was evidence of such a (mostly bilateral symmetric) quadrant loss or indentation in the superior temporal regions starting from the periphery. Here again, the usual course is a more or less pronounced symmetry. *During subsequent stages the field defects progress from the superior temporal to the inferior temporal quadrants* (crossing fibers from the superior nasal retinal quadrants!), leading to the full bitemporal hemianopia just discussed. The latter remains stationary for some time before a deterioration of other areas sets in. *Eventually, there follows a breakdown of the nasal halves of the fields, beginning with the inferior quadrants; the superior quadrants* (Figs. 3-38 and 3-39) *fre-*

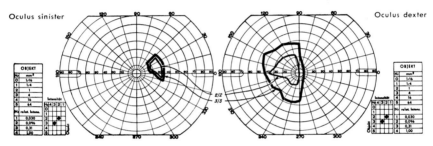

**Fig. 3-39.** Chromophobe pituitary adenoma with marked suprasellar extension. Bilateral temporal pallor of disc. Visual acuity, O.D. 0.3; O.S. 0.1. Temporal hemianopia (stage IV according to Cushing) of right eye. Island of vision in left superior nasal quadrant (stage VII according to Cushing). Tumor has reached left outer rim of chiasm!

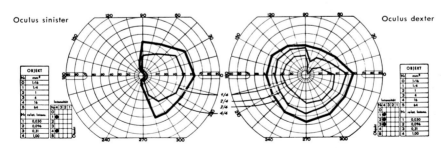

**Fig. 3-40.** Chromophobe pituitary adenoma with suprasellar extension, especially toward left optic nerve. Advanced left optic atrophy. Normal right disc. Visual acuity, O.S. finger counting at 50 cm; O.D. 1.25. Asymmetric visual fields: left temporal hemianopia with loss of macula; right beginning superior temporal quadrantanopia.

*quently remain the most enduring ones* (Cushing and Walker). Such a course is obvious if one considers that the tumor must reach a fairly large size before it can strike at the noncrossing fibers that represent the nasal field and that, because of their position at the lateral aspects of the chiasm, are better protected than the fibers at the inferior surface. *It should be emphasized again that the rather symmetric progression in the deterioration of the visual fields of the two eyes throughout the whole course of the adenoma growth is characteristic of pituitary tumor.*

In addition to these characteristic features and stages of the field changes, there are other, less pathognomonic, forms (Fig. 3-40). The field loss, for instance, may progress more rapidly in one eye than in the other. It may lead to complete amaurosis in the first eye, whereas the other eye still shows a temporal hemianopia. Such an *amaurosis of one eye with a temporal hemianopia of its fellow* occurred in one tenth of the patients in our series (16% according to Tönnis, 15.5% according to Bakay) (Fig. 3-41). Blindness of one eye and a temporal field defect in the contralateral eye can be explained either by a frontal and lateral extension of the pituitary adenoma from the chiasm to one optic nerve or by a temporal extension from the chiasm to one optic tract (the blind eye is always on the side of the extension of the tumor). However, it should be stressed here that the same picture can be produced by extrasellar tumors such

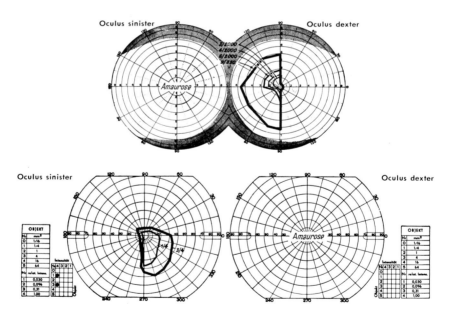

**Fig. 3-41.** Above, Chromophobe pituitary adenoma with suprasellar extension and invasion of third ventricle. Bilateral optic atrophy. Visual acuity, O.D. 0.8. Amaurosis of left eye with temporal hemianopia of right eye. Below, Enormous chromophobe pituitary adenoma with suprasellar extension. Temporal pallor of both discs, right more than left. Visual acuity, O.S. 0.5. Amaurosis of right eye with island of vision in inferior nasal quadrant of left eye.

as meningiomas of the tuberculum sellae (p. 235) or of the sphenoid ridge (p. 248) that extend into the chiasm either as primary *prechiasmal* tumors (first blindness of one eye and later temporal field defect in the contralateral eye) or as primary *postchiasmal* tumors (first homonymous hemianopia and later loss of temporal field with blindness in the eye on the side of the lesion). Thus an *amaurosis of one eye and temporal hemianopia of the other eye should be evaluated with great caution in diagnosing a pituitary tumor.* The most extensive destruction of the visual fields occurred in one of our patients with amaurosis on one side and preservation of only the inferior nasal quadrant on the other side (Fig. 3-41). In general, however, a patient with amaurosis on one side will notice disturbances on the other side relatively early.

In addition to disturbances of the peripheral field, we also find *scotomas* of varying sizes and types associated with pituitary tumors (scotomatous type of chiasmal syndrome). Traquair mentions them especially in rapidly growing tumors. Supposedly, they are not found if the tumor grows slowly or is stationary. In a review of our own cases, we found relatively few instances of central or paracentral *scotomas*, an observation in agreement with the statistics of Guillaumat and Robin. (Tönnis found them in 3.5% of patients with adenomas.)

The scotomas are important as localizing signs if they are the only manifestations of a pituitary tumor in its early stages—a type of field defect that occurs only infrequently. The quadrant or hemianopic shape of these scotomas as well as their location temporally to the vertical meridian is characteristic. Before a quadrant scotoma of the superior temporal quadrant extends into the inferior temporal quadrant, it usually merges with the blind spot. The development of such scotomas in pituitary adenomas must be interpreted as an interference of the tumor with the posterior angle of the chiasm (especially a prefixed chiasm), since the crossing macular fibers are situated near the posterior rim of the chiasm. Actually, neoplasms that attack the chiasm from the posterior rim (suprasellar tumors, craniopharyngiomas, tumors of the third ventricle) most readily cause the scotomatous type of the chiasmal syndrome. In one patient

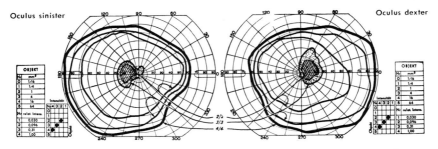

**Fig. 3-42.** Partly cystic, partly necrotic intrasellar chromophobe pituitary adenoma with compression of optic chiasm. No optic atrophy. Visual acuity, O.D. 1.25; O.S. 0.4. Bitemporal hemianopic paracentral scotomas: interference of tumor with posterior angle of chiasm. Peripheral isopters are completely intact. Scotomas are only manifestation of field defect!

with a pituitary tumor, we were able to demonstrate bitemporal hemianopic scotomas without impairment of the peripheral isopters (Fig. 3-42). Thus a central or paracentral scotoma in one or both eyes may not only be the first evidence of a pituitary tumor, but may also remain the only ocular manifestation. In general, however, the development and progress of central and paracentral scotomas parallel those of the peripheral field. Thus their diagnostic importance should not be overestimated, except as an indication of tumor interference with the posterior angle of the chiasm.

*Arcuate scotomas,* especially below the horizontal meridian, mostly unilateral, and exactly resembling those in chronic simple glaucoma, have been described in pituitary tumors by different authors (Kearns, Salassa, Kernohan, and MacCarty; Rucker; Dubois-Poulsen; Hoyt). They are interpreted as a pressure effect of the anterior cerebral and anterior communicating arteries on the superior part of the optic nerves and chiasm. Hoyt concludes from these observations that some arcuate fiber organization must persist even in decussating fiber projections within the chiasm. Central and paracentral scotomas require very careful perimetry or campimetry for early detection and exact follow-up; in this connection, we call special attention to the cardinal value of *static perimetry* (Harms; Aulhorn).

One should be mindful of the fact that some authors talk about "scotomas" of pituitary tumors if the peripheral isopters are still completely intact while the intermediate or central isopters already show a distinct quadrant or hemianopic temporal defect. Some patients under our observation showed an initial indentation of the central isopters in the superior temporal quadrant. During the course of growth of the tumor a gradual corresponding indentation of the peripheral isopters resulted in a regular quadrant defect (Fig. 3-43). Also, parts (especially temporal) of the field may become separated to form isolated islands ("ilot temporal"). During the later development of the tumor, they also become extinct (see Fig. 5-9).

In our patients, we observed only a single case of an asymmetric *homonymous hemianopia* (according to Tönnis, in 2% of patients with "chromophobe" adenomas) with the entire half of the field of one eye and three quadrants of the

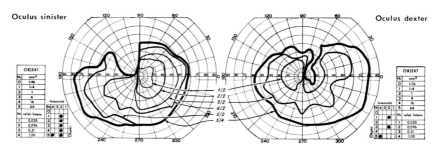

**Fig. 3-43.** Intrasellar and suprasellar chromophobe pituitary adenoma with large cyst. Bilateral temporal pallor of discs, more on right side. Visual acuity, O.D. 0.1; O.S. 1.0. Asymmetric bitemporal superior quadrantanopia of peripheral as well as central isopters as initial stage of chiasmal syndrome. Right upper temporal field remnant may break off to form "ilot temporal."

field on the other side missing. It occurred in a patient with a huge pituitary tumor with pronounced extension into the retrochiasmal space. It must be assumed that mainly one optic tract was damaged in this case.

It may be of interest to mention that there are pituitary adenomas that cause *no defect in the visual fields.* Mundinger, Riechert, and Reisert gave a figure of about 4%, whereas Cushing and Walker and also Tönnis cited a figure of 20% in their total cases of pituitary adenomas. This is in agreement with the statistics of Guillaumat and Robin, who found among 78 cases of pituitary adenomas 14 cases of normal visual fields. These high figures for normal fields might well be reduced in the future as a result of more exact and refined perimetry (for instance, static perimetry!), but also because of more extensive and refined endocrinologic examinations of patients suspected of having this lesion.

There is a certain relationship between the size of the field defect and the extent of the tumor. However, it should be emphasized that *in the case of pituitary adenomas the relationship between the size of the tumor and that of the field defect depends on the position of the chiasm relative to the diaphragma sellae* (Fig. 3-44). Under normal conditions a pituitary adenoma must expand approximately 2 cm in the superior direction before its pressure against the chiasm produces symptoms of a field defect. If the chiasm is fixed anteriorly or posteriorly, the tumor must reach an even larger size in order to produce visual field changes. In some instances, pituitary adenomas may assume an enormous *extrasellar extension* (Jefferson). They may expand into one of the following various directions: toward the sphenoid sinus, toward the hypothalamus, toward the temporal region, toward the cavernous sinus, posteriorly

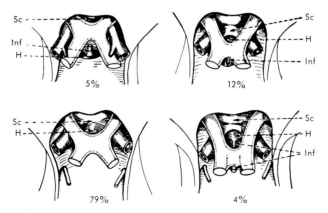

**Fig. 3-44.** Normal variants in topographic relationship between chiasm on one hand and pituitary gland and sella turcica on other hand. *Sc,* Chiasmal sulcus; *Inf,* infundibulum; *H,* pituitary gland. *5%,* Chiasm above tuberculum sellae; *12%,* chiasm wholly over sellar diaphragm; *79%,* posterior rim of chiasm above dorsum sellae; *4%,* chiasm on and behind dorsum sellae. (After de Schweinitz; from Kyrieleis.)

into the infratentorial region, and anteriorly into the frontal region (Fig. 3-45). The various neurologic symptoms characteristic for each particular area thus are added to the chiasmal syndrome. Whereas a suprasellar extension of the pituitary adenoma is quite frequent (in 70% of the cases according to Tönnis), as it is actually responsible for the chiasmal syndrome, a *parasellar extension through the thin wall of the cavernous sinus* is rare (Weinberger, Adler, and Grant; Cairns). In such cases the result may be *extraocular muscle pareses*, especially those supplied by the oculomotor and sixth nerves, with the patients occasionally reporting a corresponding diplopia (Fig. 3-46). We have

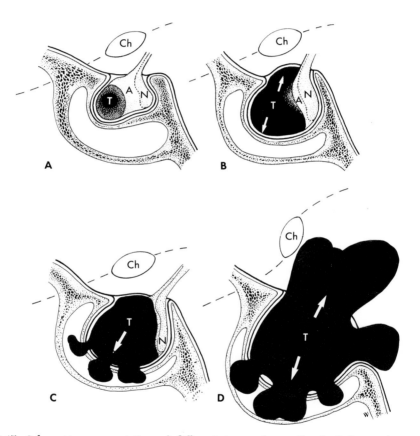

**Fig. 3-45.** Schematic representation of different types of growth of pituitary adenomas. **A,** Microadenoma, normal position of sellar diaphragm, normal size of sellar area. **B,** Enclosed adenoma with intrasphenoidal and suprasellar expansion, bulging of floor of sella against sphenoid sinus, elevation of sellar diaphragm against intracranial cavity, increase of volume of sellar area. **C,** Locally invading adenoma: dura and bone of sellar floor are destroyed and infiltrated by tumor protruding into sphenoidal sinus. **D,** Diffusely invading adenoma: tumor destroys and traverses dura and bone of sellar floor, sellar diaphragm, and anterior, posterior, and lateral walls of sella. Note displacement of chiasm. *T,* Pituitary adenoma (tumor); *A,* adenohypophysis; *N,* neurohypophysis; *Ch,* chiasm.

observed this in about one fourth of the patients with pituitary tumors (10% according to Tönnis, 7% according to Bakay). Twice the extrasellar lateral expansion resulted in an actual *cavernous sinus syndrome* (p. 39) with involvement of the third, fourth, fifth (facial neuralgia or anesthesia), and sixth cranial nerves. If the tumor produces a stasis within the cavernous sinus, it causes a more or less pronounced *exophthalmos* on the same side. In one of our patients a pituitary tumor extended into the third ventricle, causing an internal hydrocephalus with occlusion of both foramina of Monro and, at the same time, a severe psychoorganic syndrome.

Sometimes combined with bitemporal field defects in pituitary adenomas (and also in other chiasmal lesions) one may observe a so-called *see-saw nystagmus,* a peculiar dissociated vertical nystagmus consisting of rising of one eye and falling of the other combined with torsional movements of both eyes (Maddox; Mark, Smith, and Kjellberg).

It has already been mentioned that *eosinophilic adenomas show much less tendency for extrasellar extension and an associated compression of the chiasm* (Davidoff). We have observed visual field changes five times among 23 patients with acromegaly (36% according to Tönnis, 41% according to Bakay) (Fig. 3-47). There were two instances of bitemporal superior quadrant defects and

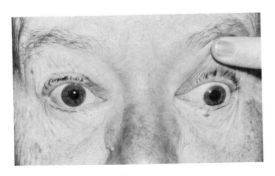

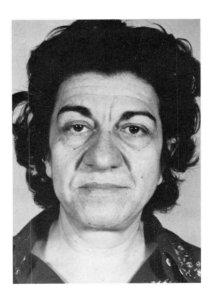

**Fig. 3-46**                          **Fig. 3-47**

**Fig. 3-46.** Left oculomotor nerve paralysis in case of chromophobe pituitary adenoma extending into cavernous sinus. Ptosis and outward and downward displacement of left eye caused by palsy of left internal and superior rectus muscles.

**Fig. 3-47.** Distinct acromegaly (enlargement of head, superciliary ridges, nose, and lower jaw) in woman with eosinophilic pituitary adenoma.

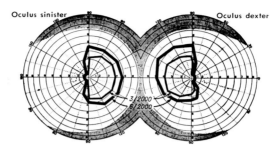

**Fig. 3-48.** Eosinophilic pituitary adenoma with suprasellar extension. Acromegaly. Visual acuity, O.D. 0.1; O.S. 0.5. No definite optic atrophy. Symmetric bitemporal hemianopia with sparing of macula.

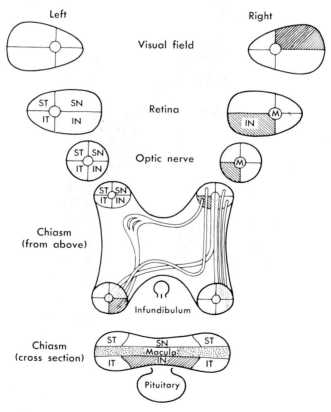

**Fig. 3-49.** Schematic representation of fiber distribution in visual pathway from retina to chiasm. Note relationship between inferior nasal (*IN*) fibers (corresponding to superior temporal visual field areas) and pituitary in cross section of chiasm.

one of a complete bitemporal hemianopia with sparing of the macula (Fig. 3-48).

This may be the opportune place to clarify in a few words the *relationship between the visual field defects and the tumor effect on the chiasm*. It has already been mentioned that the relationship between the size of the tumor and the nature of the field defect depends on the position of the chiasm relative to the diaphragma sellae. If the chiasm is in a normal position (lying above the sella turcica), bitemporal hemianopia results, indicating a lesion of the entire midline of the body of the chiasm. If the chiasm is fixed posteriorly, one or both optic nerves may be involved, and if the chiasm is fixed anteriorly, one or both tracts may be affected.

The fundamental anatomic basis for the clinical sign of bitemporal hemianopia is the separation of crossing fibers (in the midline of the chiasm) and uncrossed fibers (at the lateral edge of the chiasm) (Fig. 3-49). However, regional anatomy, intrinsic nerve fiber organization, and physiology of the chiasm are still incompletely understood even today and therefore our ability to interpret the visual defect on this basis is still limited. In this connection, we would like, in agreement with Hoyt, to call attention to the numerous existing diagrams of the chiasm that depict the fiber organization of the chiasm in schematic form but at the same time contain much conflicting and misleading information. Hoyt, an expert in chiasmal pathology, comes to the conclusion that existing diagrams (including his own) are not completely satisfactory and must be applied with caution in correlating clinical data with neuropathologic conditions (Fig. 3-50). Moreover, the mechanism by which pituitary tumors and other tumors originating from structures surrounding the chiasm produce chiasmal damage is still incompletely understood. It certainly must consist of various factors. Deformation, flattening, and stretching of the chiasm are the purely mechanical consequences of extrinsic tumor pressure. Whether such a mechanical distortion of the chiasm is really responsible for the visual field defects is not certain. Such a distortion is usually manifest before defects in the visual fields become evident. It is not even established whether direct contact of the tumor with the chiasm is necessary for the production of visual field defects. It is most probable that factors other than nerve fiber compression might be involved in the bitemporal hemianopia produced by pituitary tumors. It is a fact that despite numerous variations in the normal anatomy of the chiasm and great variation in the degree and pattern of chiasmal distortion, the resulting visual field defect, bitemporal hemianopia, remains monotonously the same. Also, the often observed rapid recovery of vision and visual fields after decompression of the chiasm suggests that nerve compression cannot be the only mechanism responsible. *Of great and often underestimated importance seems to be the arterial blood supply and its impairment by the growing tumor.* After extensive autopsy examinations, Bergland and Ray come to the conclusion that the optic chiasm receives an arterial blood supply from a *superior group of vessels* (derived from the anterior cerebral arteries) that spares the central chiasm and from an *inferior group of vessels* (derived from the internal carotid artery, the posterior cerebral artery, and the posterior communicating artery). The decussating fibers in the central chiasm receive their arterial supply only from the inferior group. During pituitary tumor surgery, these authors found the inferior group of vessels commonly distorted and compressed (the superior group is not affected) and therefore conclude that the bitemporal field defects caused by these tumors result from ischemia rather than from neural compression (Fig. 3-51).

Classic *bitemporal hemianopia* in its full development indicates a lesion of the entire midline of the chiasm, in other words, a total functional interruption of crossing projections. *Bitemporal superior field defects* indicate involvement of fibers in the anterior chiasmal notch by the expanding tumor and impairment of conduction from the inferior nasal retinas. *Bitemporal hemianopic scotomas* alone or associated with inferior field defects indicate involvement of the posterior chiasmal notch where the macular projections occupy a large area of the transverse bar of the chiasm. The clinical observation that chiasmal field defects can be recognized in the central field at the same time or even before they are present in the peripheral fields is not easily understood and must, apart from diffuse pressure effects, be the result of disturbances of the arterial blood supply.

Gradual development of *blindness in one eye* (or central scotoma or temporal hemianopic

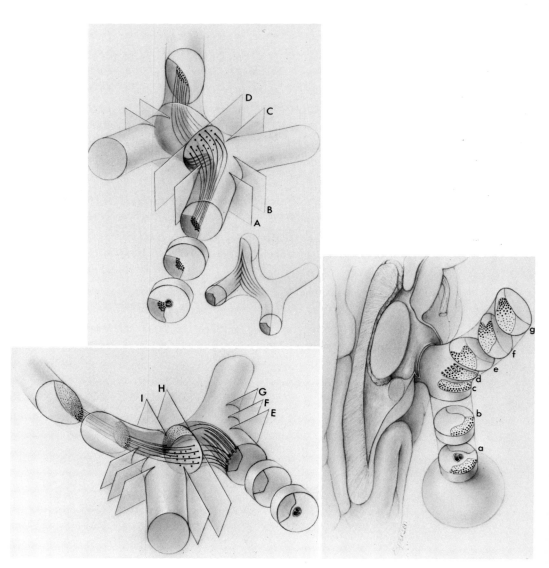

**Fig. 3-50.** Visual fiber anatomy of chiasm, as determined from Nauta's axon degeneration studies (Hoyt) in primates. Top, Inferior crossed extramacular retinal projections passing posteriorly into lateral optic tract of opposite side. Left, Superior crossed extramacular retinal projections passing posteriorly through chiasm (forming posterior inferior notch) and entering inferior medial optic tract of opposite side. Right, Uncrossed extramacular retinal projections undergoing inversion. Superior uncrossed projection takes medial position in optic tract. Large-caliber axons drop down into inferior optic tract (large black dots); smaller caliber axons rise into medial dorsal optic tract (small dots). Corresponding position of superior uncrossed quadrant projection (stippled) and inferior uncrossed projection (unstippled) are demonstrated at different levels in optic nerve, *a* and *b;* in chiasm, *c* and *d;* and in optic tract, *e, f,* and *g.* (From Hoyt, W. F., and Luis, O.: Arch. Ophthalmol. **70:**69, 1963.)

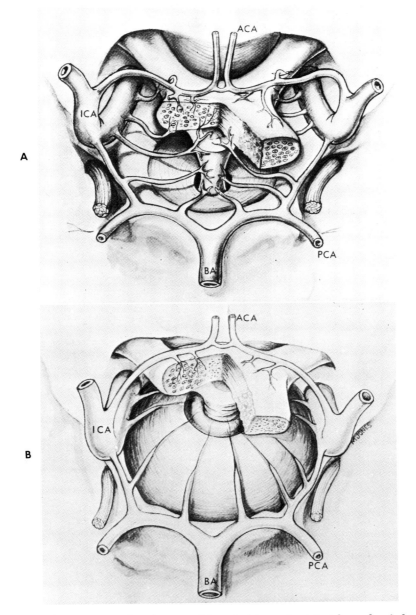

**Fig. 3-51. A,** Chiasmatic visual pathway and its arterial supply. Arterial supply of chiasm can be divided into superior and inferior groups. Superior group of vessels is derived from anterior cerebral arteries, *ACA,* and spares central chiasm. Inferior group of vessels is derived from internal carotid artery, *ICA;* posterior cerebral artery, *PCA;* and posterior communicating artery. Central chiasm containing decussating fibers derives arterial supply only from inferior group of vessels. *BA,* Basilar artery. **B,** Chiasmatic visual pathways distorted by pituitary tumor. Inferior group of vessels is distorted and compressed: thus central chiasm, containing decussating fibers, becomes ischemic. Superior group of vessels is not affected by tumor and lateral portions of chiasm retain their arterial supply. (From Bergland, R., and Ray, B. S.: J. Neurosurg. **31:**327, 1969.)

"junction" scotoma) and *later development of a temporal upper defect in the contralateral eye* point to a lesion of the intracranial segment of one optic nerve and an interruption of the anterior knee fibers at the junction of the optic nerve and the chiasm. Such pictures are also produced by prechiasmal tumors.

A lesion at the junction of the medial optic tract and the chiasm produces an *inferior quadrant defect in the contralateral temporal field* (superior crossing fibers) and a *small ipsilateral nasal field defect*, in other words, a sort of incongruous homonymous hemianopia. Hoyt has found this type of field defect in patients with glioma of the anterior third ventricle. *Homonymous hemianopia with additional loss of the temporal field* (and eventually blindness) *of the eye on the side of the lesion* indicates the extension of a tumor from the tract into the chiasm and is characteristic for postchiasmal tumors.

*Total temporal hemianopia in one eye with no temporal defect in the other eye* may also be observed in pituitary tumors (5.5% according to Tönnis) and must indicate a chiasmal lesion. However, such a defect, indicating involvement of all the crossing fibers only from one side, is difficult to explain and must be related to some peculiar pattern of chiasmal distortion by the growing tumor.

*Binasal hemianopias* are occasionally observed in patients with pituitary tumors. They are no longer regarded as a direct affection of the uncrossed fibers of both lateral chiasmal rims but rather as the result of a compression of these lateral rims by the carotid arteries, anterior cerebral arteries, or their communicating branches. However, they occur mostly in patients with infratentorial tumors (p. 290), tumors of the third ventricle (p. 276), or chiasmal arachnoiditis (p. 261).

Ipsilateral nasal hemianopia combined with an upper temporal defect in the contralateral eye (eventually associated with ipsilateral scotoma and reduction of central vision as a sign of optic nerve involvement) points to an ipsilateral lesion of the lateral margin of the chiasm. In such a case the superior temporal defect can be explained by the lateral position of the inferior crossed fibers from the optic nerve within the chiasm and the proximal parts of the contralateral optic tract.

In extremely rare instances, pituitary tumors may cause *horizontal hemianopias*. So far, there has been no satisfactory explanation for the pathogenesis of this phenomenon. They occur much more frequently in patients with chiasmal arachnoiditis or aneurysm of the circle of Willis (p. 322) or following traumas to the skull.

These reflections on some of the relations between the development and type of the visual field defect and the topographic position of the tumor with regard to the chiasm are helpful

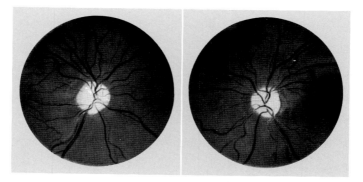

**Fig. 3-52.** Primary complete optic atrophy with distinct outlines in chromophobe pituitary adenoma with suprasellar extension (same patient as shown in Fig. 3-33). Temporal and nasal halves of both discs appear chalk white, are distinctly outlined, and are at level of retina. There is not yet atrophic excavation. Slight narrowing of arteries. Veins are normal. Capillaries on disc are missing completely. Papillomacular fiber pattern cannot be demonstrated in red-free light. Left illustration corresponds to right eye and right illustration to left eye.

in suggesting that part of the chiasm in which the tumor exerts a maximum of interference. This area, however, is not necessarily identical with the location of the main body of the tumor (Figs. 3-45 and 3-50).

The fundus changes associated with pituitary tumors can be best paraphrased as *primary simple optic atrophy*. There are gradual transitions from a partial pallor (sometimes a yellowish tint) to a snow-white, completely atrophic disc (Fig. 3-52). The disc characteristically is sharply outlined in all stages and surrounded by normal vessels. Papilledemas are extremely rare (occurring only in cases of secondary internal occlusive hydrocephalus). This is understandable if one bears in mind that patients with pituitary tumors, because of early visual disturbances, seek treatment long before the tumors reach a size where they could cause signs of an increased intracranial pressure. The atrophy is of the descending type (retrograde axonal degeneration). It is always bilateral. The involvement of the optic nerve may show the following variations: a uniform pallor of the entire disc (the most frequent form), a more pronounced pallor on the nasal side (atrophy of the nasal crossing fibers), and a more pronounced temporal pallor (in the case of a previously existing physiologic temporal pallor or excavation of the disc).

Frequently, the degree of atrophy differs in the two eyes. If, in addition to the chiasmal lesion, the optic nerve is involved (for instance, amaurosis of one eye and temporal hemianopia on the other side), the atrophy is particularly severe on the ipsilateral side. In extreme stages the atrophy causes not only pallor, but also an atrophic, pearly white crater, with the cribriform plate visible on its ground (with steep walls and a deep depression but not cupping of the disc margins, as in glaucoma!). In the one case, this pallor is caused by the ischemia of the disc structure; in the other case, it is the result of the secondary glial tissue proliferation that replaces the destroyed nerve fibers. It should be stressed that *there is no absolute relation between the degree of optic atrophy and the central vision. It is particularly characteristic for pituitary tumors that the optic atrophy lags behind the loss of vision.* The vision may have already failed considerably, yet the discs may show normal color. Evidently, the retrograde atrophy and glial proliferation have not yet extended to the nerve head.

In patients with unquestionable loss of vision and suspected bitemporal visual field losses, examination of the papillomacular bundle in red-free light (Vogt; Hoyt) may already demonstrate signs of atrophy (that is, absence of the striated pattern of the papillomacular fibers that normally is distinctly visible). We have observed *optic atrophy* in the majority of our patients; however, this is always seen *with a distinct difference between the two sides*, which usually corresponded to the difference in the visual acuity rather than the field defects. As mentioned before, the field defects in patients with pituitary tumors are rather symmetric. Although the lag of optic atrophy behind the loss of vision is the rule, the reverse (that is, pallor of the discs without marked loss of vision) is observed occasionally. *A pallor of the disc need not necessarily be identical with a func-*

*tional loss of the nerve fibers. The morphology of a pale disc may permit certain prognostic conclusions.* If, for instance, the pallor of the disc is combined with atrophic excavation, the outlook for recovery of the visual function after extirpation of the pituitary tumor is generally poor. If there is merely pallor of the disc without marked wasting of the nerve tissue, the chances for restoration of the visual function after surgical intervention are much better.

In order to give the degree of atrophy of the optic nerve a numerical value, Kestenbaum suggests counting the vessels passing over the margin of the disc. In normal eyes the number of vessels passing over the margin is fairly constant: four to five arteries, four to five veins, and about 10 small vessels. In primary optic atrophy the number of arteries and veins remains unchanged, but the number of the small vessels is diminished to seven, six, or even as few as three and thus represents a numeric measure of the degree of the pallor, allowing one to judge the development of optic nerve damage.

The *fluorescence angiogram* of primary simple optic atrophy is quite characteristic: the disc remains unstained and dark throughout all phases (which is in contrast to the fluorescence of the surrounding choroid). Even reactive glial tissue may show no staining if the atrophy of the vessels of the nerve head has progressed far enough.

*Pupillary changes* are rare among our patients with a pituitary chiasmal syndrome. *In those with marked unilateral loss of vision the pupil on the involved side shows a diminished direct reaction to light. The Marcus Gunn pupillary phenomenon is decidedly positive* (p. 27). In patients with unilateral amaurosis the pupil in question is sometimes found to be wider than the pupil of the contralateral side and fixed to light. It shows merely a consensual light reaction. It is common experience that the pupillary reaction remains intact longer than the visual function. Thus proof of a still-existing hemianopic pupillary reaction in an amaurotic eye with temporal hemianopia of the other eye may be an important diagnostic cue for a pituitary affection.

*The typical roentgenologic changes of the bony structure of the sella* should be briefly summarized, most of all because the general practitioner or the ophthalmologist frequently finds himself in a situation where he is the first to order and interpret a film. The characteristic roentgenologic sellar changes are as follows: *ballooning of the sella* with uniform enlargement in all diameters (observed in about one third of cases); depression and thinning of the floor of the sella, which protrudes into the sphenoidal sinus; and above all, *destructive changes at the dorsum and the anterior and posterior clinoid processes*, ranging from slight decalcification to destruction or erosion (Fig. 3-53). In patients with severe sellar changes and considerable extrasellar growth of the adenoma the optic foramina may manifest decalcification, blurring of their contours, or even destruction (Lombardi). Highly important information about shape, size, and connections of the pituitary adenoma can be gained by *pneumoencephalography* (preferably combined with tomographic techniques), revealing the encroachment on the suprasellar cisterns and the third ventricle and eventually also an indentation of the anterior horns of the lateral ventricles (Fig. 3-54). Most pituitary adenomas with a tissue density distinctly higher than brain tissue can be directly demonstrated (with or without contrast enhancing) in their suprasellar extensions by *computerized axial tomography*. It is important that roentgenologic sellar changes occur in patients with intrasellar pituitary tumors before the manifestation of visual field changes. This is in contrast to tumors of a primarily suprasellar growth, which frequently show visual field changes before roent-

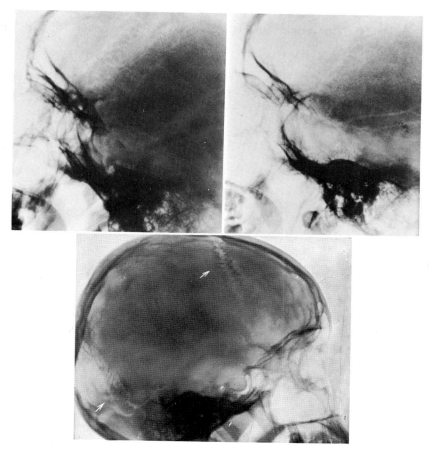

**Fig. 3-53.** Above, Roentgenogram of sella (lateral view) of 50-year-old patient with chromophobe adenoma of pituitary. Right, Enormous enlargement and ballooning of sella, thinning of sellar floor, dorsum sellae evidently destroyed, pointed appearance of tuberculum. Left, Sella of same patient 16 years before! Beginning enlargement of sella already visible. Below, Lateral view of skull of 15-year-old patient with astrocytoma of cerebellar vermis to demonstrate sellar changes in chronic increased intracranial pressure: slight enlargement of sella with normal thickness of its floor, posterior clinoid processes missing, marked osteoporosis of sella contour. Rupture of coronal and lambdoidal sutures (arrows).

genologic alterations occur. These x-ray findings are characteristic for pituitary adenoma and should not be confused with the effects of a generally increased intracranial pressure on the bony structures of the sella. The latter, as a rule, produces atrophy of the clinoid processes and the dorsum sellae as well as occasionally a certain widening of the opening of the sella (Fig. 3-53). Other neuro-ophthalmologic and purely neurologic signs should aid in the differential diagnosis of doubtful cases.

*Pituitary apoplexy* represents a syndrome characterized by intense headaches, unilateral or bilateral ophthalmoplegia, sudden occurrence of blindness in both eyes, and coma, which without surgical intervention leads to death within hours or days. Such a syndrome develops as a result of hemorrhage into a pituitary adenoma or an infarction within such a tumor. We have observed

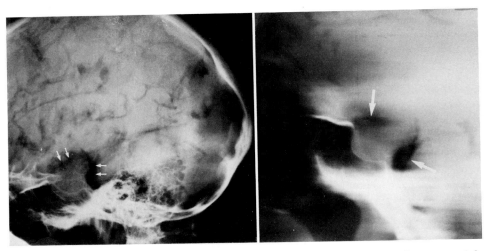

**Fig. 3-54.** Contours of pituitary adenoma growing into suprasellar space demonstrated by displacement of perichiasmatic cisterns (arrows) in ordinary pneumoencephalogram (left) and tomopneumoencephalogram (right).

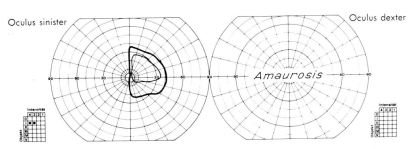

**Fig. 3-55.** Visual fields of 57-year-old patient after surgical intervention in pituitary apoplexy. Amaurosis on right side; temporal hemianopia on left side. Visual acuity, O.S., 1.0. Total disc pallor on right side; temporal disc pallor on left side.

one such patient; after operation the ophthalmoplegia disappeared within days, but one eye remained amaurotic and the other retained a complete temporal hemianopia (Fig. 3-55). Before the acute onset of the syndrome, the patient had no symptoms whatever, especially no ocular signs of his growing pituitary adenoma!

The recurrence of a chiasmal syndrome several years after successful surgery for pituitary adenoma usually indicates a tumor regrowth. In some of these cases, pneumoencephalography can reveal an *"empty sella syndrome."* The symptoms are caused by a downward movement and kinking of the optic chiasm secondary to scar formation within the sella (Olson). This scar formation as well as the visual symptoms do not occur in cases with spontaneous empty sella that is interpreted as secondary to increased cerebrospinal fluid pressure in the basal cisterns (Neelon, Goree, and Lebovitz). A bulging floor of the third ventricle resulting from obstructive hydrocephalus can cause a compression of the chiasm from above.

*In summary, it can be stated that the cardinal manifestations of the common nonhormone-secreting pituitary adenomas are chiasmal syndrome, hypopituitarism, and "ballooned" sella. The chiasmal syndrome includes the distinctive bitemporal hemianopia, which in numerous patients takes on a symmetric form. The visual field changes start in the superior temporal quadrants, usually also in a symmetric fashion. The field changes progress from the superior temporal to the inferior temporal quadrants. Only in the late stages is there involvement of the inferior nasal and, finally, of the superior nasal quadrants. The central or paracentral scotomas in the scotomatous type of chiasmal syndrome show a similar development. They may be the first and only ocular sign of a pituitary tumor! The development of amaurosis of one eye and temporal hemianopia of the other eye is a rather infrequent event. Symmetry of development and the final shape of the visual field defects are characteristic for the pituitary adenoma. The fundus changes consist of a more or less pronounced optic atrophy that, as a rule, lags behind the loss of vision; there is no direct relation between the degree of the atrophy and the loss of vision. The loss of vision may vary considerably and may progress to complete amaurosis. It is the first and most frequent ocular symptom. Complaints referring to temporal hemianopia are rare. In the case of extensive extrasellar expansion the pituitary adenoma may invade the cavernous sinus, causing extraocular muscle pareses (especially of the oculomotor and sixth nerves) or even an actual cavernous sinus syndrome. Pupillary disturbances are found mostly with severe loss of vision and especially with a unilateral amaurosis.*

After this discussion of pituitary tumor as the prototype of the sellar chiasmal syndrome, we have to consider the *differential diagnosis,* a rather complex problem because of the numerous types of tumors possible in this and the surrounding area. However, from the neuro-ophthalmologic point of view, in principle, we are always dealing with *more or less distinct modifications of a chiasmal syndrome.* Its atypical character can be summed up as *irregularity and asymmetry in its progressive development as well as in its final stage.*

### Craniopharyngiomas (suprasellar and intrasellar tumor type)

Craniopharyngiomas originate from epithelial remnants that, as vestiges of Rathke's pouch (craniopharyngeal duct), are scattered throughout the stalk of the pituitary gland (Erdheim). Such epithelial remnants are found above the diaphragma sellae on the anterior part of the infundibulum and below the diaphragm at the immediate area of transition from the stalk of the pituitary gland to the anterior lobe. Accordingly, there are craniopharyngiomas with a *primary suprasellar* and (less frequent) a *primary intrasellar origin.* The latter may show a suprasellar expansion in the course of their later development and thus form the third group, the combined intrasellar and suprasellar pharyngiomas. Craniopharyngiomas are predominantly tumors of childhood. However, they do occur in older persons up to the sixth decade. In reviewing our own series of 22 cases of craniopharyngiomas, we were surprised to find that

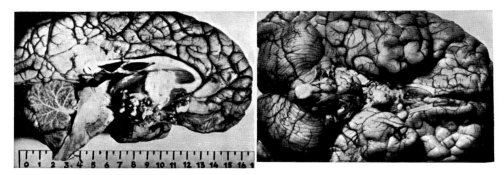

**Fig. 3-56.** Left, Median section through brain of 7-year-old girl with craniopharyngioma invading third ventricle. Right, Appearance of tumor as seen from below. Displacement and invasion of chiasm can be seen.

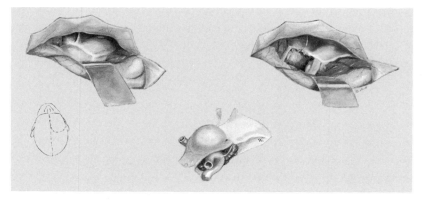

**Fig. 3-57.** Walnut-sized craniopharyngioma in region of tuberculum sellae of 41-year-old patient before and after surgical extirpation (right transfrontal osteoplastic craniotomy and extradural exposure of sellar region). Illustration in right upper corner shows right optic nerve as flattened cord. Illustration in center below shows how tumor compresses optic nerve and chiasm from above and from behind.

only one third involved adolescents and children, whereas all other patients were more than 20 years of age (according to Thiebaut, 66%!). If one considers several large series of cases in the literature, it is between the ages of 7 and 13, 20 and 25, and 60 and 65 years that most craniopharyngiomas are present. The general as well as the neuro-ophthalmologic symptomatology in children differs from that in adults (Figs. 3-56 and 3-57).

*In children and adolescents the symptoms of an increased intracranial pressure,* especially headache and vomiting, dominate the clinical picture. Tumor invasion of the third ventricle interferes with the circulation of the cerebrospinal fluid and causes an internal hydrocephalus. The head of such children is out of proportion to the size of the body. On percussion of the head, one frequently finds the typical "resonance of a cracked pot," a sign of suture ruptures. During puberty, endocrine pituitary-diencephalic disturbances (caused by an impaired development of the anterior lobe of the pituitary gland resulting from the tumor growth) produce the clinical picture of *dystrophia adiposogenitalis* (Fröhlich's type), *severe cachexia* (Simmonds' type), or *pituitary dwarfism* (Lorain's type). As a rule, there are also *hypothalamic signs* in evidence (such as, for instance, polyuria, polydipsia, and diabetes insipidus) as well as disturbances of central vegetative regulation, for instance of sleep (hypersomnia or insomnia) and temperature (hyper- or hypothermia).

In *adults* the complaints that bring the patient to a physician are not the symptoms of increased intracranial pressure but usually *visual disturbances.* In addition, adults frequently show mental disturbances and endocrine signs typical for hypopituitarism (sexual disturbances, adiposity, soft skin, loss of axillary and pubic hair, scanty growth of beard in males, etc.). There might also be hypothalamic signs in the form of polyuria, polydipsia, lethargy, hyperthermia, etc.

Some criteria regarding the *ocular signs and symptoms* can already be deduced from these introductory remarks. In *children,* especially babies, signs of increased intracranial pressure in the form of headaches, nausea, and vomiting predominate. Loss of vision is a phenomenon that occurs mostly in the later stage of the disease, but, once present, frequently progresses rapidly and even leads to blindness. There is a combined effect of compression of the chiasm and atrophy of the choked discs, with variabilities in the two factors. The parents of a child with severe impairment of vision stated that the child was unable to recognize grain while gleaning, that he ran into nettles, and that he did not look at people while talking to them. The ocular symptoms in *adults* are similar to those caused by a pituitary adenoma. In about 50% of the cases, there are *statements about loss of vision, especially on one side* (18% according to Tönnis). *In some cases, patients noted a distinct fluctuation of the visual acuity.* The frequently cystic nature of craniopharyngiomas explains such changes and may even simulate successful treatment of the visual loss caused by this tumor. Such was the case in a patient of Franceschetti and Blum; his vision in one eye improved from 0.2 to 1.0 2 weeks after retrobulbar injections of cobra venom, only to show a relapse later on. The *chances of confusing a disturbance of conductivity in the optic nerve caused by a craniopharyngioma with the signs of a retrobulbar neuritis* are great and need special consideration. In addition to making statements indicating loss of vision, the patients will often mention a corresponding constriction of the visual fields, as discussed in connection with pituitary adenomas (p. 207): a narrowing of the field to the side, the sensation of blinders, colliding with people in the street, and reading difficulties with half a word or even half a line missing. Frequently, double vision is mentioned. The underlying pareses of the extrinsic muscles are easily explained by the frequently massive extrasellar extension of these tumors or by the increased intracranial pressure.

The *ocular involvement,* especially in adults, is marked by the *chiasmal syndrome,* usually with an *asymmetric development and asymmetry in the end stage.* However, patients with the intrasellar type of craniopharyngioma may show visual field changes, which can easily be confused with those of a pituitary adenoma. In one case, we observed a typical onset in the two superior temporal quadrants combined with a temporal scotoma that extended into the blind spot (Fig. 3-58). This type of field change has been described previously in the discussion of pituitary adenomas. In not quite one fourth of our 22 patients with craniopharyngiomas, we have observed a typical *bitemporal hemianopia* (28% to 32% according to Banna, 40% to 50% according to Tönnis). However, it is important to stress again the *more or less pronounced asymmetry of the visual field defects* (Figs. 3-59 and 3-60). No vertical line separates the seeing and blind halves of the field, but the dividing line usually projects from

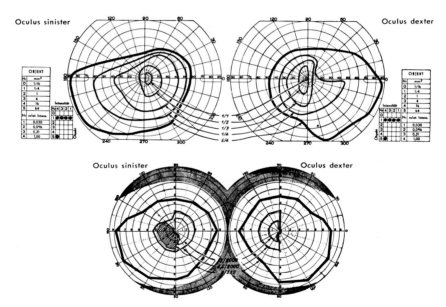

**Fig. 3-58.** Walnut-sized intrasellar craniopharyngioma near tuberculum sellae, compressing chiasm and optic nerve from anteroventral direction. One year prior to surgical intervention, loss of right visual acuity. Seven months prior to surgical intervention, right temporal hemianopia without symptoms in left eye! First signs of left field defects 2 months prior to surgery. Visual fields (above, Goldmann perimeter; below, tangent screen) taken shortly before surgery show asymmetric bitemporal hemianopia of central isopters, further advanced on right side. Peripheral isopters demonstrate similar asymmetric onset in both superior temporal quadrants. Temporal scotoma extending into blind spot on left eye. Visual acuity, O.U. 0.7; no optic atrophy.

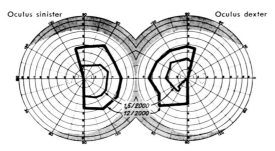

**Fig. 3-59.** Intrasellar and suprasellar craniopharyngioma of partly solid and partly cystic structure. Visual acuity, O.D. 0.8; O.S. only hand movement at 3 meters. Left disc slightly paler. Slightly asymmetric bitemporal hemianopia without sparing of macula on either side.

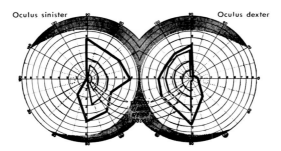

**Fig. 3-60.** Mostly intrasellar craniopharyngioma. Visual acuity, O.D. 0.25; O.S. 0.25. Bilateral optic atrophy. Bitemporal hemianopia with asymmetric development. No straight vertical dividing line. Right, Macular sparing. Left, Macular loss.

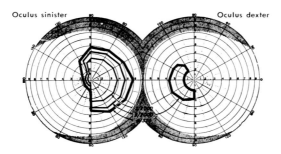

**Fig. 3-61.** Cystic craniopharyngioma in third ventricle. Visual acuity, O.D. 0.1; O.S. 0.3. Temporal optic atrophy more pronounced on right side. Bitemporal hemianopia with extreme asymmetry of visual field defects. Left, Macular sparing. Right, Kidney-shaped nasal island of visual field hugging macula.

the seeing into the blind part of the field, sparing the macula. In other cases, this dividing line deviates into the seeing part of the field, causing a macular loss. Occasionally, we have found kidney-shaped remnants of the field on the nasal side, with a peculiar hugging of the macular area (Fig. 3-61). This asymmetry may also manifest itself with one eye still showing a completely normal field and the other eye already revealing an indentation of the superior or inferior temporal quadrant (Fig. 3-62). Since craniopharyngiomas with primary extrasellar origin tend to expand into a retrochiasmal and suprachiasmal direction and to exert pressure on the chiasm from above and behind, they can be *expected to cause initial field defects in the inferior quadrants.* We made no personal observation of such a case. We do have records of two patients with *amaurosis on one side and temporal hemianopia on the other side* (33% in intrasellar craniopharyngiomas according to Tönnis) (Fig. 3-63). One patient showed a distinctly incongruous *homonymous hemianopia* (8% according to Tönnis) more suggestive of a tract lesion. Some reports in the literature (Wagener and Love; Dubois-Poulsen; Tönnis) stress the frequent and early occurrence of unilateral or bilateral central and paracentral *scotomas* in patients with

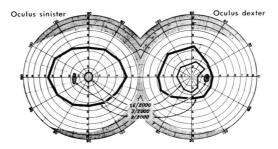

**Fig. 3-62.** Intrasellar, suprasellar, and retrosellar cystic craniopharyngioma. Visual acuity, O.D. 1.0; O.S. 0.8. Bilateral temporal optic atrophy, further advanced on left side. Beginning right temporal hemianopia with left peripheral isopters normal.

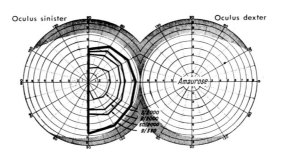

**Fig. 3-63.** Partly solid and partly cystic intrasellar and suprasellar craniopharyngioma. Visual acuity, O.S. 0.1. Complete bilateral optic atrophy with chalk-white discs. Amaurosis of right eye with temporal (strikingly symmetric) hemianopia of opposite eye.

craniopharyngioma. These observations are hardly in agreement with our experience; we have seen such scotomas (they are quite similar to the ones seen in pituitary adenomas as a consequence of compression of the crossed macular fibers in the posterior edge of the chiasm, p. 213) rather infrequently. It is evident that *it is quite difficult to prove the visual field changes in children,* especially with an increased intracranial pressure. Frequently, we have to depend here on a crude confrontation test by hand (p. 76).

In children the *predominant signs of increased intracranial pressure include more or less advanced choked discs.* These choked discs are frequently associated with a secondary optic atrophy (p. 123). Occasionally, a distinct choking is missing, but the atrophic discs show blurred or even slightly prominent margins, a quasi "forme fruste" of chronic atrophic papilledema. There are all conceivable intermediate forms and combinations between a pure atrophy and a pure papilledema. Venous and capillary stasis, tortuosity of veins, extravasations near the disc, blurring of the disc margin, and a slight prominence are infallible signs of increased intracranial pressure.

In *adults,* in whom there is a compression of the chiasm rather than the formation of a hydrocephalus, the ophthalmoscopic picture is that of a *primary optic atrophy with sharp borders.* In the section on papilledema (p. 120), we stressed that an atrophic disc, as a rule, is incapable of developing the typical signs of choking. This fact as well as the differential tendency to form a hydrocephalus must be taken into consideration in our interpretation of the difference between the fundus pictures of children and adults. Usually, there is a distinct dissimilarity in the degree of atrophy between the two eyes. Other phenomena associated with atrophy (p. 223) have been dealt with in the discussion of pituitary adenomas. They are also present here, especially a random or even inverse relation between the extent of the atrophy and the degree of loss of the visual function. *Despite normal optic discs, there may be extensive visual field defects and considerable loss of visual acuity.* In a few adults, we found a slight blurring and a trace of prominence of an atrophic disc (manifestation of an increased intracranial pressure; Seidenari).

*Disturbances of motility* involved mostly the oculomotor nerve, much more rarely the abducens. The involvement of the *oculomotor* nerve results from the parasellar expansion of the tumor—obviously into the region of the cavernous sinus. The diplopia occasionally mentioned by the patient has its objective equivalent in these muscular pareses. In one patient, we even found a bilateral oculomotor paresis. Unilateral or bilateral *sixth nerve* palsies are caused by the increased intracranial pressure and accordingly may show fluctuations. In this connection, we would like to mention that the *onset of a paralytic strabismus in a child sometimes represents one of the first symptoms of a growing craniopharyngioma!*

*Pupillary disturbances* are rather rare and occur in the case of unilateral severe impairment of vision or complete amaurosis as a diminished or even abolished direct reaction to light. There are cases of unilateral amaurosis in which the reaction to light is paradoxically retained (Walsh and Hoyt).

Once again, it should be stressed that the signs and symptoms, especially the ocular ones, associated with craniopharyngiomas may remain stationary or may even improve without any treatment because of the cystic nature of these tumors. In some cases, this has caused the understandable but *mistaken diagnosis of a unilateral or bilateral retrobulbar neuritis,* a diagnosis that seemingly was confirmed by the success of whatever therapy was employed. A tireless repeated *search for visual field defects in both eyes* is imperative in such cases; such defects may be missing in the initial stages of development of a craniopharyngioma. We observed a patient with a temporal hemianopic defect in one eye and no change whatsoever in the other eye. Only after 6 months was it possible to demonstrate a similar temporal defect in the other eye and thus substantiate the suspicion of a craniopharyngioma in the chiasmal region.

The *proof of suprasellar calcifications on the plain x-ray film* is of considerable value in the diagnosis of craniopharyngiomas (Fig. 3-64, *A*). They are present in 90% of the patients under 15 years of age and in only 40% of those over 15 years of age (Lombardi). Some of these calcifications are massive and others are quite delicate, resembling splashes. Usually they are suprasellar, only rarely intrasellar (Fig. 3-64, *A*). As a result of the decalcification and erosion of the clinoid processes and the dorsum, the sella may appear compressed. Only in the case of an intrasellar growth will there be ballooning and enlargement of the sella; its appearance resembles that seen in pituitary adenomas (p. 224). It is important to remember that in tumors with a predominantly suprasellar growth such as craniopharyngiomas *the visual field defects usually precede the roentgenologic signs.* Thus the former are of particularly great diagnostic significance. On a *computerized axial tomogram* (Fig. 3-64, *B*) a cystic craniopharyngioma can be seen directly. The diagnosis is based on the association of three types of tissue with different densities (calcified tissue, cyst, and solid tumor).

*The ocular manifestations of a craniopharyngioma can be summarized in the following manner. In children the ocular signs and symptoms of increased intracranial pressure (that is, papilledemas) dominate the picture. The bitemporal loss of the visual fields usually is difficult to demonstrate in children. As in the case of pituitary adenomas, the loss of vision is the most conspicuous sign in adults. Usually, it involves one side first, with the other side becoming impaired later. The pathologic-anatomic basis for the loss of vision is a primary optic atrophy, usually more pronounced on one side. Occasionally, minor signs of a papilledema are superimposed on the optic atrophy. The chiasmal syndrome is practically always present in adults. On the other hand, an asymmetry during the developing stages and in the end stage is typical. The characteristic visual field defect is a bitemporal hemianopia, usually with a certain asymmetry of the two halves of the field; the dividing line rarely lies in the midline, but is displaced either toward the blind or seeing part of the field. Oculomotor nerve*

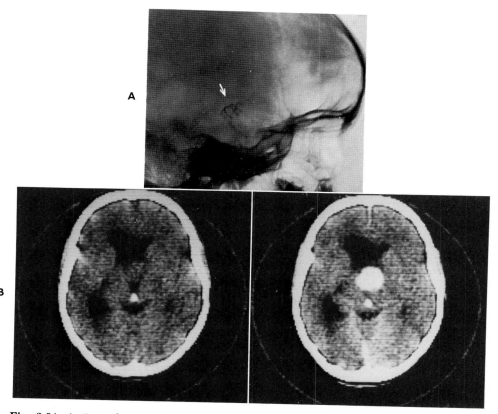

**Fig. 3-64. A,** Lateral x-ray film in patient with craniopharyngioma. Arrow indicates suprasellar calcifications. Compressed sella also present. **B,** Computerized transverse axial tomogram of craniopharyngioma. Left, Brain-identical absorption before application of contrast substance. Right, Intensive uptake of contrast substance by tumor (contrast scan). (**B** Courtesy Prof. Wuthrich, Neurological Department, Kantonsspital, Basel.)

*pareses as a sign of parasellar extension into the cavernous sinus are not so rare —at any rate, more frequent than those of the sixth nerve.*

## Meningiomas of the tuberculum sellae (suprasellar tumor type)

These tumors originate from the dura of the tuberculum sellae and its immediate surroundings (sphenoidal plane, chiasmal sulcus, anterior clinoid process, medial sphenoid ridge). A pronounced suprasellar development results in a superior and posterior displacement of the chiasm (Figs. 3-65 and 3-66). The tumors usually assume an asymmetric growth, involving at first only part of the chiasm or only one optic nerve. This causes a distinct *asymmetry of the chiasmal syndrome,* especially with amaurosis of one eye and a temporal visual field defect on the other side. The suprasellar meningiomas distinguish themselves by their *exceedingly slow growth,* which may extend over many years. Hypopituitarism or hypothalamic signs, especially in the initial stages, are extremely rare and occur only in the late stages after the tumor has reached a certain size. Compression of the third ventricle and blocking of the intraventricular foramina of Monro may cause an internal hydrocephalus during such late stages

(Cushing). In contrast to pituitary adenomas and craniopharyngiomas, there are no important roentgenologic changes of the sella turcica. Demonstration of the frequently occurring hyperostosis of the tuberculum sellae is of diagnostic importance. However, because of the paucity of nonvisual signs, suprasellar meningiomas are often misdiagnosed.

Cushing first described the picture of the chiasmal syndrome as it occurs in meningiomas of the tuberculum sellae as *"primary optic atrophy and bitemporal visual field defects with, in adults, a normal sella turcica."* In general, this definition is correct. However, it does not take into consideration the *conspicuous and characteristic incongruence of the chiasmal syndrome during its stages of development and in its final form.* Yet this phenomenon is quite pronounced in meningiomas of the tuberculum and still much more distinct than in cranio-

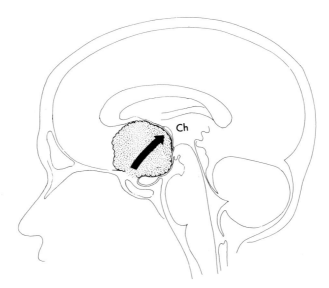

**Fig. 3-65.** Median section through skull schematically showing meningioma of tuberculum sellae displacing chiasm, *Ch*, in superior and posterior direction.

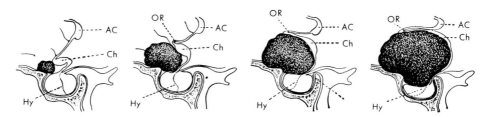

**Fig. 3-66.** Four stages in development of meningioma of tuberculum sellae demonstrating progressive deformation and compression of chiasm, which is pushed upward and backward. *AC*, Anterior commissure; *Ch*, chiasm; *OR*, optic recess; *Hy*, pituitary gland. (After Cushing and Eisenhardt.)

pharyngiomas, as the following considerations should clarify (Cushing and Eisenhardt; Hartmann; Guillaumat; Grant and Hedges) (Fig. 3-67).

The *ocular symptoms already suggest such an asymmetry;* the very first sign is always a significant *unilateral loss of visual acuity,* mostly in the form of a fog, veil, or glimmer before the eye involved first. Another characteristic symptom is a statement that the *unilateral loss of vision in one eye progresses slowly, often to complete amaurosis, yet without manifestation of any signs in the other eye.* Such signs may follow only later. Occasionally it happens that a patient is unaware of the amblyopia or amaurosis in one eye because the vision on the other side is still well preserved. The latent period between the affection of the first eye and the second eye may be years or even decades—20 years in a case we have followed up personally! *The unilateral impairment of the visual function that frequently is accompanied by a central or paracentral scotoma shows symptoms that, again, are quite similar to chronic retrobulbar neuritis*—in the broadest sense of the word.

Among 19 patients with meningioma of the tuberculum sellae, we observed three in whom the ophthalmologist who was originally consulted diagnosed a retrobulbar neuritis. In one patient a series of retrobulbar injections of tolazoline (Priscoline) seemed to cause a temporary improvement of vision. This apparently confirmed the suspected diagnosis of a retrobulbar neuritis. In another patient an optic atrophy associated with the "retrobulbar neuritis" was interpreted as being caused by multiple sclerosis. In one patient a unilateral impairment of vision improved for a short time after x-ray treatment. In this case the diagnosis of a tumor was made 15 years later and an operation finally performed. Because of unilateral loss of vision, one patient received irradiation of the pituitary region (without a convincing result) for 5 years. The first signs of loss of vision had occurred 8 years prior to the irradiation. A definite

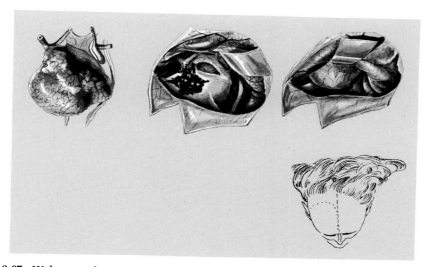

**Fig. 3-67.** Walnut-sized meningioma of tuberculum sellae in 48-year-old patient before and after extirpation (right transfrontal osteoplastic craniotomy). Small stump of tumor remains at right internal carotid artery.

diagnosis of meningioma of the tuberculum sellae and surgical intervention took place about 20 years after the occurrence of the initial symptoms in the first involved eye! Quite instructive is the history of another patient who complained of loss of vision in one eye for 9 years before a definite diagnosis was made. Throughout this period of time, he had been treated for an occupational toxic amblyopia and, accordingly, had received benefits from workmen's compensation. The tragic fact was that during this long latent period the meningioma of the tuberculum sellae resulted in amaurosis of the first involved eye and temporal hemianopia of the other eye!

The fact that impairment of vision and, with it, the field defects usually occur first only in one eye makes it understandable that subjective statements regarding these visual field defects are rather rare. The symptoms involve the temporal part of the field. The patients have the sensation of shadows, veils, a curtain, a wall, etc. on the side of the involved eye. Frequently, the patient remarks about defects only after the second eye has become involved and the first one is already amaurotic. Diplopia is rarely mentioned in the history.

*Compared with craniopharyngiomas, the asymmetry of the visual fields in patients with meningiomas of the tuberculum sellae is even more pronounced. Amaurosis of one eye with temporal hemianopia of the other eye, in our experience, is the most frequent and most characteristic sign.* We have observed this phenomenon in 12 of 19 patients. Guillaumat and Robin reported a similar ratio,

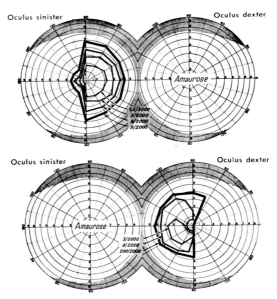

Fig. 3-68. Two cases of meningioma of tuberculum sellae with typical amaurosis on one side and temporal hemianopia on opposite side. Above, Meningioma weighing 20 gm. Complete right optic atrophy. Temporal pallor of the left disc. Visual acuity, O.S. 0.7. Left symmetric temporal hemianopia with sparing of macula. Below, Meningioma weighing 10 gm. O.S., Complete optic atrophy; O.D., incomplete optic atrophy! Visual acuity, O.D. 0.15. Slightly asymmetric right temporal hemianopia without sparing of macula.

as did Mundinger and Riechert. The explanation for this pattern is that the tumor is limited for a considerable time to one optic nerve and later extends to the median surface of the anterior angle of the chiasm, the area that contains the crossing nasal fibers of the contralateral side. Consequently, a unilateral amaurosis with temporal hemianopia of the field of the other eye is called *the syndrome of compression of the anterior angle of the chiasm.* It is *particularly characteristic for meningiomas of the tuberculum sellae* (Fig. 3-68). It must be mentioned here that the initially affected eye often progresses almost to complete blindness before a defect in the fellow eye can be noted. The temporal hemianopia of the second eye may either have a symmetric character with separation of the two halves of the field in the midline or, as happens frequently, there may be asymmetric temporal defects, with overlapping of the dividing line either into the temporal or nasal part of the field. In advanced stages the second eye may show only quadrant islands of the superior or inferior nasal field. In one patient, we

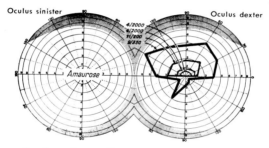

**Fig. 3-69.** Meningioma of tuberculum sellae that weighs 5 gm. Incomplete bilateral optic atrophy. Visual acuity, O.D. 0.05. Left amaurosis with right altitudinal hemianopia (partial loss in both inferior quadrants).

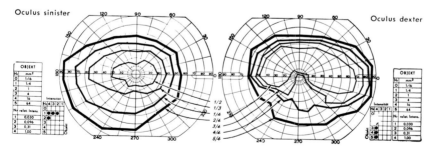

**Fig. 3-70.** Meningioma of tuberculum sellae that weighs 6 gm. Right disc shows temporal pallor. Left disc is normal. Visual acuity, O.D. finger counting at 1 meter; O.S. 1.5. Because of loss of right vision, this patient had been treated (without success) for retrobulbar neuritis! There is suggestion of asymmetric bitemporal inferior quadrantanopia. Distinct right temporal inferior quadrant defect. Left most central isopter shows indentation in inferior temporal quadrant. Involvement of right inferior nasal quadrant can be explained by extensive compression of right optic nerve confirmed during operation.

observed the onset of the temporal hemianopia in the superior temporal quadrant of the second eye. In another we noted an altitudinal hemianopia, with a horizontal dividing line and a loss of both inferior quadrants (Fig. 3-69).

In four of the 19 patients with meningiomas of the tuberculum sellae, visual field defects in both eyes could be demonstrated in the form of an extraordinarily *asymmetric, incongruous bitemporal hemianopia* (Figs. 3-70 and 3-71), occasionally with fairly large central and paracentral scotomas, often of the hemianopic type (Schlezinger, Alpers, and Weiss). For example, the asymmetry manifested itself in such a way that one eye showed a complete temporal hemianopia, with the dividing line through the point of fixation, whereas in the other eye only the inferior temporal quadrant was missing (Fig. 3-72). In the early stages of the bilateral field changes the defects of the inferior temporal quadrants seem to dominate the picture. Unilateral central or paracentral scotomas of a midline temporal hemianopic type, which are usually seen in association with peripheral temporal defects of the contralateral eye, correspond to the so-called *junction*

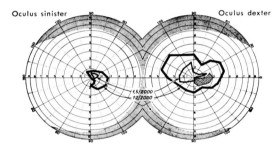

**Fig. 3-71.** Meningioma of tuberculum sellae. Primary optic atrophy with distinct margins and excavation of both discs, more on left side. Narrowing of arteries, especially on left side. Visual acuity, O.U. 0.15. Completely asymmetric, irregular bitemporal hemianopia with bizarre incongruence of remnants of visual fields. Right central-paracentral temporal scotoma of midline hemianopic character ("junction" scotoma).

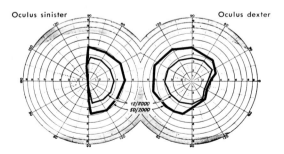

**Fig. 3-72.** Meningioma of tuberculum sellae that weighs 70 gm. Visual acuity, O.D. 1.0; O.S. 0.25. Right disc of normal color. Left disc shows temporal pallor. Asymmetric incongruous bitemporal hemianopia. Left side, Complete temporal hemianopia. Right side, Defect mostly in inferior temporal quadrant.

*scotomas* of Traquair and are typical for a lesion in the area of the optic nerve blending into the chiasm in the anterior angle of the chiasm (Fig. 3-71). As these scotomas are easily overlooked, they have to be searched for by careful (especially static) perimetry.

Just as in patients with pituitary adenomas and craniopharyngiomas, the *fundus findings* in patients with meningiomas of the tuberculum sellae are characterized by primary optic atrophy with sharply outlined discs. In line with the involvement of mainly one eye in the initial stages, a *unilateral optic atrophy or one more pronounced on one side is the rule.* The atrophy may vary in degree from partial pallor to a completely chalk-white disc with excavation (Fig. 3-52). As a rule, the atrophy lags behind the impairment of vision and the visual field defects. The latter may be present before the disc changes become manifest. In an extremely severe optic atrophy, especially with an amaurosis, there may be a narrowing of the retinal arteries and later of the veins. In such cases the caliber of the vessels is in contrast to those of the other side. Minor signs of a choked disc in the form of blurring of the margins and a slight prominence of the disc with a simultaneous atrophy of the papilla were noted once among our 19 patients—a patient with a particularly huge tumor. As a rule, there is no increased intracranial pressure, perhaps because the ocular symptoms are so alarming before the tumor grows too large. Ocular pareses were exceedingly rare in our series—one instance of a sixth nerve paresis among 19 patients.

*Pupillary disturbances* occur primarily in the first affected eye, usually as a diminished or abolished reaction to light. In a unilateral amaurosis the pupil is sometimes dilated and does not respond directly to light.

The *plain x-ray film* in meningiomas of the tuberculum sellae offers important diagnostic clues. The tumors usually do not attack the sella. Thus it appears

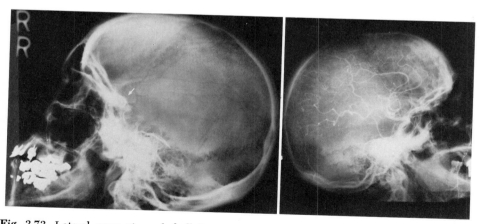

**Fig. 3-73.** Lateral x-ray view of skull in patient with meningioma of tuberculum sellae. Hyperostosis of tuberculum sellae (arrow). Carotid angiogram (right) shows characteristic elevation of anterior cerebral and anterior communicating arteries describing concave arch.

perfectly normal, at least in the initial stages. Later a decalcification and erosion of the anterior and posterior clinoid processes may be observed. Much more important from a diagnostic point of view is the *proof of hyperostosis of the tuberculum sellae or thickening of the sphenoidal plane. Occasionally there are calcifications within the tumor mass itself* (Fig. 3-73).

Cerebral arteriography is of great diagnostic help: the carotid siphon and the anterior cerebral arteries are displaced upward, forming a sort of arch, and in the venous phase, there may be a capillary "blush" staining the meningioma itself. Sometimes the ophthalmic artery is hypertrophic, indicating that it also contributes to the blood supply of the tumor (Fig. 3-73).

With contrast enhancing, most meningiomas of the tuberculum sellae can be directly visualized by *computerized axial tomography.*

*In summary, we note that a unilateral onset of ocular involvement is quite characteristic for patients with a meningioma of the tuberculum sellae. The history reveals a unilateral loss of vision that may progress to complete amaurosis. This process may extend over several years. The latent period between the involvement of the first eye and of the second eye also may be quite long. Amaurosis of one eye with temporal hemianopia of the other eye is quite characteristic for a unilateral involvement of the optic nerve and the anterior angle of the chiasm. In addition, there are asymmetric, incongruous bitemporal hemianopias, with a preponderant involvement of the inferior temporal quadrants. As a consequence of the unilateral onset of the disease, the ophthalmoscopic appearance of the optic atrophy, likewise, is unilateral or more pronounced on one side. The unilateral loss of vision, visual field changes (central scotomas!), and fundus alterations frequently cause confusion with retrobulbar neuritis. In the differential diagnosis the x-ray findings are of importance, that is, the absence of gross changes of the sella, the proof of hyperostosis of the tuberculum sellae, or actual calcification of the tumor.*

### Meningiomas of the olfactory groove (presellar tumor type)

These tumors originate from the arachnoid cells near the olfactory groove and the crista galli (Figs. 3-74 and 3-75). Although a meningioma of the olfactory groove arises in the midline, it frequently tends to grow more toward one side. According to their location, we can differentiate three groups: an anterior type with a frontal location, an intermediate type near the crista galli, and a posterior type originating near the tuberculum sellae (Cushing and Eisenhardt; David and Askenasy). The anterior and intermediate types rarely cause signs involving the visual apparatus. The posterior meningioma of the olfactory groove is most likely to press against the chiasm and the optic nerve, thus displacing and compressing these structures backward and downward. *Clinically, the most important symptom is unilateral or, later, bilateral anosmia.* During the course of several years the tumor may reach considerable size, which may lead to a more or less pronounced *psycho-organic syndrome* characterized by disturbances of memory, associations, and affect. Thus the symptomatology of these tumors frequently may convey the impression of frontal lobe tumors. The psycho-organic syndrome must be considered the result of compression of the base of the frontal lobe (Fig. 3-74).

*In patients with meningiomas of the olfactory groove the symptoms of anosmia and those of a generalized increase in intracranial pressure in the form of*

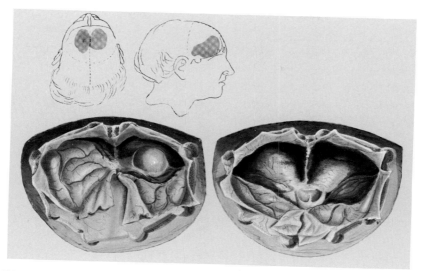

**Fig. 3-74.** Tangerine-sized bilateral meningioma of olfactory groove in 53-year-old patient before and after extirpation (bilateral frontal osteoplastic craniotomy).

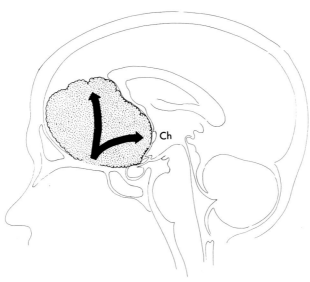

**Fig. 3-75.** Median section through skull schematically showing meningioma of olfactory groove. Compression and deformation of chiasm, *Ch*, and third ventricle.

*headache, nausea, vomiting, or vertigo usually precede the ocular symptoms.* The farther forward the meningioma originates, the later it causes ocular symptoms. As a rule, there are complaints about a unilateral *loss of vision,* with cloudiness, fogginess, and darkness of vision. Usually, loss of vision occurs first on one side and later perhaps on the other side, but it may occasionally show a bilateral onset. We observed one patient who became practically blind in both eyes before undergoing surgery. In one patient, apart from a state of confusion, generalized apathy, and loss of impulse, visual hallucinations could be recorded. There are numerous references in the literature to the fact that pregnancy (Hagedoorn) or trauma may activate the growth of meningiomas of the olfactory groove (like other meningiomas). In one patient in our series the ocular symptoms first manifested themselves shortly after trauma to the skull and progressed in both eyes to the point where there was an inability to read. In one patient the vision improved following delivery of her infant only to show further loss later.

*The visual fields and fundus findings depend to a large extent on the position and size of the tumor.* A meningioma of the olfactory groove with an anterior location that does not interfere with the optic nerve or the chiasm may assume a certain size and produce the ophthalmoscopic picture of only a generalized increase of intracranial pressure. Thus we have noted a unilateral or bilateral papilledema in about two thirds of our 16 patients with meningioma of the olfactory groove. The prominence varied from slight blurring of the disc margins to 3 diopters or more. Hemorrhages of the disc are rare. There was no correlation between the side of the tumor and the side of the more pronounced papilledema.

*During the extended course of the increased intracranial pressure the choked discs frequently undergo a chronic atrophy.* In addition to the commonly seen enlargement of the blind spot, there will be a progressive constriction of the peripheral visual field and a loss of central vision. One should always consider the possibility that mental and psychic alterations are responsible for concentrically constricted visual fields (p. 87), because a general lack of impulse and apathy may, to a large extent, cause such a defect. In our series of 16 patients, we found papilledema on one side and optic atrophy on the other side, in other words, a *Foster Kennedy syndrome,* only three times. Similar to the cases reported by Hartmann, David, and Desvignes, our patients did not always show a typical picture. One had bilateral papilledema, with one disc revealing a conspicuous atrophy. Another showed bilateral optic atrophy, but with distinct blurring and a slight prominence of the disc on one side. The third patient was a rather typical example of this syndrome, with optic atrophy on one side and a blurred and prominent nerve head on the other side. *The situation is similar to that in tumors of the frontal lobe, where we also emphasized that the Foster Kennedy syndrome manifests itself rarely in a truly typical form* (Fig. 3-78, *A*).

If a meningioma of the olfactory groove extends backward and interferes with the optic nerve and the chiasm, it causes *unilateral* or *bilateral* primary

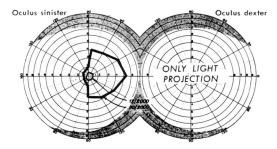

**Fig. 3-76.** Bilateral meningioma of olfactory groove with chiasmal compression. Complete optic atrophy on right side; temporal pallor on left side. Visual acuity, O.D. light localization; O.S. finger counting at 4 meters. Almost complete right amaurosis with temporal hemianopia on opposite side (syndrome of compression of anterior chiasmal angle).

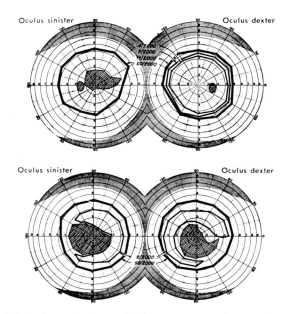

**Fig. 3-77.** Above, Bilateral meningioma of olfactory groove that weighs 65 gm and extends mainly toward left side. Bilateral papilledema of 2 to 3 diopters' elevation. In contrast to right disc, left one shows distinct pallor; atypical Foster Kennedy syndrome. Large left central and paracentral scotoma extends nasally and temporally, indicating lesion of ipsilateral optic nerve. Below, Large bilateral meningioma of olfactory groove that weighs 120 gm. Bilateral optic atrophy, more advanced on right side. Visual acuity, O.U. 0.01. Bilateral anosmia. Bilateral large central-paracentral scotomas (targets 50/2000, 9/2000). On left side, scotoma merges with blind spot (cecocentral scotoma) but does not include it on right side. Signs of lesion of both optic nerves!

optic atrophy with dissimilar involvement of the two sides. The atrophy may also show all possible gradual variations, ranging from temporal pallor to complete chalk-white atrophy with a corresponding excavation of the disc. A bilateral atrophy of equal degree is not so rare, because the tumor originates in the midline and frequently progresses in a symmetric manner toward the optic nerves and the chiasm.

Except for changes caused by papilledema, the *visual fields* in patients with meningiomas of the olfactory groove are usually quite *bizarre* and *unreliable.* It is entirely possible to find normal fields with anterior meningiomas. *Amaurosis of one eye and temporal defects of the other field* are not so rare. They are similar to those of suprasellar meningiomas (syndrome of compression of the anterior angle of the chiasm, Fig. 3-76). Actual bitemporal hemianopias are extremely rare in our series. They occur in an incomplete form, if at all. *From a diagnostic point of view the central and paracentral scotomas, with or without temporal hemianopia, are more important and characteristic.* Usually, they occur first on the side of the tumor, but may involve the other eye later. These scotomas must be regarded as the result of direct tumor pressure on one or both optic nerves. They may be confused with the consequences of chronic retrobulbar neuritis. As a rule, they are quite extensive, involving both the nasal and temporal areas, sooner or later merging with the blind spot (Fig. 3-77).

X-ray films furnish important diagnostic hints. In about one half of the patients, there are characteristic *hyperostoses along the crista galli,* sometimes also *calcifications* of the tumor itself, and occasionally a small ossification at the point of origin of the tumor. Angiography demonstrates that the anterior cerebral arteries and their branches are pushed and stretched above the floor of the anterior fossa, and sometimes there is a direct tumor stain (Fig. 3-78, *B*). Not infrequently the ophthalmic artery is seen to contribute to the vascularization of the meningioma (especially well recognized in the subtraction pictures). *Computerized axial tomography* may demonstrate the meningioma with its perifocal edema directly.

*In summary, it must be stated that the ocular signs and symptoms in patients with meningiomas of the olfactory groove have no localizing value. Some of the anterior tumors, especially the larger ones, may lead to papilledema (which usually is bilateral) or rarely to papilledema on one side (contralateral to the tumor) and to optic atrophy on the side of the tumor, that is, a Foster Kennedy syndrome (Fig. 3-78). The latter rarely appears in a typical form. If the tumor grows backward toward the optic nerve and the chiasm, it causes a unilateral or bilateral optic atrophy and loss of vision with the occurrence of large central or paracentral scotomas as well as asymmetric, atypical, and incomplete hemianopias in the case of interference with the chiasm. Usually the field defects are quite variable, bizarre, and not very reliable for diagnostic purposes. The diagnosis of such tumors is no longer based on the neuro-ophthalmologic signs, but on the two most important symptoms, that is, unilateral or bilateral anosmia*

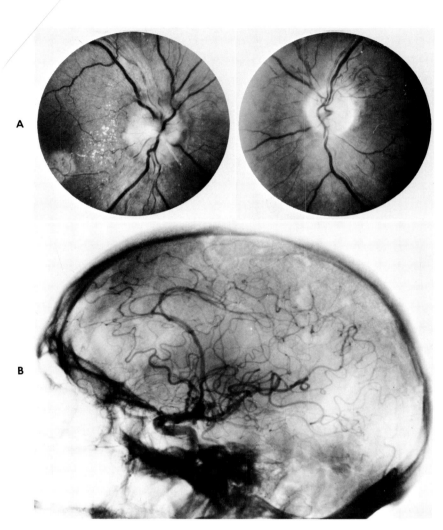

**Fig. 3-78. A,** Foster Kennedy syndrome with olfactory groove meningioma in 58-year-old patient. Papilledema with moderate elevation (1.5 diopters), distinct venous engorgement, and obscuration of all disc margins and optic cup on right side. Pallid disc with sharp margins and vessels of normal caliber in left fundus. Note signs of systemic hypertension (arterio-venous crossing phenomena, yellow deep retinal exudates, narrowing of arterioles, etc.) in both eyes. Diastolic pressure of ophthalmic arteries, O.U. 70 gm (Bailliart). Visual acuity, O.D. 0.5; O.S. 0.1. Left illustration corresponds to right eye and right illustration to left eye. **B,** Corresponding cerebral arteriogram after left carotid angiography. Dorsal displacement of anterior cerebral artery, typical curvilinear capsular vessels, compression of carotid siphon.

*and a more or less characteristic psycho-organic syndrome. In differentiating these meningiomas from those of the tuberculum sellae, one should remember that the latter, even at an early stage, lead to ocular signs and symptoms because of an upward displacement of the chiasm. Meningiomas of the olfactory groove, on the other hand, must reach considerable size before pressure from above on the optic nerves or the chiasm will impair the visual function.*

### Meningiomas of the sphenoid ridge (parasellar tumor type)

Meningiomas of the sphenoid ridge, because of their lateral position, show the greatest variance from the chiasmal syndrome in their symptomatology. Cushing and Eisenhardt distinguish three different types of manifestation of these tumors.

The first type originates in the *outer third of the sphenoid ridge* (part of the larger wing). It shows two forms with a distinctly separate symptomatology (that is, *pterional meningioma* and *meningioma "en plaque"*). The pterional meningioma grows from the pterional tip of the sphenoid ridge toward the sylvian fissure, which separates the frontal and temporal lobes. In distinct contrast to the meningioma "en plaque," it reaches considerable size before it causes any symptoms. Except for papilledema and occasional visual hallucinations (temporal lobe!), the signs and symptoms are predominantly of a nonophthalmologic nature (such as headaches, epileptic attacks, uncinate fits, central facial paresis, as

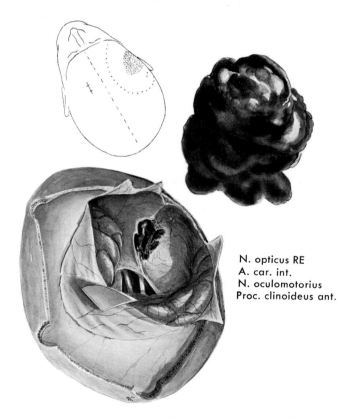

N. opticus RE
A. car. int.
N. oculomotorius
Proc. clinoideus ant.

**Fig. 3-79.** Tangerine-sized meningioma of right sphenoid ridge, middle third, in 47-year-old patient after extirpation (right frontotemporal osteoplastic craniotomy).

well as roentgenologic evidence of changes in the pterional region in the form of abnormal vascularization). In view of its important ocular symptomatology, meningioma "en plaque" will be discussed in greater detail on p. 255.

The second type includes meningiomas originating from the *middle third of the sphenoid ridge* (Fig. 3-79). The third type is of greatest interest to the ophthalmologist. It develops at the *inner third of the sphenoid ridge*, quite close to the clinoid processes and the superior orbital fissure ("clinoid type"). The middle and inner thirds of the sphenoid ridge are part of the lesser sphenoid wing.

Because of their peculiar position, usually a part of the meningiomas of the sphenoid wing extends either into the anterior or middle fossa. For this reason, they may interfere with the frontal lobe and the olfactory nerve (in the form of anosmia) or, more often, with the temporal lobe (frequently there are *uncinate fits*, but also other forms of *epileptic attacks* and fainting spells). Despite its variance with the chiasmal syndrome, the neuro-ophthalmologic symptomatology (David and Hartmann; Kearns and Wagener) is quite decisive for the diagnosis of meningiomas of the sphenoid ridge, especially the inner ridge type; even if small in size, *these tumors interfere less with the chiasm than with the optic nerve and the nerves for the extrinsic eye muscles entering the orbit through the superior orbital fissure.*

*Ocular symptoms* are almost always mentioned by patients with meningiomas of the lesser sphenoid wing.* In addition to the general symptoms of increased intracranial pressure such as headache, nausea, and vomiting, there are quite frequently statements about a *unilateral, slowly progressing loss of vision*. The loss of vision frequently is described directly. At times, patients complain about cloudy, indistinct, or blurred vision or about the appearance of a fog or shadow. These unilateral types of impaired vision should not be confused with the transient amblyopic attacks or fits of glimmering, which must be regarded as the result of an increased intracranial pressure and of a papilledema (p. 109). *In addition to loss of vision, diplopia is one of the most important symptoms.* Its pathologic basis is a paresis of the extrinsic ocular muscles, which will be discussed below. Because of the frequent involvement of the oculomotor nerve, the *double images often show a horizontal as well as a vertical separation.* Rarely are there *subjective statements concerning an exophthalmos.* In our series of 25 cases of meningiomas of the lesser sphenoid wing, patients occasionally complained about a peculiar pressure sensation, about a certain feeling of tension or swelling in the involved eye, or of an impression of pulsation in the eye or the ipsilateral temple. One patient stated that the exophthalmos occurred only during her menstrual period. Visual field changes are mentioned rarely. With meningiomas "en plaque" the patient notices a conspicuous swelling of the ipsilateral temporal region.

The *symptomatology* of meningiomas of the lesser sphenoid wing (especially the inner ridge type) permits the distinction of *two main groups of phenomena:* (1) the group that is caused by an extension of the tumor into the superior orbital fissure, producing a superior orbital fissure syndrome, and (2) the group

---

*Henceforth this abridged term will be used for meningiomas, especially of the inner third of the sphenoid ridge ("clinoidal type"). Middle ridge tumors in their later stages manifest the symptoms of inner ridge tumors. Outer ridge tumors (meningiomas "en plaque") are described separately (p. 255).

that is caused by interference of the tumor with the optic nerve (optic atrophy, visual field changes) (Fig. 3-80).

The *superior orbital fissure syndrome* that may occur in the course of the development of a meningioma of the lesser sphenoid wing is primarily characterized by *disturbances of motility of the extrinsic ocular muscles* (that is, the *abducens, oculomotor,* and *trochlear nerves*). We were able to record such disturbances of motility in about one fifth of the patients in our series. Usually a combination of various nerves is affected, with no apparent predominant involvement of one particular nerve. In addition to the orbital fissure syndrome, there is generally a *unilateral exophthalmos.* Often it is partly responsible for the impaired motility of the involved eye. Frequently, it is difficult to decide whether the impairment is caused by the affection of the extraocular nerves or the limitation of the muscle action by the exophthalmos. This exophthalmos is an extraordinarily important and frequent (30% to 40% of cases) ocular sign with meningiomas of the lesser sphenoid wing (Elsberg, Hare, and Dyke; Thorkildsen). We have observed it in a quite well-developed form in a little more than one half of our patients (Fig. 3-81). Depending on how far the tumor has progressed, the exophthalmos may range from slight, almost imperceptible degrees to quite severe forms measuring 10 to 15 mm. It may even assume the grotesque form of a protruding "chameleon eye." In extreme cases, there may be, in addition to the ordinary proptosis of the globe, a displacement, for instance, downward and outward (Figs. 1-5 and 3-82). The exophthalmos is caused by compression of the venous drainage system of the orbit and the cavernous sinus as well as (in many cases) by direct invasion of the orbit by the tumor through the orbital fissure. The venous stasis is frequently evidenced by

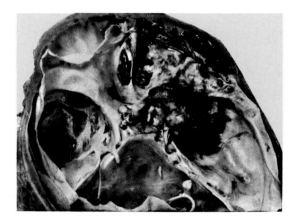

**Fig. 3-80.** Anterior and middle cranial fossae with meningioma of inner and middle ridge of right lesser sphenoid wing. Observe how tuberous tumor invades right optic nerve as well as oculomotor, trochlear, sixth, and trigeminal (ophthalmic division) nerves before their entrance into superior orbital fissure.

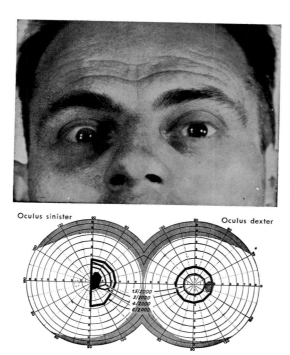

Oculus sinister                                    Oculus dexter

1.5/2000
3/2000
4/2000
6/2000

Fig. 3-81. Exophthalmos of left eye in patient with meningioma of left lesser sphenoid wing (middle ridge). Diplopia caused by slight paresis of left sixth and oculomotor nerves. Visual acuity, O.D. 1.0; O.S. 0.1. Left disc shows temporal pallor. Temporal hemianopia of left eye with central hemianopic scotoma. Slight concentric constriction of right isopters.

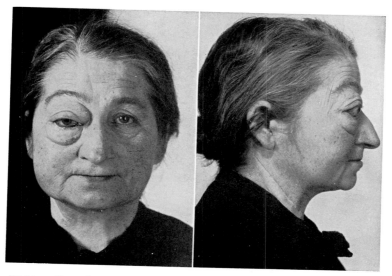

Fig. 3-82. Right unilateral exophthalmos with lid swelling and downward displacement of globe in patient with meningioma of inner third of right sphenoid ridge. Because of optic atrophy, right visual acuity reduced to light perception. Motility of right eye limited in all, especially temporal, directions.

a corresponding dilatation and tortuosity of the episcleral and conjunctival vessels as well as the vessels of the skin of the upper and lower lids.

*Part of the superior orbital fissure syndrome is a lesion of the first division of the trigeminal nerve, with hypesthesia in the area of its distribution,* especially a *diminished ipsilateral corneal reflex.* We were able to record a distinctly diminished corneal reflex (mostly in the superior and inferior quadrants) in one third of the patients in our series. *Except for the exophthalmos, the superior orbital fissure syndrome is quite similar to the cavernous sinus syndrome* (p. 39). A meningioma of the lesser sphenoid wing, especially the inner ridge type, may easily infiltrate this area. Thus it is often difficult to decide which of these two syndromes is present. Actually, the difference is only a question of definition and of little importance for a topical diagnosis.

Half of the patients in our series showed pronounced *papilledemas* that, in an overwhelming majority, were bilateral. *Often the progress of these tumors is quite slow; thus the frequent appearance of a chronic atrophic papilledema is easy to understand.* The prominence of the papilledema is often quite pronounced and reaches 4 to 5 diopters, with numerous exudates and hemorrhages on the disc. The latter may have a causal relationship to the impaired drainage of the orbital veins or the cavernous sinus. This mechanism may give rise to the conspicuous congestion of the retinal veins that we observed frequently. We have seen a *Foster Kennedy syndrome* only twice among 25 patients. (According to Cushing and Eisenhardt, it is more frequent than in frontal lobe or olfactory groove tumors.) Even these were *not typical in their appearance* but showed a slight blurring or even prominence of the atrophic disc on the tumor side. In the other half of the patients, either the discs were normal on both sides or there was a pronounced involvement of one optic nerve with unilateral *signs of atrophy* ranging in degree from a slight temporal pallor to complete optic atrophy with excavation of the disc. Including the two patients with the Foster Kennedy syndrome, we have seen a unilateral optic atrophy in one fifth of the patients in our series.

There is a great variety of visual field changes in patients with meningiomas of the sphenoid wing. This depends on whether and how much the tumor involves the optic nerve. *In slightly less than one third of our patients, we found either completely normal visual fields* or merely a slight concentric constriction and enlarged blind spots as a result of the papilledemas (Fig. 3-83). Next in frequency are unilateral visual field changes on the side of the tumor resulting from a lesion of the optic nerve. These field changes may begin either on the nasal side and progress to a *monocular nasal hemianopia* or they may involve the temporal side, leading to a *temporal hemianopia* of the involved eye. We have records of both forms in our series (Figs. 3-81 and 3-84). Occasionally, unilateral *central scotomas* (at first relative, later absolute) are seen that must be regarded as the first signs of damage to the optic nerve. The deterioration of the visual field defects may progress to *complete amaurosis on the side of the*

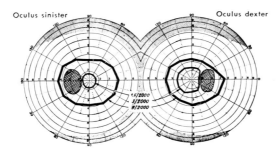

**Fig. 3-83.** Left meningioma of lesser sphenoid wing (middle and inner thirds of sphenoid ridge). Left exophthalmos. Bilateral papilledema of 3 to 4 diopters' elevation (amblyopic attacks!). No diplopia. Visual acuity, O.U. 0.7. Enormous bilateral enlargement of blind spot. Concentric constriction of visual fields. (See Fig. 1-5, p. 17, recurrence of this same tumor with invasion of orbit and development of extensive exophthalmos.)

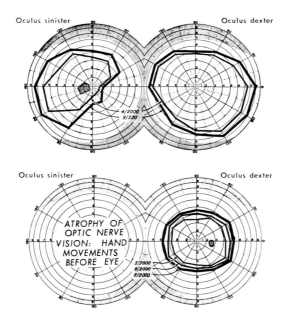

**Fig. 3-84.** Above, Meningioma of lesser left sphenoid wing (inner third) extending over orbital roof to olfactory nerve. Bilateral papilledema of 3 diopters' elevation. Visual acuity, O.D. 1.0; O.S. 0.2. Monocular left inferior nasal quadrantanopia. Right visual field normal. Paracentral temporal scotoma on left side is sign of lesion of left optic nerve! Below, Meningioma of inner third of left sphenoid ridge. Exophthalmos of 4 mm prominence on left side. No motility disturbances. Complete left optic atrophy. Right optic disc normal. Visual acuity, O.S. hand movements before eye; O.D. 1.5. Almost complete amaurosis of left eye. Right visual field normal.

*tumor,* with the field on the other side still intact (Fig. 3-84). In the later stages a temporal field defect may occur in the contralateral eye, indicating a posterior extension of the tumor and pressure on the anterior angle of the chiasm (Tönnis; Walsh and Hoyt). In one case of recurrent meningioma of the sphenoid ridge, we were even able to demonstrate bilateral, inferior-nasal, sector-shaped defects. The binasal defects seem to be based on the bearing of the tumor on the chiasm; however, one also has to consider the possibility of pressure on the lateral aspects of both optic nerves. It is an interesting and noteworthy fact that in four of a total of 25 patients with meningioma of the sphenoid ridge, there was a distinct *homonymous hemianopia* of a rather congruous form. In one patient the dividing line went through the point of fixation, and in another there was definite sparing of the macula (Fig. 3-85). We are in agreement with Dubois-Poulsen, Walsh and Hoyt, and others that these *homonymous hemianopias* (in particular those involving the superior quadrants) *result from an interference of the tumor with the temporal lobe.* However, frequently one cannot ascertain merely on the basis of the visual field findings whether or not a lesion of the optic tract is also a causal factor for such hemianopias.

*Pupillary disturbances* on the side of the tumor may be caused either by a lesion of the afferent fibers of the optic nerve or a lesion of the efferent pupillomotor fibers of the oculomotor nerve. Accordingly, there is only a disturbance of the direct or of the direct and consensual pupillary reaction to light on the tumor side, which may even assume the form of a mydriatic fixed pupil.

*The radiologic changes in meningiomas of the sphenoid wing are frequent* (40% to 60% of cases) *and quite characteristic* (Fig. 3-86). There may be an *osteomatous reaction of the lesser sphenoid wing* (especially at the site of the tumor attachment, eventually combined with narrowing of the orbital fissure and of the optic foramen), or one may find decalcification of the sphenoid ridge, pathologic enlargement of the superior orbital fissure, and decalcification of the optic foramen. Roentgenologic changes in the sella are generally minimal and

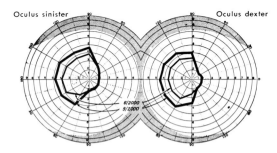

**Fig. 3-85.** Meningioma of left sphenoid outer ridge in pterional region with temporal extension. No exophthalmos. No motility disturbances. Both discs sharply outlined and of normal color. Visual acuity, O.U. 0.4 Right homonymous hemianopia with sparing of macula, sign of interference with left temporal lobe.

caused by increased intracranial pressure. Angiography helps to confirm the type and site of the tumor; in more than a third of the cases there occurs a more or less intensive tumor staining. Very often the ophthalmic artery will be found to be greatly enlarged, sending off supplying vessels to the meningioma.

The secondary hyperostosis is particularly impressive in cases of *meningioma "en plaque."* Not only does it form a thin layer on the inside of the dura, but also infiltrates it and invades the adjacent bone. For this reason, these menin-

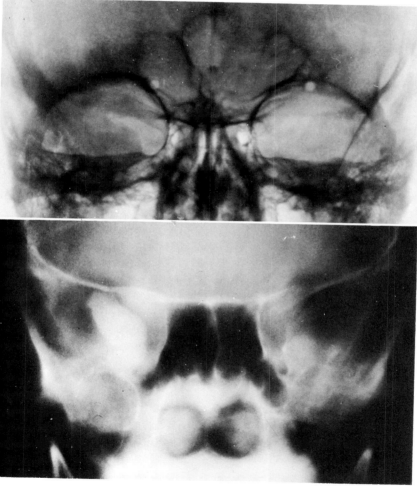

**Fig. 3-86.** Above, Anteroposterior x-ray view of orbits. Increased bone density and sclerosis of lesser and greater sphenoid wings on right side caused by meningioma of right sphenoid ridge (middle and inner third). Normal size and contour of superior orbital fissure on left side. Below, Corresponding orbital tomogram demonstrating even more distinctly hyperostosis of bone surrounding right superior orbital fissure.

giomas, despite their lateral origin in the pterional region, may produce symptoms similar to those of tuberous meningiomas of the middle and, especially, the inner third of the sphenoid ridge (that is, a combination of a superior orbital fissure syndrome with a unilateral impairment of the function of the optic nerve and an exophthalmos). A unilateral, slowly progressing, painless, and nonpulsating *exophthalmos* accompanied by a characteristic *swelling in the ipsilateral temporal region* (resulting from hyperostosis and thickening of the larger sphenoid wing) is one of the most important early signs (Fig. 3-87). In differentiating these from meningiomas of the inner third of the sphenoid ridge, Cushing stresses the more or less pronounced lid edema as well as a combined forward and downward displacement of the globe. Loss of vision and diplopia occur later and are not constant. The rare occurrence of a papilledema, even with exophthalmos of considerable degree, is characteristic for meningioma "en plaque"— a tumor that, according to Cushing, occurs almost exclusively in women between the ages of 40 and 60 years. The radiologic changes may determine the diagnosis; these consist of both erosion and bone thickening in the area of the lateral third of the sphenoid ridge and its surroundings (that is, the roof of the orbit, the lateral orbital wall, and the superior orbital fissure). *Computerized axial tomography* represents an ideal method for identification of sphenoid ridge meningiomas; they usually have a density greater than surrounding brain and their calcifications may be recognized on the computer scan before they are visible on conventional radiographs.

*In summary, we state that meningiomas of the sphenoid ridge cause ocular*

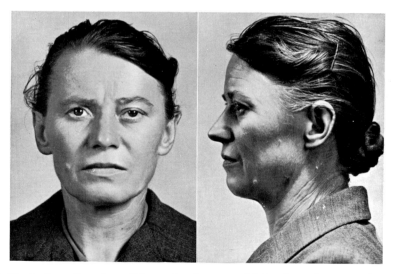

**Fig. 3-87.** Meningioma "en plaque" in pterional region of left sphenoid wing. Left exophthalmos of 5 mm prominence. No motility disturbances. Minimal left papilledema. Slight blurring of nasal margin of right disc. Visual acuity, O.U. 1.0 Palpable swelling in left temporal region.

*involvement if they expand in a mesial direction and involve the optic nerve and the superior orbital fissure. This makes it easy to deduce the characteristic signs: unilateral exophthalmos, variable pareses of the abducens, oculomotor, and trochlear nerves, and occasional hypesthesia of the ipsilateral cornea. Damage to the ipsilateral optic nerve is relatively frequent and manifests itself by a unilateral loss of vision. In such patients the visual fields show unilateral changes beginning on the temporal or nasal side progressing to unilateral temporal or nasal hemianopia or even to unilateral amaurosis. Occasionally one finds homonymous hemianopias of the congruous type—obviously caused by a lesion of the adjacent temporal lobe. A patient's complaints of double vision and diminution of vision in combination with proptosis of one eye always suggest the possibility of a meningioma of the sphenoid ridge, in addition to orbital processes (osteomas, sarcomas, angiomas, dermoids, tumors of the optic nerve, mucoceles, etc.). A painless, slowly developing exophthalmos with a palpable swelling in the ipsilateral temporal region and a later impairment of vision and ocular motility indicate a meningioma "en plaque" in the pterional region.*

In the differential diagnosis of such a syndrome, other types of tumors must, of course, be considered, tumors that occur much more rarely than meningiomas of the sphenoid ridge. We mention dermoids (we observed one case), meningiomas of the middle fossa that expand toward the sphenoid ridge, and in particular, metastatic tumors. Occasionally, one must consider the possibility of a meningioma of the sheaths of the optic nerve or a glioma of the optic nerve (p. 261).

### Differential diagnosis of tumors of the sella and its surroundings

The discussion of the various forms of sellar, suprasellar, presellar, and parasellar tumors included already a certain differential diagnosis of tumors of this particular area of the base of the skull. In our opinion, however, it would be incorrect and misleading not to consider other possible causes of a chiasmal syndrome. Although, strictly speaking, they are outside the scope of our discussion, it is essential to mention them at least briefly in order to present a complete differential diagnosis of pituitary and nonpituitary chiasmal syndromes.

In the presence of a chiasmal syndrome, one always must consider, in addition to sellar, suprasellar, presellar, and parasellar tumors, those of the chiasm itself, the so-called *gliomas of the chiasm,* as well as tumors originating in the sheaths of the optic nerve, the *meningiomas of the optic nerve,* and tumors of the optic nerve itself, such as *gliomas of the optic nerve.* Malignant tumors at the *base of the skull* (nasopharyngeal carcinomas, sarcomas, metastatic tumors) in an advanced stage may cause compression of the chiasm. As a rule, this is marked by asymmetry combined with an incomplete or complete cavernous sinus syndrome (regarding these tumors, refer to p. 268). In addition to the types of tumors just mentioned, one must also consider the rather rare *suprasellar epidermoids* (cholesteatomas or pearly tumors), as well as *specific granu-*

*lomas* (tubercles, gummas), certain *angiomas, chordomas, osteochondromas, dermoids, ectopic pinealomas, mucoceles or carcinomas of the sphenoid sinus, giant cell tumors of the sphenoid bone, trigeminal schwannomas,* and *affections caused by parasites.* These clinical conditions are so rare that their detailed discussion would be out of proportion in the overall picture. *Of greater importance in the differential diagnosis of the sellar and extrasellar tumors* are *aneurysms,* especially supraclinoid aneurysms originating from the anterior cerebral artery or the anterior communicating artery (p. 326).

Furthermore, one must always consider the possibility of an *indirect compression of the chiasm,* primarily a remote effect of a *hydrocephalus of the third ventricle* (p. 260). Finally, there is a group of inflammatory chiasmal changes (the so-called *chiasmal arachnoiditis*) that may also produce a more or less typical chiasmal syndrome. Such a differential diagnosis of the chiasmal syndrome may at first appear quite complex and difficult. Actually, it is not. We have intentionally given a very detailed discussion of the most important sellar and extrasellar tumors and their characteristics so that their differential diagnosis should create no difficulty. In addition to these neoplasms, one must primarily consider, for practical clinical purposes, aneurysms, indirect compression of the chiasm by a hydrocephalus of the third ventricle, gliomas of the chiasm, and inflammatory changes (Table 5).

**Aneurysms.** Infraclinoid and supraclinoid aneurysms of the internal carotid artery must be differentiated. The former develop in the cavernous sinus and thus usually present the picture of an ophthalmoplegia combined with an affection of the trigeminal nerve. Only by breaking through the wall of the cavernous sinus will they invade the sella and then produce the picture of a chiasmal syndrome and mimic a pituitary tumor, even with endocrine dysfunction. This happens much more frequently with *suprasellar aneurysms* of the supraclinoid section of the carotid artery that originate from the anterior cerebral or anterior communicating arteries. An important symptom that is significant for an aneurysm is the relatively early occurrence of *headaches,* mostly localized in the frontal region. Occasionally they occur in violent paroxysms. Also characteristic is the *more or less sudden appearance of visual disturbances and visual field changes,* which may be subject to *fluctuations.* One of the usual manifestations of the chiasmal syndrome in aneurysms is loss of vision, more pronounced in one eye. Sudden improvement or deterioration of vision is significant. The ophthalmoscopic picture reveals a primary optic atrophy that is usually bilateral but of distinctly different degrees in the two eyes.

*A bitemporal hemianopia of a rather asymmetric type* is the most frequent field change in aneurysms (Fig. 5-14). According to Jefferson, an inferior bitemporal quadrantanopia is more suggestive of a suprasellar aneurysm, whereas onset of the field changes in both superior temporal quadrants is more likely caused by a pituitary adenoma. There may also be amaurosis of one eye and a temporal hemianopia of the other. In the course of the disease the visual field defects may even vary, which is, apart from the tumor-progression–caused alterations, ordinarily not the case with tumors. In many cases the x-ray findings will furnish important data. Aneurysms may show a destruction of the contours of the sella and the clinoid processes, usually at first only on one side, but no enlargement of the sella. Occasionally, there are calcium deposits in the wall of the aneurysm that radiologically appear as annular streaks or small compact circles. However, such findings may be completely missing in aneurysms with a chiasmal syndrome. A definite diagnosis of an aneurysm is made by means of cerebral angiography, except in the rare case of a clotted aneurysm.

**Table 5.** Differential diagnosis of chiasmal syndrome*

| | Pituitary adenoma | Meningioma of tuberculum sellae | Craniopharyngioma | Glioma of chiasm | Aneurysm | Chiasmal arachnoiditis |
|---|---|---|---|---|---|---|
| Age | 30-50 | 30-50 | Most children, also adults | Children | As a rule, adults | All ages |
| Fundus | Primary optic atrophy | Primary optic atrophy, often more severe on one side | In children papilledema, in adults optic atrophy | Primary optic atrophy | Normal discs or optic atrophy | Unilateral or bilateral optic atrophy or papilledema |
| Visual field | Symmetric bitemporal hemianopia | Asymmetric chiasmal syndrome, often amaurosis of one eye with temporal hemianopia of the other | Asymmetric bitemporal hemianopia | Unilateral or bilateral temporal visual field defects | More or less distinct bitemporal hemianopia (fluctuations!) | Central scotomas, concentric constriction, unilateral or bilateral temporal hemianopia |
| Endocrine signs | Hypopituitarism, hyperpituitarism, or mixed | None | Hypopituitarism, perhaps also hypothalamic signs (polyuria, polydipsia, etc.) | None or hypopituitarism | None | None |
| Localization | Sellar | Suprasellar | Intrasellar and suprasellar | Suprasellar | Suprasellar (supraclinoid aneurysm), intrasellar (infraclinoid aneurysm) | Optic and chiasmal arachnoid |
| X-ray findings | Ballooning of sella, thinning of floor of sella, erosion of clinoid processes | Sella normal, hyperostosis of tuberculum sellae | Suprasellar calcifications | Unilateral or bilateral widening of optic foramen | Often negative, occasionally annular calcium shadows | Negative |

*Modified from Walsh and Hoyt.

**Indirect compression of the chiasm.** The mechanism of remote effects of distant tumors on the chiasm usually consists in the formation of a hydrocephalus of the third ventricle, with its dilated anterior wall causing damage to the chiasm by pressure from above or from behind (especially with a hypoplastic diaphragma sellae). Such a remote effect is possible with tumors of the third ventricle (p. 200), tumors of the sylvian aqueduct, and tumors of the posterior fossa (cerebellar tumors, p. 274). Klingler and Condrau, in their article on misleading signs in visual fields, reported such observations (p. 201). Characteristically, such an indirect compression of the chiasm causes a *more or less distinct bitemporal hemianopia* (Fig. 3-117) *with a more or less pronounced unilateral or bilateral loss of visual acuity.* A simultaneous increase in the intracranial pressure frequently causes signs of choking of the discs. (Papilledema is rare with pituitary adenomas!) Fluctuations in the cerebrospinal fluid pressure may be responsible for considerable improvement or deterioration of field defects and visual acuity.

In addition to the bitemporal field defects, one observes *unilateral or bilateral central scotomas, with greater frequency in the temporal halves.* The cause for the origin of such central scotomas supposedly is a downward kink of the optic nerve shortly before it enters the optic foramen as a result of the internal hydrocephalus (Mooney and McConnel) or, perhaps, an exceptional pressure by the third ventricle on the posterior rim of the chiasm (Hughes). In active hydrocephalus with third ventricle dilatation the sella can have the typical "ballooned" appearance of a pituitary adenoma. Only pneumoencephalography, ventriculography, or computerized x-ray tomography will make the correct differential diagnosis.

**Chiasmal arachnoiditis.** Despite numerous publications on this inflammatory (or posttraumatic) type of chiasmal disease, it must be considered a rare event (in agreement with Walsh and Hoyt). In our series, we have only two undisputed cases of chiasmal arachnoiditis proved after surgery. We must emphasize that this diagnosis has been made all too often, especially during the last decades. In numerous cases, it turned out that there was an occult sellar or extrasellar tumor or disseminated sclerosis.

Just as in sellar or extrasellar neoplasms, the usual onset is *loss of vision*—first in one eye and later in the other. *Characteristically, the visual field defects are quite irregular.* Likewise, their development is rather pleomorphic. These irregularities are based on the varied extent of the changes in the arachnoid, the circulatory disturbances caused by them, and a spread of the inflammatory process to the optic nerve itself. According to Bollack, David, and Puech, the most frequent and earliest signs are almost always unilateral or bi-

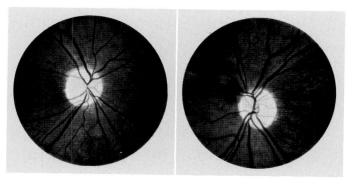

**Fig. 3-88.** Primary complete optic atrophy with distinct disc margins in chiasmal arachnoiditis, confirmed on surgical exploration of chiasmal region. Both discs are chalk white and sharply outlined. Slight excavation of central funnel. Slight narrowing of arteries. Normal veins. On both sides pattern of papillomacular bundle cannot be visualized in red-free light. Visual acuity before surgery, O.D. 1/20; O.S. 1/60. Large bilateral central scotomas. Left illustration corresponds to right eye and right illustration to left eye.

lateral *central scotomas* (sometimes of temporal hemianopic character). Next in frequency is a *concentric constriction or a unilateral or bilateral temporal hemianopia.* Much less frequent are binasal, altitudinal, or homonymous hemianopias.

The fundus changes are also quite irregular and may vary considerably in one and the same patient during different stages of the disease. Most frequently (about 50%), one finds a *primary optic atrophy* with sharply outlined disc margins (Fig. 3-88). Next in frequency is an atrophy with blurred disc margins (mixed atrophy, according to Vail). In one tenth of the patients a *papilledema* is seen that suggests a spreading of the process toward the base and an involvement of the cisterna magna. One tenth of the patients shows a perfectly normal fundus. A general neurologic examination usually is noncontributory. Other ocular signs and symptoms (paralyses of extraocular muscles, nystagmus) are quite rare. Nonocular symptoms such as headache, sleeplessness, polyuria, anosmia, amenorrhea, impotence, etc. are not very characteristic. X-ray films of the skull generally show a completely normal picture (especially a normal sella)—an extremely valuable fact in differentiating this process from others, especially from tumors in this region. Pneumoencephalography may show an irregular and deformed sellar cisterna or even an obliteration of the chiasmal or the interpeduncular cisterna.

We agree with Walsh and Hoyt that optochiasmatic arachnoiditis is a *diagnosis of exclusion* and can be readily made only at the moment of operation.

**Gliomas of the chiasm and tumors of the optic nerve.** Glioma of the chiasm is an instance of a primary tumor of the optic nerve in this particular localization. The tumors of the optic nerve can be classified into two main groups: (1) gliomas (astrocytomas or mixed astrocytoma-oligodendrogliomas) and (2) meningiomas of the optic nerve. Because of their identical or a least very similar symptomatology, both types can be discussed together.

Glioma of the chiasm, like glioma of the optic nerve (Figs. 3-89 and 3-90), is in many cases (15% according to Walsh) merely a sign of a more general affection of the peripheral and central nervous system, namely, *neurofibromatosis (von Recklinghausen's disease).* Bürki is of the opinion that an isolated primary tumor of the optic nerve may be the first or only sign of von Recklinghausen's disease. Glioma of the chiasm occurs mostly in infancy. Most of all, it must be differentiated from craniopharyngioma. As mentioned previously, there may not always be systemic signs of neurofibromatosis (Fig. 3-91). They may be completely missing. At times only "cafe au lait" spots (a so-called forme fruste of von Recklinghausen's disease) can be demonstrated on the skin. Occasionally, it may be necessary to search carefully for such skin changes among other members of the family.

Whereas glioma of the optic nerve and the chiasm is primarily a disease of infancy, *meningioma of the sheaths of the optic nerve is more likely to occur in the older age group.*

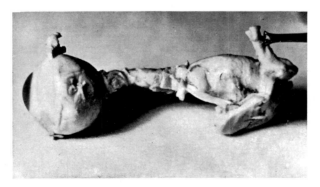

**Fig. 3-89.** Glioma of chiasm and left optic nerve. Systemic neurofibromatosis (von Recklinghausen's disease) of peripheral and sympathetic nervous system as well as glioma in medulla oblongata in 19-year-old patient.

Although we concern ourselves here only with glioma of the chiasm, it should be mentioned that a primary tumor can occur in any part of the optic nerve, that is, intraorbital, intracanalicular, or intracranial. Intraorbital optic nerve tumors tend to occur as a single focus (Figs. 3-90 and 3-92), whereas the intracranial form shows multiple foci in the chiasm and optic nerves (Fig. 3-89).

The chiasmal syndrome, as seen with gliomas of the chiasm (Martin and Cushing), is marked by a *progressive loss of vision in both eyes*, often beginning in one. *The visual field*

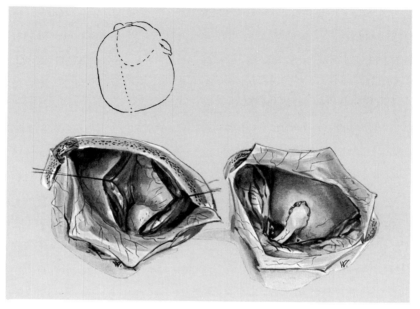

**Fig. 3-90.** Glioma of right optic nerve in 3-year-old girl before (right) and after (left) deroofing of orbit (approach via right transfrontal osteoplastic craniotomy). (See Fig. 3-92.)

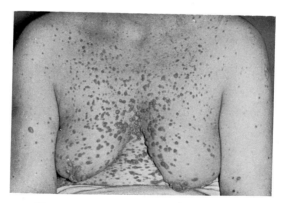

**Fig. 3-91.** Multiple neurofibromas of skin in region of breasts with neurofibromatosis (von Recklinghausen's disease) and glioma of chiasm (same patient as in Fig. 3-94).

*changes take an irregular course and differ from the ordinary type seen in the chiasmal syndrome.* There are unilateral temporal defects. In bitemporal hemianopias a certain asymmetry is the rule (Fig. 3-93). Occasionally, even homonymous hemianopias occur (Brégeat). The ophthalmoscopic appearance usually is that of a simple bilateral optic atrophy with sharp outlines of the discs (Fig. 3-94). If there are superimposed signs of increased intracranial pressure, the margins may be blurred. Marked enlargement of the tumor may embarrass the circulation of the cerebrospinal fluid. It may also produce hypothalamic signs such as drowsiness, adiposity, or polyuria.

Of utmost diagnostic importance are the radiologic findings. If the tumor has already invaded the optic canal, an *enlargement of one or both optic foramina* without decalcification can be easily demonstrated (Fig. 3-93). This sign, of course, is of greater diagnostic significance if it remains unilateral, although the bilateral optic foramen dilatation is just

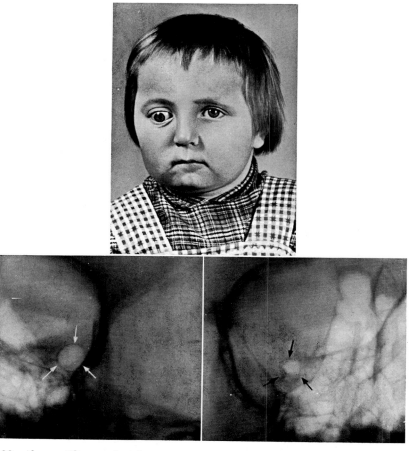

**Fig. 3-92.** Above, Glioma of right optic nerve in 3-year-old girl (see Fig. 3-90). Right exophthalmos with downward displacement of globe. Motility of right eye restricted up and out. Beginning congestion of blood vessels of upper lid and nasal aspect of bulbar conjunctiva. Right disc shows temporal pallor, blurred nasal margin, and slight elevation. Left disc normal. Below, Radiologic visualization of optic foramina, Rheese position. Right optic foramen definitely enlarged but round and of distinct outline (white arrows).

as frequently observed in cases of chiasmal glioma. Another diagnostically important change is *deformation of the sella turcica* in the form of an *omega or a pumpkin* (also called hourglass-shaped deformity) resulting from destruction of the anterior wall of the sella turcica and the lower part of the anterior clinoid processes by the tumor, which spreads along the optic nerve toward the orbit. These radiologic signs are of extraordinary importance, especially in the differential diagnosis of a craniopharyngioma. The pumpkin shape of the sella and the enlargement of the optic foramina are missing in craniopharyngiomas. The characteristic findings for the latter are the frequent suprasellar calcifications.

Expansion of a glioma of the optic nerve or chiasm toward the orbit leads to the very early development of a unilateral *exophthalmos* (Fig. 3-92). The motility of the globe in glioma is said to remain intact for a long time, whereas a meningioma supposedly causes early disturbances of the ocular movements. We have in our series three cases of primary tumors of the optic nerve, two of them gliomas in patients with von Recklinghausen's disease. The third case, a meningioma of the optic foramen with progressive unilateral loss of vision, had been considered as an essential optic atrophy, and the patient had been treated by injections. The ophthalmoscopic findings in this patient were a white atrophic disc, with a normal papilla in the other eye. A distinct dilatation of the optic foramen with thickening of the contours (reactive hyperostosis!) on one side suggested the correct diagnosis. The meningioma was extirpated, although the optic nerve had to be severed. In this connection the special value of *serial tomograms of the optic canal* in the initial and differential diagnosis of

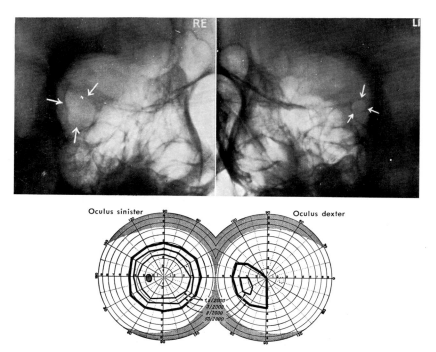

Oculus sinister                    Oculus dexter

**Fig. 3-93.** Glioma of right optic nerve and chiasm in 13-year-old boy. Slight exophthalmos and primary optic atrophy on right side. Marked loss of right vision: 0.01. Above, Radiologic visualization of optic foramina (arrows), Rheese-Goalwin position. Marked unilateral enlargement of right optic foramen. Below, Corresponding visual fields. Right temporal hemianopia with beginning destruction of upper nasal quadrant. Three years later, left temporal hemianopia and thus true chiasmal syndrome developed.

these tumors must be mentioned. Any difference of optic foramen dimension greater than 20% is presumptive evidence of an expanding lesion within the canal. Whereas gliomas of the optic nerve produce only enlargement of the optic foramen and of the canal without decalcification of its walls, meningiomas of the optic nerve may cause osteomatous thickening of the optic canal, going so far as to narrow the foramen concentrically (Fig. 3-95). *Ultrasound echography* of the orbit and *computerized axial tomography* may identify optic nerve

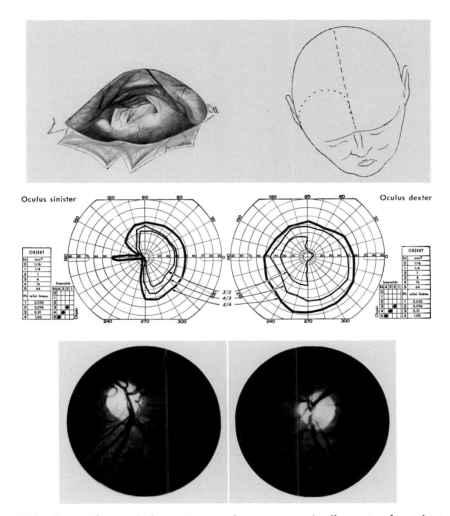

**Fig. 3-94.** Above, Glioma of chiasm in situ after exposure of sellar region by right transfrontal osteoplastic craniotomy in 25-year-old patient. Center, Asymmetric bitemporal hemianopia involving only most central isopters of right field and peripheral as well as central isopters of left field. There is peculiar spurlike remnant of left temporal field. Below, Corresponding fundus photographs, demonstrating bilateral primary optic atrophy with sharp margins. Slight venous congestion. Visual acuity strikingly well preserved: O.U. corrected to 0.9! Left illustration corresponds to right eye and right illustration to left eye.

gliomas and meningiomas in their orbital localization, even when conventional methods, including orbital arterio- or venography have been negative (Figs. 3-96 and 3-97).

In patients with a chiasmal syndrome a *granuloma* (tuberculous or syphilitic) occasionally must be considered in addition to primary tumors of the chiasm. This is illustrated by the history of a patient with an initial loss of vision of the left eye that rapidly progressed to complete amaurosis, followed by a similar course in the right eye. The left amaurosis and a right temporal hemianopia could not be explained satisfactorily. The subsequent picture was that of an acute meningitis with sudden death. Autopsy revealed a *solitary tubercle* in the intracranial section of the left optic nerve in addition to a systemic proliferating tuberculosis of various organs. The case is remarkable because of the development of an amaurosis in one eye and a temporal hemianopia in the other eye, yet without direct interference of the tubercle with the chiasm. The tubercle in the intracranial section of the left optic nerve, causing amaurosis on this side, pressed against the medial part of the right optic nerve, thus producing a temporal hemianopia (Fig. 3-98) on the right side!

A *syndrome of malignant optic glioma of adulthood* is described by Hoyt, Meshel, Lessell, Schatz, and Suckling. In contrast to the benign character of the optic and chiasmal gliomas in childhood (they have the characteristics of hamartomas), the optic gliomas of adults (malignant astrocytomas) are aggressively

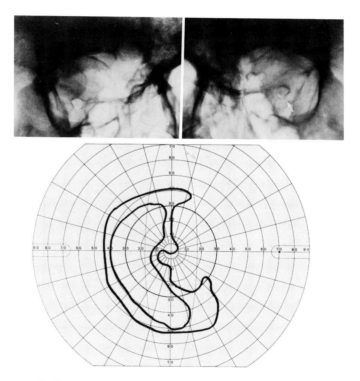

**Fig. 3-95.** Intracanalicular meningioma of left optic nerve in 62-year-old patient. Top, Irregular enlargement and densifying of walls of left optic canal (arrow). Tumor calcification within area of optic foramen. Normal configuration of right optic canal (left). Bottom, Corresponding visual field of left eye shows nasal hemianopia of irregular type with sparing of macula. Visual field of right eye intact.

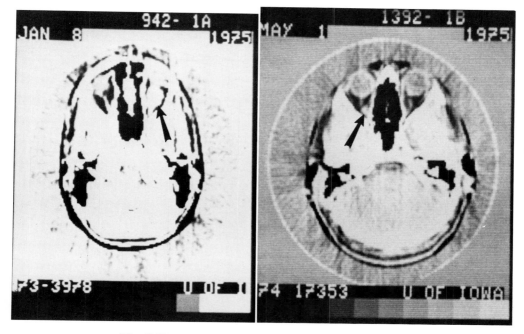

Fig. 3-96                                    Fig. 3-97

**Fig. 3-96.** Computerized axial tomogram of skull of 6-year-old boy with glioma of right optic nerve. Thickening of right optic nerve is well visible behind eye (arrow). (Courtesy Dr. F. C. Blodi, University of Iowa.)

**Fig. 3-97.** Computerized axial tomogram of skull showing small meningioma of optic nerve in left orbit. Small tumefaction at apex is well visible (arrow). (Courtesy Dr. F. C. Blodi, University of Iowa.)

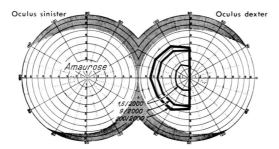

**Fig. 3-98.** Retro-orbital solitary tubercle of left optic nerve (intracranial section) in 44-year-old patient. Blindness of left eye. Temporal hemianopia without sparing of macula of right eye. No chiasmal syndrome but direct pressure of tumor on medial part of right optic nerve!

invasive and lead to death in less than 1 year. They start with the symptoms of unilateral optic neuritis, but proceed quickly to signs and symptoms of chiasmal involvement and thus to irreversible blindness. Of diagnostic importance are progressive fundus changes, that is, increasing swelling of one or both discs with superimposed occlusion of the veins initially and then of the arteries as a consequence of occlusive vascular effects of the tumor in the distal optic nerve segment. The disc swelling can assume extraordinary proportions and in some cases amount to as much as 8 to 9 diopters.

## Tumors of the cavernous sinus

In the discussion of meningiomas of the sphenoid ridge the superior orbital fissure syndrome was mentioned. Actually, it is related to the cavernous sinus syndrome. This should cause no surprise because the anatomic structures in the cavernous sinus are identical with those entering the orbit through the superior orbital fissure. *The characteristic sign of the cavernous sinus syndrome* (Foix) *is the more or less simultaneous involvement of the third, fourth, fifth, and sixth cranial nerves* (in other words, the three nerves supplying the extraocular muscles and the trigeminal nerve). The pupil may be dilated and fixed (purely oculomotor denervation) or may be small and nonreacting as a result of combined oculomotor and sympathetic denervation. In contrast to the superior orbital fissure syndrome with involvement of only the first division of the trigeminal nerve, all branches of the trigeminal nerve might be involved here. This symptomatology results from the close topographic relationship of these structures within the cavernous sinus and their proximity to the internal carotid artery (Figs. 3-99 and 3-100). According to Jefferson, one can distinguish between a *posterior cavernous sinus syndrome* (involvement of the first and second divisions of the trigeminal nerve; frequently only sixth nerve paresis) and an *anterior cavernous sinus syndrome* (only the first division of the trigeminal nerve involved, oculomotor nerve palsy alone or in association with a paresis of the fourth and the sixth nerve). This differentiation is particularly valid for aneurysms of the internal carotid artery within the cavernous sinus (Fig. 3-101) (Krayenbühl).

Our series includes 24 cases of cavernous sinus affections. Of these, not less than 18 were caused by various tumors originating from the base of the skull in this area. Two of these tumors were *neurinomas of the trigeminal nerve*, with the tumor in contact with the posterior part of the cavernous sinus. There was a characteristic history of neuralgic pains of the face, sensory disturbances, and later, numbness in the same area as well as diplopia in the later stages. Even loss of vision was mentioned. Both patients showed an incomplete cavernous sinus syndrome—only the abducens and trigeminal nerves were involved, whereas the oculomotor and trochlear nerves remained unaffected. *A total impairment of all branches of the trigeminal nerve with analgesia and anesthesia is pathognomonic for these tumors.* X-ray films in both patients showed decalcification and destruction of the ipsilateral tip of the petrous bone.

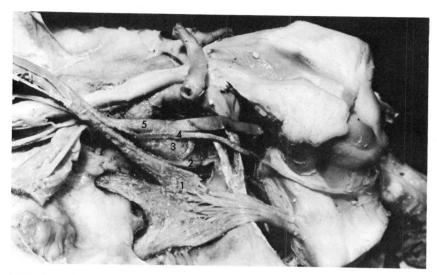

**Fig. 3-99.** Lateral view of cavernous sinus. Note intimate connection between trigeminal nerve, oculomotor nerve, trochlear nerve, and abducens nerve. *1,* Trigeminal nerve (ophthalmic branch); *2,* sixth nerve; *3,* internal carotid artery; *4,* trochlear nerve; *5,* oculomotor nerve. (Specimen of Prof. Kubic, Pathologic-Anatomic Institute of the University of Zurich.)

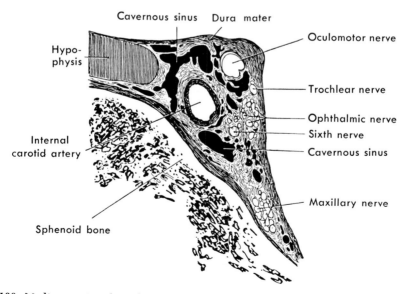

**Fig. 3-100.** Median section through cavernous sinus, hypophysis, sella turcica, internal carotid artery, and nerves of extraocular muscles. (After Corning.)

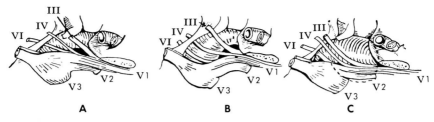

**Fig. 3-101.** Differentiation of cavernous sinus syndrome, according to Jefferson, with aneurysms of internal carotid artery within cavernous sinus. **A,** Normal. **B,** Posterior cavernous sinus syndrome. **C,** Middle or anterior cavernous sinus syndrome.

Two other cases in our series consisted of *meningiomas of the middle fossa.* These tumors are of importance because they are frequently responsible for a *lesion of the ipsilateral optic nerve.* Their symptomatology can resemble closely that of meningiomas of the sphenoid ridge. In addition to pain, ptosis, and diplopia, *characteristically* there are *complaints of unilateral loss of vision or even of a sudden blindness,* which may be mistaken for a retrobulbar neuritis. The meningiomas in our two patients extended to or even infiltrated the wall of the cavernous sinus. One originated from the sella and the other from the sphenoid ridge. The first case even showed a bilateral cavernous sinus syndrome. The second case was unusual because of an optic atrophy on the ipsilateral side and a papilledema on the contralateral side (that is, a Foster Kennedy syndrome). In both patients there was involvement of all the nerves of the extrinsic eye muscles as well as the first and second divisions of the trigeminal nerve.

Two cases of cavernous sinus syndrome caused by *chondromyxomas* or *myxomas* with parasellar or suprasellar localization were less characteristic and not so well defined. The two most severe tumors with perhaps the most malignant course originated in the nasal and retronasal space and extended to the base of the skull. One was a *round cell sarcoma of the retronasal area* and the other a lymphoepithelial *carcinoma of the nasopharyngeal area.* The first patient showed a complete bilateral cavernous sinus syndrome with bilateral amaurosis! The second showed unilateral amaurosis with protrusion of the ipsilateral globe. (Exophthalmos, extraocular muscle pareses, and loss of vision already constitute the *orbital apex syndrome,* which differs little from the superior orbital fissure and the cavernous sinus syndrome.)

An important group of tumors causing a cavernous sinus syndrome is the large number of metastatic neoplasms (seven cases), *especially metastatic carcinomas in the region of the cavernous sinus* (Fig. 3-102). Naturally, these occur mostly in patients in the older age group. Almost all of the patients initially complain of frontal or temporal headaches and also of pain or sensory disturbances in the various areas of distribution of the branches of the trigeminal nerve. In later stages, there is almost always diplopia, associated quite frequently with unilateral loss of vision. *The oculomotor nerve is invariably involved* (external

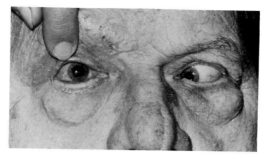

**Fig. 3-102.** Cavernous sinus syndrome in 72-year-old patient with metastatic carcinoma (lung) to right cavernous sinus. Total palsy of all branches of trigeminal nerve with analgesia and anesthesia on right side. Simultaneous involvement of third, fourth, and sixth nerves. Fixed mydriatic pupil on right side. No impairment of vision and no alteration of visual field of right eye.

and internal ophthalmoplegia and ptosis), *as are all branches of the trigeminal nerve.* In six of our seven patients the ipsilateral corneal reflex was distinctly diminished or absent. The abducens and trochlear nerves were not regularly involved. Noteworthy and, in view of the rapid growth of malignant tumors, not surprising is the relatively frequent *impairment of the ipsilateral optic nerve* in four of our seven patients. The radiologic findings showed destruction of the sella, the anterior clinoid processes, and especially the tip of the petrous bone. In five patients the metastatic carcinoma in the region of the cavernous sinus could be verified during surgery or autopsy—the primary tumors were in the breast, the bronchi, or the thyroid gland. It is not always easy to make a diagnosis without surgical exploration. However, even without evidence of a primary tumor, one should always consider a metastatic carcinoma in older people if there is a fully developed cavernous sinus syndrome with involvement of the optic nerve, a relatively rapid progress of symptoms, general cachexia, and most of all, marked roentgenologic changes in the region of the cavernous sinus and its neighborhood.

In addition to metastatic tumors, other *tumors at the base of the skull* (we cite as an example in our series a chondro-osteoma) may reach the size that could lead to a cavernous sinus syndrome. In the section on *pituitary adenomas* (p. 202), we cited two examples to discuss the possibility of the development of a cavernous sinus syndrome on the basis of an—admittedly rare—lateral extension of a pituitary tumor (Weinberger, Adler, and Grant).

In the broadest sense of the word, aneurysms are a form of tumor. In our series of 24 cases of cavernous sinus syndrome, four were caused by *aneurysms of the internal carotid artery in the region of the cavernous sinus.* Without prodromal signs, they usually set in with *pain or a sensation of numbness of the face, followed within a short period of time by diplopia with or without ptosis* (Fig. 5-8). The pain is localized in the area of distribution of the trigeminal nerve and usually is sharply demarcated. In contrast to the ordinary trigeminal neuralgia, it is not paroxysmal but constant. In addition to the subjective symptoms of irritation, it is always possible to demonstrate more or less distinct defects such as hypesthesia or hypalgesia in the area of distribution of the first, second, or even third branch of the trigeminal nerve. *Of special significance, again, is the corneal reflex that, sometimes as the only trigeminal sign, may be diminished or abolished.* Occasionally an aneurysm of unusual size may damage the ipsilateral optic nerve, causing atrophy with a corresponding loss of vision. We have records of two such cases. After their sudden onset, extraocular pareses caused by aneurysms usually remain stationary or may even regress during the further course of the disease. Not infrequently the trigeminal pain, which was quite violent at the onset, disappears. Now the hypesthetic or anesthetic zones that are so significant for the diagnosis become evident. This symptomatology actually is so typical that it almost allows a diagnosis. Radiologic proof of bony changes at the base of the skull is valuable. These bony changes consist of destruction or erosion of the mesial part of the ipsilateral lesser wing of the sphenoid and the anterior or posterior clinoid processes or of widening of the superior orbital fissure or the optic foramen. Actual proof of the aneurysm is obtained by cerebral angiography. It is interesting to note that an arteriovenous aneurysm of the internal carotid artery within the cavernous sinus (carotid-cavernous fistula) seldom causes a cavernous sinus syndrome and rarely leads to pareses of the extraocular muscles (p. 39).

In addition to tumors and aneurysms, one must consider cavernous *sinus thrombosis* as a third etiologic group in the differential diagnosis of the cavernous sinus syndrome. This picture sets in with unilateral or bilateral *proptosis, lid swelling,* and *chemosis.* Usually, there is an impairment of the three nerves supplying the extraocular muscles (including ptosis) as well as an involvement of the trigeminal nerve. A *preceding infection in the area of the head* (such as furunculosis, cellulitis of the lid, tonsillitis, maxillary or sphenoidal sinusitis, otitis) and signs of a *septicemia* make the diagnosis obvious (Weber). We have two recorded cases of cavernous sinus thrombosis; one was secondary to a septic tonsillitis and the other to an erysipelas of the face. (See Fig. 1-3.)

Quite rarely a cavernous sinus syndrome may develop secondary to *herpes zoster.*

The *painful ophthalmoplegia syndrome* (Tolosa-Hunt), characterized by retro- and supraorbital pain, paralysis of the third, fourth, sixth, and ophthalmic division of the trigeminal nerve, spontaneous remission, and tendency to recurrence, represents an inflammatory involvement (low-grade, nonspecific) of the cavernous sinus, responding promptly to corticosteroid therapy.

*In summary, it can be stated that in the majority of cases a cavernous sinus syndrome is caused by tumors. Usually these are metastatic carcinomas in the cavernous sinus or malignant tumors at the base of the skull. Sellar, suprasellar, or especially parasellar tumors likewise may produce a cavernous sinus syndrome if their expansion reaches sufficient size. Next to tumors, aneurysms must be primarily considered in the differential diagnosis. A more or less simultaneous involvement of the third, fourth, fifth, and sixth cranial nerves is characteristic for the cavernous sinus syndrome. An impairment of the ipsilateral optic nerve is frequent with malignant tumors. Besides diplopia and unilateral loss of vision, a pronounced incidence of pain and sensory disturbances in the various areas of distribution of the trigeminal nerve are characteristic. X-ray films frequently show destruction of the sella and the tip of the petrous bone.*

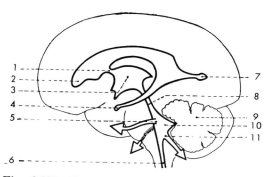

1, Interventricular foramen of Monro
2, Anterior horn of lateral ventricle
3, Third ventricle
4, Descending horn of lateral ventricle
5, Foramina of Luschka
6, Central canal of spinal cord
7, Posterior horn of lateral ventricle
8, Sylvian aqueduct
9, Cerebellum
10, Fourth ventricle
11, Median aperture of fourth ventricle
(foramen of Magendie)

**Fig. 3-103.** Diagrammatic cross section through ventricular system indicating connection openings (arrows) to subarachnoid space.

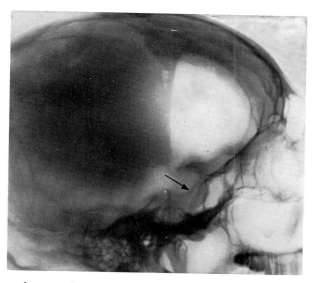

**Fig. 3-104.** Ventriculogram (lateral view) of internal hydrocephalus caused by stenosis of aqueduct in 16-year-old boy. Hydrocephalic lateral ventricle (in this illustration, only anterior part is visible) causes downward displacement of enlarged third ventricle and extension into sella turcica (arrow). Chronic atrophic bilateral papilledema. Visual acuity of both eyes reduced to 0.5. Questionable bitemporal hemianopia.

**Tumors of the third ventricle**

Tumors of the third ventricle produce early *embarrassment in the circulation of the cerebrospinal fluid* by obliteration of either the foramina of Monro (tumors in the anterior section) or the anterior opening of the aqueduct (tumors of the posterior section, Fig. 3-103). This results in the formation of an *internal hydrocephalus* (Fig. 3-104) and consequently, the appearance of symptoms of *increased intracranial pressure.* It follows that general symptoms of increased intracranial pressure (often intermittent, coming about suddenly, especially with changing of position of the head) dominate the picture for some time, especially in view of the fact that tumors within the third ventricle cause focal signs relatively late (Oldberg and Eisenhardt; Dandy). Tumors of the infundibulum produce hypothalamic and pituitary signs quite early; actually, they are *craniopharyngiomas* and should be discussed here with other tumors of the third ventricle. However, they have already been considered together with the sellar processes in view of their importance in the differential diagnosis. True tumors of the third ventricle are characterized by a rather unspecific symptomatology: bouts of occlusive hydrocephalus, sometimes accompanied by mental disorders, and falling as a result of loss of tone in the lower limbs.

It is quite characteristic that *tumors of the third ventricle predominantly cause ophthalmoscopic signs of increased intracranial pressure* (Fig. 3-105). Very frequently, there are *pronounced* papilledemas with a prominence of up to 6 diopters. *Relatively early, they change into the chronic atrophic form, with disastrous consequences for the visual acuity and the visual fields* (Fig. 3-105). *Intermittent attacks of blurred vision or even transient amaurosis,* mostly combined with paroxysmal headache, nausea, or vomiting, occur characteristically in colloid cysts of the third ventricle and its area, often related in a peculiar way to changes in the position of the head (Dandy). With the head bent to the side the vision may suddenly disappear, and with the head in an erect or backward position, it may come back gradually. The intermittent headaches can be explained by paroxysmal blocking of the foramina of Monro, but not the loss of vision. The latter has to be interpreted on the basis of intermittent pressure of the dilated third ventricle on the chiasm and the optic nerves. Diplopia as a result of lesions of the sixth nerve is often seen at the stage of confirmed increase in intracranial pressure.

In addition to the general symptoms of increased intracranial pressure, there may be *local signs and symptoms referable to the chiasm:* a tumor in the anterior part of the third ventricle and the infundibulum may exert direct pressure on the chiasm, or a tumor in the posterior part may cause a hydrocephalic dilation of the ventricle, whose anterior wall compresses the chiasm (Hughes) (Figs. 3-104 and 3-106). In both instances the result will be a *more or less asymmetric chiasmal syndrome with bitemporal hemianopia and primary optic atrophy,* or secondary atrophy after papilledema. The visual fields in patients with tumors of the third ventricle show a rather asymmetric appearance. Usually, there is first an involve-

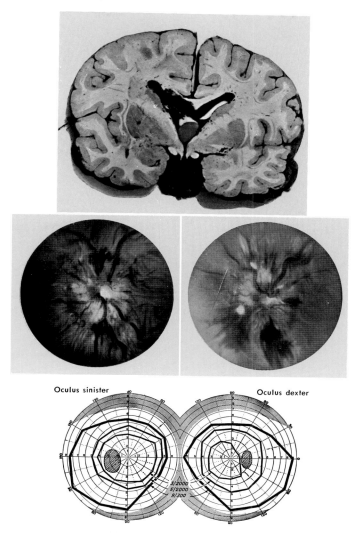

Oculus sinister                    Oculus dexter

**Fig. 3-105.** Plexus cyst in third ventricle with internal hydrocephalus in 43-year-old patient. Above, Frontal section through brain. Center, Fully developed papilledemas with marked prominence of 5 to 6 diopters. Numerous hemorrhages. White spots. Extension of edema into adjacent retina (radial folding). Left illustration corresponds to right eye and right illustration to left eye. Below, Corresponding visual fields. Enormous enlargement of both blind spots. Suggestion of right temporal hemianopia in area of central isopter (beginning chiasmal syndrome?).

ment of the upper fibers of the chiasm, causing *mostly initial inferior temporal hemianopias*. Frequently, the compression embarrasses the posterior rim or the chiasm and thus often causes *central scotomas*. One may also observe vertical or binasal hemianopias with tumors of the third ventricle (François). A tumor at the floor of the third ventricle in one of our patients caused temporal hemianopia on one side and loss of the inferior nasal quadrant on the other side. In another, a hemangioma in the third ventricle caused an almost symmetric bitemporal hemianopia (Fig. 3-107). A lateral extension of the tumor toward the thalamus

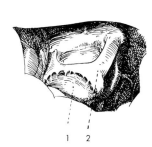

**1,** Anterior wall (lamina terminalis) of dilated third ventricle
**2,** Chiasm and right optic nerve

1  2

**Fig. 3-106.** Dilation of third ventricle and compression of chiasm and right optic nerve in internal hydrocephalus caused by stenosis of aqueduct in 48-year-old patient. Distinct chiasmal syndrome. Bilateral optic atrophy. Asymmetric bitemporal hemianopia. Visual acuity reduced to O.D. finger counting at 1 meter; O.S. 0.6.

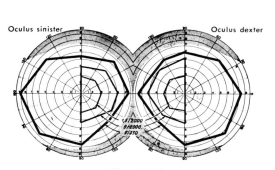

Oculus sinister    Oculus dexter

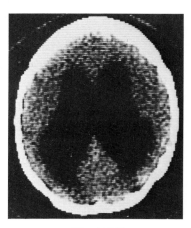

**Fig. 3-107**            **Fig. 3-108**

**Fig. 3-107.** Cystic hemangioma in rostral part of third ventricle in 29-year-old patient. Visual acuity, O.D. 0.15; O.S. 0.3. No optic atrophy. No radiologic changes of sella turcica. Slight asymmetric bitemporal hemianopia of central isopters without sparing of macula.
**Fig. 3-108.** Computerized transverse axial tomogram of internal hydrocephalus caused by aqueduct stenosis: enormous dilatation of lateral and third ventricles, which are directly visualized by sharp limits between brain substance and cerebrospinal fluid (higher density structure of brain contrasted against lower density of cerebrospinal fluid).

or the suprachiasmatic visual pathways may produce a homonymous hemianopia. If a tumor in the posterior part of the third ventricle grows upward toward the tectal area, the result may be a Parinaud syndrome (p. 280), characterized by light-near dissociation of the pupillary reaction and vertical gaze palsy.

The most frequently observed tumors of the third ventricle are colloid cysts, ependymomas, plexus papillomas, and epidermoid cysts.

*In summary, tumors of the third ventricle cause general signs and symptoms of increased intracranial pressure and thus papilledemas at a relatively early stage. The latter soon change to the chronic atrophic form, with its disastrous sequelae for the visual functions. Intermittent and paroxysmal headaches produced or relieved by alterations in the position of the head are sometimes accompanied by corresponding intermittent loss and recovery of vision. A direct pressure effect by the tumor in the anterior part of the third ventricle or an indirect effect caused by an internal hydrocephalus leads to asymmetric chiasmal syndromes with loss of vision and optic atrophy (possibly combined with choking) and to quite irregular visual field defects (mostly in the form of an incomplete bitemporal hemianopia). Such a chiasmal syndrome frequently can only be differentiated from the other forms previously discussed by means of encephalography, ventriculography, or computerized x-ray tomography, which permits proof of an internal hydrocephalus.*

*Dilatation of the third ventricle with consequent pressure on the chiasm and production of a chiasmal syndrome (incomplete bitemporal hemianopia, unilateral central scotoma with temporal hemianopia in the opposite eye, unilateral amaurosis with temporal hemianopia in the other eye, always choked discs) occurs also in the late stages of posterior fossa lesions (tumors of the cerebellum and the cerebellopontine angle), in pinealomas, in obliterations of the sylvian aqueduct, and in internal hydrocephalus of any origin (Wagener and Cusick; Hughes) (p. 274) (Fig. 3-108).*

Because of their topographic position, tumors of the third ventricle may produce hypothalamic symptoms such as polyuria, polydipsia, or drowsiness. Another hypothalamic disturbance has been described by Penfield as *diencephalic autonomous epilepsy.* It is found especially in association with tumors of the third ventricle. This form of epilepsy is distinguished by attacks that set in with great restlessness and that later lead to reddening of the face and the arms, slowdown of respiration, epiphora, intense perspiration, drooling, hiccough, dilation of pupils, and tachycardia. Certain mental disturbances associated with tumors in the region of the third ventricle such as memory failure, lack of impulse, apathy, and general loss of interest should also be mentioned.

## Tumors of the thalamus

True tumors of the thalamus (glioblastomas, astrocytomas, oligodendrogliomas, angiomas) actually are rare. More often, an invision of tumors from the brain stem, the third ventricle, the midbrain, or the pineal body into the thalamus causes neurologic disturbances. For this reason the primary signs of the original tumor predominate in the symptomatology. Thus what has been called the classic *thalamus syndrome* is quite rare in tumors of the thalamus: crossed hemihypesthesia (involving more deep than superficial sensitivity), "main thalamique," hemiastereognosia, incessant or paroxysmal intolerable pain on the involved side (thalamic pain), occasional choreoathetotic movements, hemiataxia, or even a slight transient hemiparesis (Bailey).

The ocular symptoms associated with such tumors are not characteristic and, at any rate, not of localizing value. A papilledema usually occurs only in the later stages (80% according to Tönnis). Important ocular symptoms occur if the tumor expands toward the chiasm and creates a chiasmal syndrome (p. 206). There are reports of pupillary disturbances in tumors of the thalamus (Névin). One of our patients with a tumor in this region showed a difference in the size of the pupils, with a distinct decrease of the pupillary reaction of both eyes to light and in convergence. This patient also showed a distinct decrease of the corneal reflex on the contralateral side. Nystagmus (horizontal or vertical), paralysis of upward or downward gaze, and oculomotor or sixth nerve pareses are described in primary tumors of the thalamus (glioblastomas, astrocytomas, etc.) by McKissock and Paine.

A few of our patients with glioblastoma in the thalamic region show symptoms of motor and sensory hemiparesis as well as a homonymous hemianopia. It must be assumed that the tumor has invaded the internal capsule and the lateral geniculate body or the optic radiation.

### Tumors of the basal ganglia

Tumors of the basal ganglia (caudate nucleus, putamen, and pallidum) frequently show an onset with headache, followed by vomiting. The increased intracranial pressure may produce signs of cerebellar herniation, with violent pain in the neck or even extensor spasms. Usually there are pyramidal tract signs (partial or complete hemiplegia), as a rule on the contralateral side. Hemiparesthesias and other sensory disturbances have been described. Tremor, athetosis, rigidity, choreiform movements, disturbances of coordination, speech disturbances, ataxia, and memory changes are late manifestations.

It should be emphasized, by the way, that tumors of the basal ganglia frequently cannot be differentiated clinically from those of the thalamus. They are discussed separately to present an overall topographic picture.

The ophthalmologic signs and symptoms of tumors of the basal ganglia, again, are not characteristic and localizing. Papilledemas occur quite often (in about 80% of all patients). There are practically no visual field changes. Occasionally, there is an ipsilateral disturbance of the pupillary reflex. Eye muscle palsies (fourth and sixth nerves) occur in about one half of the cases (Tönnis). In isolated cases a vertical or ipsilateral horizontal gaze paresis or gaze palsy is seen (Lillie). If possible, it is important to demonstrate tumor calcifications on x-ray films of the skull, which, as a rule, makes the diagnosis easy.

### Tumors of the pineal body and the midbrain

Tumors of the pineal body and midbrain, as parts of the brain that are in close proximity, are discussed in one section because their symptomatology is quite similar. By causing pressure on the roof of the midbrain, tumors of the pineal body produce signs and symptoms quite similar to those of neoplasms with the primary site in the midbrain, especially in its cranial part. It also seems justified to discuss these tumors together from the standpoint of differential diagnosis. It is practically impossible to differentiate between tumors of the pineal body (Fig. 3-109) and the midbrain (Fig. 3-110), since, as a result of their close proximity, their signs and symptoms are quite similar.

There are numerous references in the literature (Horrax and Bailey) to the fact that *pinealomas in boys* often produce *precocious puberty,* with premature development of the sex organs, the appearance of axillary and public hair, and breaking of the voice. We have a record of precocious puberty in only one patient with a pinealoma. In three other patients, no sexual prematurity was noticeable. On the contrary, one boy showed a distinct dystrophia adiposogenitalis and one girl a marked obesity, especially of the hips and thighs. The association between pineal tumors and precocious puberty cannot be simple and direct! Three children in our series developed cerebellar symptoms such as trunk ataxia during the early stages that made it impossible for them to walk (effect of the tumor on the cerebellum or the spinocerebellar tract). The combination of cerebellar ataxia and aqueduct signs is called

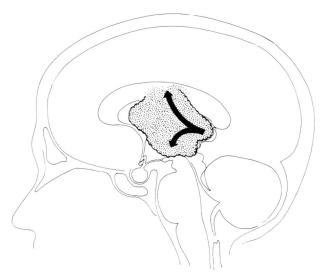

**Fig. 3-109.** Median section through skull showing pinealoma invading third ventricle. Note infiltration and compression of roof of midbrain and narrowing of sylvian aqueduct.

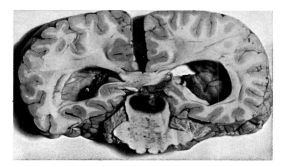

**Fig. 3-110.** Frontal section through brain with tumor (glioblastoma multiforme) in region of midbrain and aqueduct of Sylvius. Enormous internal hydrocephalus can be recognized by enlarged lateral ventricles.

*Nothnagel's syndrome.* Especially in children, the cerebellar symptoms in association with signs of increased intracranial pressure represent the first symptoms of tumors of the quadrigeminate plate (Tönnis) and thus may mislead to the diagnosis of a posterior fossa lesion. *Deafness* is another characteristic symptom resulting from involvement of the inferior colliculi. The acoustic impairment commences with the high tones. Occasionally, pinealomas produce signs and symptoms indicating impairment of the neighboring hypothalamus. They take the form of drowsiness, polyuria, polydipsia, and elevation of the body temperature. This is particularly the case if the tumor originates from vestiges of the pineal gland in the third ventricle. The symptomatology then is very similar to that of tumors of the third ventricle.

The signs and symptoms of *tumors of the midbrain* (ependymomas, spongioblastomas, astrocytomas, metastatic carcinomas) are practically identical with those of the pineal body, especially if they develop in the roof of the midbrain (that is, the region of the corpora quadrigemina) (Glaser; Globus). Affection of the red nucleus and the ipsilateral oculomotor nerve results in the well-known *Benedikt syndrome* (rhythmic tremor of the arm on the contralateral side and oculomotor paresis on the side of the lesion). If the tumor has an even more ventral position, it usually causes *Weber syndrome,* consisting of an ipsilateral oculomotor paresis with hemiplegia on the opposite side. Frequently, the tumors involve both sides. Thus a bilateral Benedikt syndrome or Weber syndrome (tetraplegia) is not rare. Deafness resulting from compression of the lateral lemniscus and a contralateral sensory disturbance caused by involvement of the median lemniscus are rather late signs of tumors of the midbrain. Rather early in the course of midbrain neoplasms are personality changes, accompanied by memory disturbances (Weber).

*In the topical diagnosis of tumors of the pineal body and midbrain, ocular signs are of decisive significance.* This can be expressed with the key phrase *Parinaud's syndrome* (Posner and Horrax; Barker; Devic, Paufique, Girard, and Guinet). It consists of *supranuclear disturbances of conjugate eye movements in the form of a vertical gaze palsy* in addition to *pupillary disturbances of the Argyll Robertson type (light-near dissociation)* and *nuclear oculomotor pareses.* This symptomatology is clear if one remembers the location of the supranuclear vertical gaze centers, the pupillary centers, and the oculomotor nuclei in the region of the midbrain, especially its periaqueductal area (see Fig. 1-12).

Accordingly, the *ocular symptoms* caused by these tumors consist of relatively early *double vision* that, as a quasi preliminary stage of the diplopia (p. 10), may be preceded by an undefined sensation of blurred vision. In our own series of 10 patients (six with pinealomas and four with tumors of the midbrain), this diplopia with vertically separated images, besides early general symptoms of increased intracranial pressure (headache and vomiting), was one of the earliest and most striking symptoms and one that caused the patient to seek medical consultation. Other symptoms such as flickering, clouds, or blackouts must be interpreted as the result of papilledemas.

*The most important and constant sign is a vertical gaze palsy.* (Horizontal conjugate gaze is always intact.) We have found it in all 10 patients in our series and in every instance as a *gaze palsy of the upward movement* (Fig. 3-111). Only in one patient was the palsy of the upward movement combined with one of the downward movement. It is characteristic that neither spontaneous and command saccadic movements nor pursuit movements, optically induced movements, and nonoptic (vestibular and otolithic) reflex movements can be executed with the eyes in this one particular direction of gaze. In rare cases only the vestibular eye movements may remain. These can be elicited by means of the caloric nystagmus or the vertical doll's head maneuver. This is the so-called Roth-Bielschowsky type of a vertical gaze palsy. However, loss of all types of conjugate eye movements, that is, the saccadic as well as the pursuit and nonoptic reflex (vestibular and otolithic) movements, is the rule. In the initial stages of a tumor of the pineal body or of the midbrain, there may be only a vertical gaze paresis that, however, soon changes to complete paralysis. Upward gaze becomes limited before downward gaze, and saccadic movements are limited before pursuit movements. In combination with a vertical gaze palsy, there may be a consequent *downward or upward conjugate deviation of the eyes* according to the nature of the palsy, also either a *ptosis* or a *retraction of the upper lids* (Collier). Occasionally, the very first sign of such a gaze paresis may be merely a vertical jerk (so to speak, gaze paretic) nystagmus in upward or, more rarely, downward gaze. Only a purely vertical gaze nystagmus is suggestive of a lesion of the midbrain, whereas a combination of horizontal and vertical nystagmus occurs in association with tumors of the vermis cerebelli (p. 285).

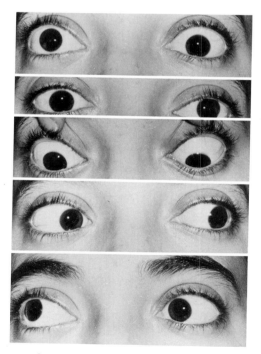

**Fig. 3-111.** Vertical gaze palsy in 25-year-old patient with arteriovenous malformation of midbrain. Inability to perform saccadic or pursuit movements upward. Note skew deviation of both eyes in attempt by patient to look up (top). Downward gaze as well as horizontal gaze to left and to right intact.

It has already been stressed in the section on gaze palsies (p. 50) that the supranuclear character of an impairment of the conjugate vertical eye movements (in other words, preservation of function of the individual nerves and their nuclei) can be proved by a positive Bell phenomenon (upward rotation of the eyes during lid closure or sleep). Such vertical gaze palsies must be caused, as we know from newer publications (Balthasar; Nashold and Gills), by lesions in the *midbrain tegmentum,* especially its lateral periaqueductal segment. The earlier doctrine that vertical gaze palsy is produced by affections of the quadrigeminate plate (colliculi) can no longer be supported. Of great importance in this connection are the stereotactic experiments of Nashold and Gills, who were able to produce the ocular signs of Parinaud's syndrome by making lesions (unilateral) in the mesencephalic tegmentum (6 to 8 mm from the midaqueductal plane). In most patients, it is impossible to demonstrate a definite oculomotor paresis in addition to a vertical gaze palsy. Hence it must be assumed that the diplopia is the result of an unequal effect of the vertical gaze palsy on the two eyes (Duke-Elder; Bielschowsky; Böhringer and Koenig). With a more detailed test for ocular motility, such a supranuclear vertical gaze palsy with an unequal effect on the two eyes (a sort of "skew deviation," as described in midbrain lesions by Bielschowsky, Hoyt, and others) will not appear as a paresis of one extraocular muscle, but as a persistent vertical divergence without essential change in the angle of strabismus in all fields of gaze (similar to a hyperphoria or a vertical concomitant strabismus). However, one should not forget that true *nuclear oculomotor palsies or pareses* do occur with tumors of the pineal gland or, in particular, the midbrain. They may be responsible for some of the phenomena of diplopia. It is characteristic for nuclear oculomotor pareses that *only one isolated muscle or just some of them of either one eye or frequently both eyes may be involved.* Interestingly enough, we could demonstrate such nuclear oculomotor pareses in only four of the 10 patients in our series. In about one fourth, there was a paresis of the levator of the upper lid (mostly bilateral), causing a slight or moderate ptosis. The diplopia may also result from a sixth nerve paresis, which quite frequently occurs in association with these types of tumors, as they tend to cause early embarrassment of circulation of the cerebrospinal fluid and, consequently, increased intracranial pressure (two of 10 patients). We observed one instance of a *nuclear trochlear palsy in the very early stages of Parinaud's syndrome* caused by a pinealoma (Jaensch). Oculomotor palsy and a typical vertical gaze palsy, in addition to the trochlear nerve palsy, developed only some time later.

Part of Parinaud's syndrome in patients with tumors of the pineal body and midbrain also involves characteristic *pupillary changes in the form of light rigidity of the pupil of the Argyll Robertson type* (light-near dissociation) on the basis of a lesion in the pretectal region, where the fibers for the light reaction from the optic tract end. We have observed such a pupillary disturbance (p. 25) in a more or less typical form in nine patients (50% according to Tönnis). Mostly it involved both sides and once only one side. Anisocoria was seen frequently, but corectopia (displaced pupils) seldom. The size of the pupils was rather larger than normal. The usual miosis of the typical Argyll Robertson pupil was quite rare. In contrast to the true Argyll Robertson phenomenon, the *light rigidity* of the pupils was *not always complete*. However, the reaction to light usually was quite markedly diminished. There may be signs of defective accommodation (Walsh and Hoyt) or accommodation spasms (producing acquired myopia) before disturbances of pupillary reaction appear. Another atypical mark of pupillary disturbance consisted of an *occasional additional impairment of the convergence reaction* (often combined with an actual *paralysis of convergence*), which is not true for the Argyll Robertson pupil (pseudo-Argyll Robertson pupil or incomplete general pupil rigidity according to Kestenbaum). We observed a paralysis of convergence in three of our 10 patients. *Convergence spasm and nystagmus retractorius*—a jerking retraction of the eyes caused by clonic convergence spasms without simultaneous relaxation of the lateral recti (cocontraction of muscles)—was found only once. Both phenomena are generally evoked on attempted upward gaze and are related. We saw one case of true convergence spasm. (The intention to look upward caused a strong convergence movement of both eyes.)

By definition, Parinaud's syndrome consists only of a vertical gaze paresis, nuclear oculomotor pareses, and pupillary disturbances. If there are, in addition, tonic convergence spasms

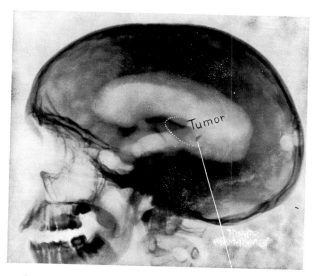

**Fig. 3-112.** Ventriculogram (lateral view) of skull of 15-year-old patient with pinealoma. Localization of tumor is indicated by calcification. Tumor caused occlusion of aqueduct, resulting in enormous internal hydrocephalus. Dilated third ventricle extends toward sella turcica. Clinical picture: typical vertical gaze palsy, pupillary disturbances of the Argyll Robertson type, and bilateral papilledema of 2 to 3 diopters' elevation.

and a nystagmus retractorius (especially in an attempt to look up), the term *"sylvian aqueduct syndrome"* is frequently used. We have seen these two signs, supposedly characteristic for the region of the sylvian aqueduct, in association with pinealomas. Thus they are of no localizing value in the differentiation of Parinaud's and sylvian aqueduct syndromes. It would be more correct to consider the latter a rare and special form (although with additional symptoms) of the former.

Because of the close proximity of these tumors to the sylvian aqueduct (Yanagida), early blockage of the aqueduct and the development of an internal hydrocephalus (Fig. 3-112), with considerable increase in intracranial pressure (headache, vomiting, uni- or bilateral sixth nerve paresis) are possible. We have observed such an event with the occurrence of markedly prominent *papilledemas* in four of a total of 10 patients. The others showed a perfectly normal fundus. On the basis of our own experience, we cannot concur with the opinion of other authors (Walsh and Hoyt; Tönnis), according to whom papilledemas occur almost invariably with such tumors. Tönnis found papilledemas in 80% of the patients in his series; one fifth of these already showed secondary optic atrophy. Twenty-five percent of all the patients with quadrigeminate plate tumors had visual disturbances; 15% already manifested amaurosis. We also were unable to record abnormal field changes in our patients, except occasional enlargement of the blind spot. Bitemporal or homonymous hemianopias caused by interference with the visual pathways have been described.

*In summary, the ocular signs and symptoms are decisive for the diagnosis of tumors of the pineal gland and the midbrain. They can be defined as the so-called Parinaud's syndrome, which consists of a vertical gaze palsy, pupillary disturbances of the true or pseudo-Argyll Robertson type, and nuclear oculomotor and trochlear palsies. Rarer additional phenomena are convergence paresis or convergence spasms and nystagmus retractorius. Occlusion of the sylvian aqueduct may cause early papilledemas as well as a nonspecific sixth nerve paresis. Parinaud's syndrome is so extraordinarily characteristic that its presence alone is convincing proof of a lesion, most often a tumor in the region of the midbrain or the pineal gland.*

*Ectopic pinealomas may involve the third ventricle, the optic chiasm, and the optic nerves (Weber; Horrax and Wyatt). From such ectopic pineal tumors a chiasmal syndrome with primary optic atrophy, bitemporal hemianopia, diabetes insipidus, and hypopituitarism may result.*

Only in rare instances will the remote effect of tumors located elsewhere cause Parinaud's syndrome. We have seen this a few times in patients with tumors of the corpus callosum and the frontal lobe, especially in association with signs of transtentorial herniation and compression of the brain stem. In the interpretation of such disturbances of the vertical gaze, utmost caution is indicated. *Lack of attention* (caused either by a psycho-organic syndrome or a disturbance of the sensorium) may lead to impairment of the conjugate upward eye movements. As a manifestation of the inhibited cooperation on the part of the patient, the vertical motors of the globe fail earlier than the lateral rotators. This is evident from the fact that even under normal conditions it is considerably more strenuous to look up than to any other direction. A *disturbed sensorium* (associated with tumors of the frontal lobe or the corpus callosum, general increase in intracranial pressure, or subarachnoid hemorrhage) makes a "vertical gaze palsy" useless of localization. A lesion of the midbrain must be differentiated from a mere lack of attention with the help of other available signs (such as pupillary signs or extraocular muscle pareses).

## INFRATENTORIAL TUMORS

Supratentorial tumors interfere primarily with the visual pathways and thus frequently produce visual field changes. For this reason the neuro-ophthalmologic symptomatology of supratentorial tumors is governed largely by the more or less characteristic visual field defects. Since direct interference with the visual tracts by infratentorial tumors is impossible, the visual field is of lessened significance in the ocular symptomatology. However, these tumors tend to affect the brain stem, the site of the nuclei of the cranial nerves, including those of the extraocular muscles and the medial longitudinal fascicle. *The picture of the ocular signs in infratentorial tumors thus is dominated by phenomena of ocular motility disturbances* of the peripheral, nuclear, or supranuclear type. Common to both supratentorial and infratentorial tumors is an increase in intracranial pressure. A prematurely embarrassed circulation of the cerebrospinal fluid in patients with infratentorial tumors produces earlier and more pronounced formation of signs of increased intracranial pressure, including papilledemas.

### Tumors of the cerebellum

The symptomatology of affections of the cerebellum can be expressed with the keywords *ataxia, asynergy, dysmetria, and hypotonia.* Depending on whether the lesion is in the hemispheres or the vermis, these signs may show somewhat different forms (Krayenbühl; deMartel and Guillaume; Stewart and Holmes). A clinical differentiation between the *syndrome of the cerebellar hemispheres* and *the syndrome of the cerebellar vermis is possible.* In children, the syndrome of the cerebellar hemispheres is caused by an astrocytoma (Fig. 3-113). In adults, it is usually caused by astrocytomas and hemangioblastomas. The syndrome of the cerebellar vermis in children is predominantly the result of a medulloblastoma (Fig. 3-114). In adolescents and adults, it may be caused by an astrocytoma, a hemangioblastoma, or other tumors. In addition to horizontal gaze nystagmus (to be discussed subsequently), the characteristic signs of the *syndrome of the cerebellar hemispheres* are hypotonia (excessive range of movements on passive ductions) of the ipsilateral extremities with atactic and dysmetric movements and a distinct tendency to fall, frequently toward the side of the lesion. Ataxia and asynergy manifest themselves in the knee-heel test and in the test for diadochokinesis (rapidly executed pronation and supination movements of the hands or arms). Dysmetria as well as asynergy and intention tremor will be evident with the finger-nose test. The *syndrome of the cerebellar vermis* usually shows vertical gaze in addition to horizontal gaze nystagmus; ataxia and dysmetria of the extremities are insignificant, whereas ataxia of the gait and trunk are very pronounced. In children with medulloblastomas the symptoms of increased intracranial pressure (such as vomiting with or without headaches, double vision, and squint) frequently precede other signs. Marked loss of weight is characteristic in children with medulloblastomas (Fig. 3-115). Only in the late stages will there be signs of herniation of the cerebellar tonsils through the foramen magnum in the form of stiffness of the neck, sensory disturbances and weakness of the extremities, and ultimately extensor spasms and respiratory paralysis. Less frequently, there is an upward herniation of the cerebellum, expanded by a tumor through the tentorial opening, thus producing midbrain symptoms such as anisocoria, disturbances of the light and convergence reaction of the pupils, and vertical gaze palsies, especially upward. In children up to 14 years of age a tumor of the cerebellar vermis interfering with the circulation of the cerebrospinal fluid, and thus causing an internal hydro-

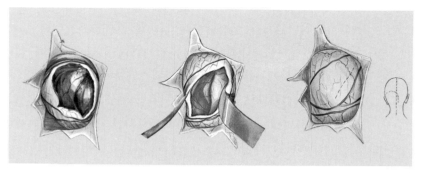

**Fig. 3-113.** Astrocytoma of caudal and lateral parts of left cerebellar hemisphere in 9-year-old boy before and after surgical extirpation (left cerebellar exploration).

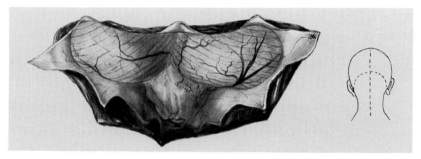

**Fig. 3-114.** Huge medulloblastoma of cerebellar vermis filling fourth ventricle in 13-year-old patient. View after cerebellar exploration.

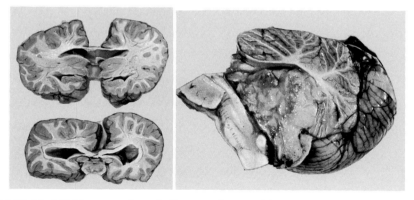

**Fig. 3-115.** Medulloblastoma of cerebellum. Occlusion of fourth ventricle and internal hydrocephalus (frontal section of brain). (Specimen from the Pathologic-Anatomic Institute of the University of Zurich.)

cephalus, will cause separation of the sutures of the skull and the characteristic "cracked-pot resonance" elicited by knocking on the head. Occasionally, a chronic internal hydrocephalus associated with cerebellar tumors may be responsible for generalized epileptic seizures.

One should not forget that the symptomatology of cerebellar tumors is largely marked by *signs and symptoms of increased intracranial pressure* (vomiting, headache, bradycardia, respiratory disorders). Especially with slowly growing tumors, signs attributable to the cerebellum are insignificant compared to those caused by the increased intracranial pressure. In such cases, differentiation from supratentorial tumors often is not easy, especially since herniation of the cerebellum upward or downward may produce symptoms seen in all sorts of brain tumors. The sequence in which the symptoms appear is enormously important for proper evaluation. If cerebellar signs are present in the early stages before the onset of signs of increased pressure, a cerebellar tumor should be suspected. If the cerebellar signs appear late, they are not localizing.

As far as eye symptoms are concerned, it is unnecessary to differentiate between tumors of the vermis and the hemispheres of the cerebellum. There is no essential difference between these two types of localization and their effect on the visual apparatus.

In a little more than one half of the cerebellar tumors among the 30 adults and 25 children in our series, *ocular symptoms were present that were more or less directly related to increased intracranial pressure and the formation of papilledemas.* Patients frequently complain about flickering before the eyes, temporary blurring, and a peculiar quivering or regular transient amblyopic attacks (p. 109). Exceptionally frequent (45% according to Tönnis) are statements about a *diminution of vision* (usually bilateral). One patient stated that he saw his surroundings as through a "scraped-off" mirror. At times the loss of vision (usually bilateral) and a corresponding concentric constriction of the visual field (evidence of an incipient atrophy of a chronic papilledema, p. 125) are the *very first symptoms that bring the patient to the physician and perhaps to the ophthalmologist.* The cerebellar signs are still absent or are present only in a very minor form. We have records of a few patients with cerebellar tumors who consulted an ophthalmologist first and in whom a diagnosis of bilateral papilledema led to referral to the neurosurgeon for further evaluation. The history reveals, in addition to loss of vision and obscurations, occasional double vision (30% according to Tönnis) and photophobia. The anatomic basis for the *diplopia* is a nonspecific, usually unilateral, sixth nerve paresis related to the increased intracranial pressure. Accordingly, the two images usually show horizontal separation. Diplopia and manifest strabismus (in addition to loss of vision, headache, and vomiting) are also among the first signs and symptoms of a cerebellar tumor that bring the patient to the physician or ophthalmologist. The ocular symptoms of patients with cerebellar tumors are actually absolutely nonspecific and should be regarded merely as the result of increased intracranial pressure.

One of the most frequent and perhaps earliest ocular signs of cerebellar tumors (especially in progressive cases) is *nystagmus.* We found it in practically all of the patients in our series. Its absence in slowly progressive tumors is, however, reported (Walsh and Hoyt). This *cerebellar nystagmus* is a jerk nystagmus (p. 53). It usually has the character of a central vestibular nystagmus, sometimes also of a symmetric, asymmetric, horizontal, or vertical gaze nystagmus. The cerebellar nystagmus is predominantly horizontal in nature, rarely horizontal rotary. It may be spontaneous with the eyes in the primary position or, more frequently, appear only during lateral movements, with the quick phase in the direction of gaze. In unilateral cerebellar lesions the amplitude varies with the direction of gaze. Despite some exceptions, it can be stated generally that *the direction of gaze associated with the coarser form of nystagmus corresponds to the side of the lesion. The nystagmus with cerebellar tumors is sometimes characteristically dissociated,* which means that the direction or amplitude of the oscillations is greater in one eye than in the other (Cogan). It is also said to vary with the position of the head. If the tumor has a mesial location (for instance, in the vermis), there may be a purely vertical gaze nystagmus either caused by direct pressure on the floor of the fourth ventricle and thus the posterior longitudinal bundle or by a remote effect on the midbrain tectal or pretectal area. It also indicates a considerable anterior extension of the tumor from the posterior fossa anteriorly. This nystagmus is particularly noticeable in upward gaze. Among our own series, we have observed vertical gaze nystagmus (also usually in combination with horizontal nystagmus) almost exclusively in patients with tumors of the cerebellar vermis, especially in those with medulloblastoma (seven times) (Fig. 3-115). Twice it was noticed in patients with large tumors of the hemisphere that tended to expand toward the midline. It is still questionable whether nystagmus associated with cerebellar tumors represents truly a cerebellar sign or whether it is caused by a remote effect on the brain stem.

Like the nystagmus of tumors of the pons and the cerebellopontine angle, cerebellar nystagmus belongs to the group of so-called *central nystagmus* (p. 58) (Kestenbaum). It may assume the character of a central vestibular, symmetric or asymmetric, horizontal, or vertical gaze nystagmus. The central vestibular nystagmus, a result of disturbed connections between the cerebellum and the vestibular nuclei, has a horizontal-rotary character. It shows first-, second-, or third-degree intensity. In contrast to peripheral vestibular nystagmus, it is permanent. As a rule, it is not associated with acoustic disturbances or dizziness. The symmetric or asymmetric gaze nystagmus is purely horizontal; it is missing in the primary position and it becomes manifest only in gaze to the right or left, its intensity increasing as the terminal positions are reached. It is caused by a remote effect of the cerebellar process on the brain stem structures. If vertical gaze nystagmus is an only sign, it is suggestive of a median lesion (vermis) with remote effect on the midbrain tectal or pretectal area. If there is a simultaneous horizontal nystagmus in the lateral positions of gaze, a vertical nystagmus is only one of the components of a severe symmetric gaze nystagmus and has therefore no importance of its own. Undoubtedly, these various components of a central nystagmus in cerebellar tumors merge, making their analysis difficult at times. For practical and clinical purposes, it is sufficient to consider the criteria of cerebellar nystagmus previously outlined.

Some of the rarer phenomena of motility disturbances associated with cerebellar tumors are *horizontal gaze pareses* and *dissociated movements,* as seen in two patients in our series. Such manifestations must be regarded as the effect of a tumor on the pons or pressure on the floor of the fourth ventricle. (If the dissociation alternates, the lesion lies in both hemispheres.) One example of dissociated ocular movements is the *"skew deviation,"* or the Hertwig-Magendie syndrome: one eye turns down and in and the other up and out. The dissociation remains unchanged in all directions of gaze. The side of the cerebellar lesion corresponds to the eye that is turned down.

With cerebellar tumors, one may sometimes observe *ocular dysmetria, flutterlike oscillations, opsoclonus,* and disturbed pursuit movements in the sense of *cogwheel eye movements.* However, it is quite uncertain whether these signs are caused by the primary cerebellar involvement or a secondary affection of the brain stem, although it is generally assumed that the cerebellum provides a continuous correction of eye movements (Eccles).

*Ocular dysmetria* (Cogan), obviously an analogy to the dysmetria of the limbs, is characterized by an overshoot in saccadic eye movements and a subsequent correction by several oscillations when the eyes have to change from one fixation point to another one. With unilateral lesions the overshoot is generally greatest on looking toward the side of the lesion.

*Flutterlike oscillations,* like dysmetria (according to Cogan), are typical of cerebellar lesions. These are intermittent horizontal oscillations of the eyes lasting only seconds and induced mostly by changes in fixation.

*Opsoclonus* represents a sequence of saccadic eye movements unrelated to any specific stimulus (mostly horizontal) and thus a disruption of the microsaccadic system (Gay, Newman, Keltner, and Stroud).

*Cogwheel eye movements* (saccadic following) are jerky, inaccurate pursuit movements, probably in relation to the cerebellar hypotonia. (See discussion of gaze palsies.) Other damage to the pursuit system that manifests itself in cerebellar disease is absent or greatly decreased *optokinetic nystagmus.*

Other ocular signs to be discussed are only nonspecific signs of an increased intracranial pressure. *Sixth nerve pareses* occur in about one fifth of the patients —interestingly, *mostly in unilateral,* rarely in bilateral form. These sixth nerve pareses are seen with particular frequency in association with tumors of the cerebellar vermis. Thus one cannot assume a relationship between the side of the tumor and a unilateral sixth nerve paresis. We maintain that, in the case of cerebellar tumors, such pareses belong to the *general signs of an increase in the intracranial pressure,* although a certain direct or indirect pressure effect on the brain stem and the abducens nuclei cannot be ruled out. Of 55 patients with cerebellar tumors, 50 showed *bilateral papilledemas.* There was a particularly marked prominence, with numerous hemorrhages and exudates, in those with tumors of the vermis. It is significant that these papilledemas occur in a relatively early stage because of the well-known tendency of cerebellar tumors to compress the fourth ventricle and thereby to interfere with the circulation of the cerebrospinal fluid. In fact, general signs of increased intracranial pressure frequently first manifest cerebellar neoplasms. *Numerous papilledemas in cerebellar tumors, especially those of the vermis, already show distinct evidence of beginning atrophy at the first examination.* There is a grayish white discoloration of the disc, at first narrowing of the arteries and later of the veins, and together with loss of vision (progressing occasionally to blindness; 10% according to Tönnis), also a concentric constriction of the visual fields (p. 125 and Fig. 2-16).

Except for an enlargement of the blind spot caused by the choked disc, the visual fields generally are not characteristic in patients with cerebellar tumors. There are references in the literature (Wagener and Cusick; Weinberger and Webster) pointing out the possibility of various field defects as the indirect result of an increased intracranial pressure or an internal hydrocephalus (Fig. 3-115). We have seen such *visual field changes very rarely*. A patient with hemangioblastoma of the vermis showed an unquestionable *homonymous hemianopia* with sparing of the macula (Fig. 3-116). Another patient with hemangioma of the vermis showed a temporal hemianopia on one side and slight concentric constriction of the field on the other side. In a patient with an astrocytoma in the region of the vermis, there was a superior bitemporal quadrant defect. *Bitemporal defects in cases of cerebellar tumors naturally must be regarded as a remote effect,* most likely *pressure on the chiasm* from above and behind *by a dilated third ventricle caused by internal hydrocephalus* (p. 274). This also explains the occurrence of central scotomas (the macular fibers are situated at the posterior angle of the chiasm!) reported by a number of authors (Walsh and Hoyt and others). Cushing and Walker describe the occurrence of *binasal hemianopias* in patients with cerebellar tumors. They are of the opinion that a dilated third ventricle displaces the optic nerves laterally and presses them against the carotid arteries. It is difficult to find an explanation for homonymous field defects associated with cerebellar tumors except as a direct insult to one occipital lobe as a result of supratentorial expansion. At any rate, it can be stated that *a bitemporal, mostly asymmetric hemianopia, combined with pronounced papilledemas, is suspicious of a tumor in the cerebellar or infratentorial region* (Fig. 3-117). The significance of visual field changes in cerebellar tumors, however, is small, considering their rare occurrence. On closer scrutiny, especially bitemporal visual field defects are much rarer in association with cerebellar neoplasms than is generally assumed (Fig. 3-117). Walsh and Hoyt observed homonymous defects more often than bitemporal defects.

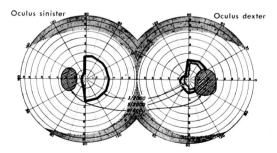

**Fig. 3-116.** Hemangioblastoma in caudal section of cerebellar vermis in 38-year-old patient. Bilateral papilledema of 2 diopters' prominence with marked venous congestion and numerous massive hemorrhages. Visual acuity, O.D. 1.0; O.S. 0.5. Amblyopic attacks! Enormous bilateral enlargement of blind spot. Left homonymous hemianopia with sparing of macula.

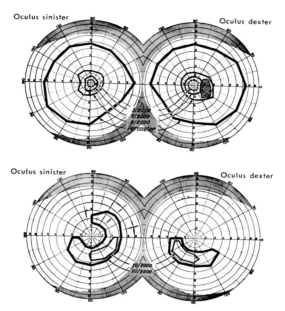

Fig. 3-117. Above, Astrocytoma in lateral part of left cerebellar hemisphere extending to cerebellopontine angle in 19-year-old patient. Beginning atrophy of bilateral papilledema. O.D. 3 diopters' elevation; O.S. 4 diopters' elevation. Visual acuity, O.U. 1.0. Concentric constriction of central isopters with suggestion of beginning bitemporal hemianopia. Marked enlargement of right blind spot. Below, Astrocytoma of cerebellar vermis extending to roof of fourth ventricle in 11-year-old girl. Beginning left papilledema. Normal right disc. Considerable internal hydrocephalus! Completely asymmetric bitemporal hemianopia with loss of right superior nasal quadrant and left kidney-shaped field remnants hugging macula.

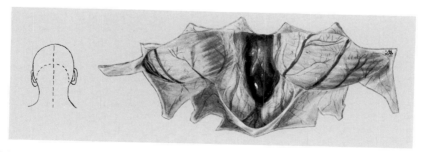

Fig. 3-118. Walnut-sized hemangioblastoma of cerebellar vermis in 57-year-old patient after bilateral cerebellar exploration.

An occasional observation of a *unilateral diminished corneal reflex* must be explained as a pressure effect on the trigeminal nerve in the region of the cerebellopontine angle. The facial and acoustic nerves usually are involved at a later stage.

*Hemangioblastomas make up a significant number of tumors of the cerebellar hemispheres* (Fig. 3-118). In our series of 55 patients, we observed three instances of a simultaneous retinal angiomatosis, examples of the so-called *von Hippel–Lindau* disease (Craig, Wagener, and Kernohan; Danis; Martin; and others). A relationship between the occurrence of angiomas in the retina and the cerebellum is known to be loose: *retinal angiomas occur much more rarely and very infrequently in association with cerebellar hemangioblastomas.* Nevertheless, it is important to search carefully for angiomas of the retinal periphery (Traquair) in cases of similar cerebellar tumors.

Generally, the *retinal angiomas* tend to be located in the fundus periphery (seldom at the macula or the disc). They have a distinctly globular and quite prominent shape. Markedly

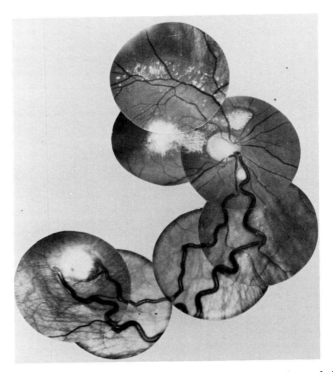

**Fig. 3-119.** Angiomatosis retinae in von Hippel–Lindau disease (with cerebellar hemangioblastoma). Composite fundus photographs. Spherical retinal angioma in right periphery of fundus is covered almost completely by grayish white exudate. Tumor is fed by markedly dilated and tortuous vessels (artery above, vein below). Retinopathy in form of foci of fatty degeneration to side and below disc.

dilated veins and arteries feed these angiomas, which can be distinguished only in the early stages. The hemangiomas appear as reddish globular structures in the fundus periphery. There may be a multiplicity of foci, predominantly in the lower parts of the retina. Frequently, the angiomas are surrounded and eventually covered by a grayish white exudate (Fig. 3-119). Similar exudates accompany the enormously dilated and tortuous vessels. Massive recurrent retinal hemorrhages are frequent. As a rule, there is a more or less distinct retinal detachment in the later stage of growth of these tumors, which tends to mask the original picture and makes the diagnosis more difficult. An early diagnosis of the retinal angiomas is quite essential because it is frequently possible to destroy them with electro- or photocoagulation if a retinal detachment has not yet developed. Such a procedure will prevent a secondary retinal detachment. In one of our patients, electrocoagulation of such a retinal angioma was successful in one eye. The patient completely lost the sight in the other eye as a result of a retinal detachment and a secondary complicated cataract.

*The ocular signs and symptoms associated with cerebellar tumors can be summarized as follows. Most of them are the result of an early increase in the intracranial pressure. Choked discs are almost always present and usually quite distinct. They cause flickering, foggy vision, and amblyopic attacks. Relatively early, they develop atrophy, with loss of vision and concentric contraction of the visual fields. An outstanding ocular sign is nystagmus of the central vestibular type, which usually has a horizontal direction but may have a vertical component with tumors of the cerebellar vermis. As a rule, this nystagmus is coarser toward the tumor lesion than toward the opposite side. Ocular dysmetria, flutter, opsoclonus, and cogwheeling represent further oculomotor disorders associated with cerebellar tumors. Nonspecific unilateral or bilateral sixth nerve pareses resulting from the increased intracranial pressure account for diplopia mentioned by the patient. Unilateral sixth nerve pareses are more frequent than the bilateral form. Visual field changes associated with cerebellar tumors are quite rare. They are not the result of a direct effect on the visual pathways but a remote effect via a dilated third ventricle and compression of the chiasm. Most common are unilateral temporal or bitemporal field defects. Occasional homonymous hemianopias are difficult to interpret. In rare cases a combination of a cerebellar and a retinal hemangioblastoma represents an example of von Hippel–Lindau disease. On the x-ray film, increased intracranial pressure manifests itself by demineralization (atrophy of the dorsum sellae), secondary enlargement of the structures of the sella turcica, and eventually also by intensified digital markings and in children by suture diastasis.*

## Tumors of the fourth ventricle

Actually, tumors of the cerebellar vermis cause signs and symptoms very similar to those of neoplasms of the fourth ventricle (ependymomas, choroid plexus papillomas) (Figs. 3-120 to 3-123). The characteristic picture includes *early increase of intracranial pressure with bilateral choked discs, coarse horizontal gaze nystagmus in the lateral terminal positions,* and *severe trunk ataxia.* If the tumors originate from the floor of the fourth ventricle, there may be the additional *signs of disturbances of this area,* that is, facial palsy, a diminished corneal reflex on one side, or even a disturbed coordination of the ocular movements (Craig and Kernohan). In fourth ventricle tumors (also in third and lateral ventricle tumors), one may occasionally observe *Bruns' syndrome,* which is characterized by attacks of headache, vomit-

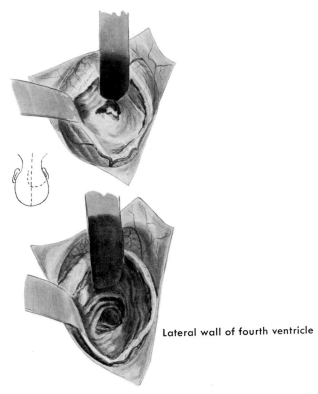

Lateral wall of fourth ventricle

**Fig. 3-120.** Solid, partly cystic, walnut-sized papilloma of plexus of fourth ventricle in medial and caudal section of left cerebellar hemisphere in 57-year-old patient before and after extirpation via left cerebellar exploration.

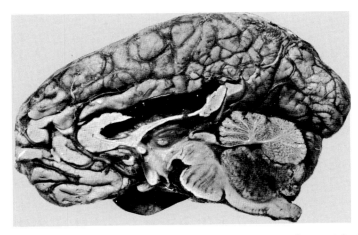

**Fig. 3-121.** Median section through brain with ependymoma of fourth ventricle in 64-year-old patient. (Specimen from the Pathologic-Anatomic Institute of the University of Lausanne.)

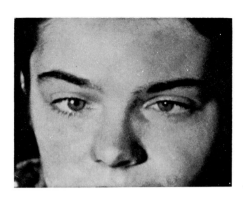

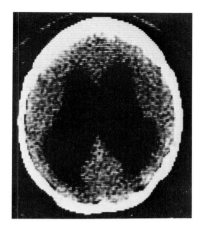

**Fig. 3-122**                     **Fig. 3-123**

**Fig. 3-122.** Unclassified benign glioma originating from floor of fourth ventricle. Horizontal gaze palsy to both sides. Convergence spasm of globes on command to look to side or up.
**Fig. 3-123.** Computerized transverse axial tomogram of internal hydrocephalus in 29-year-old patient with astrocytoma of fourth ventricle. Excellent illustration of increased ventricular size (dark areas).

ing, vertigo, and transient blindness produced by changes of position of the head. Between the attacks, there is freedom from symptoms, but the head usually remains in a fixed position.

Our one patient showed very early disturbances of the extraocular muscles, which were said by his acquaintances to give him a "funny look." Detailed analysis of the ocular motility revealed a *severe horizontal gaze palsy to both sides.* Also, peculiarly, a pronounced *convergence spasm* occurred when the patient was asked to look up or to the side (Fig. 3-122). We shall discuss these supranuclear motility disturbances in more detail in connection with tumors of the pons (p. 300), which produce similar gaze disorders. Our patient also showed very severe papilledemas of the chronic type. There were early episodes of amaurosis fugax as a form of amblyopic attacks (Fig. 3-123).

## Tumors of the cerebellopontine angle

By far the greatest number of tumors of the cerebellopontine angle consists of *acoustic neurinomas* (87% according to Tönnis), which most often originate from the neurilemma of the vestibular nerve near the internal porus acusticus (Fig. 3-124). The site of these tumors produces characteristic signs and symptoms that can be summarized as a *combination of signs of lesions of the fifth, sixth, seventh, and eighth cranial nerves with cerebellar symptoms* (Cushing; Edwards and Paterson; Lundberg). For a correct diagnosis, it is of the utmost importance to note the chronologic development of the various signs. *One of the early symptoms is intermittent or constant tinnitus,* combined at the same time or in later stages with progressive *hearing loss.* This loss of hearing progresses to almost complete deafness. About 70% of acoustic tumors demonstrate consistent or typical retrocochlear test findings. Although the tumor originates in the vesibular part of the acoustic nerve, there are usually no initial vestibular disturbances because of the slow progress of the tumor. As a rule, they are secondary to acoustic signs and symptoms and take the form of unsteadiness, vertigo (similar to that in Ménière's disease), and nystagmus. During the later stages of development of the tumor an uncertain gait appears, which probably indicates damage to the cerebellum. Much later there is involvement of the other cranial nerves in the region of the cerebellopontine angle mentioned previously. The *facial nerve* is impaired quite frequently. It first shows signs of irrita-

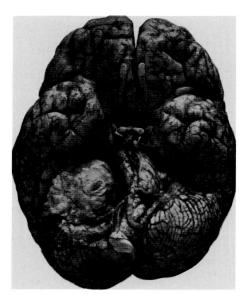

**Fig. 3-124.** Right acoustic neurinoma with distinct displacement of brain stem toward left side. (Specimen from the Pathologic-Anatomic Institute of Basel.)

tion in the form of spasms or twitching (for instance, blepharospasm). Later a peripheral facial palsy may be seen. *Trigeminal symptoms* manifest themselves as paresthesias (such as numbness or a dead feeling in parts of the face), later as slight neuralgias in the area of distribution of the trigeminal nerve. An important sequel of a trigeminal lesion is a diminished or abolished corneal reflex on the ipsilateral side, as will be described in greater detail subsequently. There may be additional symptoms indicating impairment of the ninth, tenth, eleventh, and twelfth cranial nerves with a corresponding increase in size of the tumor. Predominant are disturbances of deglutition and articulation. As a rule, the appearance of lesions involving the cranial nerves is accompanied by *signs implicating the cerebellum,* such as cerebellar ataxia, tendency to fall toward the tumor side, and other disturbances of coordination (p. 285). Apart from cerebellar signs and symptoms in this stage, there are also *brain stem* signs and symptoms such as hemiparesis (contralateral), hemianesthesia (contralateral), and Babinski's sign. The last stage is that of *increased intracranial pressure* caused by hydrocephalus produced by closure of the sylvian aqueduct. Headache, papilledema, and palsies of the sixth nerve are the common features of this stage.

As a rule, the acoustic neurinoma is unilateral. Occasionally, it may occur as a bilateral lesion and then is part of a systemic von Recklinghausen's disease (neurofibromatosis). In such cases, one should search for neurofibromas of the skin or the characteristic "café au lait" spots. Besides acoustic neurinomas, any expansive process in the angle between the petrous bone, tentorium, and pons may produce similar symptoms (for instance, meningiomas, primary cholesteatomas [epidermoid cysts], arachnoiditis of the pontocerebellar cistern, gliomas of the pons, or even cerebellar tumors).

Our own series includes 31 tumors of the cerebellopontine angle. Of these, 25 were acoustic neurinomas (Fig. 3-125) (23 unilateral, two bilateral) and six tumors of a different nature, such as meningioma, astrocytoma of the cerebellar hemisphere, medulloblastomas, and angiomas. Although it is evident from this

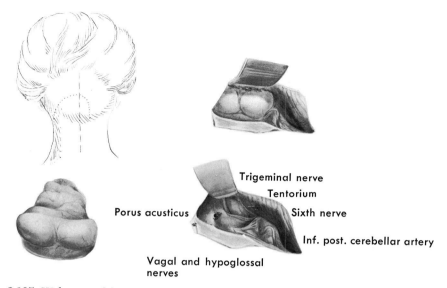

**Trigeminal nerve**

**Tentorium**

**Porus acusticus**    **Sixth nerve**

**Inf. post. cerebellar artery**

**Vagal and hypoglossal nerves**

**Fig. 3-125.** Walnut-sized left acoustic neurinoma in 44-year-old patient before and after radical extirpation via left cerebellar exploration and exposure of left cerebellopontine angle.

discussion that the early diagnosis of acoustic tumors must be made on the basis of hearing disturbances, the *ocular symptomatology* has a certain significance (Best). It can be briefly summarized as *nystagmus, blepharospasm and facial nerve palsy* (seventh nerve), *disturbances of the corneal reflex* (fifth nerve), *and sixth nerve pareses.* Generally, signs of increased intracranial pressure are missing until the late stages. Consequently, *choked discs* are usually found rather late and only in about one half of the patients.

In the later stages, among the most frequent *ocular symptoms* in patients with tumors of the cerebellopontine angle are blurred vision, flickering before the eyes, and occasional amblyopic attacks—all phenomena directly related to increased intracranial pressure. Next in frequency is *double vision.* It may either be more pronounced during violent attacks of headaches or noticeable only during these attacks. Because of its etiology (sixth nerve pareses), the diplopia is usually horizontal. It is interesting to note that *defects of the facial nerve* may also assume a subjective character. For instance, some patients stated that one eye had become larger and could not be closed as well as usual; it showed frequent inflammations (lagophthalmic keratitis!). Some patients also noted an annoying blepharospastic twitching in one eye. The *trigeminal symptoms* involve less the eye itself than the sense of touch of the skin surrounding it, especially the forehead and cheek: a peculiar sensation of numbness, a feeling of swelling of the eye, and, rarely, a neuralgic pain in the area of distribution of the trigeminal nerve.

An early and most constant *ocular sign is nystagmus.\** This is a *horizontal jerking gaze nystagmus, usually of greater amplitude in its excursions with gaze toward the side of the tumor than toward the opposite side.* In some instances, we have seen, in addition to this horizontal nystagmus, a rotary or, with eyes up, even a vertical component. The fact that nystagmus observed in association with tumors of the cerebellopontine angle is persistent and does not disappear (as does peripheral vestibular nystagmus caused by a lesion of the labyrinth or the vestibular nerve) suggests that it is less the result of a lesion of the vestibular nerve than a phenomenon of involvement of the brain stem or the cerebellar peduncles. In other words, this is a *central type* of nystagmus similar to the one seen in association with cerebellar tumors (p. 287). This is equally true for the frequent occurrence of a vertical component (that is, a remote effect on the midbrain tectal or pretectal area), especially if it appears as an isolated phenomenon and without horizontal nystagmus. In large acoustic neurinomas, there is frequently a bilateral nystagmus (Bruns' type): horizontal gaze paretic nystagmus to the side of the tumor and vestibular jerk nystagmus away from the tumor.

A visible involvement of the *ophthalmic branches of the facial nerve* manifested itself in only four of our 31 patients in the form of a distinctly widened lid fissure, although a general facial paresis could be demonstrated in almost all of the patients at an early date. In one patient the facial palsy was so pronounced that he was unable to close the eye on the involved side (in other words, a true lagophthalmos). This eye was the site of repeated inflammatory episodes in the form of a lagophthalmic keratitis. (See p. 12 and Fig. 1-3.)

One of the signs of trigeminal disturbance is a *diminished or abolished ipsilateral corneal reflex. It is known to become extinguished before sensory disturbances of corresponding skin areas can be demonstrated.* We have found this important ocular sign in a more or less distinct form among 29 of our 31 patients. *It plays an important part in the diagnosis of tumors of the cerebellopontine angle.* The involvement of the corneal reflex may show varying gradations from slight diminution to complete anesthesia of the cornea. Often it can be demonstrated at first only in either the upper or lower quadrant (more frequently in the upper one). For testing of the corneal sensitivity, see p. 21.

In a little more than one third of our patients a *unilateral sixth nerve paresis* on the side of the tumor could be demonstrated (caused by the increased intracranial pressure rather than direct tumor growth). This was the anatomic basis for the symptoms of double vision. In the initial stage, these sixth nerve pareses are often minor and cannot be demonstrated by pure clinical examination of motility. It is then imperative to use the red-green glass test to render the separation of the two images more distinct (p. 34). Conjugate gaze palsies (mostly of the horizontal type) are extremely rare. They are caused by compression of the brain stem.

---

*For detection of subclinical nystagmus and for analysis of the response of the vestibular apparatus to caloric stimulation, electronystagmography (p. 56) is of great value.

It has been mentioned previously that ocular signs of increased intracranial pressure such as *papilledemas* are present *in a little more than one half of the patients.* We observed all stages from slight blurring of the nasal and temporal disc margins to a fully developed choked disc of several diopters' elevation. As in patients with cerebellar tumors, but much less prevalent, we found hemorrhages, white exudates, and frequently a beginning atrophy—a sign of transition into chronic atrophic papilledema.

Visual field changes are extremely rare in patients with tumors of the cerebellopontine angle. Once we found concentric constriction of both fields resulting from chronic atrophic papilledemas and once a suggestion of homonymous hemianopia. Bitemporal or binasal defects as described in association with cerebellar tumors could never be demonstrated here. As a result of their lateral position, these tumors are less likely to interfere with the circulation of the cerebrospinal fluid and to produce internal hydrocephalus with dilation of the third ventricle (and subsequent chiasmal compression) than are cerebellar tumors, especially neoplasms of the vermis with their mesial position.

Even for the ophthalmologist, it may be of interest and importance to know that on x-ray films (Stenvers' projection) 70% to 80% of patients with acoustic neuromas show more or less pronounced *enlargement of the internal auditory canal,* progressing in later stages to erosion and even destruction of the whole petrous bone pyramid (Tönnis; Graf; Hitselberger).

*The ocular signs and symptoms of tumors of the cerebellopontine angle can be summarized as follows. The trigeminal and facial nerves are involved relatively early. A lesion of the trigeminal nerve manifests itself in the eye as a diminished or abolished corneal reflex on the ipsilateral side—one of the most frequent and most constant signs of tumors of the cerebellopontine angle. Less common is a facial palsy, especially widening of the lid fissure or actual inability to close the lids (lagophthalmos). One of the most important ocular signs is horizontal jerk nystagmus, usually coarser with gaze toward the tumor rather than to the opposite side. Sixth nerve pareses appear relatively late, with more extensive growth of the tumor. Ocular signs of increased intracranial pressure in the form of choked discs (nonspecific for this site) occur in a little more than one half of all patients. However, it must be remembered that the diagnosis of acoustic tumors is based on nonocular symptoms, among which tinnitus and progressive hearing loss are the most important ones.*

## Tumors of the pons and the medulla oblongata

Because of the extremely close topographic relationship between the pons and the medulla oblongata, it is hardly necessary to present tumors of these two structures as separate entities, especially since their neurologic symptoms are strikingly similar (Foerster; Horrax and Buckley). These symptoms can be divided into six groups, which ensue from the close proximity of various systems in the pons and the medulla oblongata (Kaufmann): (1) cranial nerves (fifth to twelfth), (2) their internuclear or supranuclear tracts, (3) the cerebellar system with its connections, (4) the pyramidal system, (5) the long sensory tracts, and (6) the important fact that a group of signs either are present in a bilateral form or some of them alternate between the two sides (for instance, impairment of the cranial nerves and horizontal gaze palsy on one side, lesions of the pyramidal and the long sensory tracts on the other side).

In summary, it can be stated that tumors of the pons and the medulla oblongata (glioblastomas, astrocytomas, hemangiomas, ependymomas) are distinguished by signs involving the right and left sides as well as by a *combination of signs involving cranial nerves at the level of the tumor, with early signs of pyramidal and sensory tract disorders* (often together with ataxia, dysmetria, and horizontal and vertical nystagmus). It is also characteristic for tumors of this region that, in contrast to tumors of the midbrain, an increased intracranial pressure occurs relatively late (Fig. 3-126).

The ocular symptomatology of tumors of the pons and the medulla oblongata is mostly distinguished by *nuclear and supranuclear disturbances of the eye movements, especially of abduction and horizontal conjugate movements* (13 cases). In addition to vomiting, *disturbances of ocular motility are among the very first symptoms and signs of a tumor of the pons or the medulla oblongata.* Next in frequency are disturbances of the equilibrium.

Quite frequently the history reveals an annoying and confusing horizontal *diplopia.* It is caused by a nuclear, usually ipsilateral sixth nerve paresis (in seven of our 13 patients). Only in three patients (and in the late stages) could a paresis of isolated muscles supplied by the oculomotor nerve be demonstrated in addition to a sixth nerve paresis.

Of greater localizing value than sixth nerve pareses are *horizontal gaze palsies,* which occurred in one half of our patients, three times in unilateral form (the globes could not be rotated past the midline) and three times in bilateral form (the globes remained in a primary parallel for convergent position) (Fig. 3-122). The anatomic basis is a *lesion in the center for conjugate lateral movements in the pons* (the paramedian pontine reticular formation) (Fig. 1-12). It is characteristic for horizontal gaze palsies associated with lesions in the pons (Santha) that all the various forms of gaze movements (that is, saccadic, pursuit, optically elicited, and vestibular movements) are involved. A unilateral horizontal gaze palsy is toward the side of the lesion. If there is a *compensatory*

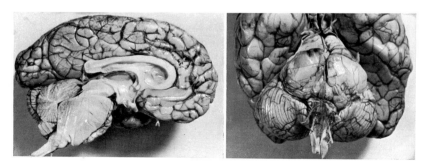

**Fig. 3-126.** Glioblastoma multiforme of pons. Left, Median section through brain. Right, Tumor seen from base of skull. (Specimen from the Pathologic-Anatomic Institute of the University of Zurich.)

*deviation of the eyes, it is toward the opposite side.* We have observed one such case. Characteristically, compensatory conjugate deviation associated with pontine tumors is permanent in contrast to the deviation associated with cortical or subcortical lesions of the frontal optomotor centers of the hemispheres and the frontomesencephalic pathways, where we have a relatively rapid compensation, apparently from the contralateral side. Likewise, a horizontal gaze palsy caused by a lesion of the frontomesencephalic fibers is frequently marked by a turning of the head toward the side of the lesion. This phenomenon is missing in patients with pontine horizontal gaze palsies. Generally in patients with tumors of the pons, *only the horizontal conjugate eye movements are paralyzed. Vertical gaze palsies are not part of this picture, but are a distant sign of a lesion in the midbrain* (p. 281). Only in one patient could we demonstrate a vertical gaze palsy in addition to a horizontal gaze lesion. Obviously, this was a sign of expansion of the tumor toward the region of the midbrain or, at least, of a remote effect. Internuclear ophthalmoplegias could not be observed.

Rarely, only one side of the pons is affected by a tumor; in such cases, sixth nerve palsy and homolateral peripheral facial palsy may be associated with a crossed hemiplegia (Millard-Gubler syndrome). If there is in addition a homolateral gaze palsy (to the side of the lesion), the *syndrome is that of Foville-Millard-Gubler.*

A lateral lesion of the pontine tegmentum may lead to the phenomenon of the pontine *"skew deviation,"* which is characterized by a divergence of the eyes in the vertical plane with the eye on the side of the lesion lower than the other eye. Sometimes the lower eye shows intorsion, the higher one extorsion. Such a skew deviation in association with a pontine tumor must not be confused with an isolated palsy of a vertically acting single ocular muscle! Allerand reports paroxysmal skew deviation in a case of unilateral astrocytoma of the pons.

Hoyt describes still another motility disturbance in patients with metastatic tumors of the pons: *ocular bobbing,* characterized by jerky vertical conjugate movements of the eyes (downward movement more rapid than upward), seldom disconjugate or even uniocular. Conjugate lateral gaze is abolished simultaneously with such bobbing of the eyes.

Next to horizontal gaze palsies, *central nystagmus is an almost constant sign* in patients with tumors of the pons. We found it recorded in 12 of 13 cases of pontine tumors. Mostly *it is horizontal* (seven cases), frequently a combination of horizontal and vertical (four cases), and very rarely purely vertical (one case). In five patients, nystagmus manifested itself in combination with a horizontal gaze palsy. Most authors explain the vertical nystagmus as a pressure effect on the region of the quadrigeminate plate (respectively, on the midbrain tectal or pretectal area). The horizontal nystagmus, which is of the central type, must be interpreted as caused by a lesion of the vestibular nuclei or their connections with the cerebellum or brain stem structures. Kaufmann is correct in stressing a relationship between horizontal gaze palsies and horizontal nystagmus. He considers them similar phenomena, *the nystagmus representing a quasi incomplete form of an impaired supranuclear gaze movement.* On this basis, such disturbances of the horizontal motility could be demonstrated in all 13 patients in our series—eight times in bilateral form.

The *nystagmus* observed in association with tumors of the pons also belongs to the *central type* (p. 58). As mentioned previously, it is horizontal, or horizontal-vertical, with no rotary component. Characteristic for this "pontine nystagmus" is its asymmetry, which we could observe almost invariably among our patients (asymmetric gaze nystagmus). With the eyes straight, there usually is no nystagmus. It increases in intensity as the eyes are turned toward the side of the lesion. If the eyes are turned toward the opposite side, they have to be moved for some distance before the nystagmus becomes manifest, and then only to a lesser extent. The asymmetric gaze nystagmus is pathognomonic for an intrapontine lesion (with an involvement of the ipsilateral medial longitudinal fascicle). With medullary tumors and lesions, there are sometimes associated *downbeat nystagmus,* (one eye moves vertically and the other horizontally) and *periodic alternating nystagmus* (alternation of direction of horizontal jerk nystagmus).

An involvement of the *trigeminal nerve with impairment of the corneal reflex* could be observed in nine of our 13 patients. The corneal reflex was either diminished or completely abolished. In one half of the patients this defect was unilateral and in the other half bilateral.

As mentioned already, *the late appearance of signs of increased intracranial pressure is characteristic for pontine tumors.* Papilledema was rare among our patients. We have seen it in only four of 13 patients. It is important to state that three of these four patients had pontine tumors with a pronounced expansion into the fourth ventricle.

*The ocular symptomatology of tumors of the pons and the medulla oblongata can be summarized as follows. Dominating the picture are the characteristic supranuclear horizontal gaze palsies. They must be regarded as an extraordinarily important localizing sign. In almost all instances there is a horizontal jerk nystagmus of the central type—either as an isolated sign or combined with a horizontal gaze palsy. Occasionally this nystagmus is horizontal-vertical. In addition to these supranuclear motility disturbances, we frequently find isolated, mostly unilateral, nuclear sixth nerve pareses. Pareses of the oculomotor nerve are seen rarely. A trigeminal lesion, which occurs frequently with tumors of this area, manifests itself in the form of a diminished or abolished corneal reflex. Choked discs are extremely rare in association with true pontine tumors. They appear late and mostly if the tumor expands toward the fourth ventricle, causing embarrassment of the circulation of the cerebrospinal fluid. Cranial nerve palsies together with conjugate horizontal gaze palsies in the absence of papilledema should always be regarded as suggestive of brain stem tumor in the pons or medulla.*

# FOUR

## Relationship between type of tumor and ocular signs and symptoms

Our diagnostic endeavors are, on one hand, to determine the *location* of a brain tumor and, on the other hand, to diagnose, if at all possible, the *type of tumor* before surgical intervention. On the basis of the general neurologic symptomatology and with the help of numerous methods of examination (pneumoencephalography, ventriculography, cerebral angiography, electroencephalography, brain scanning, echoencephalography, computerized axial tomography, and others), this can be frequently accomplished in quite a satisfactory manner. It should be stated at the outset of this brief chapter that ocular signs and symptoms occasionally may help to confirm the diagnosis of the type of tumor but that, as a rule, such symptoms and signs alone can never establish such a diagnosis. This is particularly true for tumors of the hemispheres, but it is also true for those of the brain stem and the cerebellum. The situation is somewhat different for tumors of the sellar region and its surroundings. As discussed in the preceding chapter, it is actually possible in certain cases to determine the type of tumor (such as a pituitary adenoma, a craniopharyngioma, a meningioma of the sphenoid ridge, and others) from a more detailed analysis of the ocular signs and symptoms. Even here, such a diagnosis cannot be accomplished with absolute certainty, despite our detailed and discriminate neuro-ophthalmologic diagnostic technique. The following statements will be limited to some general remarks that are not particularly aimed at diagnosing the type of tumor from the ocular signs and symptoms, but that merely stress the relationship between the type of tumor and the development of the ocular disturbances. Tumors with characteristic and localizing neuro-ophthalmologic signs and symptoms (such as pituitary adenomas, craniopharyngiomas, gliomas of the chiasm, meningiomas of the sphenoid ridge, acoustic neurinomas, etc.) will not be considered or discussed further.

One of the most frequent types of brain tumor is *glioblastoma multiforme* (Fig. 3-126). It is a highly malignant tumor noted for its rapid growth. It occurs in the hemispheres as well as in the basal ganglia and brain stem. The rapid and expansive growth of this tumor produces an alarming cerebral picture in a relatively short time. It is significant that the rapidly developing neurologic local symptoms are complicated by early psychic disturbances in the form of a psycho-organic syndrome. Disturbances of the sensorium appear soon and progress from drowsiness to somnolence and coma. Statistical evaluation of our material shows that papilledemas are observed in about 50% of patients with glioblastoma, in contrast to about 65% of those with more slowly growing tumors (for instance, meningiomas). Although the difference is not significant, it seems that papilledemas in patients with rapidly growing tumors (such as, for instance, glioblastoma multiforme) occur somewhat less frequently than in those with slowly growing tumors. In the differential diagnosis of glioblastomas one must primarily consider subdural and epidural hematomas, brain abscesses, and cerebral metastases. They may produce a quite similar picture.

Resembling glioblastoma multiforme in malignancy are *medulloblastomas*, the prototype of childhood tumors, which are located predominantly in the cerebellar vermis (sometimes also in the cerebellar hemisphere and the pons). In the discussion of cerebellar tumors (p. 285), it has been mentioned that medulloblastomas have a striking tendency to invade the fourth ventricle and thus to cause an internal hydrocephalus. Thus symptoms of an increased intracranial pressure dominate the picture in the early stages of the disease: headaches, vomiting, the early appearance of pronounced papilledemas, and unilateral or bilateral sixth nerve palsies. In the latter case, even a direct pressure effect on the nuclear region may be assumed, especially with an associated peripheral facial palsy. Occasionally, medulloblastomas form metastases (for instance, in the spinal cord or the chiasm). They may then cause a chiasmal syndrome and eventually blindness. A chiasmal syndrome may also result from medulloblastomas, with their tendency to embarrass the circulation of the cerebrospinal fluid via an early dilation of the third ventricle with compression of the chiasm (p. 274 and Fig. 3-115).

The malignant and rapidly growing glioblastomas and medulloblastomas contrast with the relatively slowly progressing *astrocytomas*, the favorite localization sites of which are the hemispheres, the brain stem, and the cerebellum (also called cerebellar spongioblastoma). In accordance with the slow growth of astrocytomas of the hemispheres (Fig. 3-9), the neurologic symptoms dominate the picture. In contrast to glioblastomas, psychic changes are of rather secondary importance. It seems that, just as with meningiomas, papilledemas occur somewhat more frequently in patients with astrocytomas of the hemispheres than in patients with rapidly growing tumors (for instance, glioblastomas). The situation is, however, different with astrocytomas of the cerebellar hemispheres (Fig. 3-113). They cause rapid development of an internal hydrocephalus and, consequently, early increased intracranial pressure with pronounced papilledemas, which soon become atrophic. Not all, but most of our patients with cerebellar astrocytomas show papilledemas. *Oligodendrogliomas* are also slowly growing tumors that are localized especially in the hemispheres (frontal lobe), the basal ganglia, and in young patients in the thalamus. Apart from the local neurologic symptoms, they frequently produce epileptic attacks, which may be their only symptoms for a long time.

In the discussion of cerebellar tumors (p. 292), we mentioned the interesting relationship between cerebellar hemangioblastomas and retinal angiomas in *von Hippel–Lindau disease* (Fig. 3-119). In our series, we have three patients with this combination of angiomatosis retinae and cerebellar hemangioblastoma. This relationship is quite loose. Nevertheless, one should keep in mind the possibility of a cerebral hemangioma in patients with cerebellar symptoms who show a retinal angioma. More rarely, *hemangioblastomas* occur also in the pons and the medulla oblongata.

Regarding pituitary adenomas, craniopharyngiomas, and acoustic neurinomas, the reader is referred to the appropriate sections in Chapter 3 (pp. 202, 228, and 295). These tumors show a quite specific neuro-ophthalmologic symptomatology that to some extent is of localizing value.

Among the tumors with extracerebral development are the *meningiomas,* some of which (parasagittal meningiomas, meningiomas of the falx, suprasellar meningiomas, meningiomas of the olfactory groove, meningiomas of the sphenoid ridge) have also been discussed in Chapter 3 (pp. 199, 235, 242, and 248). These tumors are noted for their extraordinarily slow growth, which may extend over many years. Their clinical symptomatology shows a correspondingly slow and gradual progress. Signs and symptoms of increased intracranial pressure as well as psychic changes and sensory disturbances may be absent for a long time. It is important for the general practitioner and the ophthalmologist to remember that meningiomas show hyperostoses, bone erosions, or actual tumor calcifications on a plain x-ray film of the skull. It has been stressed in Chapter 3 (p. 201) that certain meningiomas (for instance, those of the parasagittal region) may cause misleading visual field defects as a result of a remote effect that is still not properly understood (Klingler and Condrau). Possibly this results from the slow growth of these tumors or possibly from their extracerebral expansion, which does not involve actual brain substance but merely causes its displacement (Fig. 3-30).

Special forms of tumor that have to be considered frequently are cerebral *metastatic carcinoma* and, more rarely, cerebral *metastatic sarcoma* (Dandy; Livingston, Horrax, and Sachs; Scheid). Unless there are multiple, disseminated foci, the neurologic symptomatology of cerebral metastases does not differ from that of primary brain tumors. Frequently, proof of the primary tumor is not possible. The following criteria suggest a metastasis to the brain: rapid development of cerebral symptoms, a disproportionate preponderance of psychic disturbances, a random appearance of new neurologic focal symptoms pointing to a site different from the original focus, a marked increase in the sedimentation rate, and general cachexia (Minkowski). However, in the differential diagnosis one must always consider a chronic subdural hematoma, a rapidly growing glioblastoma, and a brain abscess. Only proof of the primary tumor can make the diagnosis certain. Ocular signs of increased intracranial pressure (that is, papilledemas) are frequent but by no means characteristic. Nonspecific sixth nerve pareses caused by increased intracranial pressure seem to be exceedingly rare in association with metastatic carcinomas of the brain (Minkowski). In men the primary tumor is mostly a carcinoma of the lung, and in women, carcinoma of the breast. Much rarer are hypernephromas, melanomas, malignant tumors of the thyroid, and carcinomas of the prostate. According to Weber, cerebral metastases occur far more frequently in men than in women. Usually they occur in the hemispheres immediately beneath the cortex (Fig. 4-1).

In comparison to these tumors, *chordomas, teratomas, cholesteatomas* (epidermoids), *dermoid cysts, parasites,* and *granulomas* are less frequently located in the brain. Their symptomatology is not specific but depends largely on the site of the growth. Granulomas of the brain are almost always tuberculous (tuberculoma), rarely syphilitic (gumma). The picture of a cerebral *tuberculoma* differs very little from other brain tumors. Febrile or subfebrile temperatures and tuberculous foci in other organs are of little diagnostic help. Brain tubercles usually are multiple but may occur in solitary form. They are said to occur mostly in the cerebellum but may occur in the hemispheres. In the latter location, they rarely cause symptoms and signs of intracranial pressure. Very rarely a solitary tubercle may develop in the chiasm or optic nerve. This was demonstrated once in our series, a patient with a tubercle in the extraorbital portion of the optic nerve causing ipsilateral amaurosis and contralateral temporal hemianopia (Fig. 3-98).

It should be worthwhile to discuss once more bilateral *papilledema and its relationship to the site and type of tumor* (see Table 3, p. 99). Tumors of the

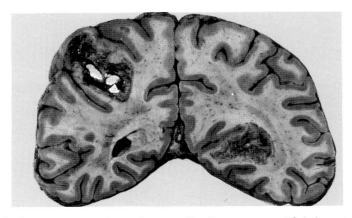

**Fig. 4-1.** Multiple metastases to brain from small cell carcinoma of left lung in 50-year-old patient. (Specimen from the Pathologic-Anatomic Institute of the University of Lausanne.)

**Table 6.** Distribution of cases with primary optic atrophy by site and type of brain tumors (according to Tönnis)*

| Type of tumor | Frontal | Temporal | Corpus callosum | Brain stem | Base | Pontine angle | Proximity of sella | Vessels | Totals |
|---|---|---|---|---|---|---|---|---|---|
| Spongioblastoma | 1 | | | 14 | | | 19 | | 34 |
| Oligodendroglioma | 1 | 1 | | | | | 1 | | 3 |
| Astrocytoma | | 1 | | 2 | | | | | 3 |
| Ependymoma | 1 | | | 3 | 1 | | 3 | | 8 |
| Neurinoma | | | | | | 3 | | | 3 |
| Meningioma | | | | | 35 | 1 | 26 | | 62 |
| Sarcoma | | | | | 2 | | | | 2 |
| Pituitary adenoma | | | | | | | 234 | | 234 |
| Craniopharyngioma | | | | | | | 64 | | 64 |
| Epidermoid | | | 1 | 1 | 1 | 1 | 5 | | 9 |
| Aneurysm | | | | | | | | 9 | 9 |
| Metastases | | | | | 1 | | | | 1 |
| Abscesses | 1 | 1 | | 1 | | | | | 3 |
| Other tumors | | | 2 | 4 | 7 | | 1 | | 14 |
| Totals | 4 | 3 | 3 | 25 | 47 | 5 | 353 | 9 | 449 = 14.8% |

*From a total of 3033 cases of intracranial tumors.

third and fourth ventricle and the lateral ventricles as well as of the cerebellum most frequently cause papilledema, whereas tumors of the area of the sella produce papilledema least often. Papilledema is also relatively infrequently produced by tumors of the base of the skull, the pontine angle, and the brain stem. Among the tumors of the hemisphere, those of the occipital lobe produce papilledema most frequently, then follow those of the temporal lobe, and least frequently those of the parietal lobe. Table 3 also shows the *difference in frequency of papilledema produced by various types of tumors.* Medulloblastoma most often (in 80% of the cases) produces papilledema, and this type of tumor is frequently found in the cerebellum. Then follow ependymomas and meningiomas (the latter, apart from papilledema, also producing secondary atrophy) and astrocytomas and oligodendrogliomas. Rapidly growing glioblastomas produced papilledema in only 50% of the patients in our series. (This differs markedly from the results of other authors, for instance, Tönnis who found a frequency of 80%.) Neurinomas occupy a position in the middle (75% according to Tönnis).

Approximately one sixth of all brain tumors produce primary optic atrophy. According to the data in Table 6, which were calculated by Tönnis, we find that the tumors close to the sella and the tumors of the base of the skull most frequently show such an atrophy. Pituitary adenomas, craniopharyngiomas, and spongioblastomas of the brain stem and hypothalamus are the types of tumors that most often produce primary optic atrophy. Tumors of the frontal and temporal lobe also have to be considered. Always, however, optic atrophy is the result of a direct compression of the optic nerve or chiasm either by the tumor itself or by other tissues in the area of the basal cisterns that have been shifted.

*Finally, we should consider those brain tumors that do not cause ocular involvement (9.9%).* Again, we would like to refer to a table containing data cal-

**Table 7.** Cases without ocular involvement (according to Tönnis)*

| Lesions | Number of cases |
|---|---|
| Cerebral tumors | 170 |
|     Frontal | 84 |
|     Temporal | 20 |
|     Parietal | 59 |
|     Occipital | 3 |
|     Corpus callosum and lateral ventricles | 4 |
| Cerebellar tumors | 7 |
| Brain stem tumors | 4 |
| Tumors of base of brain | 1 |
| Pontine angle tumors | 15 |
| Tumors close to sella | 37 |
| Multiple tumors | |
| Vessels | 67 |
| Total | 301 = 9.9% |

*From a total of 3033 cases of intracranial tumors.

culated by Tönnis (Table 7). Knowledge of such tumors and the site of such lesions is of greater importance than may be apparent on first glance. Such tumors are not diagnosed for a considerable period of time. These patients suffer from seizures, whereas symptoms of increased intracranial pressure occur much later. Among these tumors are especially neoplasms of the vessels and secondly tumors of the hemispheres, mostly of the frontal and the parietal lobes. Tumors of the cerebellum and the brain stem will only occasionally develop without affecting the visual system. The same is true, perhaps to a somewhat lesser extent, for tumors of the area of the sella and the pontine angles.

Following the discussion of the various types of tumors, it might be of interest to learn something about their relative distribution. Weber has compiled the following data based on 1645 cases at the Neurosurgical Clinic of the University of Zurich.

| | | |
|---|---:|---:|
| Gliomas and paragliomas | | 842 |
|     Angiogliomas | 9 | |
|     Astroblastomas | 65 | |
|     Astrocytomas (hemispheres) | 139 | |
|     Astrocytomas (cerebellum, pons, midbrain) | 67 | |
|     Ependymomas | 26 | |
|     Glioblastomas multiforme | 318 | |
|     Gliomas (unclassified) | 92 | |
|     Medulloblastomas | 70 | |
|     Oligodendrogliomas | 28 | |
|     Pinealomas | 10 | |
|     Spongioblastomas | 15 | |
|     Sympathicoblastoma | 1 | |
|     Gangliocytoneurinomas | 2 | |
| Meningiomas | | 253 |
| Metastases | | 135 |
| Pituitary adenomas | | 95 |
| Craniopharyngiomas | | 44 |
| Neurinomas (108 of acoustic nerve) | | 110 |
| Hemangiomas (all cerebellar) | | 39 |
| Papillomas | | 10 |
| Teratomas, cholesteatomas, dermoid cysts | | 16 |
| Chordomas and chondromyxomas | | 8 |
| Other rare forms (reticuloma, colloid cyst, lymphoendothelioma) | | 3 |
| Brain abscesses | | 60 |
| Granulomas (20 tuberculous, 1 gumma, 6 nonspecific) | | 27 |
| Parasites | | 3 |
| Total | | 1645 |

*In conclusion, one can say that about 10% of brain tumors do not cause ocular signs or symptoms. The occurrence of papilledema depends much more on the site and speed of growth of the tumor than on its histologic nature and its volume. Primary optic atrophy is to be found above all in tumors close to the sella and at the base of the skull. Supratentorial tumors frequently produce visual field changes, whereas the ocular signs in infratentorial tumors are motility disturbances of the peripheral, nuclear, or supranuclear type.*

# FIVE

## Pseudotumor cerebri, subdural hematomas, brain abscesses, and aneurysms

It was stated in the introduction to this book that subdural hematomas, brain abscesses, and aneurysms are not brain tumors in the true sense of the word. However, it would be a mistake to exclude them here because they play an important part in the differential diagnosis of brain tumors. Whereas the general neurologic symptoms and signs are preeminent in patients with subdural hematomas and brain abscesses, the situation is quite different with some cerebral aneurysms. At times a topical diagnosis can be made merely on the basis of ocular signs. In this connection, we would like to call attention also to the peculiar self-limited disease *pseudotumor cerebri* that sometimes simulates a cerebral neoplasm.

### PSEUDOTUMOR CEREBRI

The term "pseudotumor cerebri" is used for those somewhat obscure cases in which the patients have bilateral papilledema and increased intracranial pressure but negative neurologic and general physical findings. Also characteristic are the normal-sized or small ventricles found on ventriculography (therefore no signs of obstructing hydrocephalus) or on computerized axial tomography. A multitude of other names has been used for this syndrome, among which are "benign intracranial hypertension," "serous meningitis," "meningeal hydrops," and "otitic hydrocephalus." This disease occurs in young to middle-aged adults (especially in obese young women) and is characterized by headaches, sixth nerve palsy, papilledema (Fig. 5-1), occasionally field defects, and rarely blindness (resulting from chronic atrophic papilledema). The affection lasts for weeks or sometimes for months and generally has a good prognosis as long as damage does not result from atrophy secondary to the papilledema. The pathogenesis of the syndrome is either a hypersecretion or an obstruction of the outflow of cerebrospinal fluid (combined with swelling of the brain). There are indications, at least in some of the patients, that a thrombosis of the sagittal or lateral sinuses is involved. Otitis media or a chronic mastoid infection, especially in chil-

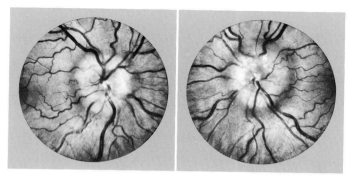

**Fig. 5-1.** Papilledema in 35-year-old patient with pseudotumor cerebri caused by use of contraceptive pills. Distinct increase of diameter of disc, blurred margins, mushroomlike prominence of about 2 diopters, and slight venous engorgement. Visual acuity, O.U. 1.0. Enlargement of both blind spots. No visual field defects. Increase of cerebrospinal fluid pressure up to 250 to 300 cm $H_2O$.

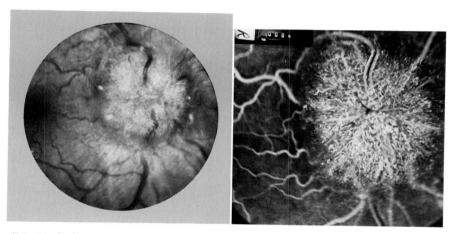

**Fig. 5-2.** Papilledema in 45-year-old patient with cerebral pseudotumor of unknown origin. Left, Normal black-and-white fundus photograph of mushroomed, blurred, and edematous disc (prominence of 3 diopters). Right, Fluorescein angiogram of same disc showing enormous capillary stasis (including irregularities of caliber and microaneurysm-like dilatation of capillaries) in early venous phase.

dren, may be the preceding cause of such a thrombosis. The pseudotumor syndrome may be observed also at the time of menarche, during pregnancy, in Addison's disease (Walsh), after prolonged corticosteriod therapy, after vitamin A intoxication, in hypoparathyroidism, in hematologic disorders, and following the use of oral contraceptives (Walsh, Clark, Thompson, and Nicholsen). It is to be noted that there still remains 15% to 20% of all patients with benign intracranial hypertension who cannot be placed in any known category (Greer) (Fig. 5-2).

## SUBDURAL HEMATOMAS

Although the clinical picture of *chronic subdural hematoma* (Figs. 5-3 and 5-4) varies a great deal, certain general guiding principles can be stated. Following a more or less pronounced trauma to the head (which may not always be mentioned spontaneously in the history), there are attacks of headache, which increase in frequency and during later stages are associated with psychic disturbances and personality changes. These are memory disturbances, lassitude, apathy, loss of energy, later disturbances of the sensorium, disorientation, and finally coma. The clinical picture may fluctuate. Improvements may alternate with relapses. There is a striking discrepancy between the severity of the general signs and symptoms of increased intracranial pressure and the insignificance of focal signs and symptoms. As a rule, the interval between trauma and onset of the alarming symptoms of the disease lasts from 4 to 8 weeks. In the differential diagnosis, all types of brain tumors (in particular, glioblastoma multiforme and brain abscess), encephalitis, and cerebral arteriosclerosis must be considered.

In addition to traumatic chronic subdural hematoma (caused by the rupture of bridging veins traversing the subdural space from the cerebral cortex to the undersurface of the dura), there is also spontaneous subdural hematoma. It is caused either by an *idiopathic internal hemorrhagic pachymeningitis* (capillary proliferation of a telangiectatic type) or an *inflammatory internal hemorrhagic pachymeningitis*. The symptomatology of the traumatic and the spontaneous types of chronic subdural hematoma is alike, particularly since there are mixed or transitional forms.

*Subdural hematoma of early childhood* usually is the result of trauma, especially a severe birth trauma. Generalized epileptic attacks with unconsciousness, vomiting, irritability, restlessness, and stupor are outstanding signs. In addition to defective physical and mental development, there is an abnormal increase in the size of the head, with marked bulging of the large fontanel and suture ruptures. In about one fourth of the patients, ophthalmoscopic examination reveals diffuse retinal hemorrhages but rarely secondary optic atrophy or papilledema.

The following statements concerning neuro-ophthalmologic signs and symptoms associated with *chronic subdural hematoma* are based on 50 cases from the Neurosurgical Clinic of the University of Zurich (Krayenbühl and Noto). Only

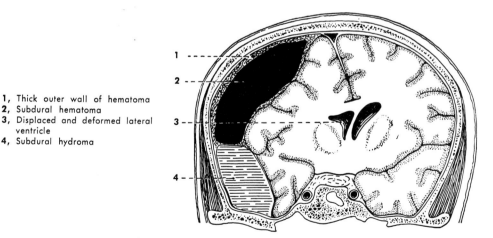

1, Thick outer wall of hematoma
2, Subdural hematoma
3, Displaced and deformed lateral ventricle
4, Subdural hydroma

**Fig. 5-3.** Diagrammatic illustration (frontal section) of chronic subdural hematoma and hydroma with compression of involved part of brain and displacement of lateral ventricles. (After Dandy.)

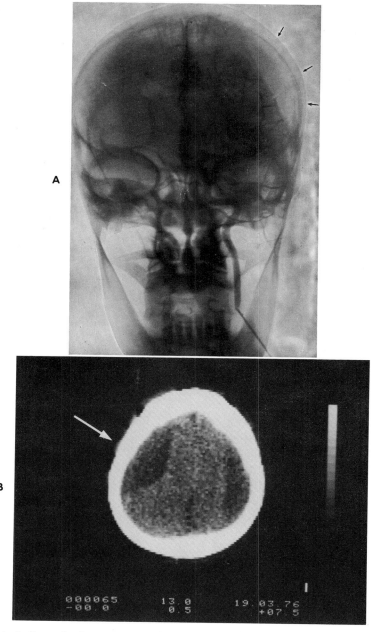

Fig. 5-4. **A,** Left cerebral arteriogram of 36-year-old patient with bilateral chronic subdural hematoma of traumatic origin. Anteroposterior exposure. Massive displacement of left sylvian vessels away from cranial vault. Arteriography renders displaced surface of hemisphere visible as oblique line (cortical arteries and veins mark surface of brain). Contents of left hematoma, 100 ml! **B,** Computerized transverse axial tomogram showing chronic subdural hematoma of traumatic origin on left side (arrow). (**B** courtesy Prof. Dr. med. Spiess, Zurich).

11 of the 50 patients showed *papilledemas,* which were in no way characteristic. The elevation may vary in degree from slight blurring to fully developed and markedly prominent choked discs. Occasionally the ipsilateral choked disc is more pronounced than the one on the opposite side. However, this sign is not dependable for purposes of localization (p. 96). It is interesting that even subdural hematomas, in certain localizations, can produce *visual field defects* (Govan and Walsh; Maltby). Among our own series, we observed contralateral homonymous hemianopia in one patient with a parieto-occipital hematoma and homonymous quadrantanopia in two patients with the hematomas in the frontal and frontotemporal positions. However, such cases concern very large space-occupying lesions. The homonymous field defects may be explained on the basis of disorders of circulation within the posterior cerebral artery (with subsequent occipitocortical infarctions) produced by the herniation of the hippocampal gyrus through the tentorium notch (see discussion of transtentorial herniation syndrome, p. 161). A homonymous field defect in a patient with subdural hematoma may represent an important lateralizing sign, even more reliable than homolateral pupil dilatation (Maltby).

Of some localizing significance are *pupillary changes,* most of all the *unilateral mydriasis and light rigidity that, as a rule, occur on the ipsilateral side* (de Quervain). This must be considered as a lesion of the peripheral oculomotor nerve, which is pressed against the tentorial ridge by protruding portions of the brain or compressed by the posterior cerebral or the superior cerebellar arteries. The damage to the oculomotor nerve forms part of the transtentorial herniation syndrome (see p. 161 and Fig. 2-51). The value of a unilateral mydriasis and light rigidity is diminished by its relatively rare occurrence (in Krayenbühl's series of 50 patients there were only three cases). More frequent and thus of greater diagnostic value is a simple *anisocoria,* which occurs in about one half of the patients. The side of the wider pupil, which still reacts to light, usually corresponds to the side of the hematoma (79% according to McKissock, Richardson, and Bloom). If both pupils are rigid and small, a bilateral hematoma should be considered according to Krayenbühl. Obviously, this miosis is a sign of irritation to the oculomotor nerve (that is, the very early stage of a transtentorial herniation syndrome). A paralysis of the trochlear nerve (one case in 50 patients) as well as the sixth nerve (six cases in 50 patients) apparently is based on the same mechanism. These extrinsic eye muscle pareses account for the diplopia observed in about one third of the patients. It has been previously mentioned that *the transtentorial herniation syndrome is by no means pathognomonic for a subdural hematoma—it occurs also with tumors.* Conjugate deviations of the eyes away from the lesion, ptosis on the side opposite to the hematoma (Govan and Walsh), nystagmus, and even palsy of upward gaze have been described as additional disturbances of ocular motility.

*Acute subdural hematoma,* which usually is traumatic in origin, can be distinguished from the chronic type by its decidedly more violent symptoms. Because of the usually severe cerebral trauma, the patient is either unconscious from the outset or becomes progressively more somnolent. Only rarely is an initial brief unconsciousness interrupted by a brief lucid interval. Sooner or later the unconsciousness, accompanied by vomiting and headaches, sets in again and progresses to a coma (with decrease of pulse rate, rapid respiration, and eventually Cheyne-Stokes breathing).

Pupillary disturbances associated with *traumatic acute subdural hematoma* (Kennedy and Wortis) are more frequent and more pronounced. Anisocoria is found in up to 70% of the patients. Mydriasis of one pupil is usually associated with light rigidity and is generally on the side of the hematoma. Bilateral light rigidity of the pupils is a prognostically unfavorable sign. It is caused either by a bilateral tentorial herniation reaction or a lesion of the brain stem. In the latter case, it may be combined with extensor spasms. A complete ophthalmoplegia is occasionally observed.

Similar ocular symptoms and signs are seen in association with *epidural hematomas,* which usually are the sequel of a traumatic rupture of the middle meningeal artery. The trauma usually causes a skull fracture. After a brief lucid interval (with or without preceding unconsciousness immediately following the trauma), symptoms and signs of rapidly increasing intracranial pressure become apparent that, without neurosurgical intervention, result in coma and eventual death. An ipsilateral mydriasis and light rigidity as signs of an "uncal" syndrome (transtentorial herniation) do occur here, too. Anisocoria is even more frequent than with acute subdural hematomas. Its localizing value is diminished by the fact that the mydriasis, which is usually ipsilateral to the hematoma, occasionally is on the opposite side in the case of simultaneous edema of the brain on the other side. Pressure on the cavernous sinus may cause congestion of the ipsilateral globe as well as pareses or paralyses of isolated extraocular muscles. Retinal hemorrhages can occur if there is a simultaneous subarachnoid hemorrhage (Woodhall, Devine, and Hart).

## BRAIN ABSCESSES

During the *acute stage, signs of a systemic infection* (such as high fever, somnolence to coma, leukocytosis, increased sedimentation rate) and perhaps some focal signs dominate the picture. During the *chronic stage* the symptomatology is less specific and could be mistaken for that of a subdural hematoma or any brain tumor, especially glioblastoma multiforme. As a rule, the general condition of the patient is poor. Leukocytosis and a toxic count, an in-

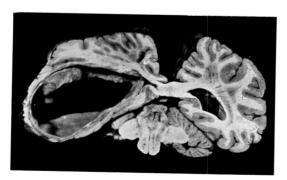

**Fig. 5-5.** Multiple brain abscesses in patient with bronchiectases. Frontal section. Firm membranous wall surrounds large left cavity of abscess. (Specimen from the Pathologic-Anatomic Institute of the University of Zurich.)

creased sedimentation rate, and bradycardia suggest an abscess. Blood-borne metastatic brain abscesses favor the hemispheres. Dissemination into the basal ganglia, the brain stem, or the cerebellum is rare. If the abscess is the result of an otitis media, it usually locates in the temporal or occipital lobe or in the cerebellum (Fig. 5-5).

The ocular symptomatology associated with brain abscesses varies according to the location of the abscess. In a frontal abscess, chemosis of the ipsilateral conjunctiva and exophthalmos with or without orbital infection are possible. Retrobulbar neuritis on the ipsilateral side and papilledema on the opposite side have been described several times in the literature as an atypical Foster Kennedy syndrome (Gros and Cazaban). *Papilledema* is particularly frequent and pronounced with an abscess in an occipital location. As a rule, it is not very characteristic (Lillie; Porto). There is no definite relationship between the size of the abscess and the severity of papilledema. Homonymous visual field defects are possible in an abscess with a temporal or occipital location. We have observed a patient with a chronic encapsulated abscess in the occipital lobe with complete homonymous hemianopia without sparing of the macula. The frequency of papilledema in patients with brain abscess is quite similar to that in patients with brain tumors, depending more or less on the location of the abscess. Chronic brain abscesses produce papilledema more frequently than acute brain abscesses; Weber found choked discs in 15 of 23 patients with chronic abscesses, but only in seven of 26 patients with acute abscesses. Papilledema usually is minimal or absent in patients with cerebellar abscesses (Colemann), because the gravity of the morbid abscess results in death or leads to surgical intervention before a true papilledema has a chance to develop. According to Colemann, there is no definite relationship between the side of the abscess and the extent of the swelling of the papilla.

It is frequently difficult to differentiate an acute brain abscess clinically from *a thrombophlebitis of the cortical veins or an intracranial sinus*. In the latter case, there are frequently bilateral choked discs that are identical to those occurring in patients with a brain tumor or a brain abscess (see discussion of pseudotumor cerebri, p. 310).

Ocular signs and symptoms in patients with *subdural empyemas* and *abscesses* are not very characteristic and diagnostically without much significance. They are quite similar to

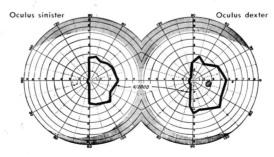

**Fig. 5-6.** Temporal-occipital subdural empyema on right side of 55-year-old patient. Hematogenous infected subdural hematoma. Left homonymous hemianopia with sparing of macula. Visual acuity, O.D. 1.25; O.S. 0.9.

those associated with subdural hematoma (p. 312). What is more, subdural empyemas may originate from a metastatic infection of a chronic subdural hematoma (Fig. 5-6).

*Extradural abscesses*, originating most frequently from mastoiditis, may produce *Gradenigo's syndrome*, which is characterized by paresis of the homolateral sixth nerve, pain in the distribution of the fifth nerve (usually ophthalmic division), and sometimes ipsilateral corneal anesthesia (p. 21).

## INTRACRANIAL ANEURYSMS

In certain tumor sites (for instance, the chiasmal region and the cavernous sinus), aneurysms always must be considered in the differential diagnosis in addition to true tumors. A large number of aneurysms are accompanied by typical ocular signs and symptoms, which may be of localizing significance. Thus we believe it is important to discuss this form of "tumors" briefly. With due consideration to the extensive literature on the subject (Cushing and Bailey; Dandy; Jefferson; Walsh and Hoyt; and others), we plan to follow more or less the important monographs of Krayenbühl and Yasargil. At the same time, we want to consider some of our own cases.

In principle, two forms of aneurysms can be distinguished: (1) the *paralytic type* (increase in the size of the aneurysm and fine extravasations into the sur-

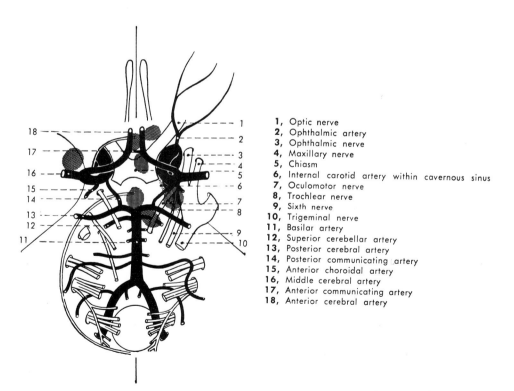

1, Optic nerve
2, Ophthalmic artery
3, Ophthalmic nerve
4, Maxillary nerve
5, Chiasm
6, Internal carotid artery within cavernous sinus
7, Oculomotor nerve
8, Trochlear nerve
9, Sixth nerve
10, Trigeminal nerve
11, Basilar artery
12, Superior cerebellar artery
13, Posterior cerebral artery
14, Posterior communicating artery
15, Anterior choroidal artery
16, Middle cerebral artery
17, Anterior communicating artery
18, Anterior cerebral artery

**Fig. 5-7.** Diagrammatic illustration of base of skull and position of large cerebral arteries and cranial nerves. Shaded round areas indicate saccular cerebral aneurysms at typical areas of predilection for arteries of base of brain.

**Table 8.** Symptomatology of intracranial aneurysms*

| Location | Signs and symptoms | | |
|---|---|---|---|
| | Ocular | Trigeminal | Other |
| *Infraclinoid aneurysms* | | | |
| Aneurysm of internal carotid within cavernous sinus | Unilateral ophthalmoplegia, especially of third nerve (rarely optic atrophy with loss of vision and field defects) | Intense pain in area of first, second, and third branches of trigeminal nerve; hypesthesia and hypalgesia in same area (sensation of numbness) | Violent headache (generally sudden onset); destructions in region of lesser sphenoid wing and clinoid processes; enlargement of superior orbital fissure |
| Posterior syndrome | Mostly only paresis of sixth nerve | Involvement of all sensory and motor fibers of trigeminal nerve | |
| Middle syndrome | Complete ophthalmoplegia | Involvement of first and second branch | |
| Anterior syndrome | Paresis of third nerve or complete ophthalmoplegia | Involvement of first branch | |
| Intrasellar aneurysm of internal carotid artery within cavernous sinus | Chiasmal syndrome with asymmetric bitemporal hemianopia; sudden onset; fluctuations of visual field defects; occasionally ophthalmoplegia | Negative | More or less pronounced headaches; no roentgenologic evidence of enlargement of sella |
| *Supraclinoid aneurysms* | | | |
| Aneurysm of anterior cerebral and anterior communicating arteries | More or less atypical chiasmal syndrome (bitemporal inferior quadrantanopia); unilateral or bilateral loss of vision, subject to fluctuations; possible optic atrophy | Negative | With exception of olfactory nerve, cranial nerves remain intact; aneurysm frequently apoplectic in type |
| Aneurysm of middle cerebral artery | Homonymous hemianopia | Negative | Convulsive seizures; hemiparesis; hemianaesthesia; aphasia |

*Modified after Franceschetti.

rounding area result in pressure effects on certain cranial nerves and, consequently, a neurologic syndrome similar to that of a brain tumor) and (2) the *apoplectic type* (as the name indicates, the apoplectic type is typified by the picture of a single or recurrent subarachnoid hemorrhage). However, in reality the paralytic and apoplectic types often form a clinical entity: eye muscle

**Table 8.** Symptomatology of intracranial aneurysms—cont'd

| Location | Signs and symptoms | | |
|---|---|---|---|
| | Ocular | Trigeminal | Other |
| | *Supraclinoid aneurysms*—cont'd | | |
| Aneurysm of carotid–posterior communicating artery junction | Partial or complete oculomotor palsy with mydriasis and disturbance of accommodation | Negative except pain in forehead and eye; neuralgic pain of ophthalmic branch | Sudden onset of unilateral headache, pain in forehead or eye ("ophthalmoplegic migraine"); with severe pain in neck, aneurysm located in posterior part of posterior communicating artery |
| Aneurysm of posterior cerebral artery | Possibly homonymous hemianopia (optic tract or radiation!) | Negative | Possibly Weber's syndrome |
| Aneurysm of basilar and vertebral artery | Possible bilateral abducens or oculomotor pareses | | Frequently no symptoms whatsoever; occasionally bulbar, pyramidal, or cerebellar signs; this aneurysm frequently belongs to apoplectic type |

palsies, for instance, arise in an apoplectic manner together with subarachnoid hemorrhage.

**Paralytic type**

It is the paralytic type of aneurysm that, because of the pressure effect on the cranial nerves (especially those of the extrinsic eye muscles), often gives rise to characteristic neuro-ophthalmologic syndromes that deserve consideration within the scope of our discussion (Fig. 5-7). Various groups of syndromes, to be discussed here, can be distinguished (Table 8).

**Aneurysms of the internal carotid artery within the cavernous sinus (intracavernous carotid aneurysms)**

In principle, the neurologic and especially the neuro-ophthalmologic signs and symptoms of an aneurysm of the internal carotid artery within the cavernous sinus (also named intracavernous carotid aneurysm) correspond to those of tumors of the cavernous sinus, as described in detail in Chapter 3, p. 268. The more or less simultaneous involvement of the third, fourth, fifth, and sixth cranial nerves is characteristic for the *cavernous sinus syndrome*. According to Jefferson, posterior, middle, and anterior cavernous sinus syndromes can be distinguished, depending on the impaired nerves (Fig. 3-101). The cavernous sinus syndrome resulting from an aneurysm sets in with *pain of the face (also behind the eye) or a sensation of numbness and is followed shortly by diplopia—with or without ptosis.* The pain usually is sharply demarcated in the area of distribution of the trigeminal nerve. In contrast to an ordinary trigeminal neuralgia, it is persistent rather than paroxysmal. In addition to these symptoms of irritation, it is always possible to demonstrate more or less distinct defects such as hypesthesias or hypalgesias in the area of distribution of the three branches of the trigeminal nerve. Of particular significance is the *corneal reflex; its decrease or loss may be the only trigeminal sign.* There is frequently a paresis of only the sixth nerve (Fig. 5-8) in association with the posterior cavernous sinus syndrome, whereas the oculomotor, trochlear, and sixth nerves may be involved simultaneously with the middle and anterior forms. *The oculomotor nerve is most frequently paralyzed.* Ptosis and internal ophthalmoplegia frequently are part of this characteristic picture (because of the simultaneous involvement of the oculo-sympathetic fibers surrounding the carotid artery, the pupil may be small, although fixed). A true exophthalmos is possible. Occasionally an aneursym of unusual size and anterior extension may injure the ipsilateral optic nerve, causing atrophy with corresponding loss of vision and field defects (on the plain x-ray film erosion of the optic foramen!). During the further course of the disease,

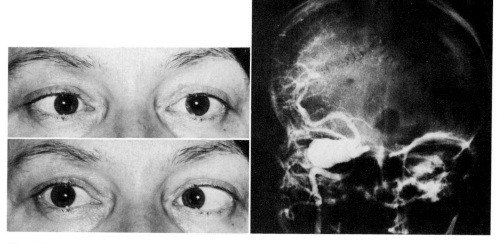

**Fig. 5-8.** Aneurysm of right internal carotid artery within cavernous sinus in 34-year-old patient. Left, Right sixth nerve palsy: with eyes turned right, right globe cannot be rotated past midline. Right hypesthesia in area of first and second branch of trigeminal nerve. Slight decrease of right superior and inferior corneal reflexes. Right, Arteriogram (anteroposterior view) after right internal carotid arteriography. Enormous saccular aneurysm of internal carotid artery within cavernous sinus.

these signs of paralysis—after their sudden onset—may remain stationary or even may recede to a certain extent. (Aberrant third nerve regeneration may be observed.) This symptomatology actually is so typical that it almost permits the diagnosis. The final proof is the arteriographic demonstration of the aneurysm, which fails only in rare instances of spontaneous thrombosis of the aneurysm. As previously mentioned, tumors in the region of the cavernous sinus and the medial cranial fossa must always be considered in the differential diagnosis.

### Intrasellar aneurysms of the internal carotid artery

A break of an *intracavernous aneurysm of the internal carotid artery* (infra-clinoid portion) through the medial wall of the cavernous sinus with intrasellar expansion may cause a more or less typical chiasmal syndrome. It results from direct compression of the chiasm by the aneurysm—usually more pronounced on one side, which causes a certain *asymmetry of the chiasmal syndrome* (Jefferson). This is the reason why in such cases the bitemporal hemianopia is rather irregular and asymmetric as compared with that in patients with pituitary tumors (p. 258 and Fig. 5-9). There are also reports of amaurosis of one eye with tem-

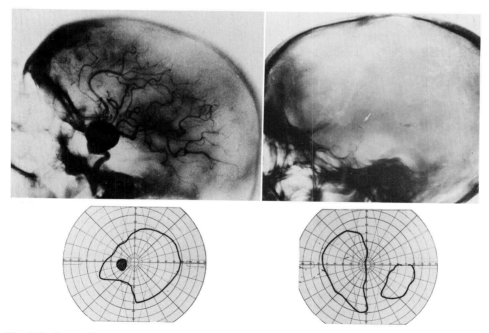

**Fig. 5-9.** Intrasellar aneurysm of infraclinoid portion of right internal carotid in 51-year-old patient. Above, Right internal carotid angiogram showing huge infraclinoid aneurysm of internal carotid above syphon (left). Shell-like calcifications corresponding to calcified walls of huge suprasellar aneurysm in suprasellar region (right). Below, Corresponding visual fields show bitemporal hemianopia of asymmetric nature (on both sides preservation of islands within bitemporal half). Visual acuity, O.D. 0.5; O.S. 0.8. No pallor of discs.

poral or nasal hemianopia of the other eye. Frequently, *the visual field defects vary in the same patient during different stages of the disease* (Klingler). Just as in patients with the chiasmal syndrome associated with pituitary tumors, there is a characteristic unilateral or bilateral loss of vision. With an aneurysm, however, it is greater in one eye. It is particularly significant that the *visual disturbance often appears suddenly and is frequently associated with headaches. Sudden deterioration as well as improvement of vision is typical for an aneurysm.* In most patients, ophthalmoscopic examination reveals a bilateral primary optic atrophy with a sharp outline of the disc margin. As a rule, it is more distinct on one side.

*The sudden appearance of a visual disturbance in the form of a chiasmal syndrome and associated with headaches or perhaps even with pareses or paralyses of extraocular muscles (cavernous sinus affection!) is highly suggestive of an intrasellar aneurysm.* The absence of an enlarged sella on the x-ray film is important in differentiating an aneurysm from a pituitary tumor, although in the later stages destructive changes in the sella (enlargement of the entrance of the sella, atrophy of the posterior clinoid processes and the dorsum sellae) may occur. Arteriographic proof of an intrasellar aneurysm is not always possible (thrombosis!). Definite proof is often (50%) obtained only on surgical exploration.

The other possible mechanism of a chiasmal syndrome is that of *suprasellar aneurysms* of the supraclinoid portion of the carotid artery (p. 258). They originate from the anterior cerebral or the anterior communicating arteries (Fig. 5-10).

*Aneurysms of the proximal segment of the internal carotid artery* generally grow to a considerable size and may show extension toward the midline, with displacement of the chiasm laterally and upward. Therefore this form of aneurysm may also produce chiasmal syndromes. Ipsilateral blindness and temporal field defects in the contralateral eye are the most common findings.

*Aneurysms at the internal carotid bifurcation,* if large enough and if extending anteriorly and medially, may involve the chiasm and produce the symptomatology of a suprasellar tumor with bitemporal field defects (Krayenbühl). Posterior and medial extension of such an aneurysm leads to compression of the optic tract (incongruent homonymous hemianopia), and posterior and inferior extension may involve the oculomotor nerve (Fig. 5-11).

### Intracranial aneurysms of the ophthalmic artery

Intracranial aneurysms of the ophthalmic artery, also termed supraclinoid or carotid-ophthalmic aneurysms, originate from the junction of the ophthalmic artery with the intracranial internal carotid artery. They are rare. (Krayenbühl and Yasargil found only seven such aneurysms among 290 intracranial aneurysms.) Because of their site in the immediate neighborhood of the optic nerve, these aneurysms produce signs of optic nerve compression that may mimic the

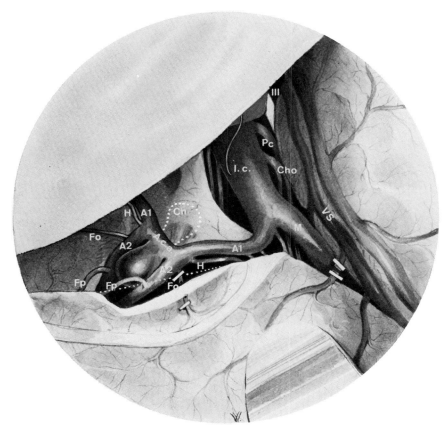

**Fig. 5-10.** Diagrammatic representation of anterior communicating artery complex and chiasmatic region. *Aca,* anterior communicating artery; *A1,* proximal segment, *A2,* distal segment; *Ch,* chiasm; *Cho,* anterior choroidal artery; *Ic,* internal carotid artery; *Pc,* posterior communicating artery; *VS,* sylvian vein; *III,* oculomotor nerve. Schematic representation shows possible relationship between aneurysm of anterior communicating artery (dotted line) and superior surface of chiasm. (From Yasargil, M. G., Fox, I. L., and Ray, M. W.: In Krayenbühl, H., editor: Advances in technical standards in neurosurgery, Vienna, 1975, Springer Verlag.)

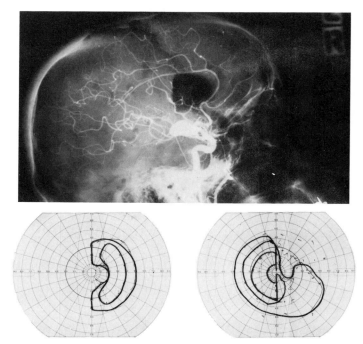

**Fig. 5-11.** Aneurysm of supraclinoid portion of left internal carotid before its bifurcation in 56-year-old patient who suffered from acute decrease of vision of left eye. Above, Left internal carotid angiogram showing partially thrombosed aneurysm of supraclinoid portion of left internal carotid. Below, Corresponding visual fields show asymmetric bitemporal hemianopia, affecting temporal superior quadrant on right side only. Rapid development of chiasmal syndrome. Visual acuity, O.D. 0.5; O.S. hand movements. First diagnosis was "retrobulbar neuritis" of left eye probably caused by temporal arteritis.

symptoms of *retrobulbar neuritis.* The usual symptomatology of intracranial aneurysm of the ophthalmic artery is a scotoma in one eye that progresses to a loss of the nasal field on the involved side (Fig. 5-12). Later, there appears an upper temporal depression of the contralateral field and finally blindness on the side of the aneurysm. This sequence of visual field defects is caused by the compression first of one optic nerve and then of the lateral side of the chiasm by the upward-growing aneurysm. Erosion of the anterior clinoid and the intracranial portion of the optic canal may be visible on x-ray films (Fig. 5-13).

**Aneurysms of the middle cerebral artery**

Aneurysms of the middle cerebral artery, originating most frequently from the trifurcation of the middle cerebral artery, may, even unruptured, cause homonymous hemianopia apart from hemiparesis and convulsive seizures. More often the homonymous field defects are associated with intracerebral hemorrhage (hemiplegia, hemianesthesia, aphasia). Large aneurysms of the middle cerebral

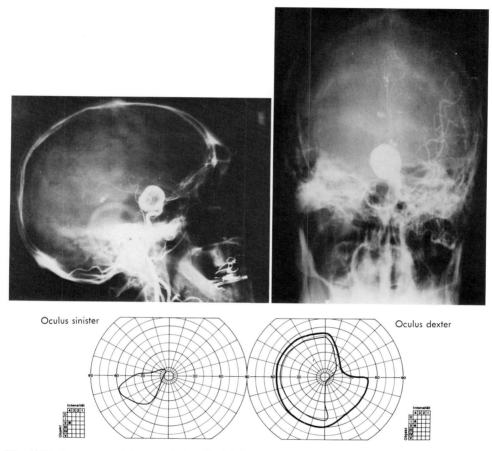

**Fig. 5-12.** Aneurysm of dorsomedial wall of left internal carotid at origin of ophthalmic artery in 32-year-old patient. Arteriogram of left internal carotid artery (lateral and anteroposterior views) after angiography of left internal carotid artery. Progressive decrease of vision particularly of left eye. Visual acuity, O.D. 0.2; O.S. hand movements. Visual fields show superior temporal quadrantanopia on right side. Loss of nasal quadrants and superior temporal quadrant on left side.

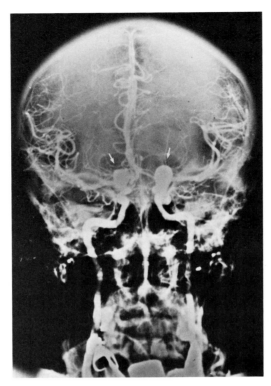

**Fig. 5-13.** Bilateral saccular aneurysms of internal carotid arteries (arrows) at origin of ophthalmic artery in 31-year-old patient. Subarachnoid bleeding, aphasia, and hemiparesis on right side. No visual symptoms.

artery sometimes can be visualized on the plain x-ray film by the curvilinear calcifications of their walls (Fig. 5-13).

### Aneurysms of the anterior cerebral and anterior communicating arteries

Although the majority of aneurysms of the anterior cerebral and anterior communicating arteries belong to the apoplectic type that leads to subarachnoid hemorrhages, a paralytic form may occur in this location. Like the intrasellar intracavernous aneurysm, this suprasellar form is marked by *a more or less atypical chiasmal syndrome. Sudden onset of bitemporal field defects with a certain preponderance on one side and fluctuations or actual improvement of impaired vision* are of diagnostic significance for such an aneurysm. Sometimes visual loss may be slowly progressive (as in any suprasellar tumor) and be accompanied by progressive optic atrophy (Fig. 3-52) of both discs. According to Jefferson, onset of the visual field defects in both inferior temporal quadrants is suggestive of a suprasellar aneurysm, provided the other signs and symptoms suggest an aneurysm. Sometimes the visual symptoms consist only in a relatively *acute loss*

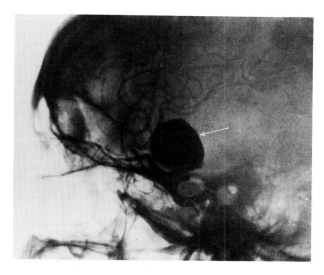

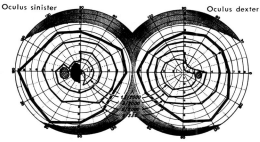

Oculus sinister             Oculus dexter

**Fig. 5-14.** Suprasellar aneurysm of left anterior cerebral and anterior communicating arteries in 46-year-old patient. Above, Arteriogram (lateral view) after left cerebral angiography. Walnut-sized saccular aneurysm of anterior communicating artery at sella entrance (giant aneurysm). Below, Bitemporal superior quadrantanopia with paracentral temporal scotoma of hemianopic type of left field. Visual acuity, O.D. 1.0; O.S. 0.05. Both discs unchanged. X-ray film of skull normal. No endocrine disturbances. (From Krayenbühl, H.: Schweiz. Arch. Neurol. Psychiatr. **47:**155, 1941.)

*of vision in one eye* preceding the subarachnoid hemorrhage by days, weeks, or years. In contrast to the intrasellar intracavernous aneurysm, the cranial nerves (except the olfactory nerve) remain intact (Fig. 5-14).

## Aneurysms of the carotid–posterior communicating artery junction

Aneurysms of the carotid–posterior communicating artery junction favor a location very close to or directly at the point where the posterior communicating artery branches off the internal carotid artery (Alpers and Schlezinger) (Fig. 5-15). Characteristic symptoms and signs are *sudden appearance of unilateral head-ache, pain in the forehead or the eye, and the simultaneous or slightly delayed appearance of a partial or complete oculomotor palsy with ptosis, mydriasis, and*

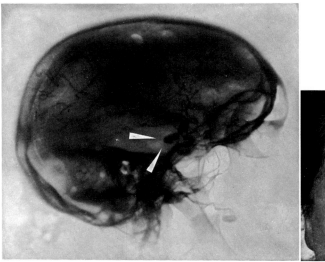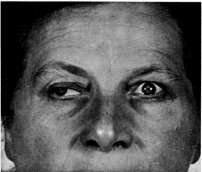

**Fig. 5-15.** Saccular aneurysm of right carotid–posterior communicating artery junction in 48-year-old patient. Left, Arteriogram (lateral view) after right cerebral angiography. Irregularly shaped lentil-sized aneurysm of posterior communicating artery. Normal configuration of vascular tree of middle cerebral artery. Anterior and posterior cerebral arteries not filled. Right, Corresponding clinical picture. Right oculomotor paresis with partial ptosis. Right globe in divergent position.

*paresis of accommodation* (Jefferson). Usually the pupil is rigid to light and mydriatic. The intense unilateral headaches at the onset of the disease are localized in the forehead or the eye and must be regarded as a trigeminal disturbance in the area of distribution of the ophthalmic nerve. Objective sensibility disturbances can be demonstrated very rarely—mostly as a slight decrease of the ipsilateral superior corneal reflex. This form can be differentiated from an aneurysm of the internal carotid artery within the cavernous sinus by the minimal impairment of the trigeminal nerve and its limitation to the oculomotor nerve.

A *sudden unilateral oculomotor paralysis (ptosis, exotropia, dilated, fixed pupil) associated with violent ipsilateral headaches, pain in the forehead, or pain in the eye* should always arouse suspicion of an aneurysm of the carotid–posterior communicating artery junction (Fig. 5-16). This is particularly true, since an isolated peripheral oculomotor palsy (Fig. 1-8) is actually rarely associated with a tumor at the base of the skull; because of its expansion, it would involve other structures, especially other cranial nerves. Hoyt is right in this connection, emphasizing that in an isolated oculomotor palsy caused by aneurysm the pupil is always involved and that "pupillary sparing" practically excludes the aneurysmatic etiology. In rare instances a peripheral oculomotor paralysis may be caused by an aneurysm of the posterior part of the posterior communicating artery. It should be considered if the oculomotor palsy is not accompanied by trigeminal

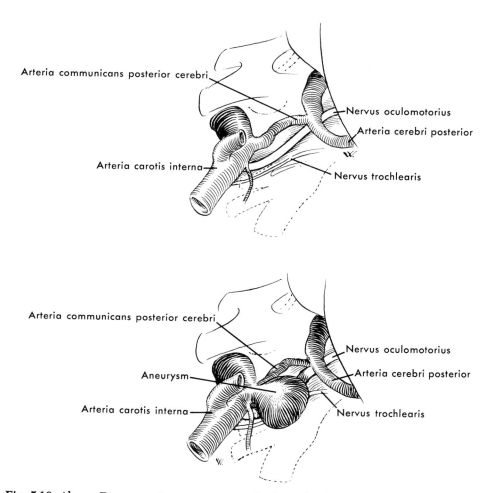

**Fig. 5-16.** Above, Diagrammatic representation of relationship between oculomotor nerve and posterior communicating artery. Below, Aneurysm of posterior communicating artery compressing oculomotor nerve.

pain but by severe pain in the neck. It should be stressed here that *frequently the picture of the so-called ophthalmoplegic migraine may be simulated by such aneurysms* (Sjöqvist; Frankel; Patrikios). The acute event of the oculomotor palsy can be preceded by neuralgic or migrainelike pains for months or years.

### Aneurysms of the posterior cerebral artery

Aneurysms of the posterior cerebral artery are extremely rare. According to Jefferson, a thrombosis of the aneurysm and the posterior cerebral artery producing an ischemic infarct of the occipital lobe or a compression of the optic tract by the aneurysm may cause a *homonymous hemianopia.* Apart from homonymous field defects, *Weber's syndrome* (third nerve palsy and contralateral hemiplegia), similar to acute occlusive vascular disease, may occur as a focal sign before the rupture of the aneurysm (Jamieson; Hanafee and Jannetta).

### Aneurysms of the basilar and vertebral arteries

The clinical diagnosis of an aneurysm of the basilar artery is difficult (Fig. 5-17). Frequently, there are no signs or symptoms. Occasionally, there is the syndrome of an acute or chronic bulbar paralysis. Krayenbühl found a bilateral sixth nerve paresis in a patient with a vertebral aneurysm (Fig. 5-18). The oculomotor nuclei are in the area immediately adjacent to the bifurcation of the basilar artery. Thus bilateral oculomotor pareses are possible. Frequently, these aneurysms are of the apoplectic type and may cause massive subarachnoid hemorrhages. After these have been absorbed, bilateral paralyses of extrinsic eye muscles may manifest themselves. Large basilar aneurysms may produce pyramidal signs, horizontal gaze palsy, nystagmus, and cerebellar or cerebellopontine angle signs.

#### Apoplectic type (subarachnoid hemorrhage)

The symptomatology of the apoplectic type of aneurysm is determined by an *acute subarachnoid hemorrhage.* The picture is extremely characteristic. The onset is marked by *violent frontal or occipital headaches and vomiting, followed in about one third of the patients by unconsciousness* lasting minutes, several hours, or days. In addition to the severe meningeal symptoms, there are usually bilateral pyramidal signs. Lumbar puncture reveals a characteristic *hemorrhagic cerebrospinal fluid.* Actually, any aneurysm (saccular or arteriovenous) outside the cavernous sinus can cause such an acute subarachnoid hemorrhage.

What has been said about subarachnoid hemorrhage is applicable also to *intracerebral hemorrhages,* which can also be produced by rupture of saccular or arteriovenous aneurysms. The blood escaping from these aneurysms may either flow into the subarachnoid space or into the substance of the brain itself.

It is of interest from the neuro-ophthalmologic point of view that a subarachnoid or intracerebral hemorrhage may cause grave ocular changes, although in a relatively small number of patients (Ballantyne; Paton; Cardarello; and

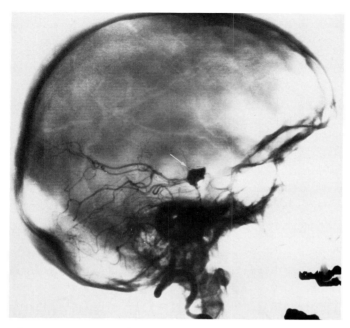

**Fig. 5-17.** Saccular aneurysm of basilar artery (arrow) in 36-year-old patient. Arteriogram (sagittal view) after right vertebral angiography.

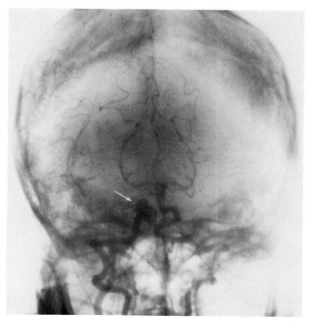

**Fig. 5-18.** Aneurysm of right vertebral artery (arrow) in 49-year-old patient. Arteriogram (anteroposterior view) after right vertebral angiography.

others). *Papilledema* (Griffith, Jeffers, and Fry), repeatedly mentioned in the literature as occurring in patients with subarachnoid hemorrhages, is rather rare (about 20%) and is seen mostly in the late stages of the disease and usually is moderate in degree (Fig. 5-19). Much more important are *intraocular hemorrhages,* which may result in considerable impairment of the visual acuity. At first, such hemorrhages are either *retinal* (either punctate or forming concentric circles around the disc) or *preretinal* (with a typical horizontal level), between the retina and hyaloid membrane. The preretinal hemorrhages after some days frequently tend to spread into the *vitreous* (Drews and Minckler; Wagener and Foster). In such cases, more or less extensive vitreous hemorrhages make an ophthalmoscopic examination impossible. Loss of vision following a subarachnoid hemorrhage may be caused by such vitreous hemorrhages (Terson's syndrome). In a small number of patients who show no evidence of vitreous or retinal hemorrhages, the loss of vision must be interpreted as being caused by acute circulatory disturbances (ischemic or hemorrhagic) in the region of the optic nerve or chiasm resulting from the subarachnoid hemorrhage. The retinal peripapillary hemorrhages may be unilateral or bilateral. The preretinal hemorrhages, with their tendency to spread into the vitreous, are mostly bilateral. Retinal and vitreous hemorrhages occur also with severe intracranial hemorrhages from any cause.

A communicating *internal hydrocephalus* has been known to occur as a sequel of a *recurrent subarachnoid hemorrhage* (Krayenbühl). This is associated with a disturbance of the absorption of the cerebrospinal fluid and an increase in the intracranial pressure. These patients occasionally develop papilledema that can be so marked that it may progress to a secondary atrophy with its deleterious consequences for visual function.

The pathogenesis of these retinal and preretinal hemorrhages is still quite controversial. It is generally assumed (MacDonald) that the cause of these hemorrhages is more or less the

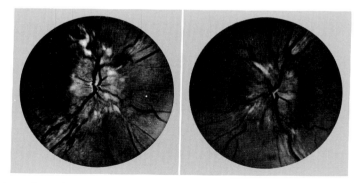

**Fig. 5-19.** Bilateral papilledema after subarachnoid hemorrhage from aneurysm in 26-year-old patient. Enlargement, edematous swelling, and elevation (2.5 diopters) of both papillae with hemorrhages and white spots. Bilateral venous congestion. Bending of vessels at disc margins. Radial folding of retina adjacent to disc. Left illustration corresponds to right eye and right illustration to left eye.

same as that of the hemorrhages in papilledema (that is, an obstruction of the central retinal vein at the site where it pierces the sheath of the optic nerve after emerging from the latter). A block of the venous drainage causes the characteristic hemorrhages in the area of distribution of the central retinal vein (that is, the retina and, secondarily, the preretinal space). At any rate, it is an accepted fact that in subarachnoid hemorrhages the extravasations, which may reach the sheaths of the optic nerve, can never enter the intraocular space because the intervaginal space of the nerve forms a cul-de-sac–like termination near the bulbus wall. As a result of his investigations, Ballantyne comes to the conclusion that obstruction of the central retinal vein cannot be blamed solely for the retinal and preretinal hemorrhages. He assumes an additional embarrassment of the venous drainage channels of the globe and orbit in their entirety, the cause of which is a sudden increase in the intracranial pressure resulting from the subarachnoid hemorrhage. It may be possible that the intracranial hypertension not only causes venous stasis in the retina, but also a considerable hyperemia in the territory of the ophthalmic artery. Therefore the rupture of the vessels of the retina is the effect of both the venous stasis and arterial hyperemia (Brueckner, Bloch, and Wolff-Wiesinger).

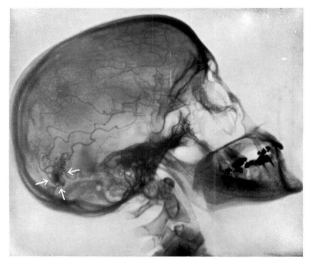

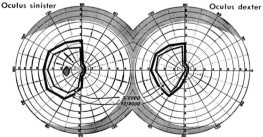

Oculus sinister    Oculus dexter

**Fig. 5-20.** Arteriovenous aneurysm in left occipital region of 32-year-old patient. Above, Arteriogram (lateral view) after left cerebral angiography. Two strong branches of posterior cerebral artery lead to arteriovenous vessel convolution (arrows) in lateral and middle region of left occipital lobe. Below, Right homonymous hemianopia with sparing of macula. Visual acuity, O.U. 0.5. Patient had unformed visual hallucinations in form of fire balls!

**Arteriovenous aneurysms**

The arteriovenous aneurysm may also assume the form of the apoplectic type (that is, a subarachnoid or intracerebral hemorrhage). The general neurologic symptomatology of the nonapoplectic type depends on the location of the aneurysm. Frequently, its site is a hemisphere, with predilection for the area of the middle cerebral artery. (Dandy; Weber; Olivecrona and Ladenheim), the location being pial, pial and dural, or extracranial.

Eighty-five percent of the cerebral arteriovenous aneurysms are supratentorial (Krayenbühl and Yasargil). Subarachnoid hemorrhage is one of the initial symptoms. Headache, epileptic seizure of the jacksonian type, and intellectual and psychic disorders are frequent signs and symptoms. Transient attacks of monocular blindness, unformed photopsias, or transient homonymous hemianopias are occasional initial ocular signs. *The most common ophthalmologic complication of supratentorial arteriovenous aneurysm is homonymous hemianopia* (some times bilateral, causing cerebral blindness). Here we would like to call attention to our observation of a patient with homonymous hemianopia with an occipital arteriovenous aneurysm (Fig. 5-20).

Intracranial arteriovenous malformations occasionally may be associated with *retinal arteriovenous aneurysms* (Fig. 2-45) and arteriovenous malformations in the orbit, the optic nerve, the maxilla, the pterygoid fossa, and the mandible *(Wyburn-Mason syndrome)*. The cerebral arteriovenous aneurysms in this syndrome generally involve the basofrontal area, the sylvian fissure, the midbrain, or the posterior fossa. We have observed a patient with Parinaud's syndrome (upward gaze palsy) resulting from an arteriovenous angioma within the roof of the midbrain.

*The arteriovenous aneurysm of the internal carotid artery within the cavernous sinus,* also called carotid-cavernous fistula (traumatic or spontaneous) (Fig. 5-21), *is especially interesting from the neuro-ophthalmologic point of view.* In contrast to the saccular aneurysm of the cavernous sinus (intracavernous aneurysm), this arteriovenous aneurysm does not result in a cavernous sinus syndrome (Dandy; Walsh; Kaeser).

Our own series includes 13 cases of arteriovenous aneurysms of the internal carotid artery within the cavernous sinus, nine of them proved by angiography. Their symptomatology can be summarized as follows. The most important sign is *exophthalmos* (Fig. 5-22), which usually occurs unilaterally (on the side of the fistula). Contralateral exophthalmos may follow in about one third of the cases days or weeks later. The exophthalmos may be pulsating (three of 13 cases). The pulsation is synchronous with the radial pulse (Martin and Mabon; Sugar and Meyer). A characteristic *bruit synchronous with the pulse* can be heard with the stethoscope in the frontotemporal region or directly over the eye. It disappears on compression of the carotid artery in the area of the neck. Often this noise is noted by the patient himself and may disturb his sleep. In case of pronounced exophthalmos, there may be additional motility disturbances, mostly

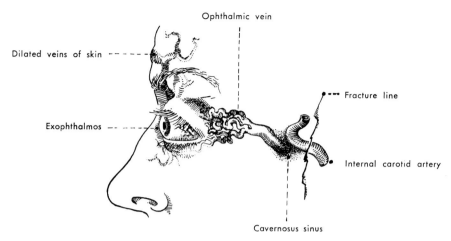

Ophthalmic vein

Dilated veins of skin

Fracture line

Exophthalmos

Internal carotid artery

Cavernosus sinus

**Fig. 5-21.** Diagrammatic illustration of development of venous stasis and exophthalmos after traumatic arteriovenous aneurysm of internal carotid artery within cavernous sinus (carotid-cavernous fistula). Rupture in internal carotid artery following fracture of base of skull led to shunt with cavernous sinus and, consequently, impairment (that is, stasis) in area of drainage of ophthalmic vein. Pulse wave of internal carotid artery is transmitted to globe: pulsating exophthalmos. (After Dandy.)

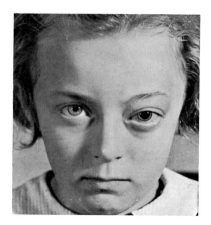

**Fig. 5-22.** Traumatic arteriovenous aneurysm of left internal carotid artery within cavernous sinus (carotid-cavernous fistula) of 8-year-old girl. Left exophthalmos measuring 4 mm with minimal pulsation of corneal apex. Distinct congestion of conjunctival and episcleral veins. Marked prominence of veins in left upper lid and left temporal region. Pulse-synchronous bruit with maximum over left eye and left temple. Compared with right side, left retinal veins are distinctly congested and tortuous. Visual acuity, O.U. 1.0. Trauma: small steel rib of umbrella penetrated left orbit.

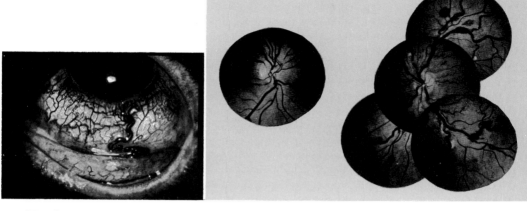

**Fig. 5-23.** Traumatic arteriovenous aneurysm of internal carotid artery within cavernous sinus (carotid-cavernous fistula) of 43-year-old patient. Left, Appearance of left exophthalmic bulbus with enormous venous congestion of conjunctival as well as, in particular, episcleral veins. Large tortuous vessel in 5:30 o'clock position. Right, Fundus photographs demonstrating enormous congestion of left retinal veins with patches of retinal hemorrhages. O.S., Beginning papilledema. Right fundus normal. Visual acuity, O.D. 1.0.; O.S. 0.25.

sixth nerve pareses, more rarely oculomotor pareses (lesions of the nerves within the cavernous sinus). Signs of the latter are an occasional ptosis of the upper lid and mydriatic pupils fixed to light. The arteriovenous shunt causes *venous stasis*, which manifests itself in dilated conjunctival veins (with chemosis), dilated veins of the lids (with lid swelling), dilated scleral veins, and especially dilated retinal veins with retinal hemorrhages (Fig. 5-23). Ophthalmoscopically, there is frequently slight choking of the disc, which changes to optic atrophy with blurred disc margins (two of 13 cases) at a later stage. There are no visual field changes or loss of vision in the initial stages. They develop at a later stage (impaired retinal circulation, secondary glaucoma either as a result of an increase in episcleral venous pressure or neovascular proliferation in the anterior chamber angle), an important fact in the differential diagnosis of intraorbital and perhaps intrasellar aneurysms. The neuro-ophthalmologic syndrome of an arteriovenous shunt between the internal carotid artery and the cavernous sinus is so characteristic that it permits a clinical diagnosis. Definite proof, however, can be obtained only by means of cerebral angiography (Fig. 5-24). *It is most important to differentiate this arteriovenous aneurysm from tumors of the orbit or a possible meningioma of the sphenoid wing. Next in importance are tumors at the base of the skull, which may create a superior orbital fissure syndrome.* Although exophthalmos and motility disturbances may occur in association with tumors as well as with arteriovenous aneurysms, the extensive venous congestion, the pulsation of the exophthalmos, and the bruit synchronous with the pulse are

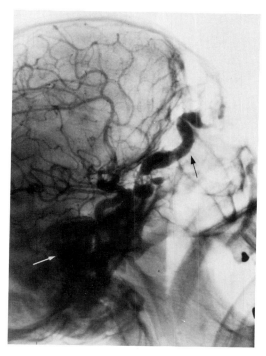

**Fig. 5-24.** Arteriogram (lateral view) after left internal carotid angiography. Large arterio-venous aneurysm (white arrow) of left internal carotid artery within cavernous sinus (carotid-cavernous fistula). Retrograde congestion of orbital veins, especially superior orbital vein (black arrow). Arteriogram of patient shown in Fig. 5-23.

missing in patients with tumors. Their presence will aid in drawing the right con-clusion.

Finally, it must be mentioned that pulsating exophthalmos may be produced also by aneurysms of the ophthalmic artery or by arteriovenous malformations within the orbit. In the differential diagnosis the orbital varix (intermittent exoph-thalmos syndrome) must also be considered. *For correct diagnosis of carotid–cavernous sinus fistulas, there is no doubt that bilateral serial carotid angi-ography (including orbital angiography) supplemented by subtraction technique represents the method of choice.*

# SIX

## Summary

The purpose of this book has been to present the ocular signs and symptoms seen in association with brain tumors. The book is based on the 8150 cases of brain tumors on record at the Neurosurgical Clinic at the University of Zurich. Personal experience in the evaluation of these cases is emphasized.

The special methods of the neuro-ophthalmologic examination in patients suspected of having a brain tumor receive consideration in Chapter 1. The first section of that chapter is devoted to the *history and the symptoms* as reported by the patients. These symptoms consist of visual field disturbances, disturbances of primitive and higher visual functions, photopsias, hallucinations, mind blindness, cortical blindness, alexia, agraphia, disturbances of motility (especially diplopia), pain, photophobia, and others. The *objective examination* includes the external aspect of the globe (lid fissure, exophthalmos, pupils), corneal sensitivity, pupils and pupillary reactions, motility (extraocular palsies, gaze palsies, nystagmus), fundus, visual acuity, color sense, dark adaptation, and finally visual fields (gross methods, perimeter, tangent screen, general pathology of visual fields). The special technique and the importance of the neuro-ophthalmologic examination justify this detailed and comprehensive presentation.

Chapter 2 concerns itself with the *general signs and symptoms of increased intracranial pressure* in patients with brain tumors. The ocular signs consist of *papilledema, extraocular pareses, transtentorial herniation syndrome,* and rarely *exophthalmos.* First the frequency of papilledemas is discussed. Then the ophthalmoscopic appearance of fully developed papilledema is described in detail. The symptoms associated with it, especially amblyopic attacks, are considered. The ways of diagnosing incipient papilledema, including the behavior of the retinal vessels (blood pressure, fluorescein angiography), are discussed. There is a separate section on unilateral papilledema and its differential diagnosis as well as chronic atrophic papilledema with its grave significance for vision and the visual fields. The pathologic anatomy of the disc and pathogenesis of papilledema are summarized. The *differential diagnosis of papilledema,* with its great importance in the neuro-ophthalmology of brain tumors and especially its significance in *papillitis, the disc edema of malignant hypertension,* and *various congenital anomalies* (drusen, pseudoneuritis, pseudochoked disc) are considered. In addition to papilledema, increased intracranial pressure causes nonspecific *extraocular muscle pareses,* especially a unilateral sixth nerve paresis. Another result of increased intracranial pressure is the *transtentorial herniation syndrome*—a compression of the oculomotor nerve by protruding brain substance at the tentorial notch results in unilateral mydriasis and rigidity to light. In later stages, there may be ptosis and paralysis of the extrinsic muscles supplied by the oculomotor nerve. *Exophthalmos* caused by a general increase in the intracranial pressure is mostly bilateral. A unilateral exophthalmos should be interpreted rather as a focal sign, as for instance, invasion of the orbit by the tumor.

In Chapter 3 the local signs and symptoms of brain tumors are presented from a topographic point of view. In order to present a true scope of the ocular involvement in relation to other neurologic signs, a brief summary of general neurologic syndromes for each location under discussion is included. The brain tumors are divided into supratentorial and infratentorial groups. The *supratentorial group* includes tumors of the hemispheres (frontal, temporal, parietal, and occipital lobes), the pituitary region, the anterior and middle fossae, the third ventricle, the thalamus, the basal ganglia, the midbrain with the sylvian aqueduct, and the pineal body. The infratentorial group involves cerebellar tumors (cerebellar spheres and vermis), the cerebellopontine angle, the pons, and the medulla oblongata. The fourth ventricle is considered in detail in the discussion of tumors of the cerebellar vermis. No special summary of the ocular symptomatology of the various tumor sites is given, since a brief summary of these symptoms is presented following each topographic description.

In Chapter 4 the *relationship between the type of tumor and the ocular signs and symptoms* is discussed. Some tumor types produce a very characteristic ocular symptomatology (for instance, pituitary adenomas, craniopharyngiomas, chiasmal gliomas, and others). In addition, there are numerous tumor types with a neuro-ophthalmologic symptomatology that does not depend on their histologic structure but merely on their localization. There is a discussion of the characteristics of glioblastoma multiforme, astrocytoma, oligodendroglioma, medulloblastoma, hemangiomas, and meningiomas. A special section deals with metastatic tumors to the brain, a special type of brain tumors. If there are specific ocular signs or symptoms, they are always considered in connection with these special types of tumors.

Chapter 5 considers tumorlike changes, an important group from the standpoint of differential diagnosis that always must be considered in the discussion of ocular symptomatology. Included are *pseudotumor cerebri, subdural hematomas, brain abscesses,* and, in the broadest sense of the word, *aneurysms.* Subdural hematomas are notable especially because of unilateral pupillary disturbances (mydriasis, possibly light rigidity, as in the transtentorial herniation syndrome). The ocular symptomatology of brain abscesses does not differ essentially from that of other tumors. Of important localizing value, however, are the ocular signs and symptoms of various forms of cerebral aneurysms; because of their close vicinity to cranial nerves, they result in characteristic syndromes. We mention especially aneurysms of the internal carotid artery within the cavernous sinus (cavernous sinus syndrome), intrasellar and suprasellar aneurysms (chiasmal syndrome) aneurysms of the middle cerebral artery (homonymous hemianopia), and aneurysms of the carotid–posterior communicating artery junction (peripheral oculomotor paralysis). In addition to the paralytic type of aneurysm, there is an apoplectic form, which is characterized by an *acute subarachnoid hemorrhage*. The ocular changes associated with such subarachnoid hemorrhages consist of retinal and especially vitreous hemorrhages.

The importance of ocular signs and symptoms in brain tumors is underlined by the fact that a little more than 50% of patients with brain tumors show ocular involvement in one form or another. These signs are not merely insignificant accompanying manifestations but in many cases important initial symptoms. Frequently, they point to a general increase in the intracranial pressure. Very often, they are extremely valuable as localizing signs or symptoms.

# Literature

## Abbreviations of journals used in the bibliography

| | |
|---|---|
| Acta Med. Scand. | Acta medica scandinavica, Stockholm |
| Acta Neurochir. | Acta neurochirurgica, Vienna |
| Acta Neurol. Scand. | Acta neurologica scandinavica, Copenhagen |
| Acta Ophthalmol. | Acta ophthalmologica, Copenhagen |
| Acta Soc. Ophthalmol. Jpn. | Acta Societatis ophthalmologicae Japonicae, Tokyo |
| Adv. Ophthalmol. | Advances in Ophthalmology, Basel |
| Allg. Z. Psychiatr. | Allgemeine Zeitschrift für Psychiatrie und ihre Grenzgebiete, Berlin |
| Am. J. Ophthalmol. | American Journal of Ophthalmology, Chicago |
| Am. J. Roentgenol. Radium Ther. Nucl. Med. | American Journal of Roentgenology, Radium Therapy and Nuclear Medicine, Springfield, Ill. |
| Ann. Oculist. | Annales d'oculistique, Paris |
| Ann. Ottalmol. | Annali di ottalmologia, Parma |
| Ann. R. Coll. Surg. Engl. | Annals of the Royal College of Surgeons of England, London |
| Annee. Ther. Clin. Ophthalmol. | Année thérapeutique et clinique en ophtalmologie, Marseille |
| Arch. Augenheilk. | Archiv für Augenheilkunde, Munich |
| Arch. Dis. Child. | Archives of Disease in Childhood, London |
| Arch. Klin. Chir. | Archiv für klinische Chirurgie, Berlin |
| Arch. Neurol. Psychiatr. | Archives of Neurology and Psychiatry, Chicago |
| Arch. Oftalmol. B. Air. | Archivos de oftalmologia de Buenos Aires, Buenos Aires |
| Arch. Ophtalmol. | Archives d'ophtalmologie, Paris |
| Arch. Ophthalmol. | Archives of Ophthalmology, Chicago |
| Arch. Otolaryngol. | Archives of Otolaryngology, Chicago |
| Arch. Pathol. | Archives of Pathology, Chicago |
| Arch. Soc. Oftalmol. Hispano-Am. | Archivos de la Sociedad oftalmológica hispano-americana, Madrid |
| Atti Soc. Oftalmol. Ital. | Atti della Società oftalmologica italiana, Rome |
| Ber. Dtsch. Ophthalmol. Ges. | Bericht deutsche ophthalmologische Gesellschaft, Munich |
| Boll. Oculist. | Bollettino d'oculistica, Bologna |
| Br. J. Ophthalmol. | British Journal of Ophthalmology, London |
| Br. J. Surg. | British Journal of Surgery, Bristol |
| Brain | Brain; Journal of Neurology, London |
| Bull. Neurol. Inst. N.Y. | Bulletin of the Neurological Institute of New York, New York |
| Bull. N.Y. Acad. Med. | Bulletin of the New York Academy of Medicine, New York |

| | |
|---|---|
| Bull. Soc. Belge Ophthalmol. | Bulletin de la Société belge d'ophtalmologie, Brussels |
| Bull. Soc. Fr. Ophthalmol. | Bulletins et mémoires de la Société française d'ophtalmologie, Paris |
| Bull. Soc. Ophthalmol. Fr. | Bulletin des Sociétés d'ophtalmologie de France, Paris |
| Circulation | Circulation; Journal of the American Heart Association, New York |
| Confin. Neurol. | Confinia neurologica, Basel |
| Doc. Ophthalmol. | Documenta ophthalmologica, The Haag |
| Dtsch. Med. Wochenschr. | Deutsche medizinische Wochenschrift, Stuttgart |
| Dtsch. Z. Nervenheilk. | Deutsche Zeitschrift für Nervenheilkunde, Berlin |
| Encephale | L'Encéphale, Paris |
| Ergeb. Physiol. | Ergebnisse der Physiologie, Biologischen Chemie und experimentellen Pharmakologie, Berlin |
| Eye Ear Nose Throat Mon. | Eye, Ear, Nose and Throat Monthly, Chicago |
| Folia Ophthalmol. Jpn. | Folia ophthalmologica Japonica, Osaka |
| Fortschr. Geb. Roentgenstr. Nuklearmed. | Fortschritte auf dem Gebiete der Roentgenstrahlen und der Nuklearmedizin, Stuttgart |
| G. Ital. Oftalmol. | Giornale italiano di oftalmologia, Florence |
| Graefe. Arch. Ophthalmol. | Albrecht von Graefe's Archiv für Ophthalmologie, Berlin |
| Helv. Med. Acta | Helvetica medica acta, Basel |
| Helv. Paediatr. Acta | Helvetica paediatrica acta, Basel |
| Helv. Physiol. Pharmacol. Acta | Helvetica physiologica et pharmacologica acta, Basel |
| Int. Arch. Allerg. Appl. Immunol. | International Archives of Allergy and Applied Immunology, Basel |
| Int. Ophthalmol. Clin. | International Ophthalmology Clinics, Boston |
| J.A.M.A. | The Journal of the American Medical Association, Chicago |
| J. Med. Lyon | Journal de médecine de Lyon |
| J. Nerv. Ment. Dis. | Journal of Nervous and Mental Disease, Baltimore |
| J. Neurosurg. | Journal of Neurosurgery, Chicago |
| Klin. Monatsbl. Augenheilkd. | Klinische Monatsblätter für Augenheilkunde, Stuttgart |
| Lancet | Lancet, London |
| Lyon Med. | Lyon médical, Lyon |
| Mayo Clin. Proc. | Mayo Clinic Proceedings, Rochester, Minn. |
| Minerva Oftalmol. | Minerva oftalmologica, Torino |
| Monatsschr. Psychiatr. Neurol. | Monatsschrift für Psychiatrie und Neurologie, Basel |
| Neuro-chirurgie | Neuro-chirurgie, Paris |
| Neurology | Neurology, Minneapolis |
| Nord. Ophthalmol. Tidsskr. | Nordisk ophthalmologisk tidsskrift, Copenhagen |
| Ophthal. Lit. | Ophthalmic Literature, London |
| Ophthalmologica | Ophthalmologica, Basel |
| Praxis | Praxis, Bern |
| Proc. All-India Ophthalmol. Soc. | Proceedings of the All-India Ophthalmological Society, Madras |
| Proc. R. Soc. Med. | Proceedings of the Royal Society of Medicine, London |
| Radiol. Med. | La radiologia medica, Turin |
| Radiology | Radiology, Syracuse, N.Y. |
| Rass. Ital. Ottalmol. | Rassegna italiana di ottalmologia, Turin |
| Rev. Esp. Otoneurooftalmol. Neurocir. | Revista española de oto-neuro-oftalmologia y neurocirurgia, Valencia |
| Rev. Méd. Suisse Romande | Revue médicale de la Suisse Romande, Lausanne |
| Rev. Otoneuroophtalmol. | Revue d'oto-neuro-ophtalmologie, Paris |
| Riv. Otoneurooftalmol. | Rivista oto-neuro-oftalmologica, Bologna |
| Schweiz. Arch. Neurol. Neurochir. Psychiatr. | Schweizer Archiv für Neurologie, Neurochirurgie und Psychiatrie, Zurich |
| Schweiz. Med. Wochenschr. | Schweizerische medizinische Wochenschrift, Basel |

| | |
|---|---|
| Sist. Nerv. | Sistema nervoso, Milan |
| Surg. Gynecol. Obstet. | Surgery, Gynecology and Obstetrics, Chicago |
| Trans. Am. Acad. Ophthalmol. Otolaryngol. | Transactions; American Academy of Ophthalmology and Otolaryngology, Rochester, Minn. |
| Trans. Am. Ophthalmol. Soc. | Transactions of the American Ophthalmological Society, New York |
| Trans. Ophthalmol. Soc. U.K. | Transactions of the Ophthalmological Society of the United Kingdom, London |
| Tunis. Med. | Tunisie médicale, Tunis |
| Wien. Klin. Wochenschr. | Wiener klinische Wochenschrift, Vienna |
| Z. Augenheilk. | Zeitschrift für Augenheilkunde, Berlin |
| Zentralbl. Chir. | Zentralblatt für Chirurgie, Leipzig |
| Zentralbl. Gesamte Ophthalmol. | Zentralblatt für die gesamte Ophthalmologie und ihre Grenzgebiete, Berlin |
| Zentralbl. Neurochir. | Zentralblatt für Neurochirurgie, Leipzig |

## Handbooks, textbooks, & monographs

Adler, F. H.: Textbook of ophthalmology, Philadelphia, 1950, W. B. Saunders Co.

Adrogue, E.: Neurologia ocular, Buenos Aires, 1942, El Ateneo.

Altenburger, H.: Die raumbeengenden Krankheiten des Schädelinnern. In Bergmann and Staehelin, editors: Handbuch der inneren Medizin, Berlin, 1939, Julius Springer, vol. 5, pt. 1.

Ambrose, J.: Computerized transverse axial scanning (tomography). II. Clinical application, Br. J. Radiol. 46:1023-1047, 1973.

Amsler, M., Brückner, A., Franceschetti, A., Goldmann, H., and Streiff, E. B.: Lehrbuch der Augenheilkunde, Basel, 1954, S. Karger AG.

Ashworth, B.: Clinical neuro-opthalmology, Oxford, 1973, Blackwell Scientific Publications, Ltd.

Bailey, P.: Die Hirngeschwülste (deutche Übertragung), Stuttgart, 1951, Ferdinand Enke Verlag.

Bailey, P., Buchmann, D. N. P., and Bucy, P. C.: Intracranial tumors of infancy and childhood, Chicago, 1939, University of Chicago Press.

Bailliart, P.: La circulation rétinienne à l'état normal et à l'état pathologique, Paris, 1923, Gaston Doin & Cie.

Bailliart, P., Coutela, C., Redslob, E., and Velter, E.: Traité d'ophthalmologie, Paris, 1939, Masson & Cie, Editeurs.

Behr, C.: Auge und Zentralnervensystem, Zentralbl. Gesamte Ophthalmol. **45:**1, 1940.

Bender, M. B.: Ophthalmoneurology. In Progress in neurology and psychiatry, New York, 1946, Grune & Stratton, Inc.

Berens, C.: The eye and its diseases, Philadelphia, 1949, W. B. Saunders Co.

Berens, C., and Zuckermann, J.: Diagnostic examination of the eye, Philadelphia, 1946, J. B. Lippincott Co.

Bergstrand, H., Olivecrona, H., and Tönnis, W.: Gefässmissbildungen und Gefässgeschwülste des Gehirns, Leipzig, 1936, Georg Thieme Verlag KG.

Best, F.: Die Augenveränderungen bei den organischen nicht entzündlichen Erkrankungen des Zentralnervensystems. In Schieck, F., and Brückner, A., editors: Kurzes Handbuch der Ophthalmologie, Berlin, 1931, Julius Springer, vol. 6.

Bing, R.: Allgemeine Anatomie, Physiologie, Pathologie und Symptomatologie des Gehirnes. In Bergmann and Staehelin: Handbuch der inneren Medizin, Berlin, 1939, Julius Springer, vol. 5, p. 33.

Bing, R.: Kompendium der topischen Gehirn- und Rückenmarkdiagnostik, Basel, 1945, Schwabe & Co.

Bing, R.: Lehrbuch der Nervenkrankheiten, Basel, 1945, Schwabe & Co.

Bing, R., and Brückner, R.: Gehirn und Auge, Grundriss der Neuro-Ophthalmologie, Basel, 1954, Schwabe & Co.

Bodechtel, G.: Differentialdiagnose neurologischer Krankheitsbilder, ed. 2, Stuttgart, 1974, Georg Thieme Verlag KG.

Bonamour, G., Brégeat, P., Bonnet, M., and Juge, P.: La papille optique, Paris, 1968, Masson & Cie, Editeurs.

Brégeat, P.: L'oedème papillaire, Paris, 1956, Masson & Cie, Editeurs.

Bumke, O., and Förster, O.: Handbuch der Neurologie, Berlin, 1936, Julius Springer, vol. 14.

Cabanis, E. A.: Transverse axial tomography with a computer (EMI Scanner); a new era in neuroradiology, Ann. Oculist. **207:** 413-429, 1974.

Cattaneo, D.: Oftalmoangioscopia, Bologna, 1947, L. Cappelli.

Cogan, D. G.: Neurology of the visual system, Springfield, Ill., 1968, Charles C Thomas, Publisher.

Cushing, H.: Intrakranielle Tumoren, Berlin, 1935, Julius Springer.

Cushing, H., and Bailey, P. B.: Tumors arising from the blood vessels of the brain: angiomatous malformations and hemangioblastomas, Springfield, Ill., 1928, Charles C Thomas, Publisher.

Cushing, H., and Eisenhardt, L.: Meningiomas: their classification, regional behavior, life, history, surgical end results, Springfield, Ill., 1938, Charles C Thomas, Publisher.

Dandy, W. E.: Intracranial arterial aneurysms, Ithaca, N.Y., 1944, Comstock Publishing Co., Inc.

Dandy, W. E.: Surgery of the brain, Hagerstown, Md., 1945, W. F. Prior Co., Inc.

Davidson, S. I.: Aspects of neuro-ophthalmology, London, 1974, Butterworth & Co. (Publishers), Ltd.

Dubois-Poulsen, A.: Le champ visuel, Paris, 1952, Masson & Cie, Editeurs.

Duke-Elder, S., editor: System of ophthalmology, vol. 1-14, St. Louis, 1958-1973, The C. V. Mosby Co.

Duke-Elder, S., and Scott, G. I.: Neuroophthalmology. In Duke-Elder, S., editor: System of ophthalmology, vol. 12, St. Louis, 1971, The C. V. Mosby Co.

Duke-Elder, S., and Wybar, K.: Ocular motility and strabismus, London, 1973, Henry Kimpton.

Focosi, M.: Le paralisi dei muscoli oculomotori estrinseci, Rome, 1948, Abruzzini.

Fulton, J. F.: Physiology of the nervous system, London, 1943, Oxford University Press.

Gerlach, J.: Grundriss der Neurochirurgie, Stuttgart, 1967, J. F. Steinkopf Verlag GMBH.

Gerlach, J., and Simon, G.: Erkennung, Differentialdiagnose und Behandlung der Geschwülste und Entzündungen der Schädelknochen. In Olivecrona, H., and Tönnis, W., editors: Handbuch der Neurochirurgie, Berlin, 1962, Julius Springer, pp. 211-366.

Guillaumat, L., Morax, P. V., and Offret, C.: Neuro-ophthalmologie, Paris, 1959, Masson & Cie, Editeurs.

Guillot, P., Saraux, H., and Sedan, R.: L'exploration neuroradiologique en ophtalmologie, Paris, 1966, Masson & Cie, Editeurs.

Harrington, D. O.: Visual fields. A textbook and atlas of clinical perimetry, ed. 3, St. Louis, 1971, The C. V. Mosby Co.

Havener, W. H., and Gloeckner, S. L.: Introductory atlas of perimetry, St. Louis, 1972, The C. V. Mosby Co.

Hess, R.: Elektroencephalographische Studien bei Hirntumoren, Stuttgart, 1958, Georg Thieme Verlag KG.

Hounsfield, G. N.: Computerized transverse axial scanning (tomography). I. Description of system, Br. J. Radiol. **46:**1016-1022, 1973.

Hoyt, W. F., and Beeston, D.: The ocular fundus in neurologic disease, St. Louis, 1966, The C. V. Mosby Co.

Huber, A., and Rintelen, F.: Neuro-ophthalmologie, Basel, 1973, S. Karger AG.

Hughes, B.: The visual fields, Oxford, 1954, Blackwell Scientific Publications, Ltd.

Hughes, B.: The visual fields: a study of the applications of quantitative perimetry to the anatomy and pathology of the visual pathways, Springfield, Ill., 1954, Charles C Thomas, Publisher.

Jentzer, A.: Klinische Neurochirurgie. In Brunner et al., editors: Lehrbuch der Chirurgie, Basel, 1949, Schwabe & Co., pp. 659-778.

Kehrer, F.: Die Allgemeinerscheinungen der Hirngeschwülste, Leipzig, 1931, Georg Thieme Verlag KG.

Kershner, C. M.: Blood supply of the visual pathway, Boston, 1943, Meador Publishing Co.

Kestenbaum, A.: Clinical methods of neuroophthalmologic examination, London, 1947, William Heinemann, Ltd.

Krayenbühl, H.: Allgemeine hirnchirurgische Diagnostik und Therapie. In Brunner et al., editors: Lehrbuch der Chirurgie, Basel, 1949, Schwabe & Co., pp. 605-658.

Krayenbühl, H., and Richter, W.: Die cerebrale Angiographie, Leipzig, 1952, Georg Thieme Verlag KG.

Krayenbühl, H., and Yasargil, G. M.: Die zerebrale Angiographie, Stuttgart, 1965, Georg Thieme Verlag KG.

Krieg, W. J. S.: Functional neuroanatomy, Philadelphia, 1942, The Blakiston Co.

Kuntz, A.: A textbook of neuroanatomy, Philadelphia, 1942, Lea & Febiger.

Kyrieleis, W.: Klinik der Augensymptome bei Nervenkrankheiten, Berlin, 1954, Walter de Gruyter & Co.

Lauber, H.: Das Gesichtsfeld, Berlin, 1944, Julius Springer.

Lhermitte, J.: Les hallucinations, Paris, 1951, Gaston Doin & Cie.

Lindenberg, R.: Neuropathology involving the lateral geniculate bodies, the optic radiation and the calcarine cortex. In Smith, J. L., editor: Neuro-ophthalmology, St. Louis, 1965, The C. V. Mosby Co., vol. 2.

Lindenberg, R., Walsh, F. B., and Sacks, J. G.: Neuropathology of vision: an atlas, Philadelphia, 1973, Lea & Febiger.

Lombardi, G.: Radiology in neuro-ophthalmology, Baltimore, 1967, The Williams & Wilkins Co.

Lyle, J. D.: Neuro-ophthalmology, Springfield, Ill., 1945, Charles C Thomas, Publisher.

Malbran, J.: Campo visual normal y patologico, Buenos Aires, 1936, El Ateneo.

McLean, A. J.: Intracranial tumors. In Bumke and Foerster, editors: In Handbuch der Neurologie, Berlin, 1936, Julius Springer, vol. 14.

Mifka, P.: Die Augensymptomatik bei der frischen Schädelhirn-Verletzung, Berlin, 1968, Walter de Gruyter & Co.

von Monakow, C.: Die Lokalisation im Grosshirn und der Abbau der Funktion durch kortikale Herde, Munich, 1914, J. F. Bergmann.

Moniz, E.: Diagnostic des tumeurs cérébrales et épreuve de l'encéphalographie artérielle, Paris, 1931, Masson & Cie, Editeurs.

Moniz, E.: Die zerebrale Arteriographie und Phlebographie, Berlin, 1940, Julius Springer.

Mumenthaler, M.: Neurologie, ed. 3, Stuttgart, 1974, Georg Thieme Verlag KG.

Netter, F. H.: The Ciba collection of medical illustrations. Nervous system, Summit, N.J., 1953, Ciba Pharmaceutical Products, Inc., vol. 1.

Nielsen, J. M.: A textbook of clinical neurology, New York, 1946, Paul B. Hoeber, Inc.

Olivecrona, H.: Chirurgische Behandlung der Gehirngeschwülste. In von Fedor, K., editor: Die spezielle Chirurgie der Gehirnkrankheiten, Stuttgart, 1941, Ferdinand Enke Verlag, vol. 3.

Olivecrona, H., and Tönnis, W.: Handbuch der Neurochirurgie, Berlin, 1954, 1955, etc., Julius Springer.

Ostertag, B.: Anatomie und Pathologie der raumfordernden Prozesse des Schädelbinnenraumes. Neue Deutsche Chirurgie, Stuttgart, 1941, Ferdinand Enke Verlag, vol. 50.

Ottonello, P., and Vassura, G. W.: Neuro-oftalmologia, Bologna, 1959, L. Cappelli.

Polyak, S.: The retina, Chicago, 1941, University of Chicago Press.

Rasmussen, A. T.: The principal nervous pathways, New York, 1941, Macmillan, Inc.

Rea, R. L.: Neuro-ophthalmology. ed. 2, St. Louis, 1941, The C. V. Mosby Co.

Rucker, W. C.: The interpretation of visual fields, American Academy of Ophthalmology and Otolaryngology, ed. 3, Omaha, 1957, Douglas Printing Co.

Sachs, E.: Diagnosis and treatment of brain tumors, St. Louis, 1931, The C. V. Mosby Co.

Sachs, E.: Diagnosis and treatment of brain tumors and care of the neurosurgical patient, St. Louis, 1949, The C. V. Mosby Co.

Sachsenweger, R.: Neuroophthalmologie, Stuttgart, 1976, Georg Thieme Verlag KG.

Scheid, W.: Lehrbuch der Neurologie, Stuttgart, 1966, Georg Thieme Verlag KG.

Schieck, F., and Brückner, A.: Kurzes Handbuch der Ophthalmologie, Berlin, 1930-1932, Julius Springer.

Smith, J. L., editor: Neuro-ophthalmology, St. Louis, 1964, 1965, 1967, 1968, 1969, 1970, 1972, 1973, The C. V. Mosby Co., vols. 1-7.

Spiegel, E. A., and Sommer, I.: Neurology of the eye, ear, nose and throat, New York, 1944, Grune & Stratton, Inc.

Streiff, E. B.: Krankheiten des Nervensystems. In Amsler, M., et al., editors: Lehrbuch der Augenheilkunde, Basel, 1954, S. Karger AG, p. 829.

Töndury, G.: Angewandte und topographische Anatomie, Zürich, 1949, Fretz & Wasmuth.

Tönnis, W.: Die Chirurgie des Gehirns und seiner Häute. In von Kirschner-Nordmann, editor: Die Chirurgie, Munich, 1948, Verlag Urban & Schwarzenberg.

Tönnis, W.: Diagnostik der intrakraniellen Geschwülste. In Olivecrona, H., and Tönnis, W., editors: Handbuch der Neurochirurgie, Berlin, 1962, Julius Springer, vol. 4, pt. 3, pp. 1-579.

Traquair, H. M.: An introduction to clinical perimetry, London, 1949, Henry Kimpton.

Troncoso, M. U.: Internal disease of the eye: an atlas of ophthalmoscopy, Philadelphia, 1942, F. A. Davis Co.

Tschermack-Seysenegg, A.: Einführung in die physiologische Optik, Berlin, 1947, Julius Springer.

Uhthoff, W.: Die Augenveränderungen bei den Erkrankungen des Gehirnes. In Graefe-Saemisch: Handbuch der gesamten Augenheikunde, Leipzig, 1915, Wilhelm Engelmann, vol. 11, pp. 1143-1375.

Vinken, P. J., and Bruyn, G. W., editors: Handbook of clinical neurology, New York, 1974, American Elsevier Publishing Co., Inc., vol. 16-18.

Walsh, F. B., and Hoyt, W. F.: Clinical neuro-ophthalmology, Baltimore, 1969, The Williams & Wilkins Co.

Weinstein, P.: Ophthalmologische Differentialdiagnose bei Gehirntumoren, Budapest, 1972, Akadémiai Kiado.

Wilbrand, H., and Saenger, A.: Handbuch der Neurologie des Auges, Munich, 1900-1922, 1927, J. F. Bergmann.

Wilson, S. A.: Neurology, Baltimore, 1940, The Williams & Wilkins Co.

Wolff, E.: The anatomy of the eye and orbit, London, 1933, H. K. Lewis & Co., Ltd.

Youmans, J. R.: Neurological surgery, a comprehensive reference guide to the diagnosis and management of neurosurgical problems, Philadelphia, 1973, W. B. Saunders Co., vol. 1-3.

Zülch, K. J.: Die Hirngeschwülste, Leipzig, 1951, Johann Ambrosius Barth.

Zülch, K. J.: Biologie und Pathologie der Hirngeschwülste. In Olivecrona, H., and Tönnis, W., editors: Handbuch der Neurochirurgie, Berlin, 1956, Julius Springer, vol. 3.

# CHAPTER ONE

## Methods of neuro-ophthalmologic examination in patients with suspected brain tumors

### History and symptoms

Amsler, M., and Huber, A.: Allgemeine Symptomatologie. In Amsler, M., et al., editors: Lehrbuch der Augenheilkunde, Basel, 1954, S. Karger AG, pp. 53-67.

Bay, E.: Analyse eines Falles von Seelenblindheit, Dtsch. Z. Nervenheilk. 168:1-23, 1952.

Bender, M. B., and Feldman, M.: The so-called "visual agnosias," Brain 95:173-186, 1972.

Bender, M. B., and Furlow, L. T.: Phenomenon of visual extinction of homonymous fields and psychologic principles involved, Arch. Neurol. Psychiatr. 53:29-33, 1945.

Bender, M. B., and Kahn, R. L.: Afterimagery in defective fields of vision, J. Neurol. Neurosurg. Psychiatry 12:196-204, 1949.

Bender, M. B., and Kanzer, M. G.: Metamorphopsia and other psychovisual disturbances in a patient with tumor of the brain, Arch. Neurol. Psychiatr. 45:481-485, 1941.

Bender, M. B., and Savitsky, N.: Micropsia and teleopsia limited to the temporal fields of vision, Arch. Ophthalmol. 29:904-908, 1943.

Benson, D. F., Segarra, J., and Albert, M. L.: Visual agnosia-prosopagnosia: a clinico-pathologic correlation, Arch. Neurol. 30:307-310, 1974.

Best, F.: Über optische Agnosie, Klin. Monatsbl. Augenheilkd. 116:14-18, 1950.

van Bogaert, L.: Sur les hallucinations visuelles au cours des affections organiques du cerveau (Contributions à l'étude du syndrome des hallucinations lilliputiennes), Encephale 21:657-679, 1926.

Clark, W. E. L.: Visual centres of brain and their connexions, Physiol. Rev. 22:205-232, 1942.

Critchley, M.: The problem of awareness

or nonawareness of hemianopic field defects, Trans. Ophthalmol. Soc. U.K. **69**:95, 1949.

Critchley, M.: Metamorphopsia of central origin, Trans. Ophthalmol. Soc. U.K. **69**: 111-121, 1949.

Critchley, M.: Types of visual perseveration: "Paliopsia" and "illusory visual spread," Brain **74**:267-299, 1951.

Cushing, H.: Trans. Am. Neurol. Assoc., p. 374, 1921.

Duensing, F.: Beitrag zur Frage der optischen Agnosie, Arch. Psychiatr. Nervenkr. **188**: 131-161, 1952.

Duke-Elder, S.: Textbook of ophthalmology, vol. 4, Neurology of vision, St. Louis, 1949, The C. V. Mosby Co.

Esper, M. L. E.: Visual agnosia, Trans. Ophthalmol. Soc. U.K. **92**:735-739, 1972.

Ethelberg, S., and Jensen, V. A.: Obscurations and further time-related paroxysmal disorders in intracranial tumors, Arch. Neurol. Psychiatr. **68**:130, 1952.

Fischer-Brügge, K.: Das Klivuskanten-Syndrom, Acta Neurochir. **1**:36, 1951.

Förster, O.: Über Rindenblindheit, Arch. Ophthalmol. **36**:94-108, 1890.

Goldstein, K., and Gelb, A.: Psychologische Analysen hirnpathologischer Fälle auf Grund der Untersuchungen Hirnverletzter, Leipzig, 1920, Johann Ambrosius Barth.

Hecaen, H., de Ajuriaguerra, J., and Massonnet, J.: Les troubles visuo-constructifs par lésion pariéto-occipitale droite, Encephale **40**:122-178, 1951.

Henschen, K.: Klinische und anatomische Beiträge zur Pathologie des Gehirns, Upsala, 1890-1922.

Hess, W. R.: Die graphische Darstellung von Bewegungsstörungen der Augen mit Beispieltafeln zur Diagnose von Augenmuskellähmungen, Arch. Augenheilkd. **70**: 10, 1912.

Horrax, G.: Visual hallucinations as a cerebral localizing phenomenon, with special reference to their occurrence in tumors of the temporal lobes, Arch. Neurol. Psychiatr. **10**:532, 1923.

Horrax, G., and Putnam, T. J.: Distortion of the visual fields in cases of brain tumor; the field defects and hallucinations produced by tumors of the occipital lobe, Brain **55**:499-523, 1932.

Krayenbühl, H.: Primary tumors of the root of the fifth cranial nerve, Brain **59**: 337, 1936.

Lebensohn, J. E., and Bellows, J.: The nature of photophobia, Arch. Ophthalmol. **12**:380-390, 1934.

Lhermitte, J.: Les fondements anatomo-physiologiques de certaines hallucinations visuelles, Confin. Neurol. **9**:43-57, 1949.

Lhermitte, J., and Ajuriaguerra, J.: Hallucinations visuelles et lésions de l'appareil visuel, Ann. Med. Physiol. **94**:321-351, 1936.

Lhermitte, J., and Ajuriaguerra, J.: Psychopathologie de la vision, Paris, 1942, Masson & Cie, Editeurs.

Lippmann, O.: Paralysis of divergence due to cerebellar tumor, Arch. Ophthalmol. **31**: 299, 1944.

Lisch, K.: Cerebrale Metamorphopsie, Graefe. Arch. Ophthalmol. **141**:554-558, 1940.

Lotmar, F.: Zur Kenntnis der herdanatomischen Grundlagen leichterer optischagnostischer Störungen, Schweiz. Arch. Neurol. Neurochir. Psychiatr. **42**:299, 1938.

Lunn, V.: Über mangelnde Wahrnehmung der eigenen Blindheit (Anton's Symptom). Eine Übersicht und klinische Studie, Acta Psychiatr. Neurol. **16**:191-242, 1941.

Lyle, T. K.: Eye symptoms and signs caused by intra-cranial lesions, Ann. R. Coll. Surg. Engl. **7**:316, 1950.

Magitot, A.: Photophobie, Ann. Oculist. **174**: 817-832, 1937.

Masson, C. B.: The disturbances in vision and in visual fields after ventriculography, Bull. Neurol. Inst. N.Y. **3**:190-209, 1933.

McKendree, C. A., and Doshay, L. J.: Visual disturbances of obscure etiology, produced by focal intracranial lesions implicating optic nerve; study of 6 cases of optic nerve compression with proven lesions, Bull. Neurol. Inst. N.Y. **5**:223-246, 1936.

Mooney, A. J., Carey, P., Ryan, M., and Bofin, P.: Parasagittal parieto-occipital meningioma with visual hallucinations, Am. J. Ophthalmol. **59**:197-205, 1965.

Moretti, G.: Su alcun rilievi a proposito della cosidetta sindromo di Anton, Riv. Otoneurooftalmol. **38**:605-609, 1963.

de Morsier, G.: Les hallucinations, Rev. Otoneuroophthalmol. **16**:241-352, 1938.

de Morsier, G., and Fellmann, H.: Disorders of body sensation caused by traumatic encephalopathy; some remarks on the pathogenesis of visual hallucinations (les troubles du schéma corporel dans l'encéphalopathie traumatique), Schweiz. Arch. Neurol. Neurochir. Psychiatr. **70**:42-47, 1952.

Nielsen, J. M., and FitzGibbon, J. P.: Agnosia, apraxia, aphasia: their value in cerebral localization, Bull. Los Angeles Neurol. Soc., 1936.

Nielsen, J. M., and von Hagen, K. O.: Three cases of mind blindness (visual agnosia): one due to softening in occipital lobes (autopsy), one due to anterior poliomyelitis (non-fatal), one due to drugs (transient), J. Nerv. Ment. Dis. 84:386-398, 1936.

Orlando, R., and Arndt, M.: La agnosia optica, Neuropsiquiatria 2:36-63, 1951.

Paillas, J. E., Alliez, J., and Tamalet, J.: Sur la valeur localisatrice des hallucinations visuelles paroxystiques, Ann. Med. Psychol. 2:473, 1949.

Parkinson, D., Rucker, C. W., and McCraig, K. W.: Visual hallucinations associated with tumors of occipital lobe, Arch. Neurol. Psychiatr. 68:66, 1952.

Quensel, F.: Die Erkrankungen der höheren optischen Zentren. In Schieck, F., and Brückner, A., editors: Kurzes Handbuch der Ophthalmologie, Berlin, 1931, Julius Springer, vol. 6, p. 324.

Renard, G.: Les hémianopsies: recherche et valeur diagnostique, Presse Med. 58:174-177, 1950.

Riese, W.: Craniopharyngiome chez une femme âgée de 57 ans; hallucinations visuelles et auditives; deuxième note sur la genèse des hallucinations survenant chez les malades atteints de lésions cérébrales, Rev. Neurol. 82:137-139, 1950.

Riley, H. A., Yaskin, J. C., Riggs, M. E., and Torney, A. S.: Bilateral blindness due to lesions in both occipital lobes, N.Y. State J. Med. 43:1619, 1943.

Sanford, H. S., and Blair, H. L.: Visual disturbances associated with tumors of the temporal lobe, Arch. Neurol. Psychiatr. 42: 21, 1939.

Savitsky, N., and Madonick, M. J.: Arch. Neurol. Psychiatr. 53:135, 1945; 55:232, 1946.

Seitelberger, F.: Über zerebrale Metamorphopsie, Wien. Med. Wochenschr. 102: 980-983, 1952.

Souter, W. C.: Visual disturbances of central origin. In Berens, C., editor: The eye and its diseases, Philadelphia, 1949, W. B. Saunders Co.

Tarachow, S.: Clinical value of hallucinations in localizing brain tumors, Am. J. Psychiatry 97:1434-1442, 1941.

Thiébaut, F., Guillaumat, L., and Brégeat, P.: L'hémianopsie relative, Bull. Soc. Fr. Ophtalmol. 60:73-80, 1947.

Triska, H. I.: Amaurose und Tumor Cerebri, Wien. Med. Wochenschr. 103:323-326, 1953.

Tyler, H. R.: Cerebral disorders of vision. In Smith, J. L., editor: Neuro-ophthalmology, St. Louis, 1968, The C. V. Mosby Co., vol. 4, pp. 266-281.

Vogel, P.: Die Bedeutung der Anamnese für die Diagnostik der Hirntumoren, Dtsch. Med. Wochenschr. 2:1277-1281, 1938.

Walsh, F. B., and Hoyt, W. F.: Aphasia, apraxia, agnosia, alexia. In Clinical neuro-ophthalmology, Baltimore, 1969, The Williams & Wilkins Co., pp. 98-119.

Weinberger, L. M., and Grant, F. C.: Visual hallucinations and their neuro-optical correlates (review), Arch. Ophthalmol. 23: 166-199, 1940.

Wernicke, E.: Der aphasische Symptomenkomplex, Breslau, 1874.

Wilbrand, H.: Seelenblindheit als Herderscheinung, Wiesbaden, 1887.

Wilbrand, H.: Die hemianopischen Gesichtsfeldformen und das optische Wahrnehmungszentrum, Wiesbaden, 1890.

**External aspect of the eyes**

Cushing, H.: The meningiomas, Brain 45: 282, 1922.

Elsberg, C. A., Hare, C. C., and Dyke, C. H.: Unilateral exophthalmos in intracranial tumors with special reference to its occurrence in meningiomas, Surg. Gynecol. Obstet. 55:681, 1932.

Uhthoff, W.: Die Augenveränderungen bei den Erkrankungen des Gehirns. In Graefe-Saemisch: Handbuch der gesamten Augenheilkunde, Leipzig, 1915, Wilhelm Engelmann, vol. 11, p. 1143.

**Corneal sensitivity**

Boberg-Ans, J.: Corneal sensitivity with special reference to clinical methods of examination (in Danish with an English summary), M.D. Thesis, Copenhagen, 1952.

von Frey, M.: Physiologische Sensibilitätsprüfungen, Verh. Dtsch. Ges. Inn. Med., pp. 19, 74, 1925.

von Frey, M., and Strughold, H.: Weitere Untersuchungen über das Verhalten von Hornhaut und Bindehaut des menschlichen Auges gegen Berührungsreize, Z. Biol. **84:** 321, 1926.

Kearns, T. P.: The neuro-ophthalmologic examination. In Smith, I. L., editor: Neuro-ophthalmology, Springfield, Ill., 1964, Charles C Thomas, Publisher, vol. 1.

Pannabecker, C. L.: Keratitis neuroparalytica: corneal lesions following operations for trigeminal neuralgia, Arch. Ophthalmol. **32:** 456-463, 1944.

Skrzypczak, J.: Der Kornealreflex und seine Bedeutung für die topische Hirntumordiagnostik, Klin. Monatsbl. Augenheilkd. **152:**465-475, 1968.

Weve, H.: Prüfung der Hornhautsensibilität. In Amsler, M., et al., editors: Lehrbuch der Augenheilkunde, Basel, 1954, S. Karger AG, p. 34.

### Pupils and pupillary reactions

Adie, W.: Complete and incomplete forms of the benign disorder characterized by tonic pupils and absent tendon reflexes, Br. J. Ophthalmol. **16:**449-461, 1932.

Adie, W.: Tonic pupils and absent tendon reflexes: a benign disorder sui generis: its complete and incomplete forms, Brain **55:** 98-113, 1932.

Adler, F. H., and Scheie, H. G.: The site of the disturbance in tonic pupils, Trans. Am. Ophthalmol. Soc. **38:**183, 1940.

Argyll Robertson, D.: Four cases of spinal miosis; with remarks on the action of light on the pupil, Edinburgh Med. J. **15:**487, 1869.

Barrios, R. R.: Diagnosis of localization of Claude Bernard-Horner's syndrome, Arch. Oftalmol. B. Air. **18:**629, 1943.

Bing, R., and Franceschetti, A.: Die Pupille. In Schieck, F., and Brückner, A., editors: Kurzes Handbuch der Ophthalmologie, Berlin, 1931, Julius Springer, vol. 6, p. 80.

Bolsi, D.: Rilievi clinici e nosologici sulla sindrome di Adie, Riv. Otoneurooftalmol. **27:**361-366, 1952.

Borgmann, H.: Basic data for clinical pupillography. I. The influence of light stimuli on the pupil reaction, Albrecht von Graefes Arch. Klin. Ophthalmol. **184:**291-299, 1972.

Bourbon, O. P.: An improved pupillometer, Am. J. Ophthalmol. **25:**1107, 1942.

Bürki, E.: Zur differentialdiagnostischen Bedeutung der reflexorischen Pupillenstarre, Schweiz. Med. Wochenschr. 34:774, 1937.

Demmler, P.: Pupillenstörungen bei Hirntumoren und ihre, Beziehungen zu anderen Schädigungen des Sehorgans, Arch. Psychiatr. **107:**701-710, 1938.

Dressler, M., and Wagner, H.: Über das Adiesche Syndrom, Schweiz. Arch. Neurol. Psychiatr. **39:**246; **40:**50, 1937.

Druault-Toufesco: Sur ce que peut apprendre l'examen des pupilles, Bull. Soc. Fr. Ophtalmol. **65:**62-66, 1952.

Duke-Elder, S.: Textbook of ophthalmology, St. Louis, 1938, 1949, The C. V. Mosby Co., vols. 2, p. 1156, and 4, pp. 3733-3805.

Dynes, J. B.: Adie's syndrome: its recognition and importance, J.A.M.A. **119:**1493, 1942.

Edinger, L.: Vorlesungen über den Bau der nervösen Zentralorgane des Menschen der Tiere, Leipzig, 1911, F. W. C. Vogel.

Fanta, H., and Reisner, H.: Argyll Robertsonsches Syndrom bei suprasellärem Tumor, Klin. Monatsbl. Augenheilkd. **121:**63-68, 1952.

Faure-Beaulieu, M., Christophe, J., and Isorni, P.: Pupillary areflexia and Parinaud's syndrome, Rev. Neurol. **73:**29, 1941.

Fischer-Brügge, K.: Das Kliuskanten-Syndrom, Acta Neurochir. **2:**36-68, 1951.

Foerster, O., and Gagel, O.: Z. Ges. Neurol. Psychiatr. **88:**1, 1932.

Foerster, O., Gagel, O., and Mahoney, W.: Über die Anatomie und Pathologie der Pupillarinnervation, Verh. Dtsch. Ges. Inn. Med. **48:**386, 1936.

Gunn, R. M.: Retrobulbar neuritis, Lancet **2:**412, 1904.

Harms, H.: Entwicklungsmöglichkeiten der Perimetrie, Graefe. Arch. Ophthalmol. **150:** 28, 1950.

Harms, H.: Hemianopische Pupillenstarre, Klin. Monatsbl. Augenheilkd. **118:**133-147, 1951.

Hartmann, E.: Les pupilles dans les traumatismes et les tumeurs cérébrales, Rev. Neurol. **69:**646-656, 1938.

Hess, C.: Untersuchungen zur Physiologie und Pathologie des Pupillenspieles, Arch. Augenheilkd. **60:**327-389, 1908.

Horner, F.: Über eine Form von Ptosis, Klin. Monatsbl. Augenheilkd. **7:**193-198, 1869.

Inciardi, J. A.: A routine for diagnosing abnormal pupils, Dis. Eye Ear Nose Throat 2:219, 1942.

Ingvar, S.: The pathogenesis of the Argyll Robertson phenomenon, Johns Hopkins Med. J. 43:363, 396, 1928.

Jackson, E.: A simple pupillometer, Am. J. Ophthalmol. 25:871, 1942.

Jackson, H.: Lancet 1:11, 1894.

Jaensch, P. A.: Pupille, Handbuch der Neurologie, Berlin, 1936, Julius Springer, vol. 4.

Jaensch, P. A.: Grenzgebiet der Ophthalmologie und Neurologie; Pupille, 1933-1937, Fortschr. Neurol. Psychiatr. 10:366-384, 1938.

Jaffe, N. S.: Localization of lesions causing Horner's syndrome, Arch. Ophthalmol. 44:710-728, 1950.

Jefferson, G.: The tentorial-pressure cone, Arch. Neurol. Psychiatr. 40:857, 1938.

Kearns, T. P.: The neuro-ophthalmologic examination. In Smith, J. L., editor: Neuro-ophthalmology, Springfield, Ill., 1964, Charles C Thomas, Publisher, vol. 1.

Kehrer, F.: Die Kuppelungen von Pupillenstörungen mit Aufhebung der Sehnervenreflexe (Adie-Syndrom, Pupillotonie, Pseudotabes, konstitutionelle Areflexie.), Leipzig, 1937, Georg Thieme Verlag KG.

Kennedy, F., Wortis, H., Reichard, J. D., and Fair, B. B.: Adie's syndrome, Arch. Ophthalmol. 19:68-80, 1938.

Kerr, F. W. L.: The pupil: functional anatomy and clinical correlation. In Smith, J. L., editor: Neuro-ophthalmology, St. Louis, 1968, The C. V. Mosby Co., vol. 4, p. 49.

Krayenbühl, H., and Noto, G.: Das intrakranielle subdurale Hämatom, Bern, 1949, Hans Huber.

Langdon, H. M.: Three cases of Argyll Robertson pupil, apparently non-luetic, Am. J. Ophthalmol. 23:331, 1940.

Leathart, P. W.: The tabetic pupil, Br. J. Ophthalmol. 25:111, 1941.

Leathart, P. W.: The tonic pupil syndrome, Br. J. Ophthalmol. 28:60, 1942.

Levatin, P.: Pupillary escape in disease of the retina or optic nerve, Arch. Ophthalmol. 62:768, 1959.

Loewenfeld, I. E.: The Argyll Robertson pupil, 1869-1969: a critical survey of the literature, Surv. Ophthalmol. 14:199-299, 1969.

Lowenstein, O.: Pupillography: its significance in clinical neurology, Arch. Neurol. Psychiatr. 44:227, 1940.

Lowenstein, O.: Clinical pupillary symptoms in lesions of the optic nerve: optic chiasm and optic tract, Arch. Ophthalmol. 52:385, 1954.

Lowenstein, O., and Friedman, E. D.: Pupillographic studies: present state of pupillography; its method and diagnostic significance, Arch. Ophthalmol. 27:969-993, 1942.

Lowenstein, O., and Friedman, E. D.: Adie's syndrome (pupillotonie, pseudotabes), Arch. Ophthalmol. 28:1042-1068, 1942.

McKinney, J. M., and Frocht, M.: Adie's syndrome: a nonluetic disease simulating tabes dorsalis, Am. J. Med. Sci. 199:546, 1940.

Morone, G., and Trimarchi, F.: Pupillographia, Atti Soc. Oftalmol. Ital. 53:423-487, 1971.

Nathan, P. W., and Turner, J. W. A.: Argyll Robertson's pupil: efferent pathway for contraction, Brain 65:343, 1942.

Pagliarani, N.: On the localizing value of Foerster's pharmacodynamic test in lesions of the cervical sympathetic, Proceedings of the Sixteenth International Congress on Ophthalmology, London, 1950, vol. 1, pp. 375-380.

de Quervain, F.: Die starre Pupillenerweiterung in der Diagnostik der Schädel- und Hirntraumen, Schweiz. Med. Wochenschr. 1:75, 1935.

Rook, J. T.: Adie's syndrome, Arch. Ophthalmol. 29:936, 1943.

Rosen, E.: Adie's syndrome, Arch. Ophthalmol. 30:553, 1943.

Rutkowski, P. C., and Thompson, H. S.: Mydriasis and increased intraocular pressure. I. Pupillographic studies, Arch. Ophthalmol. 87:21-24, 1972.

Schachter, M.: Pupillary disturbances in the course of cerebral tumors, Confin. Neurol. 5:298, 1943.

Schaefer, W. D., and Richter, G.: The significance of the mecholyl test for the diagnosis of tonic pupil, Ber. Dtsch. Ophthalmol. Ges. 71:554-557, 1972.

Scharfetter, F.: Mydriasis und Lichtstarre, Schweiz. Arch. Neurol. Neurochir. Psychiatr. 96:386-392, 1965.

Scheie, H. G.: Site of disturbance in Adie's syndrome, Arch. Ophthalmol. 24:225-237, 1940.

Schwab, R. S.: Differential diagnosis between Argyll Robertson and Adie's myotonic pupil, Am. J. Ophthalmol. 23:456, 1940.

Sears, M. L.: The cause of the Argyll Robertson pupil, Am. J. Ophthalmol. **72:** 488-489, 1971.

Stern, H. J.: A simple method for the early diagnosis of abnormalities of the pupillary reaction, Br. J. Ophthalmol. **28:**275, 1944.

Thompson, H. S.: Afferent pupillary defects. Pupillary findings associated with defects of the afferent arm of the pupillary light reflex area, Am. J. Ophthalmol. **62:**860-873, 1966.

Thompson, H. S.: Medikamentöse Pupillendiagnostik. In Dodd, E., and Schrader, K., editors: Die normale und gestörte Pupillenbewegung, Munich, 1973, J. F. Bergmann.

Turner, E. A.: Pupillary inequalities in man, Brain **68:**98, 1945.

Walsh, F. B., and Hoyt, W. F.: The pupil in neurologic diagnosis. In Clinical neuroophthalmology, Baltimore, 1969, The Williams & Wilkins Co.

Wernicke, C.: Hemianopische Pupillen-Reaktion, Virchows Arch. (Pathol. Anat.) **56:** 397, 1872.

Westphal, A.: Weiterer Beitrag zur Pathologie der Pupille, Neurol. Zentralbl. **32:**517, 1913.

Weve, H.: Vorrichtung zur Untersuchung der hemianopischen Pupillarreaktion, Klin. Monatsbl. Augenheilkd. **61:**140, 1918.

Weve, H.: Untersuchung der Pupille. In Amsler, M., et al., editors: Lehrbuch der Augenheilkunde, Basel, 1954, S. Karger AG, p. 10.

Wilson, S. A. K.: Some problems in neurology. I. The Argyll Robertson pupil, J. Neurol. Psychopathol. **2:**1-25, 1921.

Wilson, S. A. K., and Gerstle, M.: The Argyll Robertson sign in mesencephalic tumors, Arch. Neurol. Psychiatr. **22:**9-18, 1929.

Wormser, P.: Die Reaktion der Pupille auf Pharmaka nach Unterbrechung der sympathischen Pupillenbahn, Confin. Neurol. **8:** 5, 249, 1947-1948.

**Motility of the eyes (extraocular muscle palsies, palsies of conjugate eye movements, nystagmus)**

Alpers, B. J.: Partial paralysis of upward gaze (incomplete Parinaud syndrome), Confin. Neurol. **15:**1-12, 1942.

Aragones-Olle, J. M., and Obach-Tuca, J.: Contribucion al estudio electronistagmografico, con registro simultaneo de la actividad de los musculos del cuello, durante las pruebas vestibulares caloricas en los tumores endocraeneales, Rev. Esp. Otoneurooftalmol. Neurocir. **25:**378-397, 1966.

Arganaraz, R.: Nystagmus, conjugate deviations and paralyses of associated movements in cerebral diseases, Arch. Oftalmol. B. Air. **17:**113-123, 1942.

Bach-y-Rita, P., Collins, C. C., and Hyde, J. E., editors: The control of eye movements, New York, 1971, Academic Press, Inc.

Bárány, R.: Zur Klinik und Theorie des Eisenbahnnystagmus, Arch. Augenheilkd. **88:**139, 1921.

Behr, C.: Die Erkrankungen der Augennerven. In Schieck, F., and Brückner, A., editors: Kurzes Handbuch der Ophthalmologie, Berlin, 1931, Julius Springer, vol. 6, p. 156.

Bender, M. B., and Savitsky, N.: Paralysis of divergence, Arch. Ophthalmol. **23:**1046-1051, 1940.

Beres, C., and MacAlpine, P. T.: Motor anomalies of the eye. In Berens, C., editor: The eye and its diseases, Philadelphia, 1949, W. B. Saunders Co.

Best, F.: Localization of cerebral lesions producing disturbances of homolateral eye movements, Arch. Ophthalmol. **144:**25-40, 1941.

Bielschowsky, A.: Lectures on motor anomalies of eyes; paralysis of conjugate movements of eyes, Arch. Ophthalmol. **13:**569-583, 1935.

Bielschowsky, A.: Disturbances of vertical motor muscles, Acta Ophthalmol. **16:**235-270, 1938.

Bielschowsky, A.: Lectures on motor anomalies; paralysis of individual eye muscles: abducens-nerve paralysis, Am. J. Ophthalmol. **22:**357-367, 1939.

Bielschowsky, A.: Lectures on motor anomalies; oculomotor nerve paralysis and ophthalmoplegias, Am. J. Ophthalmol. **22:** 484-498, 1939.

Bielschowsky, A.: Lectures on motor anomalies; supranuclear paralyses, Am. J. Ophthalmol. **22:**603-613, 1939.

Bird, A. C., and Sanders, M. D.: Defects in supranuclear control of horizontal eye movements, Trans. Ophthalmol. Soc. U.K. **90:**417-432, 1970.

Björk, A., and Kugelberg, E.: Motor unit activity in the human extraocular muscles,

Electroencephalogr. Clin. Neurophysiol. **5:** 271, 1953.

Blodi, F. C., and Van Allen, M.: Electromyography of extraocular muscles in fusional movements, Am. J. Ophthalmol. **44:** 136-144, 1957.

van Bogaert, L.: Contribution anatomoclinique à l'étude du nystagmus optique, Rev. Otoneurooculist. **5:**793, 1927.

Böhringer, H. R., and Koenig, F.: Die diagnostische Bedeutung der vertikalen Blicklähmung, Ophthalmologica **125:**357, 1953.

Breinin, G. M.: The electrophysiology of extraocular muscle, Toronto, 1962, University of Toronto Press.

Breinin, G. M.: Research in strabismus. In Vision and its disorders, Bethesda, 1967, National Institute of Neurological Diseases and Blindness, Monograph No. 4, pp. 50-64.

Cairns, H.: Peripheral ocular palsies from neuro-surgical point of view, Trans. Ophthalmol. Soc. U.K. **58:**464-482, 1938.

Cawthorne, T., Dix, M. R., and Hood, J. D.: Recent advances in electronystagmographic technique with special reference to its value in clinical diagnosis. In Smith, J. L., editor: Neuro-ophthalmology, St. Louis, 1968, The C. V. Mosby Co., vol. 4, pp. 81-109.

Chamlin, M., and Davidoff, L. M.: Divergence paralysis with increased intracranial pressure, Arch. Ophthalmol. **46:**145-147, 1951.

Chandy, J., and Isaiah, P.: Ophthalmoplegia —a clinical study, Indian J. Surg. **15:**268-274, 1953.

Cogan, D. G.: Neurology of ocular muscles, Springfield, 1956, Charles C Thomas, Publisher.

Cogan, D. H., and Loeb, D. R.: Optokinetic response and intracranial lesions, Arch. Neurol. Psychiatr. **61:**183, 1949.

Coppez, L.: Nystagmus, Ophthalmologica **104:**102-120, 1942.

Coppez, H., and Buys, E.: Graphic records of nystagmus, Ophthalmoscope, 1909.

Cords, R.: Die Bedeutung des optischmotorischen Nystagmus für die neurologische Diagnostik, Dtsch. Z. Nervenheilk. **84:**125, 1925.

Cranmer, R.: Nystagmus related to lesions of the central vestibular apparatus and the cerebellum, Ann. Otol. **60:**186-196, 1951.

Cushing, H.: Strangulation of the nervi abducentes by lateral branches of the basilar artery in cases of brain tumor, with an explanation of some obscure palsies on the basis of arterial obstruction, Brain 33:204-235, 1910-1911.

Daroff, R. B., and Hoyt, W. F.: Supranuclear disorders of ocular control systems in man. In Bach-y-Rita, P., Collins, C. C., and Hyde, J. E., editors: The control of eye movements, New York, 1971, Academic Press, Inc., pp. 175-235.

Daroff, R. B., and Troost, B. T.: Upbeat nystagmus, J.A.M.A. **225:**312, 1973.

DeJong, R. N.: Nystagmus: appraisal and classification, Arch. Neurol. Psychiatr. **55:** 43-56, 1946.

Delplace, M.-P., Rossazza, C., and Larmande, A. M.: The optokinetic test and its topographical value in hemispheric lesions, Rev. Otoneuroophthalmol. **46:**149-154, 1974.

De Recondo, J.: Les mouvements conjugés oculaires et leurs diverses modalités d'atteinte, Paris, 1967, Masson & Cie, Editeurs.

De Recondo, J.: Etude générale des paralysies de la motilité conjuguée oculaire: élements de définition; les paralysies internucléaires), Rev. Otoneuroophtalmol. **44:**9-24, 1972.

Dichgans, J., and Bizzi, E.: Cerebral control of eye movements and motion perception, Bibliotheca Ophthalmologica, No. 82, Basel, 1972, S. Karger AG.

Druckman, R., Ellis, P., Kleinfeld, J., and Waldman, M.: Seesaw nystagmus, Arch. Ophthalmol. **76:**668-675, 1966.

Duke-Elder, S., and Scott, G. I.: Neuro-ophthalmology. In Duke-Elder, S., editor: System of ophthalmology, vol. 12, St. Louis, 1971, The C. V. Mosby Co.

Enoksson, P.: Internuclear ophthalmoplegia and paralysis of horizontal gaze, Acta Ophthalmol. **43:**697-707, 1965.

Esslen, E., and Papst, W.: Die Bedeutung der Elektromyographie für die Analyse von Motilitätas störungen der Augen, Bibl. Ophthalmol. **57:**1, 1961.

Fink, W. H.: Etiologic considerations of vertical muscle defects, Am. J. Ophthalmol. **36:**1427, 1551, 1953.

Fox, J. C.: Disorders of optic nystagmus due to cerebral tumors, Arch. Neurol. Psychiatr. **28:**1007-1029, 1932.

Fox, J. C., and Holmes, G.: Optic nystagmus and tumors, Brain **49:**333, 1926.

Franceschetti, A.: Le diagnostic des paralysies des différents muscles oculaires, Bull. Soc. Fr. Ophtalmol. **5:**471-498, 1936.

Franceschetti, A., and Blum, J. D.: Motilitätsstörungen des Auges. In Amsler, M., et al., editors: Lehrbuch der Augenheilkunde, Basel, 1954, S. Karger AG.

Franceschetti, A., Monnier, M., and Dieterle, P.: Electronystagmography in the analysis of congenital nystagmus, Trans. Ophthalmol. Soc. U.K. **72:**515, 1952.

Freeman, W.: Paralysis of associated lateral movements of the eyes, Arch. Neurol. Psychiatr. **7:**454-487, 1922.

Frenzel, H.: Spontan- und Provokations-Nystagmus als Krankheitssymptom, Berlin, 1955, Julius Springer.

Gay, A. J., Newman, N. M., Keltner, J. L., and Stroud, M. H.: Eye movement disorders, St. Louis, 1974, The C. V. Mosby Co.

Gormann, W. F., and Brock, S.: Nystagmus: its mechanism and significance, Am. J. Med. Sci. **220:**225-233, 1950.

von Graefe, A.: Symptomlehre der Augenmuskellähmungen, 1867.

Green, W. R., Hackett, E. R., and Schlesinger, N. S.: Neuro-ophthalmologic evaluation of oculomotor nerve paralysis, Arch. Ophthalmol. **72:**154-167, 1964.

Hagedoorn, A.: A new diagnostic motility scheme, Am. J. Ophthalmol. **25:**726-728, 1942.

Hallpike, C. S., Hood, J. D., and Trinder, E.: Some observations on the technical and clinical problems of electronystagmography, Confin. Neurol. **20:**232, 1960.

Hamburger, F. A.: Augenmuskellähmungen, Bücherei des Augenarztes, Heft 46, Stuttgart, 1966, Ferdinand Enke Verlag.

Harms, H.: Examination in paralysis of ocular muscles, Arch. Ophthalmol. **144:**129-149, 1941.

Hart, C. W. J.: The role of nystagmography in clinical diagnosis, Arch. Otolaryngol. **84:**631-633, 1966.

Henderson, J. W., and Crosby, E. C.: An experimental study of optokinetic responses, Arch. Ophthalmol. **47:**43-54, 1952.

Hess, W. R.: Die graphische Darstellung von Bewegungsstörungen der Augen mit Beispieltafeln zur Diagnose von Augenmuskellähmungen, Arch. Augenheilkd. **70:**10, 1912.

Holmes, G.: Palsies of the conjugate ocular movements, Br. J. Ophthalmol. **5:**241-250, 1921.

Holmes, G., and Horrax, G.: Disturbances of spatial orientation and visual attention with loss of stereoscopic vision, Arch. Neurol. Psychiatr. **1:**385, 1919.

Huber, A.: Die peripheren Augenmuskellähmungen, Ber. Dtsch. Ophthalmol. Ges. **67:**25-46, 1965.

Huber, A.: Topographische und ätiologische Analyse von Augenmuskellähmungen im Elektromyogramm, Ophthalmologica **149:**359-374, 1965.

Huber, A.: Elektromyographie der Augenmuskeln, Ophthalmologica **169:**111-126, 1974.

Huber, A., and Esslen, E.: Diagnostic des myopathies oculaires à l'aide de l'electromyographie, Bull. Soc. Fr. Ophtalmol. **80:**460-472, 1967.

Huber, A., and Meyer, M.: Die elektromyographisch-elektrookulographische Analyse peripherer und zentraler Störungen der Augenmotorik, Ophthalmologica **172:**194-204, 1976.

Jaensch, P. A.: Störungen der Augenbewegungen bei Erkrankungen des Zentralnervensystems, Fortschr. Neurol. Psychiatr. **9:**114-130, 1937.

Jayle, G. E. A.: A propos des paralysies d'origine supra-nucléaire; essai de classification, Bull. Soc. Ophthalmol. Fr. **50:**144-152, 1938.

Jung, R., and Kornhuber, H. H.: Results of electronystagmography in man; the value of optokinetic, vestibular and spontaneous nystagmus for neurologic diagnosis and research. In Bender, M. B., editor: The oculomotor system, New York, 1964, Harper & Row, Publishers.

Kestenbaum, A.: Zur Klinik des optokinetischen Nystagmus, Graefe. Arch. Ophthalmol. **124:**113, 1930.

Kestenbaum, A.: Blickbewegungen und Blicklähmungen, Confin. Neurol. **2:**121, 1939.

Kestenbaum, A.: Topical diagnosis of disturbed oculomotor motility, Am. J. Ophthalmol. **29:**94-95, 1946.

Knapp, E.: Kommt Spontan-Nystagmus bei Gesunden vor? HNO. Beih. Hals-Nasen-Ohren Heilk. **2:**17-19, 1950.

Koerner, F., and Kommerell, G.: Examination of eye movements. Its diagnostic value in neuroophthalmology, Ther. Umsch. **32:**40-46, 1975.

Kommerell, G.: Die internukleäre Ophthalmoplegie: Nystagmographische Analyse, Klin. Monatsbl. Augenheilkd. **158:**349-358, 1971.

Lancaster, W.: Fifty years' experience in ocular motility, Am. J. Ophthalmol. 24: 485, 619, 741, 1941.

Larmande, A. M., Quere, M. A., Rossazza, C., and Delplace, M. P.: Oculomotor involvement in homonymous lateral hemianopia, Arch. Ophthalmol. 32:87-95, 1972.

Leiva, A. V.: Paralisis de los nervios oculomotores, estudio de 40 casos, Arch. Soc. Cubana Oftalmol. 3:104-122, 1953.

Lenz, H.: Das Verhalten des optokinetischen Nystagmus bei einigen Fällen von Lappenresektionen, Nervenarzt 14:124-126, 1941.

Leydhecker, W.: Divergenzlähmung, Klin. Monatsbl. Augenheilkd. 123:83-86, 1953.

Ling, W., and Gay, A. J.: Optokinetic nystagmus: a proposed pathway and its clinical application. In Smith, J. L., editor: Neuro-ophthalmology, St. Louis, 1968, The C. V. Mosby Co., vol. 4, pp. 117-123.

Lippmann, O.: Paralysis of divergence due to cerebellar tumor, Arch. Ophthalmol. 31: 299, 1944.

Lutz, A.: Über die Bahnen der Blickwendung und deren Dissoziierung, Klin. Monatsbl. Augenheilkd. 70:213-235, 1923.

Lyle, D. J.: Divergence insufficiency, Arch. Ophthalmol. 52:858, 1954.

Lyle, D. J., and Mayfield, F. H.: Retraction nystagmus, Am. J. Ophthalmol. 37:177, 1954.

Lyle, T. K., and Jackson, S.: Practical orthoptics in the treatment of squint, London, 1949, H. Lewis Co.

Maddox, E. E.: Test and studies of the ocular muscles, Philadelphia, 1907, Keystone Publishing Co.

Malbrán, J.: Anomalies of the vertical movements of the eyes, Arch. Oftalmol. B. Air. 15:65-102, 1940.

Monnier, M., and Hufschmidt, H. J.: Das Elektro-Oculogramm (EOG) und Elektronystagmogramm (ENG) beim Menschen, Helv. Physiol. Pharmacol. Acta 9:348-366, 1951.

Nicolai, H.: Weitere Erfahrungen auf dem Gebiet der objektiven Sehschärfenbestimmung mit optokinetischem Nystagmus, Klin. Monatsbl. Augenheilkd. 124:81, 1954.

Norden, von G., and Preziosi, T. J.: Eye movement recordings in neurological disorders, Arch. Ophthalmol. 76:162-171, 1966.

Nordmann, J.: Considérations sur les paralysies oculo-motrices verticales, Rev. Otoneuroophtalmol. 24:152-154, 1952.

O'Brien, F. H., and Bender, M. B.: Localizing value of vertical nystagmus, Arch. Neurol. Psychiatr. 54:378-380, 1945.

Ohm, J.: Die klinische Bedeutung des optischen Drehnystagmus, Klin. Monatsbl. Augenheilkd. 68:323, 1922.

Ohm, J.: Der optische Drehnystagmus bei Augen- und Allgemeinleiden, Graefe. Arch. Ophthalmol. 114:169-191, 1924.

Ohm, J.: Zur Augenzitternkunde; über den Einfluss der gleichseitigen Halbblindheit auf den optokinetischen Nystagmus, Graefe. Arch. Ophthalmol. 135:200-219, 1936.

Parinaud, M.: Paralysie de la convergence, paralysie de la divergence, Ann. Oculist. 95:205, 1886.

Parinaud, M.: Paralysie des mouvements associés des yeux, Ann. Oculist. 175:47-66, 1938.

Rintelen, F.: Zur Kenntnis der Blickparesen, Ophthalmologica 114:325-331, 1947.

Robbins, A. R.: Divergence paralysis with autopsy report, Am. J. Ophthalmol. 24: 556-557, 1941.

Roelofs, C. O.: Optokinetic nystagmus, Doc. Ophthalmol. 7/8:579, 1954.

Roper, K. L.: Paralysis of convergence, Arch. Ophthalmol. 25:336-353, 1941.

Roussel, F.: Die Diagnostik der vertikalen Doppelbilder: (a) Koordinometer nach Hess-Lees; (b) Untersuchung nach Franceschetti, Bull. Soc. Belge Ophtalmol. 101: 439-444, 1952.

Rucker, C. W.: Nystagmus, Am. J. Ophthalmol. 2:250, 1953.

Sager, O., and Voiculescu, V.: Etudes expérimentales sur les voies cortico-oculogyres de verticalité, Folia Psychiatr. Neurol. Neurochir. Neerl. 53:394-407, 1950.

Salleras, A., Carrillo, A., and Amezuà, L.: Divergencia vertical de la mirada (Fenomeno de Hertwig-Magendie), Arch. Oftalmol. B. Air. 25:317-321, 1950.

Sanders, M. D., and Bird, A. C.: Supranuclear abnormalities of the vertical ocular motor system, Trans. Ophthalmol. Soc. U.K. 90: 433-450, 1970.

Savitsky, N., and Madonick, M. J.: Arch. Neurol. Psychiatr. 53:135, 1945; 55:232, 1946.

Scala, N. P., and Spiegel, E. A.: Mechanism of optokinetic nystagmus, Trans. Am. Acad. Ophthalmol. 43:277-303, 1938.

Schifferli, P.: Etude par enregistrement photographique de la motricité oculaire dans l'exploration, dans la reconnaissance et dans la représentation visuelles, Basel, 1953, S. Karger AG.

Schulze, F.: Electromyography in opthalmology, Leipzig, 1972, Georg Thieme Verlag KG.

Schuster, H.: Zur Pathologie der vertikalen Blicklähmung, Münch. Med. Wochenschr. **16**:497, 1921.

Sédan, J., and Séden-Bauby, S.: Principe, but, mécanisme, technique, variétés et résultats de la provocation diplopique, Rev. Otoneuroophtalmol. **21**:4, 200, 1949.

Sen Gupta, M.: Upward gaze palsy with convergence paralysis (Parinaud's syndrome) with a case report, Proc. All-India Ophthalmol. Soc. **12**:187-201, 1951.

Spaeth, E. B.: Nystagmus: its diagnostic significance, Arch. Ophthalmol. **44**:549-560, 1950.

Spiller, W. G.: Corticonuclear tracts for associated ocular movements, Arch. Neurol. Psychiatr. **28**:251, 1932.

Stadlin, W.: Hémianopsie et nystagmus optocinétique, Ophthalmologica **118**:383, 1949.

Stenvers, H. W.: On the optic (opto-kinetic, opto-motorial) nystagmus, Acta Otolaryngol. **8**:545, 1925.

Stenvers, H. W.: Die Wichtigkeit der optomotorischen Reaktionen für die klinische Diagnostik, Z. Ges. Neurol. Psychiatr. **152**:197-207, 1935.

Stenvers, H. W.: Über die klinische Bedeutung des optischen Nystagmus für die cerebrale Diagnostik, Schweiz. Arch. Neurol. Neurochir. Psychiatr. **14**:279, 1949.

Strauss, H.: Hirnlokalisatorische Bedeutung des einseitigen Ausfalls des optokinetischen Nystagmus, Z. Ges. Neurol. Psychiatr. **143**:427, 1933.

Tamler, E., and Jampolsky, A.: Electromyographic study of following movements of the eye between tertiary positions, Arch. Ophthalmol. **62**:804-809, 1959.

Teuber, H. L., and Bender, M. B.: Neuro-ophthalmology: the oculomotor system, Progr. Neurol. Psychiatr. **6**:148-178, 1951.

Torok, N., Guillemin, V., Jr., and Barnothy, J. M.: Photoelectric nystagmography, Ann. Otol. **60**:917-926, 1951.

Walsh, F. B.: Certain abnormalities of ocular movements: their importance in general and neurologic diagnosis, Bull. N.Y. Acad. Med. **19**:253-272, 1943.

Walsh, F. B., and Hoyt, W. F.: The ocular motor system. In Clinical neuro-ophthalmology, Baltimore, 1969, The Williams & Wilkins Co., pp. 130-347.

Walsh, F. B., and Hoyt, W. F.: Disorders of muscles. In Clinical neuro-ophthalmology, Baltimore, 1969, The Williams & Wilkins Co., pp. 1242-1311.

Weekers, R., and Roussel, F.: La mesure de la fréquence de fusion en clinique, Doc. Ophthalmol. **2**:130, 1948.

Weve, H.: Untersuchung der Bewegungsstörungen. In Amsler, M., et al., editors: Lehrbuch der Augenheilkunde, Basel, 1954, S. Karger AG, p. 47.

White, J. W.: What is the minimum routine examination of muscles? Arch. Ophthalmol. **24**:112-131, 1941.

Wilson, Kinnier: Cited in Rea, R. L.: Neuro-ophthalmology, 1941, The C. V. Mosby Co., p. 158.

## Fundus

Amalric, R., Bessou, P., and Aubry, J. P.: Angioscopie et angiographie rétiniennes à la fluorescéine en oto-neuro-ophtalmologie, Soc. Otoneuroophtalmol. de Toulouse, 1966.

Bailliart, P.: La circulation rétinienne à l'état normal et à l'état pathologique, Paris, 1923, Gaston Doin & Cie.

Barut, C.: Valeur séméiologique de la mesure de la pression de l'artère centrale de la rétine, Conférences Lyonnaises d'Ophtalmologie, 1968, p. 93.

Baurmann, H., and Wink, B.: Interpretation of the fluorescence of the optic nerve head. I. The normal disc, Albrecht von Graefes Arch. Klin. Ophthalmol. **182**:114-119, 1971.

Bedavanija, A.: Dynamometer-Eichkurve mit Hilfe der Applanationstonometrie, Med. Dissertation, Bonn, 1960.

Bettelheim, H.: Vergleichende ophthalmodynamometrische und ophthalmodynamographische Untersuchungen bei obliterierenden Prozessen der Karotiden, Klin. Monatsbl. Augenheilkd. **146**:801-819, 1965.

Bettelheim, H.: Experience with ophthalmodynamography in the diagnosis of carotid occlusion, Am. J. Ophthalmol. **64**:689, 1967.

Bonamour, G., and Wertheimer, J.: Valeur sémiologique de l'atrophie optique unilatérale, Ann. Oculist. **183**:199-215, 1950.

Brückner, A.: Ophthalmoskopie. In Schieck, F., and Brückner, A., editors: Kurzes Handbuch der Ophthalmologie, Berlin, 1931, Julius Springer, vol. 2, p. 862.

Charamis, J., Katsourakis, N., and Mandras, G.: The study of the cerebroretinal circulation by intravenous fluorescein injection, Am. J. Ophthalmol. **61**:1078-1080, 1966.

Duke-Elder, S., and Scott, G.: Neuro-ophthalmology. In Duke-Elder, S., editor: System of ophthalmology, vol. 12, St. Louis, 1971, The C. V. Mosby Co.

Ferrer, O.: Serial fluorescein fundus photography of retinal circulation. A description of technique, Am. J. Ophthalmol. **60**:587-591, 1965.

Gay, A. J.: Clinical ophthalmodynamometry, Int. Ophthalmol. Clin. **7**:729-744, 1967.

Hager, H.: Objektive elektrische Dynamometrie mit Hilfe des Bulbus-Orbita-Pulses, XVII. Concilium Ophthalmologicum, Belgica, 1958.

Hardy, H.: Ophthalmoscopy. In Berens, C., editor: The eye and its diseases, Philadelphia, 1949, W. B. Saunders Co., p. 174.

Hartmann, E., and Guillaumat, L.: Aspect du fond d'oeil dans les tumeurs intracrâniennes: étude statistique, Ann. Oculist. **175**:717-737, 1938.

Hollenhorst, R. W.: Ophthalmodynamometry in the diagnosis of intracerebral hypotension, Mayo Clin. Proc. **38**:532, 1963.

Horrax, G.: Importance of optic nerve atrophy in diagnosis of favorable brain tumors, Surg. Clin. North Am. **21**:903-912, 1941.

Hoyt, W. F., and Kommerell, G.: Der Fundus oculi bei homonymer Hemianopsie, Klin. Monatsbl. Augenheilkd. **162**:456-464, 1973.

Hoyt, W. F., Schlicke, B., and Eckelhoff, R. J.: Funduscopic appearance of a nerve-fibre-bundle defect, Br. J. Ophthalmol. **56**:577-583, 1972.

Hyman, B. N.: Doppler sonography. A bedside non-invasive method for assessment of carotid artery disease, Am. J. Ophthalmol. **77**:227-231, 1974.

Justice, J., and Sever, R. J.: Technique of fluorescein fundus photography. In Smith, J. L., editor: Neuro-ophthalmology, St. Louis, 1965, The C. V. Mosby Co., vol. 2, pp. 82-83.

Jütte, A., and Lemke, L.: Intravitalfärbung am Augenhintergrund mit Fluoreszein-Natrium, Bücherei des Augenarztes, no. 49, Stuttgart, 1968, Ferdinand Enke.

Keller, H., Bollinger, A., and Baumgartner, G.: Doppler ultrasound sonography in the diagnosis of occlusions and stenoses of the carotid arteries with paradoxical or absent neurological findings, J. Neurol. **207**:211-226, 1974.

Matsui, J., Koh, K., and Tashiro, T.: Studies on the fluorescence fundus photography. II. Clinical significances of the serial fluorescence fundus photography in some retinal vascular lesions, Acta Soc. Ophthalmol. Jpn. **70**:613-619, 1966. Cited in Zentralbl. Augenheilkd. **97**:430, 1967.

Niesel, P.: Ophthalmodynamometrie, Ophthalmologica **158**:342-352, 1969.

Norton, E. W. D.: Angiography of ocular fundus. In Smith, J. L., editor: Neuro-ophthalmology, St. Louis, 1965, The C. V. Mosby Co., vol. 2, pp. 62-81.

Novotny, H., and Alvis, D. L.: A method of photographing fluorescene in circulating blood in the human retina, Circulation **24**:82-86, 1961.

Raverdino, E.: Sull'importanza dei sintomi oftalmoscopici prima e dopo gli interventi per tumori endocranici, Riv. Otoneuroof-talmol. **15**:532-543, 1938.

Rintelen, F.: Zur diagnostischen Bedeutung der Dynamometrie, Klin. Monatsbl. Augenheilkd. **100**:469, 1938.

Salmon, M. L., and Gay, A. J.: Ophthalmodynamography, Int. Ophthalmol. Clin. **7**:744, 1967.

Smith, J. L., editor: Neuro-ophthalmology, Springfield, Ill., 1964, Charles C Thomas, Publisher, vol. 1.

Streiff, B., and Monnier, M.: Der retinale Blutdruck im gesunden und kranken Organismus, Berlin, 1946, Julius Springer.

Vogt, A.: Die Nervenfaserzeichnung der menschlichen Netzhaut im rotfreien Licht, Klin. Monatsbl. Augenheilkd. **66**:718, 1921.

Walsh, F. B., and Hoyt, W. F.: Optic atrophy. In Clinical neuro-ophthalmology, Baltimore, 1969, The Williams & Wilkins Co., p. 631.

Weigelin, E., and Lobstein, A.: Ophthalmodynamometry, New York, 1963, Hepner.

Wessing, A.: Fluoreszenzangiographie der Retina, Stuttgart, 1968, Georg Thieme Verlag KG.

Weve, H.: Ophthalmoskopie. In Amsler, M., et al., editors: Lehrbuch der Augenheilkunde, Basel, 1954, S. Karger AG, p. 11.

Witmer, R.: Differential diagnostische Aspekte bei retinalen Gefässtörungen und Papillenödem, Ophthalmologica **156**:313-321, 1968.

Woltman, H. W.: The ophthalmoscope in neurologic diagnosis, Mayo Clin. Proc. **26**: 226-231, 1951.

**Visual acuity**

Birkhäuser, R.: Scalae typographicae, Basel, A. E. Birkhäuser.

Brückner, A.: Die Untersuchung der Sehschärfe. In Schieck, F., and Brückner, A., editors: Kurzes Handbuch der Ophthalmologie, Berlin, 1931, Julius Springer, vol. 2, p. 921.

Busch, E., and Moller, H. U.: Ophthalmological symptoms in intracranial tumors with special reference to visual acuity, Acta Ophthalmol. **16**:453-454, 1938.

Elsberg, C. A., and Spotnitz, H.: Value of quantitative visual test for localization of supratentorial tumors of brain; preliminary report, Bull. Neurol. Inst. N.Y. **6**:411-420, 1937.

Goldmann, H.: Objektive Sehschärfenbestimmung, Ophthalmologica **105**:240-252, 1943.

Günther, G.: Objektive Sehschärfenbestimmung, Samml. Zwangl. Abh. aus d. Gebiete d. Augenheilkd., Halle a.d.S., 1950.

Holmes, G.: Disturbances of vision by cerebral lesions, Br. J. Ophthalmol. **2**:353-384, 1918.

Keeney, A. H.: Ocular examination, ed. 2, St. Louis, 1970, The C. V. Mosby Co.

Keil, F. C.: Visual acuity. In Berens, C., editor: The eye and its diseases, Philadelphia, 1949, W. B. Saunders Co.

Leinfelder, P. J.: Unilateral loss of vision in neurological disease, Am. J. Ophthalmol. **22**:1337-1342, 1939.

Lemoine, P., and Valois, G.: Les optotypes. In Bailliart, P., et al., editors: Traité d'ophtalmologie, Paris, 1939, Masson & Cie, Editeurs, vol. 2, p. 937.

Ohm, J.: Objektive Prüfung der Sehleistungen mit Hilfe der optokinetischen Augenbewegungen, Stuttgart, 1953, Ferdinand Enke Verlag.

Saraux, H., Grall, Y., Keller, J., Nou, B., and Bertrand, J. J.: The clinical value of the study of the visually evoked potentials, Ann. Oculist. **207**:201-206, 1974.

Schumann, W. P.: The objective determination of visual acuity on the basis of the optokinetic nystagmus, Am. J. Optom. **29**:575-583, 1952.

Snellen, H.: See under Brückner, A.

Weve, H.: Bestimmung der Sehschärfe. In Amsler, M., et al., editors: Lehrbuch der Augenheilkunde, Basel, 1954, S. Karger AG, p. 35.

**Color sensation**

Chance, B.: The color sense and its derangements. In Berens, C., editor: The eye and its diseases, Philadelphia, 1949, W. B. Saunders Co., p. 196.

Duke-Elder, S.: Textbook of ophthalmology, St. Louis, 1938, The C. V. Mosby Co., vol. 2, p. 1206.

Gallagher, J. R., Gallagher, C. D., and Sloane, A. E.: A critical evaluation of pseudo-isochromatic plates and suggestions for testing color vision, Yale J. Biol. Med. **15**: 79-98, 1942.

Gallagher, J. R., Gallagher, C. D., and Sloane, A. E.: A brief method of testing color vision with pseudo-isochromatic plates, Am. J. Ophthalmol. **26**:178, 1943.

Hardy, L. H., and Rand, G.: Tests for the detection and analysis of color-blindness. I. The Ishihara test, an evaluation, J. Opt. Soc. Am. **35**:268, 1945.

Hardy, L. H., and Rand, G.: Tests for the detection and analysis of color-blindness. II. The Ishihara test, comparison of editions, J. Opt. Soc. Am. **35**:350, 1945.

Hardy, L. H., and Rand, G.: Tests for the detection and analysis of color-blindness. III. The Rabkin test, J. Opt. Soc. Am. **35**:481, 1945.

Hardy, L. H., Rand, G., and Rittler, M. C.: Color vision and recent developments in color vision testing, Arch. Ophthalmol. **35**: 603, 1946.

Helmbold, R.: Der Farbensinn. In Schieck, F., and Brückner, A., editors: Kurzes Handbuch der Ophthalmologie, Berlin, 1931, Julius Springer, vol. 2, p. 295.

Hertel, E.: Stilling's Pseudo-isochromatische Tafeln, Leipzig, 1929, Georg Thieme Verlag KG.

Ishihara, S.: Tests for colour-blindness, London, 1944, H. K. Lewis & Co., Ltd.

Loken, R. D.: The color-meter: a quantitative color vision test, Am. J. Physiol. **55**:563, 1942.

Martin, L. C.: A standardized colour-vision testing lantern: transport type, Br. J. Ophthalmol. **27**:255, 1943.

Murray, E.: Color blindness: current tests and the scientific charting of cases, Psychol. Bull. **39**:165, 1942.

Murray, E.: Color vision tests. In Glasser, O., editor: Handbook of medical physics, Chicago, 1944, Year Book Medical Publishers, Inc.

Pickford, R. W.: The Ishihara test for colour blindness, Nature 153:656, 1944.

Polack, A.: Anomalies du sens chromatique. In Bailliart, P., et al., editors: Traité d' ophtalmologie, Paris, 1939, Masson & Cie, Editeurs, vol. 3, p. 339.

Schwichtenberg, A. H.: Review of color vision with some practical suggestions for medical examiners, Arch. Ophthalmol. 27:887, 1942.

Shoemaker, R. E.: The pseudoisochromatic plate test of color vision: practical application, Arch. Ophthalmol. 29:909, 1943.

Sloan, L. L.: The use of pseudo-isochromatic charts in detecting central scotomas due to lesions in the conducting pathways, Am. J. Ophthalmol. 25:1352, 1942.

Stilling, J.: Über das Sehen der Farbenblinden, Berlin, 1883.

Weve, H.: Prüfung des Farbensinnes. In Amsler, M., et al., editors: Lehrbuch der Augenheilkunde, Basel, 1954, S. Karger AG, p. 41.

Wilbrand, H.: Ophthalmologischer Beitrag zur Diagnose der Gehirnkrankheiten, Wiesbaden, 1884.

## Dark adaptation

Behr, C.: Das Verhalten und die diagnostische Bedeutung der Dunkeladaptation bei den verschiedenen Erkrankungen des Sehnervenstammes, Klin. Monatsbl. Augenheilkd. 5:193, 1915.

Bourdier, F.: Anomalies du sens lumineux. In Bailliart et al., editors: Traité d'ophtalmologie, Paris, 1939, Masson & Cie, Editeurs, vol. 3, p. 305.

Comberg, W.: Lichtsinn. In Schieck, F., and Brückner, A., editors: Kurzes Handbuch der Ophthalmologie, Berlin, 1931, Julius Springer, vol. 2, p. 172.

Della Casa, F.: Ein Adaptometer für den praktischen Arzt, Ophthalmologica 106: 143, 1943.

Gasteiger, H.: Über Störungen der Dunkeladaptation bei Sehnervenkrankheiten, Klin. Monatsbl. Augenheilkd. 78:827, 1927.

Goldmann, H.: Un nouvel adaptomètre automatique, Bull. Soc. Ophtalmol. Fr. 63: 4, 1950.

Hamburger, F. A.: Das Sehen in der Dämmerung, Berlin, 1949, Julius Springer.

Hartmann, N. B.: Testing night vision, Br. Med. J. 2:347, 1941.

Holmes, W. J.: Night vision, Arch. Ophthalmol. 30:367, 1943.

Mandelbaum, J.: Dark adaptation, Arch. Ophthalmol. 26:203, 1941.

Nagel, W. A.: Zwei Apparate für die augenärztliche Funktionsprüfung: Adaptometer und kleines Spektralphotometer, Z. Augenheilkd. 17:201, 1907.

Rutgers, G. E.: Die Dunkeladaptation bei der Opticusatrophie, Klin. Monatsbl. Augenheilkd. 71:449, 1934.

von Studnitz, G.: Physiologie des Sehens und retinale Primärprozesse, Akad. Ver.-Ges. Leipzig, 1940.

Verplanck, W. S.: Night vision, the terminal thresholds. In Berens, C., editor: The eye and its diseases, Philadelphia, 1949, W. B. Saunders Co., p. 203.

Weve, H.: Adaptationsprüfung. In Amsler, M., et al., editors: Lehrbuch der Augenheilkunde, Basel, 1954, S. Karger AG, p. 42.

Yudkin, S.: New dark adaptation tester, Br. J. Ophthalmol. 25:231, 1941.

## Visual field

Allen, T. D., and Carmann, H. F.: Homonymous hemianopic paracentral scotoma, Arch. Ophthalmol. 20:846-849, 1938.

Amsler, M.: L'examen qualitatif de la fonction maculaire, Ophthalmologica 114:248, 1947.

Amsler, M.: Quantitative and qualitative vision, Trans. Ophthalmol. Soc. U.K. 69: 397, 1949.

Aulhorn, E.: Perimetrie. In Sautter, H., editor: Entwicklung und Fortschritt der Augenheilkunde, Stuttgart, 1963, Ferdinand Enke Verlag, pp. 701-706.

Bair, H. L., and Harley, R. D.: Midline notching in the normal field of vision, Am. J. Ophthalmol. 23:183, 1940.

Bender, M. B., and Wechsler, I. S.: Irregular and multiple homonymous visual field defects, Arch. Ophthalmol. 28:904-912, 1942.

Berkeley, W. L., and Bussey, F. R.: Altitudinal hemianopia, Am. J. Ophthalmol. 33: 593-600, 1950.

Bessière, E., Rougier-Houssin, J., and Verin, P.: Contribution à la séméiologie précoce des scotomes centraux, Arch. Ophtalmol. 27:359-386, 1967.

Biemond, A.: La projection des quadrants rétiniens dans la radiation optique étudiée dans un cas d'hémianopsie bilatérale, Folia Psychiatr. Neurol. Neurochir. Neerl. **53:** 159-164, 1950.

Bjerrum, J.: About a supplementary examination of the visual field and about the field in glaucoma, Nord. Ophthalmol. Tidskr., pp. 2, 3, 11, 23, 27, 49, 1889.

Bjerrum, J.: Ein Zusatz zur gewöhnlichen Gesichtsfelduntersuchung und über das Gesichtsfeld bei Glaukom, Verh. 10. Int. Med. Kongr. Berlin **4:**66, 1890.

Bonnet, P.: Valeur sémiologique de l'hémianopsie, J. Med. Lyon **33:**587-624, 1952.

Bourbon, O. P.: Selection of the test object in perimetry, Am. J. Ophthalmol. **23:**1260, 1940.

Brückner, A.: Die Untersuchung des Gesichsfeldes. In Schieck, F., and Brückner, A., editors: Kurzes Handbuch der Ophthalmologie, Berlin, 1931, Julius Springer, vol. 2, p. 931.

Buffat, J. D.: L'hémianopsie binasale en neurochirurgie, Rev. Med. Suisse Romande **70:** 174-183, 1950.

Chamlin, M.: Visual field studies in neurosurgical problems, Eye Ear Nose Throat Mon. **31:**415-422, 1952.

Chamlin, M.: Methodology and techniques in visual field studies, Surv. Ophthalmol. **13:** 97-117, 1968.

Chamlin, M., and Davidoff, L.: The 1/2000 field in chiasmal interference, Arch. Ophthalmol. **44:**53, 1950.

Chamlin, M., and Davidoff, L. M.: Papilledema: its differential diagnosis, with special reference to minimal testing to the blind spot at two meters, Arch. Neurol. Psychiatr. **68:**213, 1952.

Comberg, U., and Lommatssch, P.: Zur Bewertung des Zentralskotomes, Klin. Monatsbl. Augenheilkd. **142:**336-347, 1963.

Cuendet, J. F., and Dufour, R.: Appréciation quantitative du champ visuel à l'aide de la planimétrie, Confin. Neurol. **14:**143, 1954.

Cushing, H.: Distortion of the visual fields in cases of brain tumor: the field defects produced by temporal lobe lesions, Brain **44:**341, 1921.

Davis, L.: The blind spots in patients with intracranial tumors, J.A.M.A. **92:**794, 1929.

D'Orio, R., and Scarinci, A.: L'Hemianopsia binasale, Riv. Otoneurooftalmol. **34:**617-659, 1959.

Dubois-Poulsen, A.: Périmétrie, campimétrie, scotométrie. In Bailliart, P., et al., editors: Traité d'ophtalmologie, Paris, 1939, Masson & Cie, Editeurs, vol. 2, p. 1011.

Dubois-Poulsen, A.: Le champs visuel, Paris, 1952, Masson & Cie, Editeurs.

Dufour, R.: Hémianopsie relative et ataxie, Confin. Neurol. **9:**413, 1949.

Duke-Elder, S., and Scott, G.: Neuro-ophthalmology. In Duke-Elder, S., editor: System of ophthalmology, vol. 12, St. Louis, 1971, The C. V. Mosby Co.

Ecker, A. D., and Anthony, E. W.: Exanopic central scotoma, a pitfall in diagnosis, J. Neurosurg. **2:**47, 1945.

Elsberg, C. A., and Spotnitz, H.: Sense of vision; Reciprocal relation of area and light intensity and its significance for localization of tumors by functional visual test, Bull. Neurol. Inst. N.Y. **6:**243-252, 1937.

Evans, J. N.: Classic characteristics of defects of visual field, Arch. Ophthalmol. **22:**410-431, 1933.

Evans, J. N.: An introduction to clinical scotometry, London, 1938, Oxford University Press.

Falconer, M. A.: Visual field changes and the value of quantitative perimetry in compression of the optic chiasm and the optic nerve, Trans. Ophthalmol. Soc. U.K. **3:**8, 1949.

Fankhauser, F., Koch, P., and Roulier, A.: On automation of perimetry, Graefe. Arch. Ophthalmol. **184:**126-150, 1972.

Fanta, H.: Das Gesichtsfeld für Bewegung und Weiss bei intrakraniellen Prozessen, Graefe. Arch. Ophthalmol. **161:**492-501, 1960.

Ferree, C. E., and Rand, G.: An illuminated perimeter with campimeter features, Am. J. Ophthalmol. **5:**455, 1922.

Ferree, C. E., and Rand, G.: Methods for increasing the diagnostic sensitivity of perimetry and scotometry with the form fields stimulus, Am. J. Ophthalmol. **13:**2, 1930.

Foerster, R.: Das Perimeter, Sitzungsber. Ophthalmol. Ges. Heidelberg, 1869, p. 411.

Forstot, S. L., Weinstein, G. W., and Feicock, K. B.: Studies with the Tubinger perimeter of Harms and Aulhorn, Ann. Ophthalmol. **2:**843-854, 1970.

François, J.: L'hemianopsie binasale, Ophthalmologica **113:**321-343, 1947.

Friedmann, A. I.: Serial analysis of changes in visual field defects employing a new instrument, to determine the activity of disease involving the visual pathways, Ophthalmologica **152**:1-12, 1966.

Goldmann, H.: Grundlagen exakter Perimetrie, Ophthalmologica **109**:57, 1945.

Goldmann, H.: Ein selbstregistrierendes Projektionskugelperimeter Ophthalmologica **109**:71, 1945.

Goldmann, H.: Demonstration unseres neuen Kugelperimeters samt theoretischen und klinischen Bemerkungen über Perimetrie, Ophthalmologica **3**:187, 1946.

Goldmann, H.: La périmétrie en oto-neuro-ophthalmologie, Confin. Neurol. **14**:102, 1954.

Guillaumat, L., and Robin, A.: Etude statistique du champ visuel dans les affections neurochirurgicales non traumatiques, Bull. Soc. Fr. Ophtalmol. **65**:5-16, 1952.

Harms, H.: Entwicklungsmöglichkeiten der Perimetrie, Graefe. Arch. Ophthalmol. **150**:28, 1950.

Harms, H.: Die praktische Bedeutung quantitativer Perimetrie, Klin. Monatsbl. Augenheilkd. **121**:683, 1952.

Harms, H.: Quantitative Perimetrie bei sellanahen Tumoren, Ophthalmologica **127**:255, 1954.

Harms, H.: Diagnostische Bedeutung der Gesichtsfelduntersuchung. In Rohrschneider, W., editor: Augenheilkunde in Klinik und Praxis, Stuttgart, 1958, Ferdinand Enke Verlag, pp. 22-49.

Harms, H.: Leitsymptom "Zentralskotom." In Sautter, H., editor: Entwicklung und Fortschritt in der Augenheilkunde, Stuttgart, 1963, Ferdinand Enge Verlag, pp. 516-539.

Harms, H., and Raabe, M.: Besondere perimetrische Methoden bei ophthalmo-neurologischen Erkrankungen, Oesterreichische Ophthalmologie Gesellschaft, Vienna, 1960, Brüder Hollinek.

Harrington, D. O.: Localizing value of incongruity in defects in the visual fields, Arch. Ophthalmol. **21**:453, 1939.

Harrington, D. O.: The visual fields, St. Louis, 1964, The C. V. Mosby Co.

Harrington, D. O.: Analysis of some unusual and difficult visual field defects, Trans. Ophthalmol. Soc. U.K. **92**:15-34, 1972.

Henschen, S. E.: Zur Anatomie der Sehbahn und des Sehzentrams, Graefe. Arch. Ophthalmol. **117**:403-418, 1926.

Holmes, G.: Disturbances of vision by cerebral lesions, Br. J. Ophthalmol. **2**:353-384, 1918.

Holmes, G., and Lister, W. T.: Disturbances of vision from cerebral lesions with special reference to the cortical representation of the macula, Brain **39**:34-73, 1916.

Huber, A.: Zur homonymen Hemianopsie nach occipitaler Lobektomie, Schweiz. Med. Wochenschr. **80**:1227, 1950.

Huber, A.: Roentgendiagnosis vs visual field, Arch. Ophthalmol. **90**:1-12, 1973.

Hughes, E. B. C.: Selected cases illustrating the value of quantitative perimetry in neurosurgical diagnosis, Trans. Ophthalmol. Soc. U.K. **63**:143-147, 1944.

Hylkema, B. S.: Klinische Anwendung der Bestimmung der Verschmelzungsfrequenz, Graefe. Arch. Ophthalmol. **146**:110, 241, 1943.

Igersheimer, J.: Zur Pathologie der Sehbahn: Über Hemianopsie, Graefe. Arch. Ophthalmol. **97**:105, 1918.

Igersheimer, J.: Binasal hemianopia, Arch. Ophthalmol. **38**:248, 1947.

Johnson, T. H.: Homonymous hemianopia: some practical points in its interpretation with report of 49 cases in which lesion in brain was verified, Trans. Am. Ophthalmol. Soc. **33**:90-113, 1935; Arch. Ophthalmol. **15**:604-616, 1936.

Kennedy, F.: Retrobulbar neuritis as an exact diagnostic sign of certain tumors and abscesses in the frontal lobe, Am. J. Med. Sci. **142**:355, 1911.

Kennedy, R. J.: Value of perimetry in brain lesions, Cleve. Clin. Q. **6**:290-303, 1939.

Kestenbaum, A.: Einfache Methode der groben Gesichtsfeldprüfung, Wien. Med. Wochenschr. **46**:2533, 1925.

Kestenbaum, A.: Wertung der neuen topischen Diagnostik der Hemianopsie, Proceedings of the Fifteenth International Congress on Ophthalmology, Cairo, 1937, vol. 4, pp. 120-123.

Klingler, M., and Condrau, G.: Lokalisatorisch irreführende Gesichtsfeldsymptome bei Hirntumoren, Ophthalmologica **120**:5, 270, 1950.

Kluyskens, J., and Titeca, J.: Examen électro-encéphalographique du champ visuel, Ophthalmologica **126**:3, 129, 1953.

Krainer, L.: Zur Anatomie und Pathologie der Sehbahn und der Sehrinde, Dtsch. Z. Nervenheilk. **141**:177-190, 1936.

Kravitz, D.: Studies of visual fields in cases of verified tumor of brain, Arch. Ophthalmol. **20**:437-470, 1938.

Krayenbühl, H.: Die Bedeutung der Gesichtsfeldbestimmung in der Diagnostik von Tumoren des Schläfen- und Hinterhauptlappens, Schweiz. Med. Wochenschr. 69: 1028-1032, 1939.

Kreiger, H. P.: Visual function in perimetrically blind fields, Arch. Neurol. Psychiatr. 65:72, 1951.

Kronfeld, P. C.: The central visual pathway, Arch. Ophthalmol. 2:709-732, 1929.

Kronfeld, P. C.: The temporal half-moon, Trans. Am. Ophthalmol. Soc. 30:431, 1932.

Meyer, A.: The connections of the occipital lobes and the present status of the cerebral visual affections, Trans. Assoc. Am. Physicians 22:7, 1907.

Miles, P. W.: Flicker fusion fields, Am. J. Ophthalmol. 33:769, 1069, 1950.

Miles, P. W.: Testing visual fields by flicker fusion, Arch. Neurol. Psychiatr. 55:39-47, 1951.

Minkowski, M.: Zur Kenntnis der cerebralen Sehbahnen, Schweiz. Med. Wochenschr. 69:990-995, 1939.

Moeller, P. M., and Hvid-Hansen, O.: Chiasmal visual field, Acta ophthalmol. 48: 678-684, 1970.

Mooney, A. J., and McConnell, A. A.: Visual scotomata with intracranial lesions affecting the optic nerve, J. Neurol. Neurosurg. Psychiatry 12:205-218, 1949.

Nachtigaeller, H., and Hoyt, W. F.: Disturbances of the visual impression in bitemporal hemianopia and shift of the visual axes, Klin. Monatsbl. Augenheilkd. 156: 821-836, 1970.

Parsons, O. A., Chandler, P. J., Teed, R. W., and Haase, G. R.: Comparison of flicker perimetry and standard visual fields in brain-damaged patients, Acta Neurol. Scand. 42:207-212, 1966.

Pasino, L.: Dati comparativi ottenuti col perimetro di Maggiore e col perimetro di Goldmann, Rass. Ital. Ottalmol. 22:318-329, 1953.

Penido Burnier, F.: Consideration on campimetry and perimetry. Paper read before the Medical Association of the Penido Burnier Institute, 1941.

Peter, L. C.: The principles and practice of perimetry, Philadelphia, 1923, Lea & Febiger.

Posner, A.: Perimetry: principles and methods, Eye Ear Nose Throat Mon. 31:378-379, 387, 1952.

Raiford, M. B.: Binasal hemianopia, Am. J. Ophthalmol. 32:99, 1949.

Riise, D.: Neuro-ophthalmological patients with bitemporal hemianopia (follow-up study of aetiology), Acta ophthalmol. 48: 685-690, 1970.

Roenne, H.: Zur Theorie und Technik der Bjerrumschen Gesichtsfelduntersuchung, Arch. Augenheilkd. 78:4, 1915.

Roenne, H.: The different types of defects of the fields of vision, J.A.M.A. 89:1860-1865, 1927.

Roenne, H.: The focal diagnostic of the visual path, Acta Ophthalmol. 16:446-453, 1938.

Rosen, L.: Contribution à l'étude des hémianopsies: symptomatologie et étiologie de 97 cas examinés à la Clinique ophthalmologiques de Bâle, entre 1925 et 1940, Confin. Neurol. 4:271, 1942.

Rubey, F.: A contribution to "sick-bed-side" perimetry, Klin. Monatsbl. Augenheilkd. 160:223-226, 1972.

Rucker, C. W.: Bitemporal defects in visual fields resulting from developmental anomalies of optic disks, Arch. Ophthalmol. 35: 546-554, 1946.

Sanford, H. S., and Bair, H. L.: Visual disturbances associated with tumors of the temporal lobes, Arch. Neurol. Psychiatr. 42:21, 1939.

Schmidt, T.: Über die Gesichtsfelduntersuchung am Goldmann-Perimeter, Klin. Monatsbl. Augenheilkd. 126:209, 1955.

Shenkin, H. A., and Leopold, J. H.: Localizing value of temporal crescent defects in visual fields, Arch. Neurol. Psychiatr. 54: 97-101, 1945.

Stenvers, H. W.: Localisation directe et localisation par image dans les champs visuels périphériques, Rev. Otoneuroophtalmol. 23:6-14, 1951.

Straub, W.: Über die binasale Hemianopsie, Acta Ophthalmol. 30:229-252, 1952.

Streiff, E. B.: Traumatismes des voies optiques, Rev. Otoneuroophtalmol. 26:356-390, 1951.

Suarez-Villafranca, M. R.: Hemianopsia binasal de localización chiasmatica, Arch. Soc. Oftalmol. Hispano-Am. 11:252-256, 1951.

Suda, K.: Interesting ocular symptoms and quantitative perimetry in brain tumors, Folia Ophthalmol. Jpn. 16:818-821, 1965.

Thiébaut, F., Guillaumat, L., and Brégeat,

P.: L'hémianopsie relative, Bull. Soc. Fr. Ophthalmol. **60**:73, 1947.

Traquair, H. M.: Perimetry and the visual pathway (Mackenzie memorial lecture), Glasgow Med. J. **133**:105-118, 1940.

Traquair, H. M.: An introduction to clinical perimetry, London, 1949, Henry Kimpton.

Traquair, H. M.: Peripheral vision and perimetry. In Berens, C., editor: The eye and its diseases, Philadelphia, 1949, W. B. Saunders Co., p. 210.

Verrey, F.: Pseudo-hémianopsie inférieure post-hémorragique, Ophthalmologica **125**: 351-356, 1953.

Walker, C. B.: Quantitative perimetry: practical devices and errors, Arch. Ophthalmol. **46**:537-561, 1917.

Wallace, T. W.: Visual-field testing without special equipment, Cleve. Clin. Q. **37**:107-110, 1970.

Walsh, F. B.: Selected visual field studies. In Smith, J. L., editor: Neuro-ophthalmology, St. Louis, 1965, The C. V. Mosby Co., pp. 84-108.

Walsh, T. J.: Temporal crescent or halfmoon syndrome, Ann. Ophthalmol. **6**:501-505, 1974.

Walsh, F. B., and Ford, F. R.: Central scotomas: their importance of topical diagnosis, Arch. Ophthalmol. **24**:500-534, 1940.

Walsh, F. B., and Hoyt, W. F.: Topical diagnosis of lesions in the visual pathways with particular reference to the visual fields. In Clinical neuro-ophthalmology, Baltimore, 1969, The Williams & Wilkins Co., p. 60.

Weekers, R., and Roussel, F.: Introduction à l'étude de la fréquence de fusion en clinique, Ophthalmologica **112**:305-316, 1946.

Westby, R. K.: Central, paracentral scotoma and intracranial tumour, Acta Ophthalmol. **41**:749-756, 1963.

Weve, H.: Untersuchung des Gesichtsfeldes. In Amsler, M., et al., editors: Lehrbuch der Augenheilkunde, 1954, S. Karger AG, p. 43.

Wiesli, P.: Eine Methode zur Frühdiagnose der bitemporalen Hemianopsie bei Hypophysentumoren, Schweiz. Med. Wochenschr. **19**:479, 1928.

Wilbrand, H.: Die hemianopischen Gesichtsfeldformen, Munich, 1890, J. F. Bergmann.

Williamson, W. P.: After-image perimetry: rapid method of obtaining visual fields, Arch. Ophthalmol. **33**:40, 1945.

Yanagida, N.: Ophthalmic symptoms of brain tumor, particularly of the visual field, Acta Soc. Ophthalmol. Jpn. **55**:836-842, 1951.

Zuckerman, J.: Perimetry, Philadelphia, 1954, J. B. Lippincott Co.

# CHAPTER TWO

## General signs and symptoms of increased intracranial pressure in patients with brain tumors

### Papilledema[*]

Adrogué, E., and Insausti, T.: Etiology of papilledema, Arch. Oftalmol. B. Air. **17**: 285, 1942.

Amsler, M.: Stauungspapille. In Amsler, M., et al., editors: Lehrbuch der Augenheilkunde, Basel, 1954, S. Karger AG, p. 686.

Amsler, M.: Neuritis nervi optici (Neuritis optica). In Amsler, M., et al., editors:

[*]A few references dealing with the blood pressure in the retinal vessels in papilledema that were cited in the text are not listed here (Coppez, Rasvan, Magitot, Pereyra, Spinelli, Gallois, Bauwens, Winthers, Ascher, Rossano, Gauddisart, Suvina, Serr, Baurmann, Marchesani). They can be found in detail in the monograph by Streiff, B., and Monnier, M.: Der retinale Blutdruck im gesunden und kranken Organismus, Vienna, 1946, Julius Springer.

Lehrbuch der Augenheilkunde, Basel, 1954, S. Karger AG, p. 689.

Amsler, M.: Papillitis. In Amsler, M., et al., editors: Lehrbuch der Augenheilkunde, Basel, 1954, S. Karger AG, p. 690.

Anastasopoulos, G.: Klinische Untersuchungen an Hirntumoren zur Frage der Entstehung der Stauungspapille, Basel, 1937, S. Karger AG.

Anderson, W. A.: Medullated nerve fibers, Trans. Ophthalmol. Soc. U.K. **62**:343, 1942.

Babel, J.: La pathogénie de la stase papillaire, Praxis **50**:3, 1948.

Bailliart, P.: La circulation rétinienne à l'état normal et pathologique, Paris, 1923, Gaston Doin & Cie.

Bailliart, P.: La circulation rétinienne, Doc. Ophthalmol. **7/8**:357, 1954.

Baumann, M.: Zur Differentialdiagnose zwischen Stauungspapille und Papillitis, Graefe. Arch. Ophthalmol. **134**:189-191, 1935.

Baurmann, H., and Wink, B.: Uncertainties in the differential diagnosis of swelling of the optic disc in fluorescein angiography, Klin. Monatsbl. Augenheilkd. **157**:533-538, 1970.

Bedell, A. J.: Ophthalmoscopical differentiation between papilledema and papillitis, South. Med. J. **30**:37-44, 1937.

Bedell, A. J.: Papilledema without increased intracranial pressure, Am. J. Ophthalmol. **25**:685, 1942.

Behr, C.: Neue anatomische Befunde bei Stauungspapille: ein weiterer Beitrag zu ihrer Pathogenese, Graefe. Arch. Ophthalmol. **137**:1-60, 1937.

Behr, C.: Zur klinischen Diagnose der Stauungspapille, Nervenarzt **10**:337-340, 1937.

Bettaies, A.: Cécité par hypertension intracrânienne, Tunisie Med. **4**:227-233, 1966.

Biemond, A.: Poliomyelitis anterior acuta mit Stauungspapillen, Psychiatr. Q. **46**:424-426, 1942.

Bietti, G. B.: Considerazioni sulla comparsa della papilla da stasi negli occhi miopi, Riv. Otoneurooftalmol. **15**:47, 1938.

Bing, R.: Stauungspapille, Arch. Neurol. Psychiatr. **39**:49-71, 1937.

Bing, R.: Zur diagnostischen Bewertung intrakranieller Drucksteigerung, Schweiz. Med. Wochenschr. **15**:407, 1942.

Bleuler, M.: Lehrbuch der Psychiatrie, Heidelberg, 1972, Springer Verlag.

Blum, J.: Disparition d'une stase papillaire hypertensive pseudo-tumorale, Rev. Otoneuroophtalmol. **19**:61-62, 1947.

Bollack, J., and Delthil, S.: Maladies de la papille. In Bailliart, P., et al., editors: Traité d'ophtalmologie, Paris, 1939, Masson & Cie, Editeurs, vol. 5, p. 673.

Bonamour, G., Brégeat, P., Bonnet, M., and Juge, P.: La papille optique, Paris, 1968, Masson & Cie, Editeurs.

Bonnet, M.: Les tumeurs de la papille, Conf. Lyon. Ophthalmol. **86**:1-27, 1966.

Braun, W.: Über familiäres Vorkommen von Drusen der Papille, Klin. Monatsbl. Augenheilkd. **94**:734-738, 1935.

Brégeat, P.: L'œdème papillaire, Paris, 1956, Masson & Cie, Editeurs.

Bregeat, P.: Surgical value of papilledema, Bull. Soc. Ophtalmol. Fr. **71**:565-577, 1971.

Brégeat, P., David, M., and Fischgold, H.: Anévrysme cirsoïde de la rétine et du cerveau; procédé d'exploration, Bull. Soc. Fr. Ophtalmol. **65**:77-85, 1952.

Brégeat, P., David, M., and Lelièvre, A.: Einige Betrachtungen zum falschen Papillenödem, Rev. Neurol. **87**:545-549, 1952.

Brock, M., and Dietz, H.: Intracranial pressure, experimental and clinical aspects, Heidelberg, 1972, Springer Verlag.

Brückner, A.: Dynamometrie. In Schieck, F., and Brückner, A., editors: Kurzes Handbuch der Ophthalmologie, Berlin, 1931, Julius Springer, vol. 2, p. 915.

Bruntse, E.: Unilateral papilledema in neurosurgical patients, Acta Ophthalmol. **48**:759-764, 1970.

Butterfield, D. L.: Types and locations of brain tumors and other space-displacing masses within the cranial cavity occurring without choked disc, N.Y. State J. Med. **465**:1935.

Bynke, H. G.: Rapid variations of the prominent optic disc. IV. Outline of the pulse curve, Acta Ophthalmol. **40**:171-180, 1962.

Bynke, H. G.: On early diagnosis and prevention of secondary optic atrophy in papilledema, Acta Ophthalmol. **44**:801-813, 1966.

Bynke, H. G., and Aberg, L.: Differentiation of papilledema from pseudopapilledema by fluorescein ophthalmoscopy, Acta Ophthalmol. **48**:752-758, 1970.

Cameron, J.: Marked papilloedema in pulmonary emphysema, Br. J. Ophthalmol. **17**:167, 1933.

Casanovas Carnicer, J.: Estasis papilar, Arch. Soc. Oftalmol. Hispano-Am. **8**:221-299, 1948.

Chalmers, J. W., and Walsh, F. B.: Hyaline bodies in the optic disks, Brain **74**:95, 1951.

Chamlin, H., and Davidoff, L. M.: Drusen of optic nerve simulating papilledema, J. Neurosurg. **7**:70-78, 1950.

Chamlin, H., and Davidoff, L. M.: Drusen of the optic nervehead: ophthalmoscopic and histopathologic study, Am. J. Ophthalmol. **35**:1599-1605, 1952.

Chamlin, H., and Davidoff, L. M.: Papilledema—its differential diagnosis, with special reference to minimal testing of the blind spot at two meters, Arch. Neurol. Psychiatr. **68**:213-232, 1952.

Champion de Crespigny, C. T.: Papilledema, Aust. Med. J. **2**:911-914, 1937.

Cohen, D. N.: Drusen of the optic disc and the development of field defects, Arch. Ophthalmol. **85**:224-226, 1971.

Cone, W., and MacMillan, J. A.: The optic nerve and papilla: cytology and cellular pathology of the nervous system, New York, 1932, Paul B. Hoeber, Inc., vol. 2, pp. 837-901.

Cordes, F. C.: Congenital and acquired anomalies of the optic disk, Arch. Ophthalmol. **23**:1063, 1940.

Cordes, F. C., and Aiken, S. D.: Papilledema (choked disk) and papillitis (optic neuritis); their differential diagnosis, J. Nerv. Ment. Dis. **99**:576-582, 1944.

Cushing, H., and Bordley, J.: Observations on experimentally induced choked disk, Johns Hopkins Med. J. **20**:95-101, 1909.

Dandy, W. E.: Papilledema without intracranial pressure (optic neuritis), Ann. R. Coll. Surg. **110**:161-168, 1939.

Davis, L.: The blind spots in patients with intracranial tumors, J.A.M.A. **92**:794, 1929.

Desvignes, P.: Les faux aspects de stase papilláire, Bull. Soc. Fr. Ophtalmol. **66**:343, 1953.

Dill, J. L., and Crowe, S. J.: Thrombosis of the sigmoid or lateral sinus: reports of thirty cases, Arch. Surg. **28**:705-722, 1934.

Doggart, J. H.: On diagnosing papilledema, Trans. Ophthalmol. Soc. U.K. **62**:141, 1942.

Dorne, P.-A., Arnaud, B., and Boudet, C.: Fluorescein angiography and the diagnosis of papilledema, Bull. Soc. Ophtalmol. Fr. **72**:797-801, 1972.

Drew, J. H., and Grant, F. C.: Polycythemia as neurosurgical problem; review with report of 2 cases, Arch. Neurol. Psychiatr. **54**:25, 1945.

Duke-Elder, S., and Scott, G.: Neuro-ophthalmology. In Duke-Elder, S., editor: System of ophthalmology, vol. 12, St. Louis, 1971, The C. V. Mosby Co.

Dunphy, E. B.: Unilateral papilledema, Am. J. Ophthalmol. **50**:1084-1087, 1960.

Dupuy-Dutemps, L.: Pathogénie de la stase papillaire dans les affections intracrâniennes, Thèse, Paris, 1900, Steinheil.

Ectors, L., and Bégaux-van Boven, C.: Glaucoma and papilledema, Ophthalmologica **180**:113-120, 1944.

Erkkilä, H.: Optic disc drusen in children, Albrecht von Graefes Arch. Klin. Ophthalmol. **189**:1-7, 1974.

Ernest, J. T., and Archer, D.: Fluorescein angiography of the optic disc, Am. J. Ophthalmol. **75**:973-978, 1973.

Ethelberg, S., and Jensen, V. A.: Obscurations and further time-related paroxysmal disorders in intracranial tumors, Arch. Neurol. Psychiatr. **68**:130, 1952.

Euzière, J., Pagès, P., Lafon, R., Cabanettes, S., and Labauge, R.: Hyperostose du canalicule optique extériorisée par une stase papillaire unilatérale et symptomatique d'une hyperostose frontale interne, Rev. Otoneuroophtalmol. **24**:331-334, 1952.

Farmilo, R. W.: Papilledema and spinal cord tumors, N.Z. Med. J. **80**:100-104, 1974.

Finke, J.: Ophthalmodynamographie. In Neurologie und Psychiatrie, Berlin, 1966, Springer Verlag.

Fischer, F.: Zur Frage sog. permanenter Stauungspapille, Klin. Monatsbl. Augenheilkd. **85**:672-673, 1930.

Foetzsch, R.: The clinical manifestations of pseudopapilledema caused by buried drusen, Nervenarzt **41**:341-347, 1970.

Freusberg, O.: Ergebnisse der Dynamometrie bei Hirntumoren, Klin. Monatsbl. Augenheilkd. **113**:279-280, 1948.

Freusberg, O., and Moellmann, D.: A oftalmodinamometria en casos de tumores cerebrais, Rev. Brasil. Oftalmol. **11**:275, 1953.

Fry, W. E.: The pathology of papilledema: an examination of 40 eyes with special reference to compression of the central vein of the retina, Am. J. Ophthalmol. **14**:874-883, 1931.

Fry, W. E., and DeLong, P.: Tumor formation at disk; report of case, Arch. Ophthalmol. **30**:417, 1943.

Galbraith, J. E., and Sullivan, J. H.: Decompression of the perioptic meninges for relief of papilledema, Am. J. Ophthalmol. **76**:687-692, 1973.

Gallais, P.: Pseudo-stase papillaire avec corps hyalins, Rev. Otoneuroophtalmol. **24**:369-372, 1952.

Ghersi, J. A., and Lara, F. D.: Contribución al conocimiento de la patogenia del edema de la papila, Rev. Asoc. Med. Argent. **64**:15-18, 1950.

Ghirardi, L., and Maione, M.: Considerazioni sull'arteriografia dell'oftalmica con speciale riguardo alla sua visualizzazione nell'ipertensione endocranica, Riv. Otoneurooftalmol. **26**:426-437, 1951.

Gibbs, F. A.: Intracranial tumor with unequal choked disk: relationship between the side of greater choking and the position of the tumor, Arch. Neurol. Psychiatr. **27**:828-835, 1932.

Gilson, M., Destexhe, B., and Comhaire-Poutchinian, Y.: Fluorescein study of drusen of the optic disc and their haemorrhagic complications, Bull. Soc. Belge Ophtalmol. **159**:643-660, 1971.

Girard, P., Devic, M., and de Gevigney, D.: Neuro-papillite œdemateuse aiguë et discopathie cervicale. Récupération de la vision et disparition de l'œdème par élongation du cou. Le syndrome "névrite optique et acroparesthésie," J. Med. Lyon **183**:161-168, 1950.

Glees, M.: Ueber Anomalien der Papillengefässe bei intrakraniellen Angiomen, Klin. Monatsbl. Augenheilkd. **130**:403, 1957.

Good, P.: Choked discs in head encephalopathy, Am. J. Ophthalmol. **24**:794-797, 1941.

Griffith, J. Q., Jr., Fry, W. E., and McGuinness, A. C.: Experimental and clinical studies in hydrocephalus, with special reference to occurrence of papilledema, Am. J. Ophthalmol. **23**:245, 1940.

Griffith, J. Q., Jr., Fry, W. E., and Roberts, E.: Studies of criteria for classification of arterial hypertension, increased intracranial pressure and papilledema, Am. Heart J. **21**:94, 97, 1941.

Griffith, J. Q., Jr., Jeffers, W., and Fry, W. E.: Papilledema associated with subarachnoid haemorrhage: experimental and clinical study, Arch. Intern. Med. **61**:880, 1938.

Gross, A. G.: The papilledema of toxic hydrocephalus, Trans. Ophthalmol. Soc. U.K. **68**:181, 1948.

Gullstrand, A.: Das vereinfachte grosse Gullstrandsche Ophthalmoskop, Klin. Monatsbl. Augenheilkd. **67**:118, 1921.

Gunn, R. Marcus: Retrobulbar neuritis, Lancet, p. 412, 1904.

Hager, H.: Die Ophthalmo-Dynamographie als Methode zur Beurteilung des Gehirnkreislaufes, Klin. Monatsbl. Augenheilkd. **142**:827-846, 1963.

Hammes, E. M., Jr.: Papilledema in optic neuritis and tumor of the brain, Med. Clin. North Am. **28**:957, 1944.

Hayreh, S. S.: Pathogenesis of oedema of the optic nerve, Ph.D. Thesis, 1965, University of London.

Hayreh, S. S., and Edwards, J.: Ophthalmic arterial and venous pressures and effects of acute intracranial hypertension, Br. J. Ophthalmol. **155**:649-663, 1971.

Hedges, T. R.: Intracranial pressure and papilledema, Trans. Ophthalmol. Soc. U.K. **89**:691-723, 1969.

Hedges, T. R.: Papilledema: its recognition and relation to increased intracranial pressure, Surv. Ophthalmol. **19**:201-223, 1975.

Hedges, T. W., and Weinstein, J. D.: The hydrostatic mechanism of papilledema, Trans. Am. Acad. Ophthalmol. Otolaryngol. **72**:741-750, 1968.

Hegner, H.: Über Stauungspapille bei Blutkrankheiten, Klin. Monatsbl. Augenheilkd. **50**:119, 1912.

Heinz, K.: Eine Methode zur Vermessung der Stauungspapille, Med. Rundschau **1**:1947.

Herzberger, E.: Papilledema due to unknown cause, Proc. Staff Meet. Beilinson Hosp. **1**:51-52, 1953.

van Heuven, J. A.: Papilledema, Trans. Ophthalmol. Soc. U.K. **58**:549-560, 1938.

Heydenreich, A., Lemke, L., and Juette, A.: Differentialdiagnose von Papillenveränderungen mit Fluorescein, Klin. Monatsbl. Augenheilkd. **162**:131-139, 1973.

Holmes, G.: Prognosis in papilledema, Br. J. Ophthalmol. **21**:337-342, 1937.

Howell, C.: The craniostenoses, Am. J. Ophthalmol. **37**:359, 1954.

Hoyt, W. F., and Beeston, D.: The ocular fundus in neurologic disease, St. Louis, 1966, The C. V. Mosby Co.

Hoyt, W. F., and Knight, C. L.: Comparison of congenital disc blurring and incipient papilloedema in red-free light—a photographic study, Invest. Ophthalmol. **12**:241-247, 1973.

Huber, A.: Einseitige Stauungspapille, Pseudoneuritis und Pseudopapillenödem, Ophthalmologica **123**:262, 1952.

Huber, A.: Papillenoedem bei Leukämien, Ophthalmologica **141**:290-300, 1961.

Igersheimer, J.: Beiträge zur Pathologie und Pathogenese der Stauungspapille, Folia Ophthalmol. Orientalia **2**:1-10, 1935.

Irisch, C. W.: Sinus thrombosis: longitudinal sinus thrombosis, Ann. Otol. **47**:402-410, 1938.

Jaensch, P. A.: Stauungspapille (Bericht über

die Jahre 1931-1935), Fortschr. Neurol. Psychiatr. **8**:387-398, 1936.

Jensen: Chorioiditis juxtapapillaris, Graefe. Arch. Ophthalmol. **69**:41, 1908.

Kafer, J. P.: Sobre un sinal oftalmoscopico de hipertensao intracraniana, Selecoes Cientificas Med. Fra. **3**:53-55, 1948.

Kapuscinski, W. J., and Baran, L.: Diagnosis of disc edema by means of fluorescein angiography of the fundus associated with the observation of the rebound pulse in the central retinal artery, Ann. Oculist. **205**: 917-926, 1972.

Keith, N. M.: Rucker, C. W.: and Parkhill, E. M.: Recession of retinal papilledema during terminal stage of malignant hypertension; report of case, Arch. Ophthalmol. **26**:240-246, 1941.

Kelley, J. S.: Autofluorescence of drusen of the optic nerve head, Arch. Ophthalmol. **92**:263-264, 1974.

Kennedy, F.: Retrobulbar neuritis as an exact sign of certain tumors and abscesses in the frontal lobe, Am. J. Med. Sci. **142**:355, 1911.

Koch, F. L. P.: Ophthalmodynamometry, Arch. Ophthalmol. **34**:234-247, 1945.

Koziak, P. H.: Craniostenosis, Am. J. Ophthalmol. **37**:380, 1954.

Kravitz, D., and Lloyd, R. S.: Dilated and tortuous retinal vessels: report of a case of congenital arteriovenous communication, Arch. Ophthalmol. **14**:591-598, 1935.

Krayenbühl, H.: Allgemeine hirnchirurgische Diagnostik und Therapie. In Brunner, et al., editors: Lehrbuch der Chirurgie, Basel, 1949, Schwabe & Co., pp. 605-658.

Kwaskowski, A.: Diagnostische Schwierigkeiten bei der Stauungspapille, Klin. Oczna **23**:63-74, 1953.

Laje Weskamp, R.: Evolución y pronostico del edema papilar, Arch. Oftalmol. B. Air. **14**:303-340, 1939.

Lambert, R. K., and Weiss, H.: Optic pseudoneuritis and pseudopapilledema, Arch. Neurol. Psychiatr. **30**:580, 1933.

Langfit, T. W.: Summary of first international symposium on intracranial pressure, Hanover, Germany, July 27-29, 1972, J. Neurosurg. **38**:541-544, 1973.

Larsson, L., and Nord, B.: Klinisk bild av retrobulbärneurit vid intrakraniella tumörer, Nord. Med. **34**:1059-1065, 1947.

Lasco, F., and Arseni, C.: La pseudonévrite optique postérieure comme manifestation

rare des néoformations intracrâniennes, Rev. Otoneuroophtalmol. **32**:385-391, 1960.

Lauber, H.: Die Entstehung der Stauungspapille, Wien. Klin. Wochenschr. **47**:1547, 1934.

Lazorthes, G., and Campan, L.: Brain edema, symptomatology, clinical forms, diagnosis and treatment. In Vinken, P. J., and Bruyn, G. W., editors: Handbook of clinical neurology, New York, 1974, American Elsevier Publishing Co., Inc., vol. 16, pp. 186-208.

Leber: In Graefe-Saemisch: Handbuch der gesamten Augenheilkunde, 1877, vol. 5, p. 778.

Leimgruber, M.: Erbforschungen über die Drusen der Sehnervenpapille, Graefe. Arch. Ophthalmol. **136**:364-376, 1936.

Leinfelder, P. J.: Choked disks and low intrathecal pressure occurring in brain tumor, Am. J. Ophthalmol. **26**:1294, 1943.

Leinfelder, P. J., and Paul, W. D.: Papilledema in general diseases, Arch. Ophthalmol. **28**:983-987, 1942.

Levatin, P.: Increased intracranial pressure without papilledema, Arch. Ophthalmol. **58**: 683-688, 1957.

Levatin, P., and Raskind, R.: Delayed appearance of papilloedema, Can. J. Ophthalmol. **8**:451-455, 1973.

Lloberas-Camino, L., Ribas-Clotet, F., and Rodríguez-Arias, B.: Sobre el diagnóstico diferencial del éstasis papilar de origin tumoral, Rev. Esp. Otoneurooftalmol. Neurocir. **11**:266-270, 1952.

Lobstein, A.: L'ophtalmodynamométrie clinique, Bull. Soc. Ophtalmol. Fr. **11**:690-692, 1959.

Love, J. G., Wagner, H. P., and Woltmann, H. W.: Tumours of the spinal cord associated with choking of the optic disk, Arch. Neurol. Psychiatr. **66**:171, 1951.

Lubow, M.: Optic disc edema revisited. In Smith, J. L., and Glaser, J. S., editors: Neuro-ophthalmology, St. Louis, 1973, The C. V. Mosby Co., vol. 7, p. 18.

Lyle, T. K.: Some pitfalls in the diagnosis of plerocephalic oedema, Trans. Ophthalmol. Soc. U.K. **73**:87, 1953.

Magitot, A. P.: How to know the blood pressure in the vessels of the retina, Am. J. Ophthalmol. **5**:777, 1922.

Mansuy, L., Rougier, J., Aimard, G., and Thierry, A.: Expérience neuro-chirurgicale de dix-sept cas d'oedème papillaire de stase de cause rare ou inconnue; avenir éloigné de ces malades, Lyon Med. **49:** 1389-1404, 1967.

Marchesani, O.: Schwierigkeiten der Diagnose der Stauungspapille bei Myopie, Arch. Psychiatr. **95:**447, 1931.

Martinez Moreno, J., and Cuevas Cancino, D.: Diferenciación clinica entre papiledema y papilitis, Boll. Hosp. Oftalmol. Mexico **5:**195-200, 1952.

Masunaga, J., and Tsukahara, I.: Metastatic adenocarcinoma of the optic disc, Folia ophthalmol. Jpn. **23:**496-504, 1972.

Matavulj, N.: Stase papillaire unilatérale d'origine intra-crânienne, Bull. Soc. Fr. Ophtalmol. **63:**19-25, 1950.

Morone, G.: Sur les facteurs oculaires qui peuvent empêcher le développement d'une stase papillaire par hypertension endocrânienne, avec considération particulière de l'influence de la myopie, Rev. Otoneuroophtalmol. **21:**1, 80, 1949.

de Morsier, G., Monnier, M., and Streiff, B.: Rev. Neurol. Belge. **6:**702, 1939.

Morton, A. S., and Parsons, J. H.: Hyaline bodies (Drusenbildungen) at the optic disk, Trans. Ophthalmol. Soc. U.K. **23:**135-153, 1903.

Nano, H. M.: Ensayo de una clasificación practica de los aspectos oftalmoscopicamente edematosos de papila, Arch. Oftalmol. B. Air. **27:**49-53, 1952.

Nottbeck, B.: Ein Beitrag zur kongenitalen Pseudoneuritis optica (Scheinneuritis), Graefe. Arch. Ophthalmol. **44:**31, 1897.

Obenchain, T. G., Crandall, P. H., and Hepler, R. S.: Blindness following relief of increased intracranial pressure. A sequel to severe papilledema, Bull. Los Angeles Neurol. Soc. **35:**147-152, 1970.

Otradovec, J., and Vladykova, J.: Haemorrhages and venous stasis in drusen of the optic disc, Ophthalmologica **161:**21-30, 1970.

Parnitzke, K. H.: Zur Bedeutung der Stauungspapille in der Hirntumordiagnostik, Dtsch. Gesund. **8:**89-91, 1953.

Paton, L.: Papilledema and optic neuritis; a retrospect, Trans. Sect. Ophthalmol. Am. Med. Assoc. pp. 98-119, 1935.

Paton, L., and Holmes, G.: The pathology of papilledema; a histological study of 60 eyes, Brain **33:**389-432, 1911.

Paufique, L., and Bonamour, G.: Aspects et diagnostic ophthalmoscopiques de la papille œdémateuse, J. Med. Lyon **658:** 433-444, 1947.

Pennybacker, J.: Papilledema due to intracranial venous obstruction, Trans. Ophthalmol. Soc. U.K. **63:**333-339, 1944.

Petrohelos, M. A., and Henderson, J. W.: Ocular findings of intracranial tumor: study of 358 cases, Am. J. Ophthalmol. **34:**1387, 1951.

Pietruschka G., and Priess, G.: Clinical importance and prognosis of drusen of the disc, Klin. Monatsbl. Augenheilkd. **162:** 331-341, 1973.

Pigassou, R.: Contribution à l'étude de la pression veneuse rétinienne, Thèse, Toulouse, 1947.

Primrose, J.: Papilledema and related eye conditions. In Vinken, P. J., and Bruyn, G. W., editors: Handbook of clinical neurology, New York, 1974, American Elsevier Publishing Co., Inc., vol. 16, pp. 270-300.

Raimondo, N.: La macchia cieca "enorme" senza papilledema, Riv. Otoneurooftalmol. **35:**288-297, 1960.

Rau, H.: Stauungspapillen bei Spinaltumoren, Beitrag zur Klinik der Liquorzirkulationsstörungen, Dtsch. Med. Wochenschr. **99:** 345, 351-354, 1974.

Redslob, E.: Sémiologie critique de la stase papillaire, Rev. Otoneuroophtalmol. **22:**1-18, 1950.

Reese, A. B.: Relation of drusen of the optic nerve to tuberous sclerosis, Arch. Ophthalmol. **24:**187, 1940.

Rehwald, E.: Die differentialdiagnostiche Bewertung der Stauungspapille vom Standpunkt des Neurologen, Med. Klin. **35:** 1108-1110, 1939.

Rentz, S.: Aneurysma racemosum retinale, Arch. Augenheilkd. **95:**84-91, 1924.

Richter, H.: Über hochgradige Stauungs papille bei bereits organisierter Sinusthrombose, HNO. Beih. Hals-Heilk. **2:**394-395, 1951.

Rintelen, F.: Zur diagnostischen Bedeutung der Dynamometrie, Klin. Monatsbl. Augenheilkd. **100:**469-471, 1938.

Rintelen, F.: Über Stauungspapille und ihre Entstehung, Schweiz. Med. Wochenschr. p. 575, 1946.

Riser, Calmettes, Garipuy, Pigassou, and Pigassou: Tension veineuse rétinienne et hypertension crânienne, Rev. Otoneuroophtalmol. **21:**1, 1949.

Riser, Couadau, and Gayral: Tension artérielle rétinienne et pression intra-crânienne mesurée par ponction sous-occipitale, Rev. Otoneuroophtalmol. **19**:371, 1947.

Riser, Géraud, Caizergues, and Dreyfus: Hypotension crânienne avec œdème papillaire et signes méningés, Rev. Otoneuroophtalmol. **21**:448, 1949.

Roberts, W. L., and Nielsen, R. F.: Uveoparotid fever with bilateral papilledema, Am. J. Ophthalmol. **28**:1252, 1945.

Rollin, A.: Mesure de la pression dans les vaisseaux rétiniens. In Bailliart, P., et al., editors: Traité d'ophtalmologie, Paris, 1939, Masson & Cie, Editeurs, vol. 2, p. 1057.

Rosselet, E.: Papilledema, Praxis **60**:605-607, 1971.

Rucker, C. W.: Defects in visual fields produced by hyaline bodies in optic disks, Arch. Ophthalmol. **32**:56-59, 1944.

Rucker, C. W.: Defects in the visual fields resulting from increased intracranial pressure, N.Y. J. Med. **49**:2417-2421, 1949.

Sadoughi, G.: La stase papillaire dans les hypotensions ventriculaires, Bull. Soc. Ophtalmol. Fr. **1**:17-23, 1950.

Salvador, J. L., Vila, E., Marco, M., and Francés, J.: Incidence of papillary stasis in expansive intracranial processes of varying localisation and nature, Arch. Soc. Esp. Oftalmol. **34**:189-202, 1974.

Samuels, B.: Histopathology of papilledema, Am. J. Ophthalmol. **21**:1242-1258, 1938.

Samuels, B.: Drusen of the optic papilla; a clinical and pathologic study, Arch. Ophthalmol. **25**:412-423, 1941.

Sanders, M. D.: A classification of papilloedema based on a fluorescein angiographic study of 69 cases, Trans. Ophthalmol. Soc. U.K. **89**:177-192, 1969.

Sanders, M. D.: Ischaemic papillopathy, Trans. Ophthalmol. Soc. U.K. **91**:371-388, 1971.

Sanders, M. D., and Fytche, T. J.: Fluorescein-angiography in the diagnosis of drusen of the optic disc, Trans. Ophthalmol. Soc. U.K. **87**:457-468, 1967.

Sanders, T. E., Gay, A. J., and Newman, N.: Haemorrhagic complications of drusen of the optic disc, Am. J. Ophthalmol. **71**:204-217, 1971.

Satanowsky de Neumann, P., and Brodsky, M.: Edemas de papila sin sintomas de hipertensión endocraneana, Arch. Oftalmol. B. Air. **28**:128-133, 1953.

Schatzmann, C.: Intrakranielle Tumoren ohne Stauungspapille, M. D. Thesis, 1971, University of Zurich.

Scheie, H. G.: Evaluation of ophthalmoscopic changes of hypertension and arterial sclerosis, Arch. Ophthalmol. **49**:117, 1953.

Schieck, F.: Über die Entstehungsart der Stauungspapille, Verh. Physikal.-Med. Ges. Würzburg **51**:121, 1926.

Schieck, F.: Beiträge zur Frage der Entstehung der Stauungspapille, Graefe. Arch. Ophthalmol. **138**:48-54, 1937.

Schieck, F.: Die ophthalmoskopische Diagnose der Stauungspapille, Graefe. Arch. Ophthalmol. **137**:203-215, 1937.

Schieck, F.: Das Wesen der Stauungspapille, Bücherei d. Augenarztes H. 12, Stuttgart, 1942, Ferdinand Enke Verlag.

Schlezinger, N. S., Waldmann, J., and Alpers, B. J.: Drusen of optic nerve simulating cerebral tumor, Arch. Ophthalmol. **31**:509-516, 1944.

Schupfer, F.: Diagnostische Schwierigkeiten und klinisches Bild der Myelinfasern in Fällen von Stauung oder Entzündung der Sehnervenpapille, Boll. Oculist. **19**:647-656, 1940.

de Schweinitz, G. E.: The relation of cerebral decompression to the relief of the ocular manifestation of increased intracranial tension, Ann. Ophthalmol. **20**:271-289, 1911.

Scott, G. I.: Optic disc oedema, Trans. Ophthalmol. Soc. U.K. **87**:733-753, 1967.

Selinger, E.: Choked disk and papillitis: differential diagnosis by the protein content of the aqueous, Arch. Neurol. Psychiatr. **33**:360-367, 1935.

Serr, H.: Die Stauungspapille in ihrer allgemein klinischen und ophthalmologischen Bedeutung, Graefe. Arch. Ophthalmol. **135**:431-450, 1936.

Simpson, T.: Papilledema in emphysema, Br. Med. J. **2**:639, 1948.

Smith, E. G.: Unilateral papilledema; its significance and pathologic physiology, Arch. Ophthalmol. **21**:856-878, 1939.

Smith, J. L.: Ophthalmodynamometric techniques. In Smith, J. L., editor: Neuroophthalmology, Springfield, 1964, Charles C Thomas, Publisher, vol. 1.

Sobanski, J.: Der Wert dynanometrischer Untersuchung für die Erklärung der Entstehung der Stauungspapille, Graefe. Arch. Ophthalmol. **137**:84, 1937.

Sokolova, O. N., Batrachenko, I. P., and Mukhamadiev, R. O.: Diagnostic value of fluorescent angiography of the retina in congestive optic papillae, Vestn. Oftalmol. **85**:39-43, 1972.

Stokes, W. H.: Racemose arteriovenous aneurysm of the retina (aneurysma racemosum arteriovenosum retinae), Arch. Ophthalmol. **11**:956, 1934.

Stopford, J. S. B.: Increased intracranial pressure, Brain **51**:485-507, 1928.

Stough, J. T.: Choking of the optic disc in diseases other than tumor of the brain, Arch. Ophthalmol. **8**:821-830, 1932.

Streiff, B.: Zwei Fälle von Allgemeinleiden mit Stauungspapille infolge Hirntumors, Klin. Monatsbl. Augenheikld. **106**:246-247, 1941.

Streiff, B.: L'ophthalmodynamométrie de Bailliart, sa valeur et sa précision, Doc. Ophthalmol. **7/8**:27, 1954.

Streiff, B., and Monnier, M.: Der retinale Blutdruck im gesunden und kraken Organismus, Berlin, 1946, Julius Springer.

Taylor, R. D., Corcoran, A. C., and Page, I. H.: Increased cerebrospinal fluid pressure and papilledema in malignant hypertension, Arch. Intern. Med. **93**:818, 1954.

Thiébaut, F., Phillippidès, D., Rohmer, F., and Mengus, M.: Stase papillaire unilatérale, Rev. Otoneuroophtalmol. **25**:303-304, 1953.

Tönnis, W.: Pathophysiologie und Klinik der intracraniellen Drucksteigerung. In Olivecrona, H., and Tönnis, W., editors: Handbuch der Neurochirurgie, Berlin, 1959, Julius Springer, vol. 1.

Tönnis, W., and Krenkel, W.: Grosshirngeschwülste ohne Stauungspapille, Acta Neurochir. **5**:458-487, 1957.

Toyama, T.: The retinal blood pressure in choked discs, Jpn. J. Ophthalmol. **3**:216-223, 1959.

Traquair, H. M.: An introduction to clinial perimetry, London, 1949, Henry Kimpton.

Uhthoff, W.: Zur Pseudoneuritis optica, Dtsch. Z. Nervenheilk. **50**:258, 1913.

Uhthoff, W.: Die Augenveräderungen bei den Erkrankungen des Gehirnes. In Graefe-Saemisch: Handbuch der gesamten Augenheilkunde, Leipzig, 1915, Wilhelm Engelmann, vol. 11, p. 1143.

Vanderlinden, R. G., and Chrisholm, L. D.: Vitreous hemorrhages and sudden increased intracranial pressure, J. Neurosurg. **41**:167-176, 1974.

Victoria, V.: Ophthalmodynamometry in papilledema, Arch. Oftalmol. B. Air. **45**:397-403, 1970.

Voisin, J.: Les signes oculaires de l'hypertension intra-crânienne, Presse Med. **58**:421, 1950.

Volhard, F.: Wesen und Behandlung des roten und blassen Hochdruckes. In von Thiel, R., editor: Gegenwartsprobleme der Augenheilkunde, Leipzig, 1937, Georg Thieme Verlag KG.

Voutres, J.: Un cas d'œdème papillaire ayant la valeur d'un signe de localisation de tumeur intracrâninne, Bull. Soc. Ophthalmol. Fr. **1**:169-171, 1949.

van Wagenen, W. P.: The incidence of intracranial tumors without "choked disk" in one years series of cases, Am. J. Med. Sci. **176**:746, 1928.

Wachholz, E.-A.: Ophthalmodynamometric findings in 10 cases of meningioma of the sphenoid, Klin. Monatsbl. Augenheilkd. **160**:430-433, 1972.

Wagener, H. P.: Drusen (hyaline bodies) of the optic disk, Am. J. Med. Sci. **210**:262-268, 1945.

Wagener, H. P., and Keith, N. M.: Diffuse arteriolar disease and hypertension, Proceedings of the Fifteenth International Congress of Ophthalmology, Cairo, 1937, vol. 1, pp. 1-86.

Walsh, F. B.: Ocular signs of thrombosis of the intracranial venous sinuses, Arch. Ophthalmol. **17**:46-65, 1937.

Walsh, T. J., Garden, J., and Gallagher, B.: Relationship of retinal venous pulse to intracranial pressure. In Smith, J. L., editor: Neuro-ophthalmology, St. Louis, 1968, The C. V. Mosby Co., vol. 4, pp. 288-292.

Walsh, T. J., Garden, J. W., and Gallagher, B.: Obliteration of retinal venous pulsations during elevation of cerebrospinal-fluid pressure, Am. J. Ophthalmol. **67**:954-956, 1969.

Walsh, F. B., and Hoyt, W. F.: Optic neuritis. In Clinical neuro-ophthalmology, Baltimore, 1969, The Williams & Wilkins Co., p. 607.

Walsh, F. B., and Hoyt, W. F.: Papilledema. In Clinical neuro-ophthalmology, Baltimore, 1969, The Williams & Wilkins Co., p. 567.

Watkins, C. H., Wagener, H. P., and Brown, R. W.: Cerebral symptoms accompanied by choked optic disks in types of blood dyscrasia, Am. J. Ophthalmol. **24**:1374, 1941.

Weber, G.: Hirnabszesse im Rahmen infektiöser intrakranieller Erkrankungen, Stuttgart, 1956, Georg Thieme Verlag KG.

Weed, L. H.: Experimental studies in intracranial pressure. The intracranial pressure in health and diseases, Baltimore, 1929, The Williams & Wilkins Co.

Weigelin, E.: Zur Genese der Stauungspapille, Ber. Dtsch. Ophthalmol. Ges. **56:** 181, 1950.

Weigelin, E.: Beurteilung des intrakraniellen Kreislaufes mit Hilfe der Netzhautarteriendruckmessung, Doc. Ophthalmol. **7/8:**183, 1954.

Weigelin, E.: Local circulation in papilledema. In Cant, J. S., editor: The optic nerve, St. Louis, 1973, The C. V. Mosby Co., pp. 137-141.

Weigelin, E., and Müller, H. K.: Über die praktische Bedeutung der Blutdruckmessung an der Zentralarterie der Netzhaut, Doc. Ophthalmol. **5/6:**357-402, 1951.

Weigelin, E., and Lobstein, A.: Ophthalmodynamometrie, Basel, 1962, S. Karger AG.

Weigelin, E., Kazuo, I., and Halder, M.: Fortschritte auf dem Gebiet der Blutdruckmessung am Auge, Fortschr. Augenheilkd. **15:**44-84, 1964.

Weiman, C. G., McDowell, F. H., and Plum, F.: Papilledema in poliomyelitis, Arch. Neurol. Psychiatr. **66:**722, 1951.

Williamson-Noble, F. A.: Venous pulsation, Trans. Ophthalmol. Soc. U.K. **72:**317-326, 1952.

Wise, G. N., Henkind, P., and Alterman, M.: Optic disc drusen and subretinal hemorrhage, Trans. Am. Acad. Ophthalmol. Otolaryngol. **78:**212-219, 1974.

Witmer, R.: Differentialdiagnostische Aspekte bei retinalen Gefässtörungen und Papillenoedem, Ophthalmologica **156:**313-321, 1968.

Witmer, R.: Differential diagnosis of papilloedema by means of fluorescent angiography, Trans. Ophthalmol. Soc. N.Z. **24:** 13-15, 1972.

Wohlwill, F.: Die Affektionen der grossen venösen Blutleiter der Dura. In Schieck, F., and Brückner, A., editors: Kurzes Handbuch der Ophthalmologie, Berlin, 1931, Julius Springer, vol. 6, pp. 17-19.

Wyburn-Mason, R.: Arteriovenous aneurysm of midbrain and retina facial naevi and mental changes, Brain **66:**163, 1943.

Yegen, V.: The importance of papilledema in the localization and diagnosis of intracranial tumours (in Turkish), Otonorooftalmol. **7:**96-116, 1952.

Zarski, S.: A case of cauda equina tumour associated with papilledema, Neurol. Neurochir. Pol. **22:**153-156, 1972.

Zülch, K. J., Mennel, H. D., and Zimmrmann, V.: Intracranial hypertension. In Vinken, P. J., and Bruyn, G. W., editors: Handbook of clinical neurology, New York, 1974, American Elsevier Publishing Co. Inc., Vol. 16, pp. 89-149.

## Pareses of extraocular muscles[*]

Collier, J.: The false localizing signs of intracranial tumour, Brain **27:**490-508, 1904.

Cushing, H.: Strangulation of the nervi abducentes by lateral branches of the basilary artery in case of brain tumor, Brain **33:** 204-235, 1910-1911.

Gassel, M. M.: False localizing signs. A review of the concept and analysis of the occurrence in 250 cases of intracranial meningiomas, Arch. Neurol. **4:**526-554, 1961.

Kirkham, T. H., Bird, A. C., and Sanders, M. D.: Divergence paralysis with raised intracranial pressure. An electro-oculographic study, Br. J. Ophthalmol. **56:**776-782, 1972.

Van Allen, M. W.: Transient recurring paralysis of ocular abduction. A syndrome of intracranial hypertension, Arch. Neurol. **17:**81-88, 1967.

Zielinski, H. W.: Paresen der äusseren Augenmuskeln bei intrakraniellen raumfordernden Prozessen, ein Ueberlick über die Beobachtungen an über 3000 Fällen, Zentralbl. Neurochir. **19:**235-251, 1959.

## Transtentorial herniation syndrome

Fischer-Brügge, K.: Das Klivuskanten-Syndrom, Acta Neurochir. **11:**36, 1951.

Hoyt, W. F.: Vascular lesions of the visual cortex with brain herniation through the tentorial incisura. Neuro-ophthalmologic considerations, Trans. Pac. Coast Otoophthalmol. Soc. **41:**301-327, 1960.

Jefferson, G.: The tentorial pressure cone, Arch. Neurol. Psychiatr. **40:**857-876, 1938.

Klintworth, G. K.: The neuro-ophthalmic manifestations of transtentorial herniation. In Smith, J. L.: Neuro-ophthalmology,

---

[*]For additional literature, see references for motility of the eyes in Chapter 1.

St. Louis, 1972, The C. V. Mosby Co., vol. 6, pp. 113-126.

Lyle, D. J.: Eye symptoms produced by tentorial herniation from increased intracranial pressure, Proceedings of the Seventeenth International Congress on Ophthalmology, New York, 1954.

McKenzie, K. G.: Extradural hemorrhage, Br. J. Surg. 26:336, 1938.

Scharfetter, F.: Mydriasis und Lichtstarre, Schweiz. Arch. Neurol. Psychiatr. 96:386-392, 1965.

Schwarz, G. A., and Rosner, A. A.: Displacement and herniation of the hippocampal gryrus through the incisura tentorii: clinicopathologic study, Arch. Neurol. Psychiatr. 46:297, 1941.

Stefani, F. H.: Optic tract compression with intracranial supratentorial increase of contents, Albrecht von Graefes Arch. Klin. Ophthalmol. 182:234-238, 1971.

Welte, E.: Zur formalen Genese der traumatischen Mydriasis. Oculomotorius-wurzelschädigung durch einseitiges Vorquellen des Uncus hippocampi, Zentralbl. Neurochir. 6:217, 1943.

**Exophthalmos**

Brain, W. R.: Neurological and general medical causes of exophthalmos, Trans. Ophthalmol. Soc. U.K. 58:27-32, 1938.

Cohn, H.: Messung der Prominenz der Augen mittels eines neuen Instruments, des Exophthalmometers, Klin. Monatsbl. Augenheilkd. 5:339, 314, 1905.

Crawford, J. S.: Proptosis in children, Trans. Can. Ophthalmol. Soc. 5:81-93, 1952.

Dixon, G. J.: Unilateral exophthalmos (proptosis), causation and differential diagnosis, Brain 64:73-89, 1941.

Elsberg, C. A., Hare, C. C., and Dyke, C. H.: Unilateral exophthalmos in intracranial tumors with special reference to its occurrence in meningiomata, Surg. Gynecol. Obstet. 55:681, 1932.

Godtfredsen, E.: Exophthalmos due to malignant tumours in the paranasal sinuses, Acta Ophthalmol. 25:295, 1947.

Hertel, E.: Ein einfaches Exophthalmomometer, Graefe. Arch. Ophthalmol. 60:171, 1905.

Knudtzon, K.: Exophthalmos and primary intracranial tumours (In Danish with an English summary), M.D. Thesis, Copenhagen, 1952, Danish Scientific Press.

Lazorthes, G., and Geraud, J.: L'exophtalmie unilatérale neurochirurgicale; analyse de 17 observations, Rev. Neurol. 83:373-379, 1950.

Morin, G., Tuset, J., Bouchacourt, A., Force, L., and Beauchamp, P.: Exophthalmie par tumeur de la fosse cérébrale moyenne, Rev. Otoneuroophtalmol. 33:270-275, 1961.

Skydsgaard, H.: Exophthalmus coincident to intracranial tumors, Acta Ophthalmol. 16:474-480, 1938.

Thurel, R.: Exophthalmie par distension de la corne temporo-sphénoïdale du ventricule latéral et refoulement de la paroi externe de l'orbite, Rev. Otoneuroophtalmol. 23:286, 1951.

Weve, H.: Exophthalmometrie und Orbitotonometrie. In Amsler, M., et al., editors: Lehrbuch der Augenheilkunde, Basel, 1954, S. Karger AG, p. 8.

Yasargil, G. M.: Die Röntgendiagnostik des Exophthalmus unilateralis, Basel, 1957, S. Karger AG.

# CHAPTER THREE

## Local signs and symptoms of brain tumors

### Reviews of local signs and symptoms in brain tumors

Abott, W. D.: Ocular symptoms in the diagnosis of tumor of the brain, Arch. Ophthalmol. 6:244, 1931.

Bardram, M., and Möller, H. U.: Diagnosis of tumours in the anterior and middle cranial fossa, Acta Ophthalmol. 30:65-96, 1952.

Behr, C.: Die Erkrankungen der Sehbahn vom Chiasma aufwärts. In Schieck, F., and Brückner, A., editors: Kurzes Handbuch der Ophthalmologie, Berlin, 1931, Julius Springer, vol. 6, p. 245.

Benda, C.: Die topische Diagnostik der Hirntumoren, Monatsschr. Psychiatr. Neurol. 93:332-354, 1936.

Best, F.: Die Augenstörungen bei Hirntumoren. In Schieck, F., and Brückner, A., editors: Kurzes Handbuch der Ophthalmologie, Berlin, 1931, Julius Springer, vol. 6, p. 563.

Bonnet, P.: Les signes ophtalmologiques des tumeurs cérébrales, J. Med. Lyon 37:511-530, 1956.

Bucy, P. C.: Early recognition of tumors of brain, Dis. Nerv. Syst. 1:356-362, 1940.

Cairns, H.: Accessory methods of diagnosis in intracranial tumor and allied diseases, Trans. Med. Soc. Lond. 58:50-74, 1935.

Cairns, H.: Ergebnisse der Behandlung der intrakraniellen Tumoren, Schweiz. Med. Wochenschr. 44:1043, 1937.

Collier, J.: The false localizing signs of intracranial tumour, Brain 27:490-508, 1904.

Coughlin, W. T.: Subtentorial tumors, South. Med. J. 30:665-674, 1937.

Cushing, H., and Walker, C. B.: Distortion of the visual fields in cases of brain tumor; binasal hemianopia, Arch. Ophthalmol. 41:559, 1912.

Dandy, W. E.: Brain tumors, general diagnosis and treatment. In Lewis, D., editor: Lewis' practice of surgery, Hagerstown, Md., 1932, W. F. Prior Co., Inc., vol. 12, pp. 443-674.

David, M.: Evolution et valeur des examens complémentaires dans le diagnostic des tumeurs intracrâniennes. Essai synthétique, Neurochirurgie 13:181-205, 1967.

Dubois-Poulsen, A.: Le champ visuel, Paris, 1952, Masson & Cie, Editeurs.

Duke-Elder, S., and Scott, G.: Neuro-ophthalmology. In Duke-Elder, S., editor: System of ophthalmology, vol. 12, St. Louis, 1971, The C. V. Mosby Co.

Evans, J. N.: An introduction to clinical scotometry, London, 1938, Oxford University Press.

Förster, O.: Über die Wechselbeziehungen von Herdsymptomen und Allgemeinsymptomen bei Hirntumor, Verh. Dtsch. Ges. Inn. Med., pp. 458-485, 1938.

Gjessing, H. G. A.: Importance of eye symptoms in diagnosis and localization of brain tumors, Trans. Ophthalmol. Soc. U.K. 54:581-602, 1934.

Globus, J. H., and Silverstone, S. M.: Diagnostic value of defects in the visual fields and other ocular disturbances associated with supratentorial tumors of the brain, Arch. Ophthalmol. 14:325, 1935.

Gorton, L. W.: Eye findings as aid in diagnosing and localization of brain tumors, New Orleans Med. Surg. J. 90:315-318, 1937.

Guillaumat, L., and Robin, A.: Statistique des modifications du champ visuel dans les affections neurochirurgicales non traumatiques. In Dubois-Poulsen, A.: Le champ visuel, Paris, 1952, Masson & Cie Editeurs.

Guillaumat, L., Morax, P. V., and Offret, G.: Neuro-ophtalmologie, Paris, 1959, Masson & Cie, Editeurs.

Hartmann, E.: Ocular symptoms in diseases of brain, spinal cord, and meninges. In Berens, C., editor: The eye and its diseases, Philadelphia, 1949, W. B. Saunders Co., p. 824.

Hartmann, E., and Guillaumat, L.: Aspect du fond d'œil dans les tumeurs intracrâniennes. Etude statistique, Ann. Oculist. 175:717-737, 1938.

Hobbs, H. E.: Visual defect as an early sign of intracranial tumor, Eye Era Nose Throat Mon. 46:602-610, 1967.

Hollwich, F.: Irrtümer beim Nachweis von Hirntumoren, Ber. Dtsch. Ophthalmol. Ges. 59:36-39, 1955.

Horrax, G., and Putnam, T. J.: Distortions of the visual fields in cases of brain tumour, Brain 55:499, 1932.

Huber, A.: Die ophthalmologische Symptomatologie der Hirntumoren. Allgemeinsymptome und supratentorielle Tumoren, Ophthalmologica 125:287-319, 1953.

Huber, A.: Eye symptoms in brain tumors, Highlights Ophthalmol. 7:3-98, 1964.

Jelsma, F.: Intracranial tumors, Kentucky Med. J. 39:203-208, 1941.

Jentzer, A.: Les tumeurs cérébrales, Helv. Med. Acta 5:6, 720, 1938.

Junius, P.: Diagnostik der Hirntumoren mit besonderer Berücksichtigung der Erscheinungen am Sehorgan, Zentralbl. Gesamte. Ophthalmol. 26:5, 273, 1932.

Kennedy, F.: Symptomatology and diagnosis of lesions of the brain, with special reference to disturbances of vision, hearing, taste, smell and speech, Trans. Am. Acad. Ophthalmol. 30:8-25, 1925.

Kraus, H.: Gutartige basale Tumoren der vorderen und mittleren Schädelgrube, Wien. Med. Wochenschr. 100:156, 1950.

Krayenbühl, H.: Hilfsmethoden der Diagnostik raumbeschränkender intrakranieller Erkrankungen, Schweiz. Med. Wochenschr. 5:89, 1937.

Krayenbühl, H.: Die Symptomatologie der Tumoren der hinteren Schädelgrube, Schweiz. Med. Wochenschr. **31**:901, 1938.

Krayenbühl, H., and Schmid, A. E.: Zur Lokalisation intrakranieller und orbitaler Dermoide, Ophthalmologica **106**:251, 1943.

Krayenbühl, H., and Weber, G.: Diagnostik und Grundzüge der Therapie der Hirntumoren im Kindesalter, Helv. Paediatr. Acta **2**:2, 115, 1947.

Lauber, H.: Das Gesichtsfeld, Munich, 1944, Bergmann & Springer.

Lobeck, E.: Über die Bedeutung des Augenbefundes für die Diagnostik und Therapie von Hirntumoren (nebst Bemerkungen über die Entstehungsweise von Zentralskotomen bei Tumoren der vorderen Schädelgrube), Graefe. Arch. Ophthalmol. **140**: 599-628, 1939.

Lyle, D. J.: Symposium on manifestations of disease affecting cerebral nerves supplying eye, ear, nose and throat due to involvement in diseases of the central nervous system, Trans. Am. Acad. Ophthalmol. **41**: 49-68, 1936.

Marburg, O.: Some remarks on tumors of the brain in childhood, Trans. Am. Neurol. Assoc. **67**:35-40, 1942.

McCulloch, R. J. P.: Eye signs in intracranial disease, Can. Med. Assoc. J. **42**: 236, 1940.

Miller, R. H., McCraig, W., and Kernohan, J. W.: Supratentorial tumors among children, Arch. Neurol. Psychiat. **68**:797-814, 1952.

Moersch, F. P., McCraig, W., and Kernohan, J. W.: Tumors of the brain in aged persons, Arch. Neurol. Psychiatr. **45**:235, 1941.

Moller, H. U.: Zur neuro-ophthalmologischen Diagnostik (in Danish), Nord. Med. **14**:1405-1409, 1942.

Monbrun, A.: Affections des voies optiques rétro-chiasmatiques et de l'écorce visuelle. In Bailliart, P., et al., editors: Traité d'ophtalmologie, Paris, 1939, Masson & Cie, Editeurs, vol. 6, p. 903.

Mooney, A. J.: Lesions of visual pathway and their relation to neuro-surgery (Mary Louise Prentice Montgomery Memorial Lecture), Ir. J. Med. Sci., pp. 315-327, 1938.

Müller, R., and Wohlfahrt, G.: Intracranial teratomas and teratoid tumours, Acta Psychiatr. Neurol. **22**:69-95, 1947.

Pandit, Y. K. C.: Intracranial space occupying lesions, Proc. All-India Ophthalmol. Soc. **13**:1-34, 1965.

Payne, F.: Neuro-ophthalmology, Arch. Ophthalmol. **50**:644-666, 1953.

Perria, L.: Sintomi oculari e tumori endocranici, Sist. Nerv. **1**:9-17, 1949.

Petrohelos, M. A., and Henderson, J. W.: The ocular findings of intracranial tumour, Trans. Am. Acad. Ophthalmol. **55**:89-98, 1950.

Petrohelos, M. A., and Henderson, J. W.: Ocular findings of intracranial tumor; study of 358 cases, Am. J. Ophthalmol. **34**:1387, 1951.

Raaf, J.: Perimetric diagnosis of intracranial tumors, Trans. Pac. Coast Otoophthalmol. Soc. **27**:131-144, 1942.

Rand, C. W., and Wagenen, R. J.: Brain tumors in childhood; review of 38 cases, J. Pediatr. **6**:322-339, 1935.

Remky, H.: Ophthalmoneurologie. Zur Diagnose von Ort und Art intrakranieller Prozesse (insbesondere Tumoren), Almanach Augenheilkd. München, pp. 107-115, 1960.

Reymond, A.: Classification anatomo-pathologique des tumeurs cérébrales, Ophthalmologica **125**:204-230, 1953.

Rintelen, F.: Die ophthalmoneurologischen Symptome und Syndrome bei infratentoriellen Hirntumoren, Ophthalmologica **125**: 320-340, 1953.

Rintelen, F.: Gesichtsfelddefekte bei Hirntumoren, Ophthalmologica **158**:451-468, 1969.

Rucker, C. W.: Neuro-ophthalmology, Arch. Ophthalmol. **44**:733, 1950.

Ruedemann, A. D.: Differential diagnosis of brain lesions; comparison by visual fields, encephalography and ventriculography, Trans. Sect. Ophthalmol. Am. Med. Assoc., pp. 32-37, 1940.

Schreck, E.: Ophthalmologische Diagnostik bei Hirntumoren, Regensb. Jb. Arztl. Fortbild. **6**:294-308, 1958.

Stender, A.: Über die Frühdiagnose von Hirntumoren, Dtsch. Med. Wochenschr. **4**: 210-213, 1953.

Tönnis, W.: Augensymptome bei 3033 Hirngeschwülsten, Ber. Dtsch. Ophthalmol. Ges. **59**:6-27, 1955.

Tönnis, W.: Diagnostik der intrakraniellen Geschwülste. In Olivecrona, H., and Tönnis, W., editors: Handbuch der Neurochirurgie, Berlin, 1962, Julius Springer, vol. 4, pt. 3, pp. 1-579.

Traquair, H. M.: An introduction to clinical perimetry, London, 1949, Henry Kimpton.

Walsh, F. B., and Hoyt, W. F.: Orbital, ocular and intracranial tumors. In Clinical neuro-ophthalmology, Baltimore, 1969, The Williams & Wilkins Co., pp. 1927-2330.

Watanabe, H.: Ophthalmologist and brain tumor, Jpn. J. Ophthalmol. 25:889-953, 1971.

Weber, G.: Zur Diagnose und Prognose intrakranieller Tumoren, Ophthalmologica 125: 231-286, 1953.

Yanagida, N.: Ophthalmic symptoms of brain tumour, particularly of the visual field, Acta Soc. Ophthalmol. Jpn. 55:836, 1951.

Yanagida, N.: Ocular symptoms of various intracranial tumours (in Japanese), Acta Soc. Ophthalmol. Jpn. 57:1377-1381, 1392-1398, 1464-1477, 1953.

**Tumors of the frontal lobe**

Bailey, P.: Syndrom des Frontallappens. Die Hirngeschwülste, Stuttgart, 1951, Ferdinand Enke Verlag, p. 214.

Botez, M. I.: Frontal lobe tumours. In Vinken, P. J., and Bruyn, G. W., editors: Handbook of clinical neurology, New York, 1974, American Elsevier Publishing Co., Inc., vol. 18, pp. 234-280.

Calmettes, L., Deodati, F., and Bec, P.: Hémianopsie horizontale et tumeur frontale, Rev. Otoneuroophtalmol. 36:175-178, 1964.

Croll, M.: Frontal lobe tumors and their ocular manifestations, Am. J. Ophthalmol. 59:206-211, 1965.

David, M., and Sourdille, G.: Sur la valeur localisatrice des signes dits de compression directe due nerf optique, en particulier du syndrome de Foster-Kennedy, dans les tumeurs cérébrales, J. Ophtalmol. 3:215, 1942.

Dilenge, D., David, M., and Fischgold, H.: Artère ophtalmique et tumeurs frontales intracrâniennes, Neurochirurgie 8:379-384, 1962.

Duke-Elder, S., and Scott, G.: Neuro-ophthalmology. In Duke-Elder, S., editor: System of ophthalmology, vol. 12, London, 1971, Henry Kimpton.

Ecker, A. D.: Concentric contraction of visual fields associated with tumor of the frontal lobe, Mayo Clin. Proc. 12:679, 1937.

François, J., and Neetens, A.: Le syndrome de Foster Kennedy et son étiologie, Ann. Oculist. 188:219-253, 1955.

Fridenberg, P.: The "Foster Kennedy" syndrome, Arch. Ophthalmol. 26:288, 1941.

Galvez Montes, J., and de Frederico Antras, A.: Sindrome de Foster-Kennedy invertido, Arch. Soc. Oftalmol. Hispano-Am. 21:225-233, 1961.

Glees, M.: Dem Foster Kennedyschen Syndrom ähnliche Veränderungen der Sehnerven durch Arteriosklerose, Klin. Monatsbl. Augenheilkd. 100:865-873, 1938.

Halpern, L.: Frontalhirnsyndrome, Monatsschr. Psychiatr. Neurol. 101:4, 239, 1939.

Holmes, G., and Fox, J. C.: Optic nystagmus and its value in the localization of cerebral lesions, Brain 49:333, 1926.

Hyland, H. H., and Botterell, E. H.: Frontal lobe tumors; clinical and physiological study, Can. Med. Assoc. J. 37:530-540, 1937.

Jenkner, F. L., and Kutschera, E.: Frontal lobes and vision, Confin. Neurol. 25:63-78, 1965.

Kennedy, F.: Retrobulbar neuritis as an exact diagnostic sign of certain tumors and abscesses in the frontal lobe, Am. J. Med. Sci. 142:355, 1911.

Kennedy, F.: A further note on the diagnostic value of retrobulbar neuritis in expanding lesions of the frontal lobes, J.A.M.A. 67:1360, 1916.

Kestenbaum, A.: Zur Klinik des optokinetischen Nystagmus, Graefe. Arch. Ophthalmol. 124:339, 1930.

Lillie, W. I.: Ocular phenomena produced by basal lesions of the frontal lobe, J.A.M.A. 89:2099-2103, 1927.

Pittrich, H.: Stirnhirngeschwülste, Arch. Psychiatr. 113:1-60, 1941.

de Recondo, J.: Les mouvements conjugués oculaires et leurs diverses modalités d'atteinte, Paris, 1967, Masson & Cie, Editeurs.

Sanders, M. D.: The Foster Kennedy sign, Proc. R. Soc. Med. 65:520-521, 1972.

Silberpfennig, J.: Contributions to problem of eye movements; disturbances of ocular movements with pseudohemianopia in frontal lobe tumors, Confin. Neurol. 4:1-13, 1941.

Skrzypczak, J.: Zur Bedeutung des Foster-Kennedy Syndroms, Klin. Monatsbl. Augenheilkd. 150:504-509, 1967.

Tönnis, W.: Geschwülste des Stirnhirns. Diagnostik der intrakraniellen Geschwülste. In

Olivecrona, H., and Tönnis, W., editors: Handbuch der Neurochirurgie, Berlin, 1962, Julius Springer, vol. 4, p. 369.

Voris, H. C., Adson, A. W., and Moersch, F. P.: Tumors of the frontal lobe: clinical observations in series verified microscopically, J.A.M.A. **104**:93-99, 1935.

Walsh, F. B., and Hoyt, W. F.: Tumors of the frontal lobe. In Clinical neuro-ophthalmology, Baltimore, 1969, The Williams & Wilkins Co., p. 2166.

**Tumors of the temporal lobe**

Bailey, P.: Syndrom des Temporallappens. Die Hirngeschwülste, Stuttgart, 1951, Ferdinand Enke Verlag, p. 246.

Barcia Goyanes, J. J.: Anatomie du lobe temporal, Rev. Otoneuroophtalmol. **22**:71-102, 1950.

Bender, M. B., and Savitsky, N.: Micropsia and teleopsia limited to the temporal fields of vision, Arch. Ophthalmol. **29**:904, 1943.

de Crinis, M.: Zur Symptomatologie der Schläfenlappentumoren, Z. Ges. Neurol. Psychiatr. **174**:169-193, 1942.

Cushing, H.: Distortion of the visual fields in cases of brain tumor: the field defects produced by temporal lobe lesions, Brain **44**:341-396, 1922.

Duke-Elder, S., and Scott, G:. Neuro-ophthalmology. In Duke-Elder, S., editor: System of ophthalmology, vol. 12, St. Louis, 1971, The C. V. Mosby Co.

Fischer-Brügge, K.: Das Klivuskantensyndrom, Acta Neurochir. **2**:36, 1951.

Fonte Barcena, A.: Visual disturbances in tumors of temporal lobe, An. Soc. Mex. Oftalmol. Otorinolaringol. **19**:1-16, 1944.

Game, J.: Temporal lobe tumors, Med. J. Aust. **1**:366-368, 1953.

Géraud, Lazorthes, Caizergues, and Ribaut: Atteinte du réflexe cornéen par méningiome temporal, Rev. Otoneuroophtalmol. **23**:169-170, 1951.

Gordon, A.: Visual field defects as a deciding diagnostic factor in lesions of temporal lobe simulating cerebellar involvement, Trans. Am. Neurol. Assoc. **60**:212-215, 1934.

Guillot, P., and Casanovas, J.: Le lobe temporal en O. N. O.: séminologie ophtalmique, Rev. Otoneuroophtalmol. **22**:2, 219, 1950.

Harrington, D. O.: Localizing value of in-congruity in defects in the visual fields, Arch. Ophthalmol. **21**:453, 1939.

Heppner, F., and Vogler, E.: Symptomatologie und Diagnostik der Schläfenlappentumoren, Wien. Klin. Wochenschr. **64**:969-976, 1952.

Horrax, G.: Visual hallucinations as a cerebral localizing phenomenon: with special reference to their occurrence in tumors of the temporal lobe, Arch. Neurol. Psychiatr. **10**:532-547, 1923.

Insausti, T., and Salleras, A.: Sintomatologia oftalmologica de los tumores temporales, Neuropsiquiatria **3**:143-157, 1952.

Kennedy, F.: The symptomatology of temporo-sphenoidal tumors, Arch. Intern. Med. **8**:317, 1911.

Koch, G.: Oculomotoriuswurzelschädigung durch einseitige Quellung des Uncus gyri hippocampi, Dtsch. Z. Nervenheilk. **159**:417, 1948.

Kolodny, A.: The symptomatology of tumours of the temporal lobe, Brain **51**:385-417, 1928.

Kravitz, D.: The value of quadrant defects in the localization of temporal lobe tumors, Am. J. Ophthalmol. **14**:781-785, 1931.

Krayenbühl, H.: Die Bedeutung der Gesichtsfeldbestimmung in der Diagnostik von Tumoren des Schläfen- und Hinterhauptlappens, Schweiz. Med. Wochenschr. **69**:43, 197, 1939.

Matavulj, N.: Syndrome ophtalmologique dans les tumeurs temporales, Rev. Otoneuroophtalmol. **22**:8, 1950.

Meyer, A.: The temporal lobe detour of the radiations, etc., Am. Neurol. Assoc. 1911; Trans. Assoc. Am. Physicians **22**:7, 1907.

Obrador Alcalde, S.: Physiologie du lobe temporal, Rev. Otoneuroophtalmol. **22**:103-120, 1950.

Paillas, J. E., and Tamalet, J.: Les glioblastomes temporaux, Marseille Chir. **2**:461-465, 1950.

Paillas, J. E., Boudouresques, J., and Tamalet, J.: Hallucinations visuelles d'origine temporale à propos de 15 observations anatomo-cliniques, Rev. Neurol. **81**:154-156, 1949.

Strobos, R. J.: Temporal lobe tumors. In Vinken, P. J., and Bruyn, G. W., editors: Handbook of clinical neurology, New York, 1974, American Elsevier Publishing Co. Inc., vol. 18, pp. 281-295.

Taveras, J. M.: Roentgenologic aspects of

the diagnosis of temporal tumors. In Smith, J. L., editor: Neuro-ophthalmology, St. Louis, 1968, The C. V. Mosby Co., vol. 4, pp. 215-229.

Thiébaut, F.: Hémianopsie relative et lobe temporal, Rev. Otoneuroophtalmol. 23:236-238, 1951.

Thurel, R.: Paralysie du moteur oculaire commun par engagement du lobe temporal, Rev. Otoneuroophtalmol. 23:285-286, 1951.

Tönnis, W.: Geschwülste des Schläfenlappens. Diagnostik der intrakraniellen Geschwülste. In Olivecrona, H., and Tönnis, W., editors: Handbuch der Neurochirurgie, Berlin, 1962, Julius Springer, vol. 4, p. 410.

Traquair, H. M.: The course of the geniculo-localcarine visual path in relation to the temporal lobe, Br. J. Ophthalmol. 6:251-259, 1922.

Walker, A. E., and Walsh, F. B.: Visual disturbances in temporal lobectomized patients. In Smith, J. L., editor: Neuro-ophthalmology, St. Louis, 1968, The C. V. Mosby Co., vol. 4, pp. 230-248.

Walsh, F. B., and Hoyt, W. F.: Temporal lobe tumors. In Clinical neuro-ophthalmology, Baltimore, 1969, The Williams & Wilkins Co., p. 2178.

Weinberger, L. M., and Grant, F. C.: Visual hallucinations and their neuro-optical correlates, Arch. Ophthalmol. 23:166-199, 1940.

**Tumors of the parietal lobe**

Bailey, P.: Syndrom des Parietallapens. Die Hirngeschwülste, Stuttgart, 1951, Ferdinand Enke Verlag, p. 230.

Cogan, D. G.: Hemianopia and associated symptoms due to parietotemporal lobe lesions, Am. J. Ophthalmol. 50:1056-1066, 1960.

David, M., and Hecaen, H.: Sur certains troubles de la latéralité du regard dans les lésions pariétales s'accompagnant de troubles de la somatognosie, Bull. Soc. Ophtalmol. Paris 1:103-105, 1947.

Duke-Elder, S., and Scott, G.: Neuro-ophthalmology. In Duke-Elder, S., editor: System of ophthalmology, vol. 12, St. Louis, 1971, The C. V. Mosby Co.

Greenblatt, S. H.: Alexia without agraphia or hemianopsia: anatomical analysis of an autopsied case, Brain 96:307-316, 1973.

Offret, G.: Modern concepts of physiology and psychophysiology of parietoccipital

lobes of brain, Arch. Ophthalmol. 6:145-172, 1946.

Penfield, W., and Rasmussen, T.: The cerebral cortex of man, New York, 1950, Macmillan, Inc.

Pouliquen, P., and Lobstein, A.: Champs visuels atypiques au cours de l'évolution d'une tumeur pariéto-temporale, Rev. Otoneuroophtalmol. 24:158, 1952.

Suchenwirth, R. M. A.: Parietal lobe tumours. In Vinken, P. J., and Bruyn, G. W.: Handbook of clinical neurology, New York, 1974, American Elsevier Publishing Co. Inc., vol. 18, pp. 296-309.

Tönnis, W.: Geschwülste des Scheitellappens. Diagnostik der intrakraniellen Geschwülste. In Olivecrona, H., and Tönnis, W., editors: Handbuch der Neurochirurgie, Berlin, 1962, Julius Springer, vol. 4, p. 406.

Walsh, F. B., and Hoyt, W. F.: Parietal lobe tumor. In Clinical neuro-ophthalmology, Baltimore, 1969, The Williams & Wilkins Co., p. 2203.

**Tumors of the occipital lobe**

Allen, I. M.: Clinical study of tumors involving the occipital lobe, Brain 53:194, 1930.

Bailey, P.: Syndrom des Occipitallappens. Die Hirngeschwülste, Stuttgart, 1951, Ferdinand Enke Verlag, p. 250.

Barkan, O., and Boyle, S. F.: Paracentral homonymous hemianopic scotoma, Arch. Ophthalmol. 14:956-959, 1930.

Bender, M. B., and Battersby, W. S.: Homonymous macular scotomas in cases of occipital lobe tumor, Arch. Ophthalmol. 60:928-938, 1958.

Bender, M. B., and Strauss, I.: Defects in visual field of one eye only in patients with a lesion of one optic radiation, Arch. Ophthalmol. 17:765-787, 1937.

Brégeat, P., Klein, M., Thiébaut, F., and Bouniol: Hémimacropsie homonyme droite et tumeur occipitale gauche, Rev. Otoneuroophtalmol. 19:238-240, 1947.

Clark, W. E. L.: The anatomy of cortical vision, Trans. Ophthalmol. Soc. U.K. 62:229, 1942.

Clark, W. E. L.: The visual centers of the brain and their connections, Physiol. Rev. 22:205, 1942.

David, H., Hecaen, R., Angelergues, R., and Magis, C.: Les tumeurs occipitales, Neurochirurgie 1:177-191, 1955.

Dubois-Poulsen, A., Magis, C., de Ajuria-guerra, J., and Hecaen, R.: Les conséquences visuelles de la lobectomie occipitale chez l'homme, Ann. Oculist. 185: 4, 305, 1952.

Duke-Elder, S., and Scott, G.: Neuro-ophthalmology. In Duke-Elder, S., editor: System of ophthalmology, vol. 12, St. Louis, 1971, The C. V. Mosby Co.

Edmund, J.: Visual disturbances associated with gliomas of the temporal and occipital lobe, Acta Psychiatr. Neurol. Scand. 29: 291, 1954.

Evans, J. N., and Browder, J.: Problem of split macula: study of visual fields, Arch. Ophthalmol. 31:43-53, 1944.

Frazier, C. H., and Waggoner, R. W.: Tumors of the occipital lobe: a review of 40 cases, Arch. Neurol. Psychiatr. 22:1096-1099, 1929.

Gassel, M. M.: Occipital lobe tumours. In Vinkel, P. J., and Bruyn, G. W., editors: Handbook of clinical neurology, New York, 1974, American Elsevier Publishing Co., Inc., vol. 18, pp. 310-349.

Halstead, W. C., Walker, A. E., and Bucy, P. C.: Sparing and nonsparing of "macular" vision associated with occipital lobectomy in man, Arch. Ophthalmol. 24:948-966, 1940.

Holmes, G. A.: Contribution to the cortical representation of vision, Brain 54:470, 1931.

Holmes, G. A., and Lister, W. T.: Disturbances of vision from cerebral lesions with special reference to the cortical representation of the macula, Brain 39:34-73, 1916.

Horrax, G., and Putnam, T. J.: Distortion of the visual fields in cases of brain tumor: the field defects and hallucinations produced by tumors of the occipital lobe, Brain 55:499, 1932.

Huber, A.: Zur homonymen Hemianopsie nach occipitaler Lobektomie, Schweiz. Med. Wochenschr. 80:1227, 1950.

Klüver, H.: Visual functions after removal of the occipital lobes, J. Psychol. 11:23, 1941.

Krayenbühl, H.: Die Bedeutung der Gesichtsfeldbestimmung in der Diagnostik von Tumoren des Schläfen- und Hinterhauptlappens, Schweiz. Med. Wochenschr. 69: 43, 197, 1939.

Le Beau, J., Wolinetz, E., and Rosier, M.:

Phénomène de persévération des images visuelles dans un cas de méningiome occipital droit, Rev. Neurol. 86:692-695, 1952.

Levenson, D. S., and Smith, J. L.: Optokinetic nystagmus and occipital lesions, Am. J. Ophthalmol. 61:753-762, 1966.

Parkinson, D., and Kernohan, J. W.: Tumours of the occipital lobe; J. Neurosurg. 7:555, 1950.

Parkinson, D., and McCraig, K. W.: Tumours of the brain, occipital lobe; their signs and symptoms, Can. Med. Assoc. J. 64: 111-113, 1951.

Parkinson, D., Rucker, C. W., and McCraig, K. W.: Visual hallucinations associated with tumors of occipital lobe, Arch. Neurol. Psychiatr. 68:66-68, 1952.

Penfield, W., Evans, J. P., and MacMillan, J. A.: Visual pathways in man; with particular reference to macular representation, Arch. Neurol. Psychiatr. 33:816-834, 1935.

Porsaa, K.: Central visual field after occipital lobectomy, Acta Ophthalmol. 22:243-250, 1944.

Putnam, T. J., and Liebmann, S.: Cortical representation of the macula lutea, with special reference to the theory of bilateral representation, Arch. Ophthalmol. 28:415, 1943.

Schweitzer, A.: Ophthalmological manifestations of lesions of the occipital lobe, Arch. Chil. Oftalmol. 28:69-77, 1972.

Stadlin, W.: Hémianopsie et nystagmus optocinétique, Ophthalmologica 118:383, 1949.

Tönnis, W.: Geschwülste des Occipitallappens. Diagnostik der intrakraniellen Geschwülste. In Olivecrona, H., and Tönnis, W., editors: Handbuch der Neurochirurgie, Berlin, 1962, Julius Springer, vol. 4, p. 417.

Walsh, F. B., and Hoyt, W. F.: Occipital lobe tumors, In Clinical neuro-ophthalmology, Baltimore, 1969, The Williams & Wilkins Co., p. 2195.

Weinberger, L. M., and Grant, F. C.: Visual hallucinations and their neuro-optical correlates (review), Arch. Ophthalmol. 23: 166-199, 1940.

**Tumors of the corpus callosum**

Bailey, P.: Syndrom des Balkens. Die Hirngeschwülste, Stuttgart, 1951, Ferdinand Enke Verlag, p. 254.

Kretschmer, H.: Callosal tumours. In Vinken,

P. J., and Bruyn, G. W., editors: Handbook of clinical neurology, New York, 1974, American Elsevier Publishing Co., Inc., vol. 17, pp. 490-554.

Walsh, F. B., and Hoyt, W. F.: Corpus callosum tumor. In Clinical neuro-ophthalmology, Baltimore, 1969, The Williams & Wilkins Co., p. 2261.

**Parasagittal meningiomas and meningiomas of falx**

Bailey, P., and Bucy, P. C.: The origin and nature of meningeal tumors, Am. J. Cancer 1:15-54, 1931.

Courville, C. B., and Abbot, K. H.: On classification of meningiomas; survey of 99 cases in light of existing schemes, Bull. Los Angeles Neurol. Soc. 6:21-31, 1941.

Custodis, E.: Meningioma der Falx und lokalisatorisch irreführendes Foster Kennedysches Syndrom, Klin. Monatsbl. Augenheilkd. 101:823-830, 1938.

Gassel, M. M.: False localizing signs. A review of the concept and analysis of the occurrence in 250 cases of intracranial meningioma, Arch. Neurol. 4:526-554, 1961.

Klinger, M., and Condrau, G.: Lokalisatorisch irreführende Gesichtsfeldsymptome bei Hirntumoren, Ophthalmological 120:270, 1950.

Krayenbühl, H.: Klinik und Therapie des intrakraniellen Meningeoms, Schweiz Med. Wochenschr. 78:841, 1948.

Marr, W. G., and Chambers, T. W.: Occlusion of the cerebral sinuses by tumor simulating pseudotumor cerebri, Am. J. Ophthalmol. 6:45-49, 1966.

Newell, F. W., and Beaman, T. C.: Ocular signs of meningioma, Am. J. Ophthalmol. 45:30-40, 1958.

Olivecrona, H.: Die parasagittalen Meningiome, Leipzig, 1934, Georg Thieme Verlag KG.

Olivecrona, H.: The parasagittal meningiomas, J. Neurosurg. 4:327, 1947.

Rucker, C. W., and Kearns, T. P.: Mistaken diagnoses in some cases of meningioma. Clinics in perimetry no. 5, Am. J. Ophthalmol. 51:15-19, 1961.

Tönnis, W.: Meningiomae. Diagnostik der intrakraniellen Geschwülste. In Olivecrona, H., and Tönnis, W., editors: Handbuch der Neurochirurgie, Berlin, 1962, Julius Springer, vol. 4, p. 39.

Vincent, C., Hartmann, E., and Le Beau, J.: Atrophie optique primitive par méningiome à distance de la région opto-chiasmatique, Zentralbl. Neurochir. 3:145, 1938.

Walsh, F. B., and Hoyt, W. F.: Parasagittal and falx meningiomas. In Clinical neuro-ophthalmology, Baltimore, 1969, The Williams & Wilkins Co., pp. 2269-2271.

**Pituitary adenomas**

Adler, F. H., Austin, G., and Grant, F. C.: Localizing value of visual fields in patients with early chiasmal lesions, Arch. Ophthalmol. 40:579-600, 1948.

Amsler, M.: Krankheiten des Chiasma. In Amsler, M., et al., editors: Lehrbuch der Augenheilkunde, Basel, 1954, S. Karger AG, p. 703.

Arganaraz, R.: Heteronymous hemianopia and intracranial tumors in the neighborhood of the chiasma, Arch. Oftalmol. B. Air. 16:349, 1941.

Asbury, T.: Unilateral scotoma as the presenting signs of pituitary tumor, Am. J. Ophthalmol. 59:510-512, 1965.

Aulhorn, E.: Perimetrie. In Sautter, H., editor: Entwicklung und Fortschritte in der Augenheilkunde, Stuttgart, 1963, Ferdinand Enke Verlag.

Bailey, P.: Das Hypophysensyndrom. Die Hirngeschwülste, Stuttgart, 1951, Ferdinand Enke Verlag, p. 73.

Bailey, P.: Syndrom des Chiasma opticum. Die Hirngeschwülste, Stuttgart, 1951, Ferdinand Enke Verlag, p. 270.

Bakay, L.: The results of 300 pituitary adenoma operations (Prof. Herbert Olivecrona's series), J. Neurosurg. 7:240-255, 1950.

Bardram, M. T.: Oculomotor paresis and non-paretic diplopia in pituitary adenomata, Acta Ophthalmol. 27:225-258, 1949.

Bergland, R., and Ray, B. S.: The arterial supply of the human optic chiasm, J. Neurosurg. 31:327-334, 1969.

Best, F.: Die Augensymptome bei Hypophysenerkrankungen. In Schieck, F., and Brückner, A., editors: Kurzes Handbuch der Ophthalmologie, Berlin, 1931, Julius Springer, vol. 6, p. 596.

Biemond, A.: Nervus opticus und chiasma, Ophthalmologica 102:287-302, 1941.

Bigorgne, J., Bigorgne, J. C., Hallot-Boyer, P., and Hermann, P.: Central scotomata in sellar and parasellar tumours, Rev. Otoneuroophtalmol. 45:185-191, 1973.

Bonamour, G., Bonnet, M., and Laffay, N.: The chiasmal syndrome occurring in pregnancy, Ann. Oculist. 204:235-256, 1971.

Borromei, A., and Palmieri, L.: Neoplasie della regione sellare; risultati neurooftalmologici postoperatori, Minerva Oftalmol. 12:65-84, 1970.

Bregeat, P.: The chiasmal syndrome in Cushing's disease, Arch. Ophthalmol. 31:389-398, 1971.

Bregeat, P.: Modern data in chiasmal syndrome, Minerva Oftalmol. 13:37-50, 1971.

Cairns, H.: Peripheral ocular palsies from the neuro-surgical point of view, Trans. Ophthalmol. Soc. U.K. 58:464, 1938.

Chamlin, M., and Davidoff, L. M.: The 1/2000 field in chiasmal interference, Arch. Ophthalmol. 44:53-70, 1950.

Chamlin, M., and Davidoff, L. M.: Symposium on pituitary tumors. II. Ophthalmologic criteria in diagnosis and management of pituitary tumors, J. Neurosurg. 19:9-18, 1962.

Chamlin, N., Davidoff, L. M., and Feiring, E. H.: Ophthalmologic changes produced by pituitary tumors, Am. J. Ophthalmol. 40:353-368, 1955.

Chiasserini, F.: Diagnostic et thérapeutique de quelques affections sellaires, Schweiz. Med. Wochenschr., p. 425, 1939.

Cullen, J. F.: Pituitary and parapituitary tumors. Value of perimetry in diagnosis, Br. J. Ophthalmol. 48:590-596, 1964.

Cushing, H.: The pituitary body and its disorders, Philadelphia, 1912, J. B. Lippincott Co.

Cushing, H., and Walker, C. B.: Chiasmal lesions with especial reference to bitemporal hemianopia, Brain 37:341-400, 1915.

Dandy, W. E.: Hypophyseal tumors. In Lewis, D., editor: Lewis' practice of surgery, Hagerstown, Md., 1937, W. F. Prior Co., Inc., vol. 12, pp. 556-605.

Davidoff, L. M.: The anamnesis and symptomatology in one hundred cases of acromegaly, Endocrinology 10:461-482, 1926.

Desvignes, P.: Le syndrome de compression directe du nerf optique intracrânien, Ann. Oculist. 174:289-308, 1937.

Duke-Elder, S., and Scott, G.: Neuro-ophthalmology. In Duke-Elder, S., editor: System of ophthalmology, vol. 12, St. Louis, 1971, The C. V. Mosby Co.

Epstein, S., et al.: Pituitary apoplexy in five patients with pituitary tumors, Br. Med. J. 2:267-270, 1971.

Fahlbusch, R., and Marguth, F.: Clinical and radiological picture in chiasmal processes, Minerva Oftalmol. 13:99-109, 1971.

Forbes, A. P., Henneman, P. H., Griswald, G. C., and Albright, F.: A syndrome characterized by galactorrhea, amenorrhea and low urinary FSH: comparison with acromegaly and normal lactation, J. Clin. Endocrinol. Metab. 14:265-271, 1954.

Franceschetti, A., and Werner, A.: Syndrome chiasmatique du à un abcès intrasellaire chronique, Rev. Otoneuroophtalmol. 29:177-182, 1957.

Franceschetti, A., Babel, J., Doret, M., and Werner, A.: A propos du syndrome chiasmatique, la fréquence de son origine non-hypophysaire; la nécessité d'un diagnostic précoce avec la névrite optique rétrobulbaire, Confin. Neurol. 16:206-207, 1956.

François, J., Hoffmann, G., and de Brabandere, J.: Le diagnostic visuel des opérations pour tumeurs hypophysaires, Ann. Oculist. 193:993-1033, 1960.

Franklin, C. R.: Visual studies in pituitary adenoma, Bull. Neurol. Inst. N.Y. 5:180-198, 1936.

Fujie, Y.: Ocular symptoms of tumors in the pituitary region. Course of visual field in the pituitary adenoma, Jpn. J. Ophthalmol. 21:1053-1060, 1967.

Gartner, S.: Ocular pathology in the chiasmal syndrome, Am. J. Ophthalmol. 34:593-596, 1951.

Gil Espinosa, M.: Über nicht hypophysäre Chiasmasyndrome, Bibliotheca Ophthalmologica, fasc. 32, Basel, 1946, S. Karger AG.

Glees, M., and Zielinksi, H.: Ueber bitemporale zentrale und parazentrale Skotome bei verschiedenen krankhaften Prozessen im Sellabereich, Klin. Monatsbl. Augenheilkd. 129:145-160, 1956.

Graham, W. V., and Wakefield, G. J.: Bitemporal visual field defects associated with anomalies of the optic discs, Br. J. Ophthalmol. 57:307-314, 1973.

di Gugliemo, G.: Diagnosi e terapia delle sindromi sellari e parasellari, Arch. Ed. Atti Soc. Ital. Chir. 44:334-413, 1938.

Guillaumat, L.: Le champ visuel dans les affections chiasmatiques, Année Ther. Clin. Ophtalmol. 11:7-190, 1960.

Hagedoorn, A.: The chiasmal syndrome and

retrobulbar neuritis in pregnancy, Am. J. Ophthalmol. **20**:690, 1937.

Harms, H.: Quantitative Perimetrie bei sellanahen Tumoren, Ophthalmologica **127**: 255-261, 1954.

Harms, H.: Leitsymptom "Zentralskotom." In Sautter, H., editor: Entwicklung und Fortschritte in der Augenheilkunde, Stuttgart, 1963, Ferdinand Enke Verlag, pp. 516-539.

Hartmann, E., and David, M.: Affections du Chiasma. In Bailliart, P., et al., editors: Traité d'ophthalmologie, Paris, 1939, Masson & Cie, Editeurs, vol. 6, p. 877.

Hedges, T. R.: Preservation of the upper nasal field in the chiasmal syndrome: an anatomic explanation, Trans. Am. Ophthalmol. Soc. **67**:131-141, 1969.

Henderson, W. R.: The pituitary adenomas, Br. J. Surg. **26**:811-911, 1939.

Hirsch, O.: Die Bedeutung des Augenhintergrundes für die Diagnose eines Hypophysentumors, Monatsschr. Psychiatr. Neurol. **117**:236-240, 1949.

Hobbs, H. E.: Visual field defects in chiasmal lesions, Trans. Can. Ophthalmol. Soc. **8**:111-121, 1956.

Hoyt, W. F., and Luis, O.: The primate chiasm: details of visual fiber organization studied by silver impregnation techniques, Arch. Ophthalmol. **70**:69-85, 1963.

Jeandelize, P., and Drouet, P. L.: L'œil et l'hypophyse, Proceedings of the Fifteenth International Congress on Ophthalmology, Cairo, 1937, vol. 1, pp. 227-400.

Jefferson, G.: Extrasellar extension of pituitary adenomas; President's Address, Proc. R. Soc. Med. **3**:433-458, 1940.

Joachim, M., Lavergne, G., Stevenaert, A., and Demanez, J. P.: Intérêt du diagnostic précoce des tumeurs hypophysaires, Bull. Soc. Belge Ophtalmol. **163**:195-202, 1973.

Karbacher, P., and Schinz, H. R.: Augensymptome bei Patienten mit Hypophysentumoren aus der Zürcher Augenklinik und dem Zürcher Röntgeninstitut von 1924-1939, Klin. Monatsbl. Augenheilkd. **103**: 541-557, 1939.

Kearns, T. P., Salassa, E. M., Kernohan, J. W., and MacCarty, C. S.: Ocular manifestations of pituitary tumor in Cushing's syndrome, Arch. Ophthalmol. **62**:242-247, 1959.

Kestenbaum, A.: Clinical methods of neuro-ophthalmologic examination, London, 1947, William Heinemann, Ltd., p. 81.

Kirkham, T. H.: The ocular symptomatology of pituitary tumours, Proc. R. Soc. Med. **65**:517-518, 1972.

Knapp, P.: Diagnostische und therapeutische Fragen bei Tumoren der Chiasmagegend, Klin. Monatsbl. Augenheilkd. **105**:401, 1940.

Knight, C. L., Hoyt, W. F., and Wilson, C. B.: Syndrome of incipient pre-chiasmal optic nerve compression, progress towards early diagnosis and surgical management, Arch. Ophthalmol. **87**:1-11, 1972.

Kraft, H.: Die Bewertung der Augenmuskelstörungen für die Differential-diagnose der Chiasmasyndrome, Ber. Dtsch. Ophthalmol. Ges. **67**:378-380, 1965.

Kravitz, D.: Visual field interpretations in chiasmal lesions, Am. J. Ophthalmol. **31**: 415, 1948.

Landolt, A. M.: Ultrastructure of human sella tumors, Acta Neurochir. Suppl. 22, 1975.

Landolt, A. M., and Hosbach, H. U.: Biological aspects of pituitary tumors as revealed by electron microscopy, Pathologica **66**:413-436, 1974.

Landolt, A. M., and Oswald, U. W.: Histology and ultrastructure of an oncocytic adenoma of the human pituitary, Cancer **31**:1099-1105, 1973.

Lillie, W. I.: Ocular phenomena in acromegaly, Am. J. Ophthalmol. **8**:32-39, 1925.

Lindenberg, R.: Neuropathology of the optic chiasma and adnexa. In Smith, J. L., editor: Neuro-ophthalmology, Springfield, Ill., 1963, Charles C Thomas, Publisher, vol. 1, pp. 385-425.

Loepp, W.: Gegenseitige Auswertung der Augen- und Röntgensymptome bei der Tumordiagnostik im Sellabereich, Berlin, 1936, S. Karger AG.

Lombardi, G.: Radiology in neuro-ophthalmology, Baltimore, 1967, The Williams & Wilkins Co.

Lyle, T. K.: Carcinoma of a parapituitary residue, Trans. Ophthalmol. Soc. U.K. **69**: 285-291, 1949.

Lyle, T. K., and Clover, P.: Ocular symptoms and signs in pituitary tumours, Trans. R. Soc. Med. **54**:611-619, 1961.

Maddox, E. E.: Symposium on nystagmus, Proc. R. Soc. Med. **1**:29-41, 1914.

Malagon Castro, V.: La exoftalmia hipofisaria, Med. Cir. Bogota **16**:255-273, 1952.

Mark, V. H., Smith, J. L., and Kjellberg, R. D.: Suprasellar epidermoid tumor. A case report with the presenting complaint of see-saw nystagmus, Neurology 10:81-83, 1960.

Martins, A. N.: Pituitary tumors and intrasellar cysts. In Vinken, P. J., and Bruyn, G. W.: Handbook of clinical neurology, New York, 1974, American Elsevier Publishing Co., Inc., vol. 17, pp. 375-439.

Matavulj, N., and Guillaumat, L.: Quelques cas d'affections de la région chiasmatique à périmétrie atypique, Bull. Soc. Ophtalmol. Fr. 7:716-728, 1951.

Meadows, S. P.: Pituitary tumors, Ann. R. Coll. Surg. Engl. 9:224, 1951.

Meadows, S. P.: Unusual clinical features and modes of presentation in pituitary adenoma, including pituitary apoplexy. In Smith, J. L., editor: Neuro-ophthalmology, St. Louis, 1968, The C. V. Mosby Co., vol. 4, pp. 178-189.

Montaldi, M., and Zingirian, M.: La perimetria mesopica, cinetica e statica nelle affezione produttive delle'ipofisi, Riv. Otoneurooftalmol. 38:15-36, 1963.

Mooney, A. J.: Perimetry and angiography in the diagnosis of lesions in the pituitary region, Trans. Ophthalmol. Soc. U.K. 72: 49, 1952.

Moreu, A.: Considerations on the ophthalmic diagnosis of hypophyseal tumors, Arch. Soc. Oftalmol. Hispano-Am. 1:181, 1942.

Mundinger, F., Riechert, T., and Reisert, P. M.: Hypophysentumoren, Hypophysektomie, Stuttgart, 1967, Georg Thieme Verlag KG.

Neelon, F. A., Goree, J. A., and Lebovitz, H. E.: The primary empty sella: clinical and radiographic characteristics and endocrine function, Medicine 52:73-92, 1973.

Nover, A.: Augensymptome bei sellanahen Tumoren, Dtsch. Med. Wochenschr. 88: 2139-2142, 1963.

Obrador, A. S.: Tumores y procesos inflamatorios de la region quiasmatica-hipofisaria, Arch. Soc. Oftalmol. Hispano-Am. 25:305-332, 1965.

Obrador, A. S.: The empty sella and some related syndromes, J. Neurosurg. 36:162-168, 1972.

O'Connell, J. E.: The anatomy of the optic chiasma and heteronymous hemianopia, J. Neurol. Neurosurg. Psychiatry 36:710-723, 1973.

Okonek, G.: Das Syndrom der Sehnervenkreuzung, Klin. Monatsbl. Augenheilkd. 116:113, 1950.

Paufique, L., and Etienne, R.: Le tuberculome du chiasma, Bull. Soc. Fr. Ophtalmol. 65: 97-109, 1952.

Pruett, R. C., and Wepsic, J. G.: Delayed diagnosis of chiasmal compression, Am. J. Ophthalmol. 76:229-236, 1973.

Ray, B. S.: Surgical lesions of optic nerves and chiasm in infants and children. In Smith, J. L., editor: Neuro-ophthalmology, St. Louis, 1967, The C. V. Mosby Co., pp. 77-99.

Remky, H.: Augensymptome bei Tumoren im Bereich des Türkensattels, Klin. Monatsbl. Augenheilkd. 150:436, 1967.

Robert, F.: L'adénome hypophysaire dans l'acromégalie gigantisme. Etude macroscopique, histologique et ultrastructurale, Neurochirurgie 19(Suppl. 2):117-162, 1973.

Robinson, J. L.: Sudden blindness with pituitary tumours. Report of three cases, J. Neurosurg. 36:83-85, 1972.

Rönne, H.: On non-hypophyseal affections of the chiasma, Acta Ophthalmol. 6:332-343, 1928.

Rougerie, M.: Paralysie unilatérale de l'accommodation, signe rélévateur d'une tumeur de l'hypophyse, Bull. Soc. Ophtalmol. Fr. 64:724-728, 1964.

Rougier, J., and Wertheimer, J.: Atypical ophthalmologic signs in hypophyseal adenomas, Rev. Otoneuroophtalmol. 46: 369-373, 1974.

Rucker, C. W.: Tumors of the region of the optic chiasm, Fourth Pan-Amer. Cong. Ophthalmol. 1:178-183, 1952.

Rucker, C. W.: Chiasmal lesions. In The interpretation of visual fields, ed. 3, 1957, American Academy of Ophthalmology, pp. 22-35.

Schneider, J. A.: Sellabrücke und Konstitution, Leipzig, 1939, Georg Thieme Verlag KG.

Siebeck, R., and Schiefer, W.: Zur Symptomatologie und Therapie sellanaher Prozesse, Klin. Monatsbl. Augenheilkd. 142: 194-212, 1963.

Smith, J. L., and Marl, V. H.: See-saw nystagmus with suprasellar epidermoid tumor, Arch. Ophthalmol. 62:280-283, 1959.

Talbot, A. N.: Pressure on chiasm, Trans. Ophthalmol. Soc. N.Z. 26:9-15, 1974.

Terrien, F.: Les troubles visuels d'origine

hypophysaire, Progr. Med., pp. 639-644, 1937.

Thomas, J. E., and Yoss, R. E.: The parasellar syndrome: problems in determining etiology, Mayo Clin. Proc. 45:617-623, 1970.

Timmerman, J. M. E. N.: The diagnosis of tumors in the region of the optic chiasma, Ophthalmologica 152:530-536, 1966.

Tiwisina, T., and Haar, H.: Die Geschwülste der Chiasmagegend im cerebralen Angiogramm, Nervenarzt 24:58-63, 1953.

Toland, J., and Mooney, A.: On the enlarged sella turcica, Trans. Ophthalmol. Soc. U.K. 93:717-731, 1973.

Tönnis, W.: Anzeigestellung zur operativen Behandlung der Geschwülste im Bereiche des Türkensattels, Klin. Monatsbl. Augenheilkd. 114:1, 1949.

Tönnis, W.: Das chromophobe Adenom. Diagnostik der intrakraniellen Geschwülste. In Olivecrona, H., and Tönnis, W., editors: Handbuch der Neurochirurgie, Berlin, 1962, Julius Springer, vol. 4, p. 165.

Tönnis, W.: Das eosinophile Adenom. Diagnostik der intrakraniellen Geschwülste. In Olivecrona, H., and Tönnis, W., editors: Handbuch der Neurochirurgie, Berlin, 1962, Julius Springer, vol. 4, p. 155.

Tönnis, W., and Rausch, F.: Sellaveränderungen bei gesteigertem Schädelinnendruck, Dtsch. Z. Nervenheilk. 171:351-369, 1954.

Tönnis, W., Friedmann, G., and Albrecht, H.: Zur röntgenologischen Differentialdiagnose der Hypophysenadenome, unter Berücksichtigung der primären und sekundären Sellaveränderungen, Fortschr. Roentgenstr. 87:678-686, 1957.

Toppel, L., Lorenz-Meyer, H., and Merte, H.-J.: The diagnosis of hypophyseal tumours from the ophthalmological point of view, Münch. Med. Wochenschr. 112:89-94, 1970.

Trobe, J. D.: Chromophobe adenoma presenting with a hemianopic temporal arcuate scotoma, Am. J. Ophthalmol. 77:388-392, 1974.

Trumble, H. C.: Pituitary tumours: observations on large tumours which have spread widely beyond the confines of the sella turcica, Br. J. Surg. 39:7, 1951.

Vercesi, G., and Gatti, E.: La paralisi del nervo oculomotore comune quale segno di esordino clinico di un adenoma ipofisario. Tre osservazioni personali, Riv. Otoneuro-oftalmol. 41:17-34, 1966.

Vogt, A.: Die Ophthalmoskopie im rotfreien Licht. In Graefe-Saemisch: Handbuch der gesamten Augenheilkunde, Leipzig, 1925, Wilhelm Engelmann, vol. 3.

Walker, A. E.: The neurosurgical evaluation of the chiasmal syndromes, Am. J. Ophthalmol. 54:563-581, 1962.

Walker, C. B., and Cushing, H.: Studies of optic nerve atrophy in association with chiasmal lesions, Arch. Ophthalmol. 45:407-437, 1916.

Walsh, F. B.: Bilateral total ophthalmoplegia with adenoma of the pituitary gland, Arch. Ophthalmol. 42:646-654, 1949.

Walsh, F. B.: Concerning the optic chiasma. Selected pathologic involvement and clinical problems. The DeSchweinitz lecture, Am. J. Ophthalmol. 50:1031-1047, 1960.

Walsh, F. B., and Hoyt, W. F.: Pituitary adenomas. In Clinical neuro-ophthalmology, Baltimore, 1969, The Williams & Wilkins Co., p. 2130.

Weber, G.: Symptomatologie und Chirurgie der sellären und suprasellären Tumoren, Ophthalmologica 149:326-342, 1965.

Weinberger, L. M., Adler, F. H., and Grant, F. C.: Primary pituitary adenoma and the syndrome of the cavernous sinus, Arch. Ophthalmol. 24:1197, 1940.

Weinstein, P.: Data concerning the ophthalmological diagnosis of hypophyseal tumors, Ophthalmologica 125:169-171, 1953.

Weskamp, C.: Contribución al diagnostico differential de los tumores hipofisarios, Arch. Oftalmol. B. Air. 28:173-181, 1953.

Weyland, R. D., McCraig, W., and Rucker, C. W.: Ungewöhnliche Krankheitsprozesse im Bereich des Chiasma, Mayo Clin. Proc. 27:505-511, 1952.

White, J. C., and Warren, S.: Unusual size and extension of a pituitary adenoma, J. Neurosurg. 2:126, 1945.

Williamson-Noble, F. A.: Die oculären Folgen gewisser Läisionen des Chiasmas, Trans. Ophthalmol. Soc. U.K. 59:627-682, 1939.

Wybar, K.: Visual field defects in chiasmal lesions, Trans. Am. Med. Assoc. Sect. Ophthalmol. 112:16-39, 1963.

Yanagida, N.: Ocular symptoms of pituitary and pontine tumours, Acta Soc. Ophthalmol. Jap. 57:1293-1305, 1953.

Young, D. G., Bahn, R. C., and Randall, R. V.: Pituitary tumors associated with acromegaly, J. Clin. Endocrinol. Metab. 25:249-259, 1965.

Zimmerman, E. A., Defendini, R., and Frautz, A. G.: Prolactin and growth hormone in patients with pituitary adenomas: a correlative study of hormone in tumor and plasma by immunoperoxidase technique and radioimmunoassay, J. Clin. Endocrinol. Metab. 38:577-585, 1974.

**Craniopharyngiomas**

Armenise, B., Regli, F., and Del Vivo, R.: I craniofaringiomi: sintomatologia oftalmologica, Ann. Ottalmol. 87:652-662, 1961.

Bailey, P.: Das Hypothalamussyndrom. Die Hirngeschwülste, Stuttgart, 1951, Ferdinand Enke Verlag, p. 105.

Banna, M.: Craniopharyngioma in adults, Surg. Neurol. 1:202-204, 1973.

Bianchi, G., Rosselet, E., and Buffat, J. D.: Cecité par craniopharyngiome et récupération fonctionelle après opération, Confin. Neurol. 17:155-162, 1957.

Bingas, B., and Wolter, M.: Augensymptome beim Kraniopharyngeom, Klin. Monatsbl. Augenheilkd. 149:275-276, 1966.

van Bogaert, L.: Le diagnostic des tumeurs suprasellaires et en particulier des tumeurs de la poche pharyngienne de Rathke, Rev. Otoneuroophtalmol. 7:645, 1929.

Brégeat, P.: Le champ visuel des cholestéatomes suprasellaires. Quelques particularités, Bull. Soc. Ophtalmol. Fr. 3:446-448, 1949.

Calmettes, L., and Déodati, F.: Les craniopharyngiomes. Symptomatologie ophtalmologique, Rev. Otoneuroophtalmol. 27:99-105, 1955.

Dandy, W. E.: Hypophyseal duct tumors. In Lewis, D., editor: Lewis' practice of surgery, Hagerstown, Md., 1936, W. F. Prior Co., Inc., vol. 12, pp. 598-605.

Dott, N. M., and Bailey, P.: A consideration of the hypophysial adenomata, Br. J. Surg. 13:314-366, 1925.

Duke-Elder, S., and Scott, G.: Neuro-ophthalmology. In Duke-Elder, S., editor: System of ophthalmology, vol. 12, St. Louis, 1971, The C. V. Mosby Co.

Erdheim, J.: Ueber Hypophysenganggeschwülste und Hirncholesteatome, S.-B. Akad. Wiss. Wien. Math.-Nat. Klin. 113:537, 1904.

Flament, J., Bronner, A., Phillippides, D., and Thiebaut, J. B.: Perimetric findings in craniopharyngioma, Rev. Otoneuroophtalmol. 43:403-408, 1971.

Franceschetti, A., and Blum, J. D.: Névrite rétrobulbaire aiguë transitoire dans un cas de tumeur cérébrale, Confin. Neurol. 11:302, 1951.

Frazier, C. H., and Alpers, B. J.: Adamantinoma of the craniopharyngeal duct, Arch. Neurol. Psychiatr. 26:905-965, 1931.

Freimann, G.: Sudden blindness and optic atrophy with craniopharyngeal pouch tumour, Am. J. Ophthalmol. 10:579, 1927.

Globus, J. H., and Gang, K. M.: Craniopharyngioma and suprasellar adamantinoma, J. Mt. Sinai Hosp. 12:220-276, 1945.

Hirsch, O., and Hamlin, H.: Symptomatology and treatment of the hypophyseal duct tumors (craniopharyngiomas), Confin. Neurol. 19:153-219, 1959.

Irsigler, F. J.: Considérations cliniques et chirurgicales sur les cranio-pharyngiomes et les kystes suprasellaires, Neurochirurgie 8:242-252, 1962.

Lombardi, G.: Radiology in neuro-ophthalmology, Baltimore, 1967, The Williams & Wilkins Co.

Love, J. G., and Marshall, T. M.: Craniopharyngiomas (pituitary adamantinomata), Surg. Gynecol. Obstet. 90:591-601, 1950.

McCritchley, D., and Ironside, R. N.: The pituitary adamantinomata, Brain 40:437-481, 1926.

Müller, R., and Wohlfahrt, G.: Craniopharyngiomas, Acta Med. Scand. 138:121, 1950.

Palomares-Petit, F., and Ley-Garcia, A.: Evolucion de la sintomatologia oftalmoneurologica en los craneofaringiomas, Arch. Soc. Oftalmol. Hispano.-Am. 22:741-774, 1962.

Pertuiset, B.: Craniopharyngiomas. In Vinken, P. J., and Bruyn, G. W., editors: Handbook of clinical neurology, New York, 1974, American Elsevier Publishing Co., Inc., vol. 18, pp. 531-572.

Rintelen, F., and Leuenberger, A.: Zur Differentialdiagnose und Therapie des Kraniopharyngeoms, Schweiz. Med. Wochenschr. 87:1189-1190, 1957.

Scheschy, H., and Benedikt, O.: Possible mistakes in diagnosing a craniopharyngioma, Klin. Monatsbl. Augenheilkd. 159:386-392, 1971.

Schulze, A.: Zur Differentialdiagnose der suprasellären Tumoren, Klin. Monatsbl. Augenheilkd. 136:166-185, 1960.

Seidenari, R.: Kraniopharyngeom bei Erwachsenen mit Stauungspapille, Osp. Magg. Milano Rev. Otol. Ecc. **18**:293-299, 1941.

Thibaut, F.: Klinik und Histologie der Kraniopharyngeome, Wien. Klin. Wochenschr. **59**:409-413, 1947.

Tönnis, W.: Kraniopharyngeome. Diagnostik der intrakraniellen Geschwülste. In Olivecrona, H., and Tönnis, W., editors: Handbuch der Neurochirurgie, Berlin, 1962, Julius Springer, vol. 4, p. 186.

Vladykova, J.: Craniopharyngioma from the ophthalmological point of view, Cs. Oftalmol. **29**:109-116, 1973.

Wagener, H. P., and Love, J. G.: Fields of vision in cases of tumor of Rathke's pouch, Arch. Ophthalmol. **29**:873, 1943.

Walsh, F. B., and Hoyt, W. F.: Craniopharyngioma. In Clinical neuro-ophthalmology, Baltimore, 1969, The Williams & Wilkins Co., p. 2157.

**Meningiomas of the tuberculum sellae**

Alfonso, G. F., and Marini, G.: I segni oculari da meningiomi del tubercolo della sela. Osservazioni di 38 casi, Boll. Oculist. **63**:524, 1964.

Bailey, P.: Syndrom des Tuberculum sellae. Die Hirngeschwülste, Stuttgart, 1951, Ferdinand Enke Verlag, p. 143.

Bird, A. C.: Field loss due to lesions at the anterior angle of the chiasm, Proc. R. Soc. Med. **65**:519-520, 1972.

Celotti, H., and Frera, C.: La sinomatologica oculare dei meningiomi del tubercolo della sella, Ann. Ottalmol. Clin. Oculist. **85**:1-13, 1959.

Coulonjou, R., Le Bozec, E., and Salaun, A.: Une erreur de diagnostic instructive: méningiome suprasellaire pris pour une arachnoïdite opto-chiasmatique, Rev. Otoneuroophtalmol. **22**:563-571, 1950.

Cushing, H.: The chiasmal syndrome of primary optic atrophy and bitemporal field defects in adults with a normal sella turcica, Arch. Ophthalmol. **3**:505-551, 704-735, 1930.

Cushing, H., and Eisenhardt, L.: Meningiomas arising from the tuberculum sellae, Arch. Ophthalmol. **1**:1-41, 168-205, 1929.

Cushing, H., and Eisenhardt, L.: Meningiomas, Springfield, Ill., 1938, Charles C Thomas, Publisher.

Desvignes, Brun, and Bounes: Sur un cas de cholestéatome suprasellaire, Bull. Soc. Ophtalmol. Paris **3**:382-385, 1947.

Duke-Elder, S., and Scott, G.: Neuro-ophthalmology. In Duke-Elder, S., editor: System of ophthalmology, vol. 12, St. Louis, 1971, The C. V. Mosby Co.

Ehlers, N., and Malmros, R.: The suprasellar meningioma. A review of the literature and presentation of a series of 31 cases, Acta Ophthalmol. (suppl.) **121**:1-74, 1973.

Finn, J. E., and Mount, L. A.: Meningiomas of the tuberculum sellae and planum sphenoidale. A review of 83 cases, Arch. Ophthalmol. **92**:23-27, 1974.

Forster, H. W., and Bouzarth, W. F.: Meningioma of the tuberculum sellae as a cause of optic atrophy, Am. J. Ophthalmol. **64**:908-910, 1967.

Grant, F. C., and Hedges, T. R., Jr.: Ocular findings in meningiomas of the tuberculum sellae, Arch. Ophthalmol. **56**:163-170, 1956.

Gregorius, F. K., Hepler, R. S., and Stern, W. E.: Loss and recovery of vision with suprasellar meningiomas, J. Neurosurg. **42**:69-75, 1975.

Guillaumat, L.: Les méningiomes suprasellaires, Paris, 1937, Gaston Doin & Cie.

Guiot, G., et al.: Méningiomes supra-sellaires rétro-chiasmatiques, Neurochirurgie **16**:273-285, 1970.

Gunn, R. M.: Retrobulbar neuritis, Lancet, p. 412, 1904.

Harms, H.: Leitsymptom "Zentralskotom." In Entwicklung und Fortschritte in der Augenheilkunde, Stuttgart, 1963, Ferdinand Enke Verlag, p. 306.

Hartmann, E.: Cas atypique de méningiome suprasellaire avec dilatation unilatérale du canal optique, Bull. Soc. Ophtalmol. Paris **3**:100, 1948.

Hartmann, E., and Guillaumat, L.: Symptomes oculaires des méningiomes suprasellaires, Ann. Oculist. **174**:1-39, 1937.

van der Hoeve, J.: Diagnosis of suprasellar tumors, Ophthalmologica **99**:258, 1940.

Jane, J. A., and McKissock, W.: Importance of failing vision in early diagnosis of suprasellar meningiomas, Br. Med. J. **2**:5-7, 1962.

Joy, H. H.: Suprasellar meningioma; report of an atypical case, Am. J. Ophthalmol. **35**:1139-1146, 1952.

Kuwajima, J.: Problem cases of intracranial tumor simulating retrobulbar neuritis, Jpn. J. Ophthalmol. **20**:1405-1411, 1966.

Lasco, F., and Arseni, C.: La pseudonévrite optique postérieure comme manifestations rare des néoformations intracrâniennes, Rev. Otoneuroophtalmol. 32:386-391, 1960.

Ley, A.: Meningiomas del "tuberculum sellae," Arch. Soc. Oftalmol. Hisp-Am. 30:241-270, 1970.

Mathewson, W. R.: Meningioma of tuberculum sellae with bitemporal hemianopia, Br. J. Ophthalmol. 30:92-102, 1946.

Mundinger, F., and Riechert, T.: Hypophysentumoren, Hypophysektomie, Stuttgart, 1967, Georg Thieme Verlag KG.

Philippidès, D., Montrieul, B., und Lévy, R.: A propos de trois cas de méningiome du tubercule de la selle, Rev. Otoneuroophtalmol. 25:16-22, 1953.

Reuter, A., and Lamprecht, J.: Zur Klinik der suprasellären Tumoren, Dtsch. Med. Wochenschr. 2:1033-1037, 1937.

Schlezinger, N. S., Alpers, B. J., and Weiss, B. P.: Suprasellar meningiomas associated with scotomatous field defects, Arch. Ophthalmol. 35:620-642, 1946.

Walsh, F. B., and Hoyt, W. F.: Meningioma of the tuberculum sellae. In Clinical neuro-ophthalmology, Baltimore, 1969, The Williams & Wilkins Co., p. 2263.

**Meningiomas of the olfactory groove**

Bailey, P.: Syndrom der Olfaktoriusrinne. Die Hirngeschwülste, Stuttgart, 1951, Ferdinand Enke Verlag, p. 150.

Bonamour, G., and Wertheimer, I.: Valeur sémiologique de l'atrophie optique unilatérale, Ann. Oculist. 183:199, 1950.

Cushing, H., and Eisenhardt, L.: Meningiomas, Springfield, Ill., 1938, Charles C Thomas, Publisher.

David, M., and Askenasy, H.: Méningiomes olfactifs, Rev. Neurol. 68:489, 1937.

David, M., and Sourdille, G.: Sur la valeur localisatrice des signes dits de compression directe du nerf optique, en particulier du syndrome de Foster Kennedy, dans les tumeurs cérébrales, J. Ophthalmol. 3:215, 1942.

Dilenge, D., and Fischgold, H.: L'angiographie orbitaire, Paris, 1968, Masson & Cie, Editeurs, p. 302.

Duke-Elder, S., and Scott, G.: Neuro-ophthalmology. In Duke-Elder, S., editor: System of ophthalmology, vol. 12, St. Louis, 1971, The C. V. Mosby Co.

Hagedoorn, A.: The chiasmal syndrome and retrobulbar neuritis in pregnancy, Am. J. Ophthalmol. 20:690, 1937.

Hartmann, E., David, M., and Desvignes, P.: Les symptômes oculaires dans les méningiomes olfactifs, Ann. Oculist. 174:505-527, 1937.

van der Hoeve, J.: Diagnosis of tumors of the suprasellar region with special reference to the Foster Kennedy syndrome, Ophthalmologica 99:258-264, 1940.

Lukasiewicz, W.: Diagnose, Differentialdiagnose und Therapie des Olfactoriusmeningeoms, M.D. Thesis, 1948, University of Zurich.

Mylius, K.: Über das Meningeom der Olfactoriusrinne, eine für den Augenarzt besonders wichtige Geschwulst, Z. Augenheilkd. 82:257, 1934.

Rohmer, F., Philippides, D., Buchheit, F., and Ben Amor, M.: Neuro-ophthalmological signs of olfactory meningiomata (21 cases), Rev. Otoneuroophtalmol. 42:335-338, 1970.

Walsh, F. B., and Hoyt, W. F.: Olfactory groove tumors. In Clinical neuro-ophthalmology, Baltimore, 1969, The Williams & Wilkins Co., p. 2175.

**Meningiomas of the sphenoid ridge**

Bailey, P.: Syndrom des Keilbeinflügels. Die Hirngeschwülste, Stuttgart, 1951, Ferdinand Enke Verlag, p. 145.

Cushing, H., and Eisenhardt, L.: Meningiomas, Springfield, Ill., 1938, Charles C Thomas, Publisher.

David, M., and Hartmann, E.: Les symptômes oculaires dans les méningiomes de la petite aile du sphénoïde, Ann. Oculist. 172:177, 1935.

Derome, P.: Les tumeurs sphéno-ethmoidales, possibilités d'exérèse et de réparation chirurgicales, Neurochirurgie vol. 18, 1972.

Doret, M.: Un cas d'hémicraniose—méningiome en plaque—avec importantes altérations du fond de l'œil, Rev. Otoneuroophtalmol. 22:460-466, 1950.

Duke-Elder, S., and Scott, G.: Neuro-ophthalmology. In Duke-Elder, S., editor: System of ophthalmology, vol. 12, St. Louis, 1971, The C. V. Mosby Co.

Elsberg, C. A., and Dyke, C. G.: Meningiomas attached to the mesial part of the sphenoidal ridge, Arch. Ophthalmol. 12:644, 1934.

Elsberg, C. A., Hare, C. C., and Dyke, C. H.: Unilateral exophthalmos in intracranial tumors with special reference to its occurrence in meningiomata, Surg. Gynecol. Obstet. **55**:681, 1932.

Fischer, E.: Paraselläre Geschwülste, Zentralbl. Chir., p. 2893, 1938.

Henderson, W. R.: Anterior basal meningiomas, Br. J. Surg. **26**:124-165, 1938.

Kearns, T. P., and Wagener, H. P.: Ophthalmologic diagnosis of meningiomas of the sphenoidal ridge, Am. J. Med. Sci. **226**:221-228, 1953.

Kennedy, F.: Retrobulbar neuritis as an exact diagnostic sign of certain tumors and abscesses in the frontal lobe, Am. J. Med. Sci. **142**:355, 1911.

Kennedy, F.: The symptomatology of temporosphenoidal tumors, Arch. Intern. Med. **8**:317-350, 1911.

Kraft, H.: Zur unterschiedlichen Symptomatologie der Keilbeinflügelmeningiome, Klin. Monatsbl. Augenheilkd. **144**:944, 1964.

Mortada, A.: Misinterpretation of sphenoidal ridge meningiomata, Br. J. Ophthalmol. **51**:829-838, 1967.

Mylius, K.: Über das Meningeom des Keilbeinflügels, Klin. Monatsbl. Augenheilkd. **113**:105-110, 1948.

Smith, J. W.: Meningioma producing unilateral exophthalmos; syndrome of tumor of pterional plaque arising from outer third of sphenoid ridge, Arch. Ophthalmol. **22**:540-549, 1939.

Thorkildsen, A.: Meningioma of the sphenoid wing with proptosis (in Norwegian), Nord. Med. **38**:1027-1028, 1948.

Tönnis, W.: Meningeome des kleinen Keilbeinflügel. Diagnostik der intrakraniellen Geschwülste. In Olivecrona, H., and Tönnis, W., editors: Handbuch der Neurochirurgie, Berlin, 1962, Julius Springer, p. 50.

Tönnis, W., and Schürmann, K.: Meningeome der Keilbeinflügel, Zentralbl. Neurochir. **11**:1-13, 1951.

Truemann, R. H.: Syndrome of meningeal fibroblastoma arising from the lesser wing of the sphenoid bone; analysis from an ophthalmologic standpoint, Am. J. Ophthalmol. **30**:1585, 1947; Arch. Ophthalmol. **38**:566, 1947.

Uihlein, A., and Weyand, R. D.: Meningiomas of anterior clinoid process as a cause of unilateral loss of vision: surgical consideration, Arch. Ophthalmol. **49**:261-270, 1953.

Walsh, F. B., and Hoyt, W. F.: Meningiomas of the sphenoid ridge. In Clinical neuro-ophthalmology, Baltimore, 1969, The Williams & Wilkins Co., p. 2266.

### Aneurysms*

Jefferson, G.: Compression of the chiasm, optic nerves and optic tracts by intracranial aneurysms, Brain **60**:444, 1937.

Rhonheimer, C.: Zur Symptomatologie der sellären Aneurysmen, Klin. Monatsbl. Augenheilkd. **134**:1-34, 1959.

Thomas, H., Tridon, P., Laxenaire, M., and Montaut, J.: Anévrisme simulant une tumeur hypophysaire avec hypopituitarism, Rev. Otoneuroophtalmol. **36**:128-135, 1964.

### Indirect compression of the chiasm

Hughes, E. B. C.: Some observations on visual fields in hydrocephalus, J. Neurol. Neurosurg. Psychiatry **9**:30, 1946.

Klingler, M., and Condrau, G.: Lokalisatorisch irreführende Gesichtsfeldsymptome bei Hirntumoren, Ophthalmological **120**:270, 1950.

Mooney, A. J., and McConnel, A. A.: Visual scotomata with intracranial lesions affecting the optic nerve, J. Neurol. Neurosurg. Psychiatry **12**:205, 1949.

### Chiasmal arachnoiditis

Bollack, J., David, M., and Puech, P.: Les arachnoïdites optochiasmatiques, Paris, 1937, Masson & Cie, Editeurs.

Hartmann, E.: Optochiasmic arachnoiditis, Arch. Ophthalmol. **33**:68, 1945.

Jacquemin, P. J., and Frippiat, M.: Les arachnoidtes opto-chiasmatiques: étude clinique de quelques cas: essai de classement de la symptomatologie et des indications thérapeutiques, Bull. Soc. Belge. Ophthalmol. **152**:550-595, 1969.

Kravitz, D.: Arachnoiditis, Arch. Ophthalmol. **37**:199-210, 1947.

Meyer, F. W.: Zur Symptomatologie der Arachnoiditis opticochiasmatica, Klin. Monatsbl. Augenheilkd. **107**:274-280, 1941.

Migliore, A., Massarotti, M., Ettorre, G., and Bozzini, S.: L'aracnoidite ottico-chiasmatica: revisione critica di 108 casi operati, Ann. Ottalmol. **96**:221-232, 1970.

Vail, D.: Optochiasmic arachnoiditis; importance of mixed type of atrophy of optic nerve as diagnostic sign, Arch. Ophthalmol. **20**:384-394, 1938.

---

*For additional literature, see references for intracranial aneurysms in Chapter 5.

**Gliomas of the chiasm; tumors
of the optic nerve**

Berkmann, N.: Three cases of tuberculoma of the chiasma, Bull. Soc. Ophtalmol. Fr. **72:**573-584, 1972.

Brégeat, P.: Les gliomes du chiasma, Thèse, Paris, 1942.

Buffat, J. D.: Tumeurs du nerf optique et neurochirurgie, Confin. Neurol. **9:**411, 1949.

Bürki, E.: Über den primären Sehnerventumor und seine Beziehungen zur Recklinghausenchen Neurofibromatose. Bibliotheca Ophthalmologica, fasc. 30, Basel, 1944, S. Karger AG.

Bürki, E.: Über den klinischen Wert der Röntgenaufnahme des Canalis opticus, Ophthalmologica **123:**243-248, 1952.

Christensen, E., and Ry Andersen, S.: Primary tumours of the optic nerve and chiasma, Acta Psychiatr. Neurol. **27:**5-16, 1952.

Chutorian, A. M., Schwartz, J. F., Evans, R. A., and Carter, S.: Optic gliomas in children, Neurology **14:**83-95, 1964.

Cogan, D. G.: Tumors of the optic nerve. In Vinken, P. J., and Bruyn, G. W.: Handbook of clinical neurology, New York, 1974, American Elsevier Publishing Co., Inc., vol. 17, pp. 35-374.

Cohen, I.: Tumours of the intracranial portion of the optic nerve, J. Mt. Sinai Hosp. **17:**738-745, 1951.

Daum, S., and Guillaumat, L.: Tumeurs de la gaine méningée du nerf optique, Rev. Otoneuroophtalmol. **21:**18, 1949.

Davis, F. A.: Primary tumors of optic nerve (phenomenon of Recklinghausen's disease); clinical and pathologic study with report of five cases and review of literauture, Arch. Ophthalmol. **23:**735-957, 1940.

Dufour, R., and Cometta, F.: Aspects radiologiques de l'orbite en ONO, Confin. Neurol. **10:**201, 1950.

Epstein, B. S., and Kulick, M.: Technique for optic foramen roentgenography, Radiology **42:**186-187, 1944.

Floris, V., and Castorina, G.: I gliomi del nervo ottico; Varietà endocranica, Riv. Neurol. **22:**799-821, 1952.

Foerster, O., and Gagel, O.: Ein Fall von sog. Gliom des Nervus opticus—Spongioblastoma multiforme ganglioides, Z. Ges. Neurol. Psychiatr. **136:**335-366, 1931.

François, J., and Rabaey, M.: Tumeurs primi-

tives du nerf optique, Acta Ophthalmol. **30:**203-221, 1952.

Glaser, J. S., Hoyt, W. F., and Corbett, J.: Visual morbidity with chiasmal glioma. Longterm studies of visual fields in untreated and irradiated cases, Arch. Ophthalmol. **85:**3-12, 1971.

Goldmann, H., and Grunthal, E.: Über einen Tumor des Sehnerven und seiner Leptomeningen bei Recklinghausenscher Krankheit, Ophthalmologica **102:**79-92, 1941.

Greenway, R.: The optic foramina, X-ray Techn. **25:**31-35, 1953.

Grote, W.: Zur Klinik und Behandlung der Tumoren des Nervus opticus und des Chiasmas, Klin. Monatsbl. Augenheilkd. **144:**841-855, 1964.

van der Hoeve, J.: Röntgenphotographie des Foramen Opticum bei Geschwülsten und Erkrankungen des Sehnerven, Graefe. Arch. Ophthalmol. **115:**355, 1925.

van der Hoeve, J.: Eye symptoms in phakamatoses (the Doyne Memorial Lecture), Trans. Ophthalmol. Soc. U.K. **52:**380-401, 1932.

Hoyt, W. F., Meshel, L. G., Lessell, S., Schatz, N. J., and Suckling, R. D.: Malignant gliomas of adulthood, Brain **96:**121-132, 1973.

Javett, S. N., and Samuel, E.: Tumor of the optic chiasm, Arch. Dis. Child. **22:**248-250, 1947.

Ingvar, A.: Primary tumors of optic nerve and their relation to Recklinghausen's disease, Acta Paediatr. **32:**262, 1945.

Katzin, H. M.: Glioma of optic nerve, J. Mt. Sinai Hosp. **11:**332, 1945.

Lloyd, L. A.: Gliomas of the optic nerve and chiasm in childhood, Trans. Am. Ophthalmol. Soc. **71:**488-535, 1973.

Löhlein, W., and Tönnis, W.: Die operative Behandlung der das Foramen opticum überschreitenden Sehnervengeschwülste, Graefe. Arch. Ophthalmol. **149:**318-354, 1949.

Love, J. G., and Rucker, C. W.: Meningioma of sheath of optic nerve, Arch. Ophthalmol. **23:**377, 1940.

Mac Carty, C. S., Boyd, A. S., Jr., and Childs, D. S., Jr.: Tumors of the optic nerve and optic chiasm, J. Neurosurg. **33:**439-444, 1970.

Mannheimer, M.: Glioma of optic nerve, Am. J. Ophthalmol. **29:**323, 1946.

Marinkovic, A.: Imagine stratigrafica dei

canali ottici, Radiol. Med. 37:987-997, 1951.

Marshall, D.: Glioma of the optic nerve as a manifestation of von Recklinghausen's disease, Am. J. Ophthalmol. 37:15, 1954.

Martin, P., and Cushing, H.: Primary gliomas of the chiasm and optic nerves in their intracranial portion, Arch. Ophthalmol. 52: 209-241, 1923.

McCraig, W., and Gogela, L. J.: Intraorbital meningiomas, Am. J. Ophthalmol. 32:1663-1680, 1949.

McCraig, W., and Gogela, L. J.: Meningioma of the optic foramen as a cause of slowly progressive blindness, J. Neurosurg. 7:44-48, 1950.

McFarland, P. E., and Eisenbeiss, J.: Glioma of the optic nerve, Am. J. Ophthalmol. 33: 463-466, 1950.

Meadows, S. P.: Optic nerve compression and its differential diagnosis, Proc. R. Soc. Med. 42:1017, 1949.

Minton, J.: Glioma of optic chiasma, Proc. R. Soc. Med. 38:594, 1945.

Montaut, J., Picard, L., Vittini, F., and Macinot, C.: Isolated optic nerve glioma. Value of early diagnosis with a view to radical excision, Rev. Otoneuroophtalmol. 43:207-214, 1971.

Nordmann, J.: Les tumeurs du nerf optique. In Bailliart, P., et al., editors: Traité d'-ophtalmologie, Paris, 1939, Masson & Cie, Editeurs, vol. 6, p. 385.

Paillas, J. E., Bonnal, J., Sedan, R., Berard-Badier, M., and Combalbert, A.: Tumeurs du chiasme, Neurochirurgie 7:278-297, 1961.

Penfield, W., and Young, A. W.: Nature of von Recklinghausen's disease and tumors associated with it, Arch. Neurol. Psychiatr. 23:320-344, 1930; Trans. Am. Neurol. Assoc. 55:319-343, 1929.

Pereira Gomes, J.: Tumors of the optic nerve; study of 13 cases in Brazil: relation to Recklinghausen's disease, Am. J. Ophthalmol. 24:1144-1169, 1941.

Pfaffenbach, D. D., Kearns, T. P., and Hollenhorst, W.: An unusual case of optic nerve-chiasmal glioma, Am. J. Ophthalmol. 74:523-531, 1972.

Ray, B. S.: Surgical lesions of optic nerves and chiasm in infants and children, In Smith, J. L., editor: Neuro-ophthalmology, St. Louis, 1967, The C. V. Mosby Co.

Rettelbach, E., and Schutzbach: Über Sehnerventumoren, ihre Beziehungen zur Neurofibromatosis Recklinghausen und ihr klinisches Krankheitsbild, Graefe. Arch. Ophthalmol. 145:179-241, 1942.

Schoen, D.: Übersichtsaufnahme beider Foramina nervi optici, Fortschr. Roentgenstr. 78:349-350, 1953.

Schwarz, K.: Zur Klinik und Anatomie der Geschwülste des Sehnerven, Graefe. Arch. Ophthalmol. 135:247-264, 1936.

Terence Myles, S., and Murphy, S. B.: Gliomas of the optic nerve and chiasm, Can. J. Ophthalmol. 8:508-514, 1973.

Tönnis, W.: Die operative Behandlung der das Foramen opticum überschreitenden Geschwülste des N. opticus, Acta Neurochir. 1:52-71, 1950.

Udvarhelyi, G. B., Khodadoust, A. A., and Walsh, F. B.: Gliomas of the optic nerve and chiasm in children, Clin. Neurosurg. 13:204-237, 1966.

Wagener, H. P.: Gliomas of the optic nerve, Am. J. Med. Sci. 237:238-261, 1959.

Wagner, F.: Beitrag, zur Frage der primären Opticusgliome, Klin. Monatsbl. Augenheilkd. 103:606, 1939.

Walsh, F. B.: The ocular signs of tumors involving the anterior visual pathway, Am. J. Ophthalmol. 42:347-377, 1956.

Walsh, F. B., and Hedges, T. R., Jr.: Optic nerve sheath haemorrhage, Trans. Am. Acad. Ophthalmol. 54:29-48, 1950.

Walsh, F. B., and Hoyt, W. F.: Primary tumors of the optic nerve and chiasm. In Clinical neuro-ophthalmology, Baltimore, 1969, The Williams & Wilkins Co., p. 2075.

Wilson, J. M., and Farmer, W. D.: Glioma of optic nerve, Arch. Ophthalmol. 23:605, 1940.

Wilson, J. M., and Farmer, W. D.: Spongioblastoma of the optic nerve: a critical review; report of 2 cases with autopsy observation in one, Arch. Ophthalmol. 23: 605-618, 1940.

## Tumors of the cavernous sinus

Aron-Rosa, D.: Utilité de la phlébographie orbitaire dans l'étude anatomique et pathologique du sinus caverneux, Bull. Soc. Ophtalmol. Fr. 66:912-916, 1966.

Clay, C., and Vignaud, J.: Syndromes du sinus caverneux, Arch. Ophtalmol. 34:165-178, 1974.

Fairclough, W. A.: Drainage in infected

cavernous sinus thrombosis, Austral. N.Z. J. Surg. 16:193-196, 1947.

Foix, C.: Syndrome de la paroi externe du sinus caverneux, Rev. Neurol. 37/38:827, 1922.

Franceschetti, Jentzer, Junet, and Doret: Deux cas d'anévrisme artério-veineux de la carotide interne dans le sinus caverneux, Rev. Otoneuroophtalmol. 19:53-54, 1947.

Godtfredsen, E.: Ophthalmologic and neurologic symptoms of malignant nasopharyngeal tumors, Acta Pathol. Microbiol. Scand. (suppl.) 55:1944.

Huber, A.: Les anévrismes de l'orbite et du sinus caverneux, Bull. Soc. Fr. Ophtalmol. 64:374, 1951.

Huber, A.: Über das Syndrom des Sinus cavernosus, Ophthalmologica 121:118, 1951.

Jefferson, G.: On the saccular aneurysms of the internal carotid artery in the cavernous sinus, Br. J. Surg. 26:267, 1938-1939.

Jefferson, G.: Concerning injuries, aneurysms and tumours involving the cavernous sinus, Trans. Ophthalmol. Soc. U.K. 73:117-152, 1953.

Kaeser, E. H.: Das arteriovenöse Aneurysma im Sinus cavernosus, Ophthalmologica 126: 237-282, 1953.

Krayenbühl, H.: Die Hirnaneurysma, Schweiz. Arch. Neurol. Psychiatr. 47:155, 1941.

McNeal, W. J., Frisbee, F. C., and Blevine, A.: Thrombophlebitis of the cavernous sinus; review of reported recoveries with special reference to thrombophlebitis of staphylococcic origin, Arch. Ophthalmol. 29:231-257, 1943.

Weber, G.: Hirnabs zesse im Rahmen infektiöser intrakranieller Erkrankungen, Stuttgart, 1956, Georg Thieme Verlag, KG.

Weinberger, L. M., Adler, F. H., and Grant, F. C.: Primary pituitary adenoma and the syndrome of the cavernous sinus, Arch. Ophthalmol. 24:1197, 1940.

**Tumors of the third ventricle**

Dandy, W. E.: Benign tumors of the third ventricle of the brain: diagnosis and treatment, Springfield, Ill., 1933, Charles C Thomas, Publisher.

Duke-Elder, S., and Scott, G.: Neuro-ophthalmology. In Duke-Elder, S., editor: System of ophthalmology, vol. 12, St. Louis, 1971, The C. V. Mosby Co.

François, M. J.: La pathogénie de l'hémi-anopsie binasale, Bull. Soc. Belge. Ophtalmol. 81:1945.

François, M. J.: L'hémianopsie binasale, Ophthalmologica 113:321, 1947.

Hughes, E. B. C.: Some observations on visual fields in hydrocephalus, J. Neurol. Neurosurg. Psychiatr. 9:30, 1946.

Jefferson, G., and Jackson, H.: Tumors of lateral and third ventricles, Proc. R. Soc. Med. 32:1105-1137, 1939.

Jentzer, A.: Les tumeurs du troisième ventricule, Schweiz. Arch. Neurol. Psychiatr. 14: 2, 1939.

Newton, T. H.: Neuroradiologic evaluation of lesions affecting the third ventricle and adjacent structures. In Smith, J. L., editor: Neuro-ophthalmology, St. Louis, 1967, The C. V. Mosby Co.

Oldberg, E., and Eisenhardt, L.: Neurological diagnosis of tumors of third ventricle, Trans. Am. Neurol. Assoc. 64:33-36, 1938.

Pecker, J., Ferrand, B., and Javalet, A.: Tumeurs du troisième ventricule, Neurochirurgie 12:7-136, 1966.

Pecker, J., Guy, G., and Scarabin, J.-M.: Third ventricle tumours. In Vinken, P. J., and Bruyn, G. W., editors: New York, 1974, American Elsevier Publishing Co., Inc., vol. 17, pp. 440-489.

Penfield, W.: Diencephalic autonomic epilepsy, Arch. Neurol. Psychiatr. 22:358-375, 1929.

Penfield, W., and Erickson, T.: Epilepsy and cerebral localization, Springfield, Ill., 1941, Charles C Thomas, Publisher.

Rand, R. W., and Lemmen, L. J.: Tumours of the posterior portion of the third ventricle, J. Neurosurg. 10:1-18, 1953.

Tönnis, W.: Tumoren im dritten Ventrikel. Diagnostik der intrakraniellen Geschwülste. In Olivecrona, H., and Tönnis, W., editors: Handbuch der Neurochirurgie, Berlin, 1962, Julius Springer, vol. 4, p. 429.

Wagener, H. P., and Cusick, P. L.: Chiasmal syndromes produced by lesions in posterior fossa, Arch. Ophthalmol. 18:887-891, 1937.

Walsh, F. B., and Hoyt, W. F.: Third ventricle tumor. In Clinical neuro-ophthalmology, Baltimore, 1969, The Williams & Wilkins Co., p. 2248.

**Tumors of the thalamus**

Arnould, G., Masingue, M., Weber, M., Picard, A., Reny, A., and Renard, M.:

Divergent strabismus revealing a thalamic tumour, Rev. Otoneuroophtalmol. **45**:455-461, 1973.

Bailey, P.: Thalamussyndrom. Die Hirngeschwülste, Stuttgart, 1951, Ferdinand Enke Verlag, p. 228.

Knapp, P., and Schwarzmann, A.: Contraction in visual fields caused by diencephalic lesion, Ophthalmologica **11**:270-278, 1946.

McKissock, W., and Paine, K. W. E.: Primary tumors of the thalamus, Brain **81**: 41-63, 1958.

Névin, S.: Thalamic hypertrophy or gliomatosis of the optic thalamus. J. Neurol. Neurosurg. Psychiatry **1**:342, 1938.

Payne, C. A.: Thalamic tumors. In Vinken, P. J., and Bruyn, G. W., editors: Handbook of clinical neurology, New York, 1974, American Elsevier Publishing Co., Inc., vol. 17, pp. 610-619.

Ranson, S. W., and Magoun, H. W.: The hypothalamus, Ergeb. Physiol. **41**:56-163, 1939.

Tönnis, W.: Tumoren des Thalamus. Diagnostik der intrakraniellen Geschwülste. In Olivecrona, H., and Tönnis, W., editors: Handbuch der Neurochirurgie, Berlin, 1962, Julius Springer, vol. 4, p. 433.

Walsh, F. B., and Hoyt, W. F.: Tumors of the thalamus. In Clinical neuro-ophthalmology, Baltimore, 1969, The Williams & Wilkins Co., p. 2221.

Weinberger, L. M., and Grant, F. C.: Precocious puberty and tumors of the hypothalamus, Arch. Intern. Med. **67**:762, 1941.

**Tumors of the basal ganglia; tumors of the pineal body and the midbrain**

Argyll Robertson, D.: Four cases of spinal myosis; with remarks on the action of light on the pupil, Edinburgh Med. J. **15**:487, 1869.

Bailey, P.: Syndrom der Epiphysengegend. Die Hirngeschwülste, Stuttgart, 1951, Ferdinand Enke Verlag, p. 282.

Balthasar, K.: Gliomas of the quadrigeminal plate and eye movements, Ophthalmologica **155**:249-270, 1968.

Barker, L. F.: Parinaud's syndrome, Am. J. Ophthalmol. **18**:827-832, 1935.

Best, F.: Erkrankungen der Vierhügel, die Zirbeldrüsengeschwülste. In Schieck, F., and Brückner, A., editors: Kurzes Handbuch der Ophthalmologie, Berlin, 1931, Julius Springer, vol. 6, p. 497, 499.

Bielschowsky, A.: Lectures on motor anomalies: paralysis of conjugate movements of eyes, Arch. Ophthalmol. **13**:569, 1935.

Böhringer, H. R., and Koenig, F.: Die diagnostische Bedeutung der vertikalen Blicklähmung, Ophthalmologica **125**:357, 1935.

Calmettes, L., and Deodati, F.: Nystagmus retractorius, Année Ther. Clin. Ophthalmol. **15**:71-91, 1964.

Collier, J.: Nuclear ophthalmoplegia. With special reference to the retraction of lids and ptosis and to lesions of posterior commissure, Brain **50**:488-498, 1927.

Devic, A., Paufique, L., Girard, P., and Guinet, P.: Syndrome de Parinaud, Ann. Oculist. **178**:199, 1945.

Foerster, O., Gagel, O., and Mahoney, W.: Die encephalen Tumoren der Oblongata, Pons und des Mesencephalons, Arch. Psychiatr. Nervenkr. **110**:1-74, 1939.

Glaser, M. A.: Tumours of the pineal body, corpora quadrigemina and third ventricle, the inter-relationship of their syndromes and their surgical treatment, Brain **52**:226-262, 1929.

Globus, J. H.: Tumors of quadrigeminate plate; clinico-anatomic study of 7 cases, Arch. Ophthalmol. **5**:418-444, 1931.

Globus, J. H.: Pinealoma, Arch. Pathol. **31**: 533-568, 1941.

Hatcher, M. A., and Klintworth, G. K.: Sylvian aqueduct syndrome, Arch. Neurol. **15**:215-222, 1966.

Horrax, G., and Bailey, P.: Tumors of the pineal body, Arch. Neurol. Psychiatr. **13**: 423-467, 1925.

Horrax, G., and Bailey, P.: Pineal pathology: further studies, Arch. Neurol. Psychiatr. **19**:394-414, 1928.

Horrax, G., and Wyatt, J. C.: Ectopic pinealomas in chiasmal region, J. Neurosurg. **4**: 309-326, 1947.

Jaensch, P. A.: Doppelseitige Trochlearisparese als einzige Motilitätsstörung bei Zirbeldrüsentumor, Z. Augenheilkd. **75**:58, 1931.

Lillie, W. I.: Homonymous hemianopia; primary signs of tumors involving lateral part of the transverse fissure, Trans. Sect. Ophthalmol. Am. Med. Assoc., pp. 200-212, 1929.

Nashold, B. S., and Gills, J. P.: Ocular signs resulting from brain stimulation and lesions in the human, Arch. Ophthalmol. **77**:609-618, 1967.

Netsky, M. G., and Strobos, R. R. J.: Neoplasms within the midbrain, Arch. Neurol. Psychiatr. **68**:116-129, 1952.

Palomar-Gollado, F., and Palomar, P. F.: Tumores cerebrales y signo de Argyll-Robertson, Arch. Soc. Oftalmol. Hispano-Am. **20**:470-477, 1960.

Pia, H. W.: Klinik, Differentialdiagnose und Behandlung der Vierhügelgeschwülste, Dtsch. Z. Nervenheilk. **172**:12-32, 1954.

Posner, M., and Horrax, G.: Eye signs in pineal tumors, J. Neurosurg. **3**:15-24, 1946.

Schultz-Zehden, W.: Augenveränderungen bei Tumoren der Vierhügelgegend, Z. Gesamte Inn. Med. **6**:8-12, 1951.

Seybold, M. E., Yoss, R. E., Hollenhorst, R. W., and Moyer, N. J.: Pupillary abnormalities associated with tumours of the pineal region, Neurology **21**:232-237, 1971.

Smith, R. A., and Montgomery, N. E.: Pineal tumors. In Vinken, P. J., and Bruyn, G. W., editor: Handbook of clinical neurology, New York, 1974, American Elsevier Publishing Co., Inc., vol. 17, pp. 648-665.

Smith, J. L., Zieper, I., Gay, A. I., and Cogan, D. G.: Nystagmus retractorius Arch. Ophthalmol. **62**:864-867, 1959.

Thiébaut, F., Philippides, D., and Buchheit, F.: Clonus rétractorius ou nystagmus retractorius, symptome neurochirurgical, Rev. Otoneuroophtalmol. **39**:72-82, 1967.

Tönnis, W.: Tumoren des Corpus striatum. Diagnostik der intrakraniellen Geschwülste. In Olivecrona, H., and Tönnis, W., editors: Handbuch der Neurochirurgie, Berlin, 1962, Julius Springer, vol. 4, p. 431.

Tönnis, W.: Geschwülste der Vierhügelgegend. Diagnostik der intrakraniellen Geschwülste. In Olivecrona, H., and Tönnis, W., editors: Handbuch der Neurochirurgie, Berlin, 1962, Julius Springer, vol. 4, p. 436.

Tönnis, W.: Geschwülste des Mittelhirns. Diagnostik der intrakraniellen Geschwülste. In Olivecrona, H., and Tönnis, W., editors: Handbuch der Neurochirurgie, Berlin, 1962, Julius Springer, vol. 4, p. 441.

Wakusawa, S.: Sylvian aqueduct syndrome and mesencephalic skew deviation, Jpn. J. Ophthalmol. **17**:154-165, 1973.

Walsh, F. B., and Hoyt, W. F.: Midbrain tumors. In Clinical neuro-ophthalmology, Baltimore, 1969, The Williams & Wilkins Co., p. 2215.

Walsh, F. B., and Hoyt, W. F.: Tumors of the basal ganglia. In Clinical neuro-ophthalmology, Baltimore, 1969, The Williams & Wilkins Co., p. 2222.

Walsh, F. B., and Hoyt, W. F.: Pineal tumors. In Clinical neuro-ophthalmology, Baltimore, 1969, The Williams & Wilkins Co., p. 2240.

Weber, G.: Tumoren der Glandula pinealis und ektopische Pinealozytome, Schweiz. Arch. Neurol. Psychiatr. **91**:473-509, 1963.

Weber, G.: Midbrain tumours. In Vinken, P. J., and Bruyn, G. W., editors: Handbook of clinical neurology, New York, 1974, American Elsevier Publishing Co., Inc., vol. 17, pp. 620-647.

Yanagida, N.: Ocular symptoms of tumor in the aqueduct of Sylvius, Acta Soc. Ophthalmol. Jpn. **57**:254-258, 1953.

Young, S., Wu, C. P., and Chen, C. S.: Pinealoma, Chin. Med. J. **68**:261-262, 1950.

**Tumors of the cerebellum**

Arseni, C., Maretsis, M., and Vasilesco, A.: La maladie de von Hippel-Lindau, Rev. Otoneuroophtalmol. **39**:174-182, 1967.

Bailey, P.: Syndrom des Kleinhirnwurms. Die Hirngeschwülste, Stuttgart, 1951, Ferdinand Enke, Verlag, p. 199.

Bailey, P.: Syndrom der Kleinhirnhemisphäre. Die Hirngeschwülste, Stuttgart, 1951, Ferdinand Enke Verlag, p. 206.

Best, F.: Die Augenstörungen bei Kleinhirnerkrankungen. In Schieck, F., and Brückner, A., editors: Kurzes Handbuch der Ophthalmologie, Berlin, 1931, Julius Springer, vol. 6, p. 510.

Biemond, A.: Cerebellar tumours. In Vinken, P. J., and Bruyn, G. W., editors: Handbook of clinical neurology, New York, 1974, American Elsevier Publishing Co., Inc., vol. 17, pp. 707-718.

Cogan, D. G.: Ocular dysmetria, flutter-like oscillations of the eyes and opsoclonus, Arch. Ophthalmol. **51**:318-335, 1954.

Cogan, D. G.: Dissociated nystagmus with lesions in the posterior fossa, Arch. Ophthalmol. **70**:361-368, 1963.

Craig, W. M., Wagener, H. P., and Kernohan, J. W.: Lindau-von Hippel disease, Arch. Neurol. Psychiatr. **46**:36, 1941.

Cushing, H., and Walker, C. V.: Distortions of the visual fields in cases of brain tumor: binasal hemianopia, Arch. Ophthalmol. **41**:559, 1912.

Danis, P.: Aspects ophthalmologiques des

angiomatoses du système nerveux, Acta Neurol. Psychiatr. Belge. **50**:615-679, 1950.

Daroff, R. B.: Ocular motor manifestations of brain stem and cerebellar dysfunction. In Smith, J. L., editor: Neuro-ophthalmology, St. Louis, 1970, The C. V. Mosby Co., vol. 5, pp. 104-118.

Delmas-Marsalet, Lafon, and Faure: Vollständiges Chiasma-Syndrom, ausgelöst durch Ventrikelhydrocephalie bei Kleinhirntumor, J. Med. Bordeaux **118**:661-664, 1941.

Eccles, J. C.: Mode of operation of the cerebellum in the dynamic loop control of movement, Brain Res. **40**:73-80, 1972.

François, J., Hoffmann, G., and Jadoul, P.: Les astrocytomes kystiques du cervelet et leurs manifestations oculaires, Confin. Neurol. **21**:307-325, 1961.

Gay, A., Newman, N., Keltner, I., and Stroud, M.: Eye movement disorders, St. Louis, 1974, The C. V. Mosby Co.

Hall, C. S.: Blood vessel tumors of brain with particular reference to Lindau's syndrome, J. Neurol. Psychopathol. **15**:305-312, 1935.

Heine, L.: Über Angiogliosis retinae mit Hirntumor, Graefe. Arch. Ophthalmol. **88**: 1914.

von Hippel, E.: Über eine sehr seltene Erkrankung der Netzhaut, Graefe. Arch. Ophthalmol., vol. 59, 1904.

von Hippel, E.: Die anatomische Grundlage der von mir beschriebenen seltenen Netzhauterkrankungen, Graefe. Arch. Ophthalmol., vol. 95, 1918.

Holmes, G.: The cerebellum of man, Brain **62**:1, 1939.

Huber, A.: Cerebrale und retinale Angiopathie, Ophthalmologica **117**:265, 1949.

Kestenbaum, A.: Mechanismus des Nystagmus, Graefe. Arch. Ophthalmol. **105**:799, 1921.

Krayenbühl, H.: Die Symptomatologie der Tumoren der hinteren Schädelgrube, insbesondere des Kleinhirns, Schweiz. Med. Wochenschr. **2**:901-905, 1938.

Lewis, P. M.: Angiomatosis retinae, Arch. Ophthalmol. **30**:250, 1943.

Lindau, A.: Studien über Kleinhirncysten. Bau, Pathogenese, Beziehungen zur Angiomatosis retinae, Acta Pathol. Scand. (Suppl. 1), p. 128, 1926.

Lindau, A.: Vascular tumors of brain, Proc. R. Soc. Med. **24**:363, 1941.

Lotmar, F.: Zur Kenntnis der Lindauschen Krankheit, Schweiz. Arch. Neurol. Psychiatr. **36**:2, 1935.

MacNab, G. H.: Lindau's disease, Proc. R. Soc. Med. **34**:324-325, 1941.

Magendie: Précis de Physiologie **3**:1, 380, 1833.

de Martel, T., and Guillaume, J.: Les tumeurs de la loge cérébelleuse (fosse cérébrale postérieure), Paris, 1934, Gaston Doin & Cie.

Martin, P.: L'angiomatose rétinocérébelleuse et sa pathologie chirurgicale, Acta Neurol. Psychiatr. Belge. **50**:457-461, 1950.

McDonald, A. E.: Lindau's disease; report of 6 cases with surgical verification in 4 living patients, Arch. Ophthalmol. **23**:564-576, 1940.

McGovern, F. H.: Angiomatosis retinae, Am. J. Ophthalmol. **26**:184, 1943.

Olson, A. K., and Pinley, C. C.: Cerebellar tumors and their clinical signs, Guthrie Clin. Bull. **17**:141, 1948.

Paillas, J. E., et al.: L'atteinte contro-latérale des nerfs crâniens au cours des tumeurs de la fosse postérieure, Rev. Neurol. **121**: 452-464, 1969.

Palin, A.: Von Hippel-Lindau's disease, Proc. R. Soc. Med. **32**:1618, 1939.

Rumbaur, W.: Angiomatosis retinae (Hippel-Lindau disease): report on a genealogic tree, Klin. Monatsbl. Augenheilkd. **106**:168, 1941.

Ryan, E. P.: Angiomatosis retinae, Arch. Ophthalmol. **23**:623, 1940.

Salorio, D. P., and Oliveros, F. R.: Papillary stasis in astrocytoma of the cerebellum, Arch. Soc. Oftalmol. Hispano.-Am. **30**:95-104, 1970.

Staz, L.: Angiomatosis retinae, Br. J. Ophthalmol. **25**:167, 1941.

Stewart, T., and Holmes, G.: Symptomatology of cerebellar tumors; a study of forty cases, Brain **27**:522-591, 1904.

Susac, J. O., et al.: Clinical spectrum of ocular bobbing, J. Neurol. Neurosurg. Psychiatry **33**:771-775, 1970.

Tönnis, W.: Geschwülste des Kleinhirs. Diagnostik der intrakraniellen Geschwülste. In Olivecrona, H., and Tönnis, W., editors: Handbuch der Neurochirurgie, Berlin, 1962, Julius Springer, vol. 4, p. 444.

Traquair, H. M.: Hemangioma of the retina, Trans. Ophthalmol. Soc. U.K. **52**:311, 1932.

Wagener, H. P., and Cusick, P. L.: Chiasmal syndromes produced by lesions in posterior fossa, Arch. Ophthalmol. **18**:887-891, 1937.

Walsh, F. B., and Hoyt, W. F.: Cerebellar tumor. In Clinical neuro-ophthalmology, Baltimore, 1969, The Williams & Wilkins Co., p. 2206.

Weinberger, L., and Webster, J. E.: Visual field defects associated with cerebellar tumors, Arch. Ophthalmol. **25**:128-138, 1941.

Wertheimer, P., Lapras, C., Wertheimer, J., Thierry, A., and Dusquesnel, J.: A propos de quelques aspects ophthalmologiques des angiomes de la fosse cérébrale postérieure, Bull. Soc. Fr. Ophtalmol. **77**:290-296, 1964.

**Tumors of the fourth ventricle**

Alpers, D. J., and Yaskin, H. E.: The Bruns syndrome, J. Nerv. Ment. Dis. **100**:115-134, 1944.

Bailey, P.: Das Syndrom des 4. Ventrikels. Die Hirngeschwülste, Stuttgart, 1951, Ferdinand Enke Verlag, p. 183.

Best, F.: Erkrankungen im Bereiche des 4. Ventrikels. In Schieck, F., and Brückner, A., editor: Kurzes Handbuch der Ophthalmologie, Berlin, 1931, Julius Springer, vol. 6, p. 500.

Craig, W. M., and Kernohan, J. W.: Tumors of fourth ventricle, J.A.M.A. **111**:2370-2377, 1938.

Walsh, F. B., and Hoyt, W. F.: Tumors of the fourth ventricle. In Clinical neuro-ophthalmology, Baltimore, 1969, The Williams & Wilkins Co., p. 2256.

**Tumors of the cerebellopontine angle**

Ageeva-Majkova, O. G.: The clinical findings in neurinoma of the eighth nerve from the oto-neurological viewpoint (in Russian), Vestn. Otorinolaringol. **12**:3-10, 1950.

Bailey, P.: Syndrom des Kleinhirnbrückenwinkels. Die Hirngeschwülste, Stuttgart, 1951, Ferdinand Enke Verlag, p. 59.

Best, F.: Die Augenstörungen bei Kleinhirnbrückenwinkelschwülsten. In Schieck, F., and Brückner, A., editors: Kurzes Handbuch der Ophthalmologie, Berlin, 1931, Julius Springer, vol. 6, p. 515.

Brunner, H.: Brain tumors and ear, Trans. Am. Acad. Ophthalmol. **40**:59-78, 1935.

Cushing, H.: Tumors of the nervus acusticus and the syndrome of the cerebello-pontile angle, Philadelphia, 1917, W. B. Saunders Co.

Edwards, C. H., and Paterson, J. H.: A review of the symptoms and signs of acoustic neurofibromata, Brain **74**:144, 1951.

Globus, J. H.: Pontofacial angle tumors, with particular reference to involvement of the acoustic nerve, Laryngoscope **51**:1119-1138, 1941.

Graf, K.: Die Kleinhirnbrückenwinkelgeschwülste, Basel, 1955, S. Karger AG.

Hitselberger, W. E.: Acoustic neurinoma diagnosis, Eye Ear Nose Throat Mon. **29**:49-54, 1967.

House, W. F., and Hitselberger, W. E.: Acoustic tumors. In Vinken, P. J., and Bruyn, G. W.: Handbook of clinical neurology, New York, 1974, American Elsevier Publishing Co., Inc., vol. 17, pp. 666-692.

Lundberg, T.: The symptomatology and diagnosis of acoustic tumours from an otological viewpoint (in Swedish), Nord. Med. **44**:1520-1523, 1950.

Lundberg, T.: Diagnostic problems concerning acoustic tumours: a study of 300 verified cases and the Békésy audiogram in the differential diagnosis, Acta Otolaryngol. (Suppl.) **99**:110, 1952.

Salgado Benavides, E.: Tumors of cerebellopontine angle, Arch. Soc. Oftalmol. Hispano-Am. **4**:75, 1944.

Schuermann, K., Brock, M., Reulen, H.-J., and Voth, D.: Brain edema, cerebellopontine angle tumors, Adv. Neurosurg., vol. 1, 1973.

Thiebaut, J. B., Philippides, D., Buchheit, F., Bronner, A., and Flament, J.: Unilateral papilloedema symptomatic of a tumor of the right cerebello-pontine angle, Rev. Otoneuroophtalmol. **43**:367-374, 1971.

Tönnis, W.: Neurinom des N. acusticus. Diagnostik der intrakraniellen Geschwülste. In Olivecrona, H., and Tönnis, W., editors: Handbuch der Neurochirurgie, Berlin, 1962, Julius Springer, vol. 4, p. 60.

Tönnis, W.: Geschwülste des Kleinhirnbrückenwinkels. Diagnostik der intrakraniellen Geschwülste. In Olivecrona, H., and Tönnis, W., editors: Handbuch der Neurochirurgie, Berlin, 1962, Julius Springer, vol. 4, p. 459.

Walsh, F. B., and Hoyt, W. F.: Cerebellopontine angle tumors. In Clinical neuro-ophthalmology, Baltimore, 1969, The Williams & Wilkins Co., p. 2229.

Winston, J.: Revision of cerebellopontile angle lesion syndrome, with analysis of vestibular findings in 34 cases of verified tumor of cerebellopontile angle, Arch. Otolaryngol. **32**:877-886, 1940.

**Tumors of the pons and medulla oblongata**

Allerand, C. D.: Paroxysmal skew deviation in association with a brain stem glioma, report of an unusual case, Neurology **12**: 520-523, 1962.

Bailey, P.: Syndrom des Hirnstammes. Die Hirngeschwülste, Stuttgart, 1951, Ferdinand Enke Verlag, p. 275.

Best, F.: Die Ponserkrankungen. In Schieck, F., and Brückner, A., editors: Kurzes Lehrbuch der Ophthalmologie, Berlin, 1931, Julius Springer, vol. 6, p. 494.

Brock, S., and Needles, W.: Tumors of the brain stem: a clinical study of 5 cases with autopsy findings, J. Nerv. Ment. Dis. **72**:531-534, 1930.

Buckley, R.: Pontile gliomas: a pathologic study and classification of 25 cases, Arch. Pathol. **9**:779, 1930.

Cogan, D. G., and Wray, S. H.: Internuclear ophthalmoplegia as an early sign of brainstem tumors, Neurology **20**:629-633, 1970.

Dandy, W. E.: In Lewis, D., editor: Lewis' practice of surgery, Hagerstown, 1936, W. F. Prior Co., Inc., vol. 12, pp. 534-556.

Daroff, R. B., and Waldman, A. L.: Ocular bobbing, J. Neurol. Neurosurg. Psychiatry **28**:375, 1965.

Fisher, C. M.: Ocular bobbing, Arch. Neurol. **11**:543-546, 1964.

Foerster, O.: Die encephalen Tumoren der Oblongata, des Pons und des Mesencephalons, Z. Neurol. Psychiatr. **168**:482-518, 1940.

Foerster, O., Gagel, O., and Mahoney, W.: Die encephalen Tumoren des verlängerten Markes, der Brücke und des Mittelhirns, Arch. Psychiatr. **110**:1-74, 1939.

Gay, A., Newman, N., Keltner, I., and Stroud, M.: Eye movement disorders, St. Louis, 1974, The C. V. Mosby Co.

Goebel, H. H., Komatsuzaki, A., Bender, M. B., and Cohen, B.: Lesions of the pontine tegmentum and conjugate gaze paralysis, Arch. Neurol. **24**:431-440, 1971.

Haire, C. C., and Wolf, A.: Intramedullary tumors of the brain stem, Arch. Neurol. Psychiatr. **32**:1230-1252, 1934.

Horrax, G., and Buckley, R.: A clinical study of the differentiation of certain pontile tumors from acoustic tumors, Arch. Neurol. Psychiatr. **24**:1217-1230, 1950.

Kaufmann, J.: Tumeurs pontines et bulbopontines, Schweiz. Arch. Neurol. Psychiatr. **64**:197, 1949.

Lassman, L. P.: Tumours of the pons and medulla oblongata. In Vinken, P. J., and Bruyn, G. W., editors: Handbook of clinical neurology, New York, 1974, American Elsevier Publishing Co., Inc., vol. 17, pp. 693-706.

Mackensen, G.: Differentialdiagnose Kleinhirnbrückwinkel—pontiner Tumor, Ber. Dtsch. Ophthalmol. Ges. **67**:430-431, 1965.

Sagebiel, J.: Intrapontine tumors; clinicopathologic study, Ohio Med. J. **33**:760-768, 1937.

Santha, K.: Zur Symptomatologie der Ponstumoren, klinisch-anatomischer Beitrag zur Kenntnis der pontinen Blicklähmung, Arch. Psychiatr. **103**:539-551, 1935.

Simon, K. A., and Gay, A. J.: Optokinetic responses in brain stem lesions, Arch. Ophthalmol. **71**:303-307, 1964.

Smith, J., David, N. J., and Klintworth, G.: Skew deviation, Neurology **14**:96-105, 1964.

Tönnis, W.: Tumoren von Pons und Oblongata. Diagnostik der intrakraniellen Geschwülste. In Olivecrona, H., and Tönnis, W., editors: Handbuch der Neurochirurgie, Berlin, 1962, Julius Springer, vol. 4, p. 442.

Walsh, F. B.: Tumors of the medulla. In Clinical, neuro-ophthalmology, Baltimore, 1947, The Williams & Wilkins Co., p. 2219.

Walsh, F. B., and Hoyt, W. F.: Gliomas of the pons. In Clinical neuro-ophthalmology, Baltimore, 1969, The Williams & Wilkins Co., p. 2216.

Wybar, K.: Disorders of ocular motility in brain stem lesions in children, Ann. Ophthalmol. **3**:645-662, 1971.

# CHAPTER FOUR

## Relationship between type of tumor and ocular signs and symptoms

Arendt, A.: Ependymomas. In Vinken, P. J., and Bruyn, G. W., editors: Handbook of clinical neurology, New York, 1974, American Elsevier Publishing Co., Inc., vol. 18, pp. 105-150.

Bailey, P.: Metastatische Tumoren. Die Hirngeschwülste, Stuttgart, 1951, Ferdinand Enke Verlag, p. 303.

Bonkalo, S.: Die Bedeutung der Hirngeschwulstart und des Geschwulstsitzes für die Entstehung der Hirnschwellung, Dtsch. Z. Nervenheilk. 149:243-253, 1939.

Dandy, W. E.: Metastatic tumors. In Lewis, D., editor: Lewis' practice of surgery, Hagerstown, Md., 1944, W. F. Prior Co., Inc., vol. 12, p. 669.

Dastur, H. M.: Tuberculoma. In Vinken, P. J., and Bruyn, G. W., editors: Handbook of clinical neurology, New York, 1974, American Elsevier Publishing Co., Inc., vol. 18, pp. 413-426.

Fahlbusch, R., and Marguth, F.: Endocrine disorders associated with intracranial tumours. In Vinken, P. J., and Bruyn, G. W., editors: Handbook of clinical neurology, New York, 1974, American Elsevier Publishing Co., Inc., vol. 16, pp. 341-359.

Finkemeyer, H., Pfingst, E., and Zülch, K. J.: The astrocytomas of the cerebral hemispheres. In Vinken, P. J., and Bruyn, G. W., Handbook of clinical neurology, New York, 1974, American Elsevier Publishing Co., Inc., vol. 18, pp. 1-48.

Gärtner, J.: Statische Untersuchungen an 654 intrakraniellen raumfordernden Prozessen: ein Beitrag zur Biologie der Hirngeschwülste, Zentralbl. Neurochir. 15:333-351, 1955.

Klingler, M., and Condrau, G.: Lokalisatorisch irreführende Gesichtsfeldsymptome bei Hirntumoren, Ophthalmologica 120:270, 1950.

Livingston, K. E., Horrax, G., and Sachs, E.: Metastatic brain tumours, Surg. Clin. North Am. 28:805, 1948.

MacCabe, J. J.: Glioblastoma. In Vinken, P. J., and Bruyn, G. W., editors: Handbook of clinical neurology, New York, 1974, American Elsevier Publishing Co., Inc., vol. 18, pp. 49-72.

Mahoney, W.: Die Epidermoide des Zentralnervensystems, Z. Ges. Neurol. Psychiatr. 155:416-471, 1936.

Minkowski, M.: Über metastatische Hirngeschwülste, Schweiz. Arch. Neurol. Psychiatr. 47:9, 1941.

Orban, T., and Födö, V.: Rindenblindheit infolge beiderseitiger Metastase im Okzipitalpol, Klin. Monatsbl. Augenheilkd. 148:700-704, 1966.

Paillas, J. E., and Pellet, W.: Brain metastases. In Vinken, P. J., and Bruyn, G. W., editors: Handbook of clinical neurology, New York, 1974, American Elsevier Publishing Co., Inc., vol. 18, pp. 201-232.

Pass, E. K.: Zur Klinik der zerebralen Karzinommetastasen, Nervenarzt, p. 385, 1939.

Rados, A.: Occurrence of glioma of retina and brain in collateral lines in same family: genetics of glioma, Arch. Ophthalmol. 35:1, 1946.

Reymond, A.: Classification anatomo-pathologique des tumeurs cérébrales, Ophthalmologica 125:204, 1953.

Rubinstein, L. J.: The cerebellar medulloblastoma: its origin, differentiation, morphological variants, and biological behavior. In Vinken, P. J., and Bruyn, G. W.: Handbook of clinical neurology, New York, 1975, American Elsevier Publishing Co., Inc., vol. 18, pp. 167-194.

Sassin, J. F.: Intracranial chordoma. In Vinken, P. J., and Bruyn, G. W.: Handbook of clinical neurology, New York, 1974, American Elsevier Publishing Co., Inc., vol. 18, pp. 151-164.

Scheid, W.: Zur Klinik der intrakraniellen Karzinommetastasen, Allg. Z. Psychiatr. 113: 66-82, 1939.

Tönnis, W.: Augensymptome bei 3033 Hirngeschwülsten, 59. Zusammenk. Dtsch. Ophthalmol. Ges., Heidelberg, 1955.

Tönnis, W.: Erscheinungsbild und Verlaufsform der verschiedenen Geschwulstarten. Diagnostik der intrakraniellen Geschwülste. In Olivecrona, H., and Tönnis, W., editors: Handbuch der Neurochirurgie, Berlin, 1962, Julius Springer, vol. 4, p. 2.

Walsh, F. B., and Hoyt, W. F.: Hematogenous metastases to the brain. In Clinical neuro-ophthalmology, Baltimore, 1969, The Williams & Wilkins Co., p. 2328.

Weber, G.: Zur Diagnose und Prognose intra-kranieller Tumoren, Ophthalmologica **125**: 231, 1953.

Zimmermann, H. M.: Vascular tumors of the brain. In Vinken, P. J., and Bruyn, G. W., editors: Handbook of clinical neurology, New York, 1974, American Elsevier Publishing Co., Inc., vol. 18, pp. 269-298.

Zülch, K.: Pathologische Anatomie der raum-fordernden intracraniellen Prozesse, Heidelberg, 1956, Springer-Verlag.

## CHAPTER FIVE

### Pseudotumor cerebri, subdural hematomas, brain abscesses, and aneurysms

#### Pseudotumor cerebri

Albrecht, H.: Stauungspapille bei nicht tu-morösen Hirnprozessen. Sammlung zwang-loser Abhandlungen aus dem Gebiete der Psychiatrie und Neurologie, Stuttgart, 1964, Gustav Fischer Verlag, Heft 26.

Bailey, P.: Contribution to the histopathology of pseudotumor cerebri, Arch. Neurol. Psychiatr. **4**:401-416, 1920.

Frazier, C. H.: Cerebral pseudotumors, Arch. Neurol. Psychiatr. **24**:1117-1132, 1930.

Greer, M.: Benign intracranial hypertension. Pseudotumor cerebri. In Vinken, P. J., and Bruyn, G. W., editors: Handbook of clinical neurology, New York, 1974, American Elsevier Publishing Co., Inc., vol. 16, pp. 150-166.

Kirkham, T. H., Sanders, M. D., and Sapp, G. A.: Unilateral papilledema in benign intracranial hypertension, Can. J. Ophthalmol. **8**:533-538, 1973.

Krayenbühl, H.: Die Bedeutung der Angio-graphie für die Diagnose der cerebralen Thrombophlebitis, Acta Neurochir. 3(Suppl.):198-201, 1955.

Marr, W. G., and Chambers, J. W.: Occlusion of the cerebral dural sinuses by tumor simulating pseudotumor cerebri, Am. J. Ophthalmol. **61**:45-49, 1966.

Meythaler, H., and Meythaler-Radeck, B.: Pseudo-tumour of the brain, Klin. Monatsbl. Augenheilkd. **163**:200-204, 1973.

Morrice, G.: Papilledema and hypervitamino-sis, J.A.M.A. **213**:1344, 1970.

Nonne, M.: Ueber Fälle von Symptomen-komplex "Tumor cerebri" mit Ausgang in Heilung (Pseudo-Tumor cerebri), Dtsch. Z. Nervenheilkd. **27**:169, 1904.

Stochdorph, O.: Zur Frage der chronischen Hirnschwellung, Arch. Psychiatr. Nervenkr. **181**:101, 1949.

Walsh, F. B.: Papilledema associated with in-creased intracranial pressure in Addison's disease, Arch. Ophthalmol. **47**:86, 1952.

Walsh, F. B., and Hoyt, W. F.: Pseudotumor cerebri. In Clinical neuro-ophthalmology, Baltimore, 1969, The Williams & Wilkins Co., p. 593.

Walsh, F. B., Clark, D. B., Thompson, R. S., and Nicholsen, D. H.: Oral contraceptives and neuro-ophthalmologic interest, Arch. Ophthalmol. **74**:628-640, 1965.

#### Subdural hematomas

Bailey, P.: Subdurales Hämatom. Die Hirn-geschwülste, Stuttgart, 1951, Ferdinand Enke Verlag, p. 354.

Bradley, K. C.: Extra-dural haemorrhage, Aust. N.Z. J. Surg. **21**:241-260, 1952.

Fischer-Brügge, K.: Das Klivuskanten-Syn-drom, Acta Neurochir. **2**:36, 1951.

Furlow, L. T.: Chronic subdural hematoma, Arch. Surg. **32**:688-708, 1936.

Govan, C. D., and Walsh, F. B.: Symptom-atology of subdural haematoma in infants and in adults: comparative study, with particular reference to the ocular signs; an observation concerning pathogenesis of sub-dural haematoma, Arch. Ophthalmol. **37**: 701-715, 1947.

Guthkelch, A. N.: Extradural haemorrhage as a cause of cortical blindness, J. Neuro-surg. **6**:180-182, 1949.

Hanke, H.: Das subdurale Hämatom, Berlin, 1939, Julius Springer, p. 180.

Heyser, J., and Weber, G.: Die epiduralen Hämatome. Med. Wochenschr. **94**:2-7, 46-52, 1964.

Klingler, M.: Das Schädel-Hirntrauma, Stutt-gart, 1961, Georg Thieme Verlag KG.

Krayenbühl, H., and Noto, G.: Das Intra-kranielle subdurale Hämatom, Bern, 1949, Hans Huber.

MacDonald, E. A.: Ocular lesions caused by intracranial hemorrhage, Trans. Am. Ophthalmol. Soc. **29**:418, 1931.

Maltby, G. L.: Visual field changes and subdural hematomas, Surg. Gynecol. Obstet. **74**:496-498, 1942.

McKissock, W., Richardson, A., and Bloom, W. H.: Subdural haematoma, a review of 389 cases, Lancet **1**:1365-1369, 1960.

Metzger, O., and Philippides, D.: Étude d'un syndrome de Parinaud au cours de l'évolution d'un hématome sous-dural chronique, Rev. Otoneuroophtalmol. **20**:377-378, 1948.

Poppe, J. L., and Strain, R. E.: Chronic subdural hematomas, Surg. Clin. North Am. **32**:791-799, 1952.

de Quervain, F.: Die starre Pupillenerweiterung in der Diagnostik der Schädel- und Hirntraumen, Schweiz. Med. Wochenschr. **1**:75, 1935.

Schörcher, F.: Über die Ursache der einseitigen Pupillenerweiterung beim epi- und subduralen Hämatom, Dtsch. Z. Chir. **248**:420, 1937.

Sunderland, S., and Bradley, K. C.: Disturbances of oculomotor function accompanying extradural haemorrhage, J. Neurol. Neurosurg. Psychiatry **16**:35-46, 1953.

Voris, H. C.: Diagnosis and treatment of subdural hematomas, Surgery **10**:447-456, 1941.

Walsh, F. B., and Hoyt, W. F.: Subdural hematoma. In Clinical neuro-ophthalmology, Baltimore, 1969, The Williams & Wilkins Co., p. 2413.

Weber, G.: Über subdurale Empyeme, Schweiz. Med. Wochenschr. **80**:51, 1349, 1950.

Weber, G., Heyser, J., Rosenmund, H., and Duckert, F.: Subdurale Hämatome, Schweiz. Med. Wochenschr. **94**:541-548, 1964.

Welte, E.: Zur formalen Genese der traumatischen Mydriasis: Oculomotoriusschädigung durch einseitiges Vorquellen des Uncus hippocampi, Zentralbl. Neurochir. **8**:217, 1943.

Woodhall, B., Devine, J. W., and Hart, D.: Homolateral dilatation of the pupil, homolateral paresis and bilateral muscular rigidity in the diagnosis of extradural hemorrhage, Surg. Gynecol. Obstet. **72**:391, 1941.

## Brain abscesses

Bailey, P.: Hirnabscess. Die Hirngeschwülste, Stuttgart, 1951, Ferdinand Enke Verlag, p. 349.

Bucy, P. E., and Weaver, T. A., Jr.: Paralysis of conjugate lateral movement of the eyes in association with cerebellar abscess, Arch. Surg. **42**:839-849, 1941.

Colemann, C. C.: Brain abscess: a review of twenty-eight cases with comment on ophthalmologic observations, J.A.M.A. **95**:568, 1940.

Cowan, A.: Ophthalmic symptoms in brain abscess, Ann. Surg. **101**:56-63, 1935.

Evans, W.: The pathology and etiology of brain abscess, Lancet **1**:1231-1235, 1931.

Grant, F. C.: Brain abscess; collective review, Int. Abstr. Surg. **72**:118-138, 1941.

Gros, C., and Cazaban, R.: Stase papillaire contro-latérale et papillite homolatérale: complication d'un abcès du cerveau d'origine fronto-sinusienne, Montpellier Med. **37**:134-137, 1950.

Krayenbühl, H., and Weber, G.: Zur Behandlung und Diagnose akuter Hirnabszesse und cerebraler Thrombophlebitiden, Acta Neurochir. **2**:281, 1952.

Lillie, W. I.: The clinical significance of choked disks produced by abscess of the brain, Surg. Gynecol. Obstet. **47**:405-406, 1928.

Lundberg, N.: Diagnostik und Behandlung der Hirnabscesse: Klinische Übersicht, Acta Otolaryngol. **29**:36-55, 1941.

Portmann, G., Pouyanne, H., Leman, P. M., and Mesnage, S. J.: Troubles oto-neuro-ophtalmologiques par abcès du cerveau de diagnostic étiologique difficile, Rev. Otoneuroophtalmol. **24**:138-141, 1952.

Porto, G.: Pappilledema in encephalic abscesses. Paper read before the Association of Medicine of the Penido Burnier Institute, 1941.

Raimondo, N.: I sintomi oculari degli acessi endocranici. Studio su 100 casi, Minerva Oftalmol. **2**:114-117, 1960.

Simonetta, B.: Osservazioni sulla terapia degli ascessi encefalici, Riv. Otoneurooftalmol. **26**:1-29, 1951.

Weber, G.: Ueber subdurale Empyeme, Schweiz. Med. Wochenschr. **80**:1349, 1950.

Weber, G.: Der Hirnabszess, Stuttgart, 1957, Georg Thieme Verlag KG.

## Intracranial aneurysms (including subarachnoid hemorrhage)

Abrahamson, L. A., and Bell, L. B.: Carotid cavernous fistula syndrome, Am. J. Ophthalmol. **39**:521-526, 1955.

Alpers, B. J., and Schlezinger, N. S.: Aneurysm of the posterior communicating artery, Arch. Ophthalmol. **42**:353-364, 1949.

Amyot, R.: Céphalée orbito-frontale et ophtalmoplégie par anévrisme carotidien intracrânien, Union Med. Can. **79**:756-761, 1950.

Bailey, P.: Aneurysma. In Die Hirngeschwülste, Stuttgart, 1951, Ferdinand Enke Verlag, p. 354.

Ballantyne, A. J.: The ocular manifestations of spontaneous subarachnoid hemorrhage, Br. J. Ophthalmol. **27**:383, 1943.

Bergouignan, Pouyanne, Arne, and Leman: Ophtalmoplégies par anévrismes artériels de la base du crâne, Rev. Otoneuroophtalmol. **25**:54-55, 1953.

Bird, A. C., et al.: Unruptured aneurysms of the supraclinoid carotid artery: a treatable cause of blindness, Neurology **20**:445-454, 1970.

Bonnet, P.: Les anévrismes artériels intracrâniens, Paris, 1955, Masson & Cie, Editeurs.

Brückner, R., Bloch, W., and Wolff-Wiesinger, L.: Zur Genese der Retina- und Opticus-Scheidenblutungen bei akuter intrakranieller Drucksteigerung, Ophthalmologica **118**:607-610, 1949.

Bynke, H. G., Efsing, H. O.: Carotid-cavernous fistula with contralateral exophthalmos, Arch. Ophthalmol. **48**:971-978, 1970.

Cardarello, G.: I sintomi oculari nell'emorragia subaracnoidea, Rass. Ital. Ottalmol. **16**:50-63, 1947.

Cardarello, G.: Ulteriore contributo allo studio dei sintomi oculari nelle emorragie subaracnoidee, Rass. Ital. Ottalmol. **18**:182-188, 1949.

Chavanne, H., and Devic, M.: Valeur sémiologique des hémorragies rétiniennes au cours de processus anévrismaux intracrâniens, Bull. Soc. Fr. Ophthalmol. **63**:39-49, 1950.

Cushing, H. W., and Bailey, P.: Tumors arising from the blood vessels of the brain, London, 1928, Baillière Tindall.

Dandy, W. E.: Carotid-cavernous aneurysms (pulsating exophthalmos). In Lewis, D., editor: Lewis' practice of surgery, Hagerstown, Md., 1936, W. F. Prior Co., Inc., vol. 3, pp. 319-323.

Dandy, W. E.: Carotid-cavernous aneurysms (pulsating exophthalmus), Zentralbl. Neurochir. **2**:77, 1937.

Dandy, W. E.: Arteriovenous aneurysms of the brain, Arch. Surg. **17**:190-243, 1938.

Dandy, W. E.: Intracranial arterial aneurysm, Ithaca, N.Y., 1944, Comstock Publishing Co.

Dandy, W. E., and Follis, R. H.: On the pathology of carotid-cavernous aneurysms (pulsating exophthalmos), Am. J. Ophthalmol. **24**:365-385, 1941.

Drews, L. C., and Minckler, J.: Massive bilateral preretinal type of hemorrhage associated with subarachnoidal hemorrhage of brain (with case report and pathologic findings), Am. J. Ophthalmol. **27**:1-15, 1944.

Duke-Elder, S., and Scott, G.: Neuro-ophthalmology. In Duke-Elder, S., editor: System of ophthalmology, vol. 12, St. Louis, 1971, The C. V. Mosby Co.

Ectros, L.: Contribution à l'étude des anévrismes intracrâniens de la carotide et de ses branches, Rev. Otoneuroophtalmol. **21**:259-285, 1949.

Enoksson, P., and Brynke, H.: Visual field defects in arteriovenous aneurysms of the brain, Acta Ophthalmol. **36**:586-600, 1958.

Fahmy, J. A.: Papilledema associated with ruptured intracranial aneurysms, Acta Ophthalmol. **50**:793-802, 1972.

Fahmy, J. A.: Fundal haemorrhages in ruptured intracranial aneurysms. I. Material, frequency and morphology, Acta Ophthalmol. **51**:289-298, 1973.

Fahmy, J. A.: Fundal haemorrhages in ruptured intracranial aneurysms. II. Correlation with the clinical course, Acta Ophthalmol. **51**:299-304, 1973.

Feld, M., and Taptas, J.: L'ophtalmoplégie dans les anévrismes artériels intracrâniens, Rev. Otoneuroophtalmol. **20**:244-249, 1948.

Frankel, K.: Relation of migraine to cerebral aneurysm, Arch. Neurol. Psychiatr. **63**:195-204, 1950.

Gerlach, J., Spuler, H., and Viehweger, G.: Ueber das Aneurysma der Orbita, Klin. Monatsbl. Augenheilkd. **140**:344-356, 1962.

Globus, J. H., and Schwab, J. M.: Intracranial aneurysms: their origin and clinical behavior in a series of verified cases, J. Mt. Sinai Hosp. **8**:547-578, 1942.

Griffith, J. Q., Jeffers, W., and Fry, W. E.: Papilledema associated with subarachnoidal haemorrhage: experimental and clinical study, Arch. Intern. Med. **61**:880, 1938.

Guidetti, B., and La Torre, E.: Carotid-ophthalmic aneurysms (a series of 16 cases treated by direct approach), Acta Neurochir. (Wien) **22**:289-305, 1970.

Hanafee, W., and Jannetta, P. J.: Aneurysm as a cause of stroke, Am. J. Roentgenol. **98**:647-652, 1966.

Heppner, F., and Lechner, H.: Diagnostische Probleme bei einem gleichzeitigen Vorkommen von Hirnaneurysma und Hirntumor, Zentralbl. Neurochir. **13**:269-275, 1953.

Holmes, J. M.: The ocular symptoms of intracranial aneurysm, Trans. Ophthalmol. Soc. U.K. **74**:549, 1954.

Huber, A.: Cerebrale und retinale Angiopathie, Ophthalmologica **117**:265, 1949.

Huber, A.: Les anévrismes de l'orbite et du sinus caverneux, Bull. Soc. Fr. Ophtalmol. **64**:347-355, 1951.

Huber, A.: Arteriography and phlebography in the diagnosis of orbital affections, Bull. N.Y. Acad. Med. **44**:409-430, 1968.

Ikui, H., Inomata, H., and Hayashi, J.: The pathogenesis of optic nerve sheath hemorrhage, J. Ophthalmol. **11**:67-78, 1967.

Insausti, E., and Matera, R. F.: Sintomas oftalmologicos de los aneurismas intracraneanos, Arch. Oftalmol. B. Air. **28**:105-127, 1953.

Irish, C. W.: Aneurysms of the cerebral vessels: with a study of 32 cases found at 12,503 consecutive necrospsies, Ann Arbor, Mich., 1940, Edwards Brothers, Inc.

Jaeger, R.: Aneurysm of the intracranial carotid artery: syndrome of frontal headache with oculomotor nerve paralysis, J.A.M.A. **142**:304, 1950.

Jamieson, K. G.: Aneurysms of the vertebrobasilar system: surgical intervention in 19 cases, J. Neurosurg. **21**:781-797, 1964.

Jefferson, G.: Compression of the chiasma, optic nerves and optic tracts by intracranial aneurysms, Brain **60**:444, 1937.

Jefferson, G.: On the saccular aneurysms of the internal carotid artery in the cavernous sinus, Br. J. Surg. **26**:267, 1938.

Jefferson, G.: Isolated oculomotor palsy caused by intracranial aneurysm, Proc. R. Soc. Med. **40**:419-432, 1947.

Jefferson, G.: Chiasmal lesions produced by intracranial aneurysms, Arch. Neurol. Psychiatr. **72**:11, 1954.

Kaeser, E. H.: Das arteriovenöse Aneurysma im Sinus cavernosus, Ophthalmologica **126**:257, 1953.

Klingler, M.: Compression des nerfs et du chiasma optique par des anévrismes, Confin. Neurol. **11**:261-270, 1951.

Kothandaram, P., Dawson, B. H., and Kruyt, R. C.: Carotid ophthalmic aneurysms. A study of 19 patients, J. Neurosurg. **34**:544-548, 1971.

Krayenbühl, H.: Das Hirnaneurysma, Schweiz. Arch. Neurol. Psychiatr. **47**:155, 1941.

Krayenbühl, H., and Richter, H.: Die zerebrale Angiographie, Stuttgart, 1952, Georg Thieme Verlag KG.

Krayenbühl, H., and Yasargil, M. G.: Die vasculären Erkrankungen im Gebiet der Arteria vertebralis und Arteria basalis, eine anatomische und pathologische, klinische und neuroradiologische Studie, Stuttgart, 1957, Georg Thieme Verlag KG.

Krayenbühl, H., and Yasargil, M. G.: Das Hirnaneurysma, Basel, 1958, J. R. Geigy.

Krayenbühl, H., and Yasargil, M. G.: Die Zerebrale Angiographie, Stuttgart, 1965, Georg Thieme Verlag KG.

Krayenbühl, H., Yasargil, M. G.: Klinik der Gefässmissbildungen und Gefässfisteln. In Gänshirt: Hirnkreislauf, Stuttgart, 1972, Georg Thieme Verlag KG, pp. 465-511.

Ley, A.: Compression of the optic nerve by a fusiform aneurysm of the carotid artery, J. Neurol. Neurosurg. Psychiatry **13**:75-86, 1950.

Lutz, A.: Ueber einige weitere Fälle von binasaler Hemianopsie, Graefe. Arch. Ophthalmol. **125**:103-124, 1930-1931.

MacDonald, A. E.: Ocular lesions caused by intracranial haemorrhage, Trans. Am. Ophthalmol. Soc. **29**:418, 1931.

MacDonald, A. E., and Korb, M.: Intracranial aneurysms (reference bibliography of 1125 cases), Arch. Neurol. Psychiatr. **42**:298-328, 1939.

Madsen, P. H.: Carotid-cavernous fistulae, a study of 18 cases, Acta Ophthalmol. **48**:731-751, 1970.

Manschot, W. A.: Subarachnoid hemorrhage; intraocular symptoms and their pathogenesis, Am. J. Ophthalmol. **38**:501, 1954.

Manschot, W. A., and Hampe, J. F.: The origin of ocular symptoms in spontaneous subarachnoid haemorrhage, Proceedings of the Sixteenth International Congress of Ophthalmology, London, 1950, vol. 1, pp. 356-368.

Martin, J. D., and Mabon, F. R.: Pulsating exophthalmos: review of all reported cases, J.A.M.A. **121**:330-335, 1943.

Mason, T. H., Swain, G. M., and Osheroff, H. R.: Bilateral carotid cavernous fistula, J. Neurosurg. 11:323-326, 1954.

Meadows, S. P.: Aneurysms of the internal carotid artery, Trans. Ophthalmol. Soc. U.K. 69:137-155, 1949.

Meves, H.: Zur Genese der Augenhintergrunudshämorrhagien bei subarachnoidalen Blutungen, Klin. Monatsbl. Augenheilkd. 106:339-342, 1941.

Milletti, M.: Gli aneurismi dei vasi cerebrali. Diagnostica clinica e terapia chirurgica, Arch. Neurochir. 1:433-656, 1952.

Moniz, E.: Die cerebrale Arteriographie und Phlebographie. Ergänzungsband zum Handbuch der Neurologie II, Berlin, 1940, Julius Springer.

Oberle, A.: Über irreführende Symptome bei Aneurysmen der basalen Hirnarterien, M.D. Thesis, 1951, University of Zurich.

Olivecrona, H., and Ladenheim, J.: Congenital arteriovenous aneurysms of the carotid and vertebral arterial systems, Berlin, 1957, Julius Springer.

Ott, T., and Cuendet, J. F.: Hémorragies sous-arachnoïdienne et rétinienne par rupture d'anévrisme artério-veineux intracrânien, Confin. Neurol. 13:3, 170-174, 1953.

Paton, L.: Ocular symptoms in subarachnoid haemorrhage, Trans. Ophthalmol. Soc. U.K. 44:110-126, 1924.

Patrikios, J. S.: Ophthalmoplégie et Migraine, Arch. Neurol. Psychiatr. 63:902-917, 1950.

Penholz, H., and Mildbraed, I.: Über die Augensymptome intrakranieller arterieller und arteriovenöser Aneurysmen und ihre Behandlung, Klin. Monatsbl. Augenheilkd. 124:179, 1954.

Pfingst, A. O., and Spurling, R. G.: Intracranial aneurysms: their role in the production of ocular palsies, Arch. Ophthalmol. 2:391-398, 1929.

Pool, L., and Potts, D. G.: Aneurysms and arteriovenous anomalies of the brain: diagnosis and treatment, New York, 1965, Harper & Row, Publishers.

Rhonheimer, C.: Zur Symptomatologie der sellären Aneurysmen; ein Beitrag zur Differentialdiagnose der Chiasmasyndrome, Klin. Monatsbl. Augenheilkd. 134:1-34, 1959.

Richardson, J. C., and Hyland, H. H.: Intracranial aneurysms: a clinical and pathological study of subarachnoid and intracerebral hemorrhage caused by berry aneurysms, Medicine 20:1-83, 1941.

Riddoch, G., and Goulden, C.: On the relationship between subarachnoid and intraocular haemorrhage, Br. J. Ophthalmol. 9:209-223, 1925.

Sands, I. J.: Diagnosis and management of subarachnoid hemorrhage, Arch. Neurol. Psychiatr. 46:973, 1941.

Schiefer, W., and Marguth, F.: Intraselläre Aneurysmen, Acta. Neurochir. 4:344-354, 1956.

Sharr, M. M., and Kelvin, R. M.: Vertebrobasilar aneurysms. Experience with 27 cases, Eur. Neurol. 10:129-143, 1973.

Sjöqvist, O.: Über intrakranielle Aneurysmen der A. carotis und deren Beziehungen zur ophthalmoplegischen Migräne, Nervenarzt 9:233-241, 1936.

Smith, D. C., Kearns, T. P., and Sayre, G. P.: Preretinal and optic nerve sheath hemorrhage: pathologic and experimental aspects in subarachnoid hemorrhage, Trans. Am. Acad. Ophthalmol. Otolaryngol. 61:201-211, 1967.

Sugar, H. S., and Meyer, S. J.: Pulsating exophthalmos, Arch. Ophthalmol. 23:1288-1321, 1940.

Thiébaut, F., and Matavulj, N.: Troubles oculaires dans quelques cas d'angiome artério-veineux du cerveau, Bull. Soc. Fr. Ophtalmol. 74:759-770, 1961.

Thomas, M. H., and Petrohelos, M. A.: Diagnostic significance of retinal artery pressure in internal carotid involvement, Am. J. Ophthalmol. 36:335, 1953.

Thompson, J. R., Harwood, D. C., and Fitz, C. R.: Cerebral aneurysms in children, Am. J. Roentgenol. Radium Ther. Nucl. Med. 118:163-175, 1973.

Troost, T. B., and Newton, T. H.: Occipital lobe arteriovenous malformations, Arch. Ophthalmol. 93:250, 1975.

Vassiliou, G., and Doris, M.: The Terson syndrome in subarachnoid haemorrhages, Bull. Soc. Hellen. Ophthalmol. 39:347-384, 1971.

Wagener, H. P., and Foster, R. F.: Ruptured intracranial aneurysm with hemorrhages into retina and vitreous, Mayo Clin. Proc. 10:225-229, 1935.

Walsh, F. B.: Diagnosis, localization and treatment of intracranial saccular aneurysms, Arch. Neurol. Psychiatr. 44:671, 1940.

Walsh, F. B.: Visual field defects due to aneurysms at the circle of Willis, Arch. Ophthalmol. **71**:15, 1964.

Walsh, F. B., and Hedges, T. R., Jr.: Optic nerve sheath hemorrhage, Trans. Am. Acad. Ophthalmol. Otolaryngol. **55**:29-48, 1950; Am. J. Ophthalmol. **34**:509-527, 1951.

Walsh, F. B., and Hoyt, W. F.: Arteriovenous aneurysm. In Clinical neuro-ophthalmology, Baltimore, 1969, The Williams & Wilkins Co., p. 1690.

Walsh, F. B., and Hoyt, W. F.: Carotid-cavernous fistula. In Clinical neuro-ophthalmology, Baltimore, 1969, The Williams & Wilkins Co., p. 1714.

Walsh, F. B., and Hoyt, W. F.: Aneurysms of the cerebral arteries. In Clinical neuro-ophthalmology, Baltimore, 1969, The Williams & Wilkins Co., p. 1737.

Walsh, F. B., and Hoyt, W. F.: Subarachnoid and intracerebral hemorrhage. In Clinical neuro-ophthalmology, Baltimore, 1969, The Williams & Wilkins Co., p. 1782.

Walsh, F. B., and King, A. B.: Ocular signs of intracranial saccular aneurysms: experimental work on collateral circulation through the ophthalmic artery, Arch. Ophthalmol. **27**:1-33, 1942.

Weber, G.: Zur Diagnose und Behandlung der arterio-venösen Aneurysmen im Bereich der Grosshirnhemisphären, Schweiz. Med. Wochenschr. **78**:629-634, 1948.

Weber, G.: Das intrazerebrale Hämatom, Schweiz. Arch. Neurol. Psychiatr. **91**:510-552, 1963.

White, J. C., and Ballantine, H. T., Jr.: Intrasellar aneurysm simulating hypophyseal tumors, J. Neurosurg. **18**:34-50, 1961.

Wyburn-Mason, R.: Arteriovenous aneurysm of mid-brain and retina, facial naevi and mental changes, Brain **66**:163-203, 1943.

Yasargil, G. M.: Die Röntgendiagnostik des Exophthalmus unilateralis, Basel, 1957, S. Karger AG.

Yasargil, M. G., Fox, J. E., and Ray, M. W.: The operative approach to aneurysms of the anterior communicating artery. In Krayenbühl, H., editor: Advances and technical standards in neurosurgery, vol. 2, Vienna, 1975, Springer Verlag KG.

Ziedses des Plantes, B. G.: Subtraktion, Stuttgart, 1961, Georg Thieme Verlag KG.

Zielinski, H. W.: Augenhintergrundsveränderungen bei intracraniellen Aneurysmen und arteriovenösen Angiomen, Ber. Dtsch. Ophthalmol. Ges. **59**:48-52, 1955.

# Index